Functional Neurology
for Practitioners of
Manual Therapy

Dedicated to:

To My Mentor
  Professor Frederick Robert Carrick

To My Wife
  Marianne

To My Children
  Justin, Brandon, Lindsay, Randi, Charli, and Warren

Commissioning Editor: **Claire Wilson**
Project Manager: **Elouise Ball**
Designer: **Charlotte Murray**
Illustrator: **Oxford Illustrations**
Illustration Manager: **Gillian Richards**

Functional Neurology
for Practitioners
of Manual Therapy

Randy W. Beck

BSc (Hons), DC, PhD

Clinic Director
Murdoch University Chiropractic Clinic
Perth, Australia

Lecturer
Clinical Diagnosis and Clinical Neurology
Division of Health Science
Murdoch University
Perth, Australia

Previously,
Clinic Director
Papakura Neurology Centre
Auckland, New Zealand

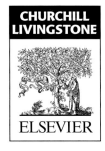

CHURCHILL
LIVINGSTONE

ELSEVIER

EDINBURGH   LONDON   NEW YORK   OXFORD   PHILADELPHIA   ST LOUIS   SYDNEY   TORONTO 2008

CHURCHILL
LIVINGSTONE
ELSEVIER

An imprint of Elsevier Limited
© 2008, Elsevier Limited. All rights reserved.

First published 2008
Reprinted 2008, 2009

ISBN: 978–0–443–10220–2

British Library Cataloguing in Publication Data
A catalogue record for this book is available from the British Library

Library of Congress Cataloging in Publication Data
A catalog record for this book is available from the Library of Congress

The
Publisher's
policy is to use
**paper manufactured
from sustainable forests**

Printed in China

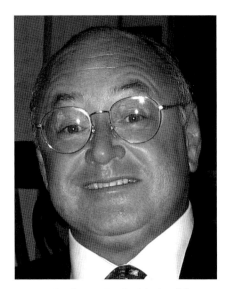

Professor Frederick Carrick

Professor Frederick Carrick is considered the founder of Functional Neurology. He has established a worldwide reputation for the successful treatment of neurological disorders that have been refractory to other treatments. His professional life has been one of sharing; a career in the service of others. His clinical skills are complemented by his ability to explain the complexities of clinical neurology in a fashion that promotes mastery. He is the recipient of a multitude of professional, governmental and societal awards, but in spite of the miracles associated with his service and the praise of patients and colleagues he remains a humble servant of humankind. His dedication to the improvement of the quality of life of all patients has been key in his ability to inspire others to embrace a journey of similar dedication. The neurological system of humankind is complex. Professor Carrick's life work has enabled an infinite number of clinicians and patients to understand it better and to utilize applications which can and do make a difference in our global society. This work has been inspired by him.

Table of Contents

1-AAD 1-amino acid decarboxylase
ACC anterior cingulate gyrus
ACh acetylcholine
ACTH adrenocorticotrophic hormone
AD Alzheimer's disease
ADP adenosine diphosphate
aMCC anterior midcingulate cortex
ANT adenosine nucleotide transferase
APP amyloid precursor protein
ATP adenosine triphosphate
AV atrioventricular
AVCN anterior ventral cochlear nucleus
AVM arteriovenous malformation
BPPV benign paroxysmal positional vertigo
cAMP cyclic AMP
CEST cognitive experiential self theory
cGMP cyclic GMP
CGRP calcitonin-gene-related-peptide
CHI closed head injury
CIEGr cellular immediate early gene responses
CIS central integrative state
CNS central nervous system
'CREB cAMP response element binding protein
CRPS complex region pain syndrome
CSF cerebral spinal fluid
CVLM caudal ventrolateral medulla
DA dopamine
DCN dorsal cochlear nucleus
DES differential emotions scale
dPCC dorsal posterior cingulate cortex
DRG dorsal root ganglion
DMN/DMV dorsal motor nucleus (of the vagus)
E epinephrine
ECF extracellular fluid
EEG electroencephalogram
EMG electromyography
EPSPs excitatory post-synaptic potentials
EWN Edinger–Westphal nucleus
FADH flavin adenine dinucleotide
FEF frontal eye fields
FOF frequency of firing
FRA flexor reflex afferent
FSH follicle-stimulating hormone
FTA-ABS fluorescent treponemal antibody
        absorption test
GABA γ-aminobutyric acid
GAD generalized anxiety disorder
GALT gut-associated lymphoid tissue
GAP growth-associated proteins

GBP Guillain–Barre polyneuropathy
GH growth hormone
GPe globus pallidus externa
GPi globus pallidus interna
GTOs Golgi tendon organs
HD Huntingdon's disease
5-HT 5-hydroxy-tryptophan
IEG immediate early genes
IML intermediolateral
IMM intermediomedial group
IPSPs inhibitory post-synaptic potentials
KS Kearn's–Sayer syndrome
LD lateral dorsal
LGN lateral geniculate nucleus
LH luteinizing hormone
LORETA low-resolution tomographic analysis
LP lateral posterior
MALT mucosa-associated lymphoid tissue
MAO-B monoamine oxidase-B
MAPK mitogen-activated protein kinase
MELAS myoclonic epilepsy with lactic acidosis and
        stroke-like episodes
MGN medial geniculate nucleus
MHC major histocompatibility complex
MLF medial longitudinal fasciculus
MRF mesencephalon reticular formation
MTLE mesial temporal lobe epilepsy syndrome
NADH nicotinamide adenine dinucleotide
NE norepinephrine
NGF nerve growth factor
NMDA N-methyl-D-aspartate
NSAIDs nonsteroidal anti-inflammatory drugs
NTS nucleus tractus solitarius
OPK opticokinetic
OR opticokinetic
OTR ocular tilt reaction
OxPhos oxidative phosphorylation
pACC pregenual anterior cingulate cortex
PAG para aqueductal grey
PET positron emission tomography
PGE2 prostaglandin E2
PKA/C protein kinase A/protein kinase C
PLRs pupil light reflexes
pMCC posterior midcingulate cortex
PMRF pontomedullary reticular formation
PNS parasympathetic nervous system
PSDC postsynaptic dorsal column
PVCN posteroventral cochlear nucleus
qEEG quality electroencephalogram

riMLF rostral interstitial nucleus of the medial longitudinal fasciculus

RMP resting membrane potential

RPR rapid plasma reagin

RSD reflex sympathetic dystrophy

RVLM rostral ventrolateral medulla

RVM rostral ventral medulla

sACC subgenual anterior cingulate cortex

SCM sternocleidomastoid muscle

SDH subdural haematoma

SNc substantia nigra pars compacta

SNr substantia nigra pars reticulata

SNS sympathetic nervous system

SP senile plaques

SSN superior salivatory nucleus

STT spinothalamic tract

SVV subjective visual vertical

TENS transepithelial electrical nerve stimulation

TMJ temporal mandibular joint

TND transneural degeneration

TSH thyroid stimulating hormone

TTA time to activation

TTF time to fatigue

TTR time to response

TTS time to summation

TTSp time to peak summation

TVP transverse process

V:A vein-to-artery ratio

VBI vertebrobasilar insufficiency

VBS vertebrobasilar stroke

VCN ventral cochlear nucleus

VDRL venereal disease research laboratory

VHCs ventral horn cells

VORs vestibulo-ocular reflexes

vPCC ventral posterior cingulate cortex

VPI ventral posterior inferior

VPL ventral posterior lateral

VPM ventral posterior medial

Dr Randy Beck has answered the need for a text specific to Functional Neurology. Clinicians worldwide have been searching for a body of knowledge specific to the breadth, depth and applications necessary for procedures that do not involve drugs or surgery and his is a textbook that takes the reader on a journey through the nervous system of humankind. It is practical in its approach to function and addresses how the nervous system works to a greater degree than a typical exploration of neuropathology. Beck promotes a clinical understanding of a complex and challenging subject in an easy-to-read format.

This is not a book to be used to review the differential diagnosis of neurological disease. Dr Beck addresses function rather than pathology, allowing the reader to gain an understanding of the neurological processes in health and disease. The work stands alone and is unique in its approach. It is current, well referenced and is sure to become a compulsory text in programs specific to neurological approaches to health. Dr Beck also includes a substantial contribution to manipulation techniques that are linked to a neurologically functional model. The techniques are well illustrated and serve the learning needs of both students and field practitioners.

It has been a great pleasure to read this text and a greater pleasure to recommend it.

Professor Frederick Carrick
Carrick Institute for Graduate Studies
Cape Canaveral, Florida

Preface

The concepts covered in this textbook are by their very nature rapidly changing. I have tried to use the most up-to-date information available and present it in a unique fashion that relates the science to the clinical application. I have chosen the content of the textbook based on the suggestions that I have received from countless students and practitioners about the diversity and difficulty of the subject matter and the need for multiple textbooks to gain a basic understanding of the subject. This textbook will hopefully reduce the number of textbooks needed to gain an overview of the subject. In-depth study of the topic will undoubtedly require the mastery of many other texts in detail that was not possible in this edition. It is important to understand that this textbook was not written to be the end of the learning process but the beginning of a wonderful life-long journey of learning. Many of the concepts and clinical applications in this text have not yet withstood the rigorous scrutiny of scientific investigation, but have been included on the basis of the clinical results that have been observed on patients by myself and several thousand clinicians around the world over for the past twenty or so years. I have attempted to include abundant references when discussing controversial concepts and direct the reader to the original articles whenever possible.

The manipulation section is not intended as an encyclopaedic collection of manipulations but as an introduction and guide to those practitioners and/or students who wish to learn a general approach to manipulation as an afferent stimulation technique as well as a motion restoration tool. I have included a quite detailed historical overview of the concepts relating to the development of emotions because I have found that far too often the connection between clinical sciences and the esoteric workings of the mind become mutually exclusive in approaches to understanding how thoughts can influence all aspects of our functionality as humans. The original concept for this text developed out of several requests from students and practitioners of various specialties that became intrigued with the concepts of functional neurology only to be frustrated and discouraged by the sheer volume of material that seemed to be exponentially multiplying yearly. The concept was born in discussions with two exceptionally talented and bright functional neurologists, Dr Kelly Holt of New Zealand and Dr Stephen Sexton of Australia, following a neurology conference weekend in Auckland, New Zealand in 2004. Further discussions with Professor Frederick Carrick of the United States developed the text into a working overview, which was submitted to Elsevier and accepted for publication.

I thank Drs Sexton and Holt for their inspiration and many suggestions concerning content, and their contribution of charts and diagrams that demonstrate complicated concepts in a clear and effective manner. I thank Claire Bonnett and Sarena Wolfaard, my editors at Elsevier, who believed in the project and continually supported me through the trials and tribulations that always arise when a project of this magnitude is undertaken. I thank the many students and practitioners who read drafts and made suggestions for the order, content, and clarity of the text. I thank my wife, Marianne, for her encouragement, love, and uncanny ability to type extremely fast, raise the children, and take care of me at the same time. Finally, I thank Professor Frederick Carrick for writing the Foreword and for his unwavering support and wisdom throughout the past several years. Ted, you are a true friend.

This book has been written in an order that allows the reader to firmly grasp the concepts necessary for the understanding of functional neurology. However, the chapters will also stand alone as review or first-time introduction.

The clinical cases are designed to be read and answered before starting the chapter to allow the reader to gauge their current state of knowledge. They can then be revisited at various times during the passage through each chapter to apply the principles learned thus far and to solidify the anatomy, functional circuits and concepts. Only after the entire chapter has been read and the case studies attempted should the answers to the case studies at the end of each chapter be consulted.

A special feature called **Quick Facts** is included in the body of the text and this will introduce new but related information or review information already presented in the text, in a brief and succinct manner. This feature will facilitate quick review of the material for examinations or periodic review.

A wide range of additional case studies are also included. The reader should read the case history and attempt to devise a differential diagnosis list and treatment approach to the patient themselves before continuing into the diagnosis and treatment sections of the case in the text. This will give the reader an idea of their level of understanding of the concepts and information that have been presented.

We are always interested in improving the presentation and effectiveness of the text material and welcome any suggestions or comments in this regard.

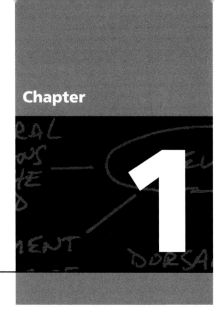

Chapter

1

Fundamental Concepts in Functional Neurology

Introduction

Much of the understanding that we have today of how human neurons function was based on the 'integrate and fire' concept formed by Eccles in the 1950s which was developed based on studies of spinal motor neurons (Brock et al 1952). In this model, spinal motor neurons integrate synaptic activity, and when a threshold is reached, they fire an action potential. The firing of this action potential is followed by a period of hyperpolarization or refraction to further stimulus in the neuron. This early integrate and fire model was then extrapolated to other areas of the nervous system including the cortex and central nervous system which strongly influenced the development of theories relating to neuron and nervous system function (Eccles 1951).

Early in the 1970s, studies that revealed the existence of neurons that operated under much more complex intrinsic firing properties started to emerge. The functional output of these neurons and neuron systems could not be explained by the existing model of the integrate and fire hypothesis (Connor & Stevens 1971).

Since the discoveries of these complex firing patterns many other forms of neural interaction and modulation have also been discovered. It is now known that in addition to complex firing patterns neurons also interact via a variety of forms of chemical synaptic transmission, electrical coupling through gap junctions, and interactions through electric and magnetic fields, and can be modulated by neurohormones and neuromodulators such as dopamine and serotonin.

With this fundamental change in the understanding of neuron function came new understanding of the functional interconnectivity of neuron systems, new methods of investigation, and new functional approaches to treatment of nervous system dysfunction.

With the emergence of any clinical science it is essential that the fundamental concepts and definitions are clearly understood. Throughout the textbook the following concepts and terms will be referred to and discussed frequently so it is essential that a good understanding of these concepts be established in the reader's mind before moving on to the rest of the text.

This chapter will constitute an introduction to the concepts below, which will be covered in more elaborate detail later in the text.

Central Integrative State (CIS) of a Neuron

The central integrative state (CIS) of a neuron is the total integrated input received by the neuron at any given moment and the probability that the neuron will produce an action potential based on the state of polarization and the firing requirements of the neuron to produce an action potential at one or more of its axons.

The physical state of polarization existing in the cell at any given moment is determined by the temporal and spatial summation of all the excitatory and inhibitory stimuli it has processed at that moment. The complexity of this process can be put into perspective when you consider that a pyramidal neuron in the adult visual cortex may have up to 12,000 synaptic connections, and certain neurons in the prefrontal cortex can have up to 80,000 different synapses firing at any given moment (Cragg 1975; Huttenlocher 1994).

The firing requirements of the neuron are usually genetically determined but environmentally established and can demand the occurrence of complex arrays of stimulatory patterns before a neuron will discharge an action potential. Some examples of different stimulus patterns that exist in neurons include the 'and/or' gated neurons located in the association motor areas of cortex and the complex rebound burst patterns observed in thalamic relay cells.

'And' pattern neurons only fire an action potential if two or more specific conditions are met. 'Or' pattern neurons only fire an action potential only when one or the other specific conditions are present (Brooks 1984).

The thalamic relay cells exhibit complex firing patterns. They relay information to the cortex in the usual integrate and fire pattern unless they have recently undergone a period of inhibition. Following a period of inhibition stimulus, in certain circumstances, they can produce bursts of low-threshold spike action potentials referred to as post-inhibitory rebound bursts. This activity seems to be generated endogenously and may be responsible for production of a portion of the activation of the thalamocortical loop pathways thought to be detected in encephalographic recordings of cortical activity captured by electroencephalograms (EEG) (Destexhe & Sejnowski 2003).

The neuron may be in a state of relative depolarization, which implies the membrane potential of the cell has shifted towards the firing threshold of the neuron. This generally implies that the neuron has become more positive on the inside and the potential difference across the membrane has become smaller. Alternatively, the neuron may be in a state of relative hyperpolorization, which implies the membrane potential of the cell has moved away from the firing threshold. This implies that the inside of the cell has become more negative in relation to the outside environment and the potential difference across the membrane has become greater (Ganong 1983) (Fig. 1.1).

The membrane potential is established and maintained across the membrane of the neuron by the flux of ions; usually sodium (Na), potassium (K), and chloride (Cl) ions are the most involved although other ions such as calcium can be involved with

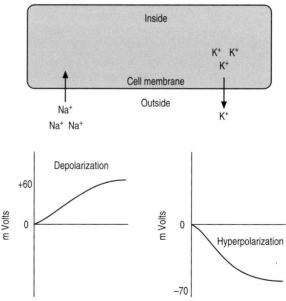

Fig. 1.1 The effects of ionic movement across the neuron cell membrane. The left side of the diagram illustrates the depolarizing effect of sodium ion movement into the cell. The right side of the diagram illustrates the hyperpolarizing effect of potassium movement out of the cell. The graphs illustrate the change in potential voltage inside the cell relative to outside the cell as the respective ions move across the membrane. Note the equilibrium potentials for sodium and potassium, +60 and −70 mV, respectively, are reached when the chemical and electrical forces for each ion become equal in magnitude.

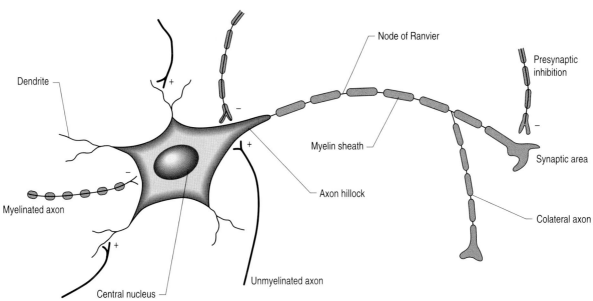

Fig. 1.2 Anatomical characteristics of a healthy neuron. The central nucleus is maintained by microtubule and microfilament production, which requires active protein synthesis. The myelin sheath is composed of oligodendrogliocytes in the central nervous system and Schwann cells in the peripheral nervous system. Note the different types of synaptic contacts illustrated from left to right: axodendritic, axosomatic, dendrodendritic, axohillonic, axoaxonic (presynaptic).

modulation of permeability. The movement of these ions across the neuron membrane is determined by changes in the permeability or ease at which each ion can move through selective channels in the membrane.

When Na ions move across the neuron membrane into the neuron, the potential across the membrane decreases or depolarizes due to the positive nature of the Na ions, which increases the relative positive charge inside the neuron compared to outside the neuron. When Cl ions move into the neuron, the neuron the membrane potential becomes greater or hyperpolarizes due to the negative nature of the Cl ions, which increase the relative negative charge inside the neuron compared to outside the neuron. The same is true when K ions move out of the neuron due to the relative loss of positive charge that the K ions possess.

The firing threshold of the neuron is the membrane potential that triggers the activation of specialized voltage gated channels, usually concentrated in the area of the neuron known as the axon hillock or activation zone, that allow the rapid influx of Na into the axon hillock area, resulting in the generation of an action potential in the axon (Stevens 1979) (Fig. 1.2).

Central Integrative State of a Functional Unit of Neurons

The concept of the CIS described above in relation to a single neuron can be loosely extrapolated to a functional group of neurons. Thus, the central integrative state of a functional unit or group of neurons can be defined as the total integrated input received by the group of neurons at any given moment and the probability that the group of neurons will produce action potential output based on the state of polarization and the firing requirements of the group.

The concept of the central integrative state can be used to estimate the status of a variety of variables concerning the neuron or neuron system such as:

- The probability that any given stimulus to a neuron or neuron system will result in the activation of the neuron, or neuron system;
- The state of prooncogene activation and protein production in the system; and
- The rate and duration that the system will respond to an appropriate stimulus.

Transneural Degeneration

The central integrative state of a neuron or neuron system is modulated by three basic fundamental activities present and necessary in all neurons.

These activities include:

1. Adequate gaseous exchange, namely oxygen and carbon dioxide exchange—this includes blood flow and anoxic and ischaemic conditions that may arise from inadequate blood supply;
2. Adequate nutritional supply including glucose, and a variety of necessary cofactors and essential compounds; and
3. Adequate and appropriate stimulation in the form of neurological communication, including both inhibition and activation of neurons via synaptic activation—synaptic activation of a neuron results in the stimulation and production of immediate early genes and second messengers within the neuron that stimulate DNA transcription of appropriate genes and the eventual production of necessary cellular components such as proteins and neurotransmitters.

Although other activities of neuron function require certain components of oxygen or nutritional supplies, the major necessity of adequate gaseous exchange and adequate nutritional intake into the neuron is to supply the mitochondrial production of adenosine triphosphate (ATP).

The mitochondria utilize a process called chemiosmotic coupling, to harness energy from the food obtained from the environment, for use in metabolic and cellular processes. The energy obtained from the tightly controlled slow chemical oxidation of food is used to membrane-bound proton pumps in the mitochondrial membrane that transfer H ions from one side to the other, creating an electrochemical proton gradient across the membrane. A variety of enzymes utilize this proton gradient to power their activities including the enzyme ATPase that utilizes the potential electrochemical energy created by the proton gradient to drive the production of ATP via the phosphorylation of adenosine diphosphate (ADP) (Alberts et al 1994). Other proteins produced in the mitochondria utilize the proton gradient to couple transport metabolites in, out of, and around the mitochondria (Fig. 1.3).

The proteins required to support neuron function, including the proteins necessary for mitochondrial function and thus ATP production described above, are produced in response to environmental signals that reach the neuron via receptor and hormonal stimulation that it receives. Thus, the types and amounts of protein present in the neuron at any given moment are determined by the amounts of oxygen and nutrients available and the amount and type of stimulation it has most recently received.

The mechanisms by which extracellular signals communicate their message across the neuron membrane to alter the protein production are discussed in Chapter 3. Here it will suffice to say that special transmission proteins called immediate early genes (IEG) are activated by a variety of second messenger systems in the neuron in response to membrane stimulus (Mitchell & Tjian 1989). Type 1 IEG responses are specific for the genes in the nucleus of the neuron and type 2 IEG responses are specific for mitochondrial DNA (Fig. 1.4).

Proteins have a multitude of functions in the neuron, some of which include cytoskeletal structure formation of microtubules and microfilaments, neurotransmitter production, intracellular signalling, formation of membrane receptors, formation of membrane channels, structural support of membranes, and enzyme production.

Needless to say, if the cell does not produce enough protein the cell cannot perform the necessary functions to the extent required for optimal performance and/or to sustain its very life.

In situations where the neuron has not had adequate supplies of oxygen, nutrients, or stimulus, the manufacturing of protein is down-regulated. This process of degeneration of function is referred to as transneural degeneration.

Initially the neuron response to this down-regulation is to increase its sensitivity to stimulus so that less stimulus is required to stimulate protein production. This essentially means that the neuron alters its membrane potential so that it is closer to its threshold

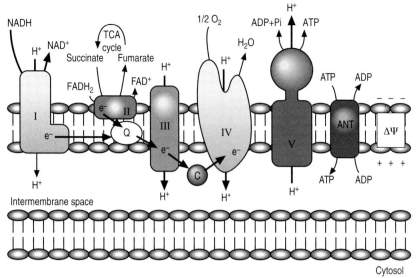

Fig. 1.3 Enzymes of oxidative phosphorylation. Electrons (e⁻) enter the mitochondrial electron transport chain from donors such as reduced nicotinamide adenine dinucleotide (NADH) and reduced flavin adenine dinucleotide (FADH$_2$). The electron donors leave as their oxidized forms, NAD⁺ and FAD⁺. Electrons move from complex I (I), complex II (II), and other donors to coenzyme Q$_{10}$ (Q). Coenzyme Q$_{10}$ transfers electrons to complex III (III). Cytochrome c (c) transfers electrons from complex III to complex IV (IV). Complexes I, III, and IV use the energy from electron transfer to pump protons (H⁺) out of the mitochondrial matrix, creating a chemical and electrical (Δψ) gradient across the mitochondrial inner membrane. Complex V (V) uses this gradient to add a phosphate (P$_i$) to adenosine diphosphate (ADP), making adenosine triphosphate (ATP). Adenosine nucleotide transferase (ANT) moves ATP out of the matrix. *From D. Wolf, with permission.*

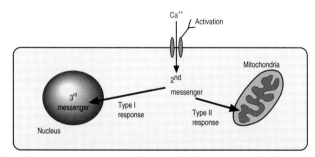

Fig. 1.4 Immediate early genes responses type I and type II. Following receptor activation the entry of calcium (Ca⁺⁺) ions into the neuron activate both type I and type II response cascades. The type I cascade involves the activation of third-order messengers that modulate the activation or inhibition of DNA in the nucleus of the neuron. The type II cascade involves the activation of third-order messengers that modulate activation or inhibition of the mitochondrial DNA of the neuron.

potential; in other words, it becomes more depolarized and becomes more irritable to any stimulus it may receive.

After a period of time if the neuron does not receive the deficient component in sufficient amounts, it can no longer sustain its state of depolarization and starts to drastically downgrade the production of protein as a last ditch effort to conserve energy and survival. At this stage, the neuron will still respond to stimulus but only for short periods as it consumes its available protein and ATP stores very quickly. In this state the neuron is vulnerable to overstimulation that may further exhaust and damage the neuron (Fig. 1.5).

The process of transneural degeneration may be one approach that determines the survival or death of neurons during embryological development where it has become quite clear that neurons that do not receive adequate stimulus do not usually survive (see Chapter 2).

The concept of transneural degeneration can also apply to systems or groups of neurons that will respond in a similar pattern to that described above when they do not receive the appropriate stimulus or nutrients that they require.

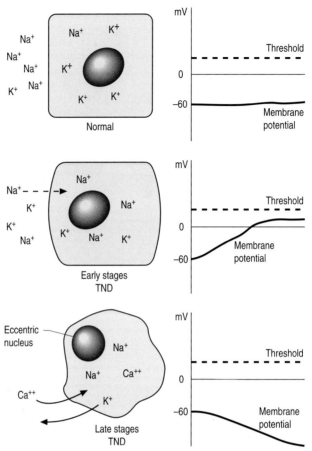

Fig. 1.5 The progression of transneural degeneration in a neuron. (Top) A normal healthy neuron with a normal distribution of sodium (Na⁺) and potassium (K⁺) ions across its membrane, resulting in a normal resting membrane potential. Note the central nucleus. (Middle) The early stages of transneural degeneration. In this stage, the Na⁺ ion concentration in the cell increases because of loss of Na⁺/K⁺ pump activity and alterations in membrane permeability, resulting in a membrane potential more positive and closer to the threshold of firing of the neuron. A neuron in this state will fire action potentials when normally inadequate stimuli is received. This inappropriate firing is called physiological irritability. The neuron will only be able to maintain the frequency of firing for short periods because of the lack of sufficient enzymes and ATP supplies before it fatigues and fails to produce action potentials. (Bottom) The neuron in the late stages of transneural degeneration. Note the eccentric nucleus, which can no longer be maintained by the degraded state of the microfilaments and microtubules. The membrane has lost its ability to segregate ions, and calcium ions have entered the neuron in high concentrations, which will eventually result in cell death. The resting membrane potential has shifted away from firing threshold, resulting in the neuron requiring excessive stimulus in order to fire an action potential.

Frequency of Firing of a Neuron or Neuron System

The frequency of firing (FOF) of a neuron is quite simply the number of action potentials that it generates over a defined period time. As a rule, the FOF is an important indicator of the central integrative state of a neuron. Neurons with high and regular FOF usually maintain high levels of energy and protein production that maintains the neuron in a good state of 'health'. One exception to this rule is a neuron that is in the early stages of transneural degeneration, in which case it will produce high FOF but only for short durations.

Time to Activation of a Neuron or Neuron System

The time to activation (TTA) of a neuron is a measure of the time from which the neuron receives a stimulus to the time that an activation response can be detected. Obviously, in clinical practice the response of individual neurons cannot be measured but the response of neuron systems such as the pupil response to light can be. As a rule, the TTA will be less in situations were the neuron system has maintained a high level of integration and activity and greater in situations were the neuron has not maintained a high level of integration and activity or is in the late stages of transneural degeneration. Again an exception to this rule can occur in situations were the neuron system is in the early stages of transneural degeneration and is irritable to stimulus and responds quickly. This response will be of short duration and cannot be maintained for more than a short period of time.

Time to Fatigue in a Neuron or Neuron System

The time to fatigue (TTF) in a neuron is the length of time that a response can be maintained during a continuous stimulus to the neuron. The TTF effectively measures the ability of the neuron to sustain activation under continuous stimuli, which is a good indicator of the ATP and protein stores contained in the neuron. This in turn is a good indication of the state of health of the neuron. The TTF will be longer in neurons that have maintained high levels of integration and stimulus and shorter in neurons that have not. TTF can be very useful in determining whether a fast time to response (TTR) is due to a highly integrated neuron system or a neuron system that is in the early stages of transneural degeneration.

For example, in clinical practice we can compare the individual responses of two pupils to light. If both pupils respond very quickly to light stimulus (fast TTR), and they both maintain pupil contraction for 3–4 seconds (long TTF) this is a good indication that both neuronal circuits are in a good state of health. If, however, both pupils respond quickly (fast TTR) but the right pupil immediately dilates despite the continued presence of the light stimulus (short TTF), this may be an indication that the right neuronal system involved in pupil constriction may be in an early state of transneural degeneration and more detailed examination is necessary.

Diaschisis

Diaschisis refers to the process of degeneration of a downstream neuronal system in response to a decrease in stimulus from an upstream neuronal system.

This reemphasizes the point that neuronal systems do not exist in isolation but are involved in highly complicated and interactive networks. Interference or disruption in one part of the network can impact other parts of the network.

For example, injury or disease affecting the cerebellum invariably also affects the activity of the contralateral thalamus and cortex.

Constant and Non-Constant Neural Pathways

All multimodal integrated neuronal systems need to receive input from a constant stimulus pathway as well as appropriate oxygen and nutrient supply in order to maintain a healthy CIS.

Constant stimulus pathways are neural receptive systems that supply constant input into the neuraxis that are integrated throughout all multimodal systems to provide the stimulus necessary for the development and maintenance of the systems. Examples of constant stimulus pathways include receptors that detect the effects of gravity or constant motion, namely the joint and muscle position receptors of joint capsules and muscle spindles of the midline or axial structures including the ribs and spinal column. Certain aspects of the vestibulocerebellar system receive constant input and are constantly active. Several neural systems contain groups of neurons that exhibit innate pacemaker depolarization mechanisms such as cardiac pacemaker cells, certain thalamic neurons, and selective neurons of the basal ganglia.

All other receptor systems are non-constant in nature, which means they are activated in bursts of activity that are not constantly maintained.

A few examples should illustrate this concept. One would think that the constant stimulus input to the cortical cells of vision would be the optic radiations from the lateral geniculate nucleus of the thalamus, which transmits the visual information received by the retinal cells to the cortex. Although it is true that most of the time these neurons are active when your eyes are open, these pathways are not active for large periods at a time, specifically about 7–8 hours per day while you sleep. These neurons are maintained in a healthy CIS by the activity generated in constant activation circuits of multimodal systems that include input via the thalamus from midline structures such as the vertebral and costal joint and muscle receptors.

Cortical neurons involved in memory may experience long periods of inactivity and only be activated to threshold when needed to supply appropriate memory information. These neurons are maintained in a high CIS by subthreshold activation supplied by complex multimodal neuron systems.

Finally, ventral horn neurons of small inactive muscles are only brought to activation occasionally when their motor units are called to action. These neurons are maintained in a high CIS by subthreshold stimulus from spinal and supraspinal multimodal neuron systems as well.

Neural Plasticity

Neural plasticity results when changes in the physiological function of the neuraxis occur in response to changes in the internal or external milieu (Jacobson 1991). In other words the development of synapses in the nervous system is very dependent on the activation stimulus that those synapses receive. The synapses that receive adequate stimulation will strengthen and those that do not receive adequate stimulation will weaken and eventually be eliminated (see Chapter 2).

The organization of the synaptic structure in the neuraxis largely determines the stimulus patterns of the nervous system and hence the way in which the neuraxis functions.

Neural plasticity refers to the way in which the nervous system can respond to external stimuli and adjust future responses based on the outcome of the previously initiated responses. In essence, the ability of the nervous system to learn is dependent on neural plasticity.

Cerebral Asymmetry (Hemisphericity)

The study of brain asymmetry or hemisphericity has a long history in the behavioral and biomedical sciences but is probably one of the most controversial concepts in functional neurology today.

The fact that the human brain is asymmetric has been fairly well established in the literature (Geschwind & Levitsky 1968; LeMay & Culebras 1972; Galaburda et al 1978; Falk et al 1991; Steinmetz et al 1991). The exact relationship between this asymmetric design and the functional control exerted by each hemisphere remains controversial.

The concept of hemispheric asymmetry or lateralization involves the assumption that the two hemispheres of the brain control different asymmetric aspects of a diverse array of functions and that the hemispheres can function at two different levels of activation. The level at which each hemisphere functions is dependent on the central integrative state of each hemisphere, which is determined to a large extent by the afferent stimulation it receives from the periphery as well as nutrient and oxygen supply. Afferent stimulation is gated through the brainstem and thalamus, both of which are asymmetric structures themselves, and indirectly modulated by their respective ipsilateral cortices (Savic et al 1994).

Traditionally the concepts of hemisphericity were only applied to the processing of language and visuospatial stimuli. Today, the concept of hemisphericity has developed into a more elaborate theory that involves cortical asymmetric modulation of such diverse constructs as approach versus withdrawal behaviour, maintenance versus interruption of ongoing activity, tonic versus phasic aspects of behaviour, positive versus negative emotional valence, asymmetric control of the autonomic nervous system, and asymmetric modulation of sensory perception, as well as cognitive, attentional, learning, and emotional processes (Davidson & Hugdahl 1995).

The cortical hemispheres are not the only right- and left-sided structures. The thalamus, amygdala, hippocampus, caudate, basal ganglia, substantia nigra, red nucleus, cerebellum, brainstem nuclei, and peripheral nervous system all exist as bilateral structures with the potential for asymmetric function.

Hemisphericity can result in dysfunction of major systems of the body including the spine. Some spinal signs of hemisphericity include:

- Subluxation;
- Spinal stiffness—increased extensor tone;
- Spondylosis;
- Intrinsic spinal weakness—decreased postural tone;
- Decreased A–P curves in cervical and lumbar spine;
- Increased A–P curves in thoracic spine;
- Increased postural sway in sagittal or coronal planes; and
- Pelvic floor weakness.

Embryological Homological Relationships

In the application of functional neurology the concept of embryological homological relationships between neurons born at the same time frequently needs to be taken into consideration.

The term embryological homologues is used to describe the functional relationships that exist between neurons born at the same time in the cell proliferation phase of development. These cells born at the same time along the length of neuraxial ventricular area develop and retain synaptic contact with each other, many of which remain in the mature functional state. This cohort of cells that remain functionally connected after migration results in groups of neurons that may be unrelated in cell type or location but fire as a functional group when brought to threshold. Dorsal root ganglion cells detecting joint motion and muscle contraction and postsynaptic neurons in the sympathetic ganglia controlling blood flow to the joints and muscles illustrate the concept. Another example includes the motor column of the cranial nerves III, IV, VI, and XII in the brainstem which act functionally as a homologous column. This concept also applies to functional areas of the neuraxis that developed from the same embryological tissues. Neuron systems that have developed from the same embryological tissues usually maintain reciprocal connections throughout their life span. For example, in the mesencephalon that is an area of the neuraxis that develops in an undifferentiated fashion, all of the functional structures would be considered embryological homologues and as such be expected to maintain reciprocal connections throughout life. This would imply that the structures in the mesencephalon such as the red nucleus, the substantia nigra, the oculomotor nucleus, the Edinger–Westphal nucleus, and the reticular neurons all maintain close functional relationships. This is in fact the case. Another spin-off from this concept is that all neuron systems developing from the same tissue remain in close reciprocal contact even after further differentiation; for example, the cortex and the thalamus, which develop from prosencephalon but further differentiate to telencephalon and diencephalon respectively, would still be considered embryological homologues. These two structures do indeed retain reciprocal connectivity throughout life. Other examples include the structures that have developed from the rhombencephalon: the cerebellum, pons, and brainstem.

Neurophysiological Excitation and Inhibition in Neural Systems

Excitation of a neuron moves the neuron membrane potential closer to threshold so that the probability of generating an action potential increases.

Inhibition of a neuron moves the membrane potential of the neuron away from its threshold potential and decreases the probability that the neuron will produce an action potential. These same concepts apply to neuron systems; however, in a neuron system several components are integrated to arrive at the final system output.

Components of a neuron system usually involve an input stimulus, a series of integration steps, and an output (Williams & Warwick 1980).

The input stimulus or output, as well as any steps in the integration portion, may be either excitatory or inhibitory in nature (Fig. 1.6).

Virtually all input from the primary afferent neurons of the peripheral nervous system and most cortical output is excitatory in nature. In order to modulate both the input to the integrator (central nervous system) and the output from the integrator the nervous system utilizes a complex array of interneuronal inhibitory strategies.

Some examples of these inhibitory strategies utilized by the nervous system include direct inhibition, feed-forward inhibition, feedback inhibition, disinhibition, feedback disinhibition, lateral inhibition, and surround inhibition.

Direct inhibition involves a hyperpolarizing stimulus to the target neuron, which results in a decreased probability that the target neuron will be brought to threshold potential and fire and action potential per unit stimulus (Fig. 1.7).

Feed-forward inhibition involves the linking of an inhibitory interneuron into a pathway that causes relative hyperpolarization of the next neuron in the pathway, resulting in a decreased probability of output activation of that pathway (Fig. 1.8).

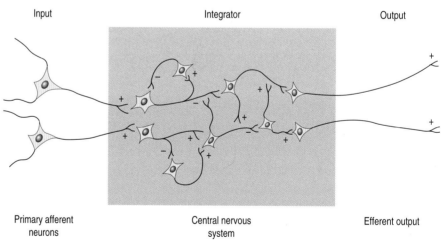

Fig. 1.6 The 'integrate and fire' model of the nervous system. The primary afferent neurons supply the sensory input to the system. The input is then integrated and modulated by the neurons of the central nervous system, which then produce the appropriate efferent or motor activation in response to the original input received.

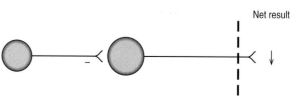

Fig. 1.7 Direct inhibition. The process of direct inhibition involves the inhibition of the downstream neuron by a neuron directly upstream, with no interneuron involvement.

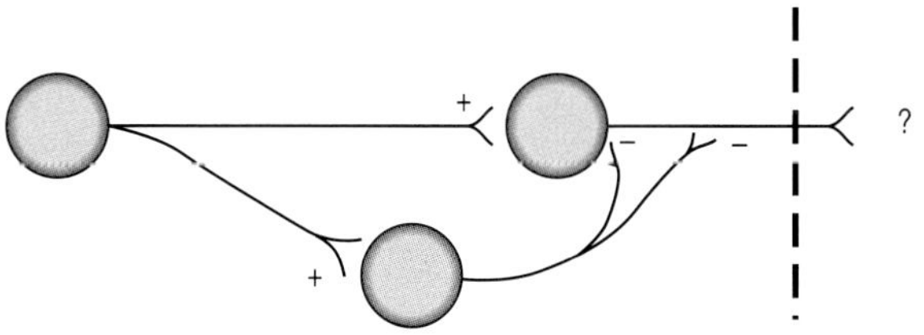

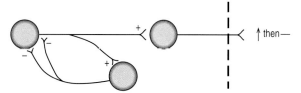

Fig. 1.8 Feedforward inhibition. The process of feedforward inhibition involves the simultaneous activation of the target neuron and an inhibitory interneuron, which in turn inhibits the target neuron.

Fig. 1.9 Feedback inhibition. Feedback inhibition involves the simultaneous stimulation of a downstream neuron and an inhibitory interneuron that in turn inhibits the original stimulating neuron.

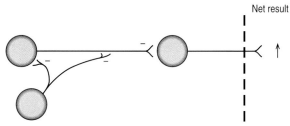

Fig. 1.10 Disinhibition. Disinhibition involves the inhibition of an inhibitory interneuron. The result of this process is a decrease inhibition of the target neuron or increased probability of firing in the target neuron.

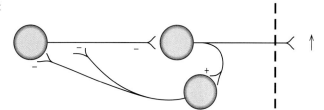

Fig. 1.11 Feedback disinhibition. Feedback disinhibition involves the stimulation of an inhibitory interneuron that in turn synapses on a primary inhibitory neuron of the target neuron. This system tends to result in a positive feedback stimulus of the target neuron and is rare in humans.

Feedback inhibition involves an inhibitory interneuron that receives stimulus from the neuron that it projects to and thus also inhibits (Fig. 1.9).

Disinhibition (inhibition of inhibition) involves two inhibitory interneurons linked in series with each other so that stimulation of the first neuron results in inhibition of the second neuron, which in turn results in decreased inhibitory output of the second interneuron to the target. The overall effect of disinhibition is an increased probability that the effector will reach threshold potential per unit stimulus (Fig. 1.10).

Feedback disinhibition involves a series of inhibitory interneurons that receive their original stimulus from the neuron that they project to; however, in this case the net result is an increase in the probability that the target neuron will reach threshold per unit stimulus (Fig. 1.11).

To illustrate these concepts the corticostriate-basal ganglio-thalamocortical neuron projection system in the neuraxis will be examined (see Chapter 11 for more detailed descriptions).

Selective pyramidal output neurons, in wide areas of cortex, project to the neostriatum (caudate and putamen) via the corticostriatal projection system. The cortical neurons are excitatory in nature to the neurons in the caudate and putamen. The neurons of the caudate and putamen project to neurons in both regions of the globus pallidus, the globus pallidus pars interna and globus pallidus pars externa, and are inhibitory in nature. For the purposes of this example we will only consider the projections to the globus pallidus pars interna. This nucleus comprises the final output nucleus of the basal ganglia, to the thalamus. (For a more complete description see Chapter 11.)

Neurons in the globus pallidus pars interna project to neurons in the thalamus and are inhibitory in nature.

The neurons in the thalamus project back to neurons in the cortex and are excitatory in nature to the cortical neurons.

Following the flow of stimulus through the system (Fig. 1.12) it can be noted that the end result is a disinhibition of the thalamus and an increased likelihood of cortical activation by thalamic neurons.

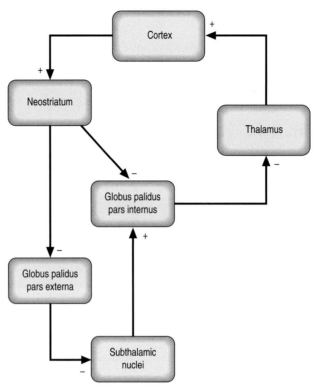

Fig. 1.12 The direct and indirect functional pathways of the basal ganglia. The input to the basal ganglia occurs via the neostriatum from the cortex. The output of the neostriatum projects to both areas of the globus pallidus, the globus pallidus pars internus (GPi) and externus (GPe). The stimulus received from the neostriatum is inhibitory on both the GPi and the GPe. The direct pathway involves the projections from the neostriatum to GPi, the projections from the GPi to the thalamus, and the projections from the thalamus to the cortex. The direct pathway results in inhibition of the inhibitory output of the GPi on the thalamus (inhibition of inhibition). This results in a gating pattern of disinhibition, or increased probability of firing of the thalamic neurons. The disinhibition of the thalamus results in increased activation of the cortical neurons. The indirect pathway involves the projections from the neostriatum to the GPe, the projections from the GPe to the subthalamic nuclei, the projections from the subthalamic nuclei to the GPi, the projections from the GPi to the thalamus, and the projections from the thalamus to the cortex. The projections from the neocortex to the GPe are inhibitory to the GPe. The projections from the GPe to the subthalamic nuclei are inhibitory to the subthalamic nuclei. Projections from the subthalamic nucleus to the GPi are excitatory and the projections from the GPi to the thalamus are inhibitory. The end result of stimulation of the indirect pathway is a gating mechanism that increases the inhibition on the thalamic neurons, which in turn results in decreased activation input from the thalamic neurons to the cortex. To summarize, stimulus of the direct pathway results in increased cortical stimulation and stimulus of the indirect pathway results in decreased cortical stimulation. The physiological impact of these pathways will be discussed in more detail in following chapters.

Neurological 'Wind-Up' in a System

Occasionally a system will experience 'wind-up', which results in the development of a hyperexcited state of activity. This is usually not ideal since the output from the system will be inappropriate per unit input. Chronic wind-up can also result in damage to individual neurons or the whole system in the following ways:

1. Overactivation of glutamate N-methyl-D-aspartate (NMDA) receptors can result in excitotoxicity in neurons because of increased intracellular Ca^{++} ion concentrations.

2. Free radical formation due to anaerobic energy production pathways may lead to damage to membrane and membrane receptor structures, or to mutations in DNA.

3. Transneural degeneration may result when intracellular protein and energy stores become inadequate to support the increased demands of hyperexcitability.

Wind-up usually occurs when either the neuron or system receives too much excitatory stimulus or normal levels of tonic inhibition malfunction. The following example will illustrate the concept.

The thalamus contains neurons that tonically generate innate excitatory potentials that project to the cortex and result in excitation of cortical neurons. Under normal conditions, modulation of this tonic excitation occurs via the inhibitory output of the globus pallidus pars interna (GPi) of the basal ganglionic circuits. However, in certain circumstances, such as an increased output of the neostriatum, which can occur with loss of inhibition from the substantia nigra pars compacta, the globus pallidus receives an increased inhibitory input from the neostriatum. This increased inhibition to the GPi reduces the inhibition received by the thalamus from the GPi. This results in an increase in the innate tonic excitation to the cortex from the thalamus, which in turn results in a hyperexcitation or wind-up of cortical neurons. This example demonstrates how inhibition of inhibition can result in hyperexcitation of a neuron system. The concept of inhibition of inhibition is very important clinically in understanding the symptoms produced in multimodal integrative systems and is encountered frequently in clinical practice.

Ablative and Physiological Dysfunctional Lesions

Ablative lesions are lesions that result in the death or destruction of neural tissues. This type of lesion commonly occurs as the result of a vascular stroke when tissues experience critical levels of hypoxia or anoxia and die as a result. Direct or indirect trauma as in the 'coup counter coup' injuries in whiplash or head trauma can also result in ablution of tissues or function. Replacement of the damaged tissue is usually very slow, if it occurs at all, and restoration of function depends on the rerouting of nerve pathways or regrowth of new synaptic connections.

Physiological lesions are functional lesions that result from overstimulation, excessive inhibition, excessive disinhibition, or understimulation of a neuronal system. Correction of these functional lesions is dependent on restoring normal levels of activation to the involved systems. The results are usually apparent relatively quickly and can occur almost immediately in some cases.

Often the symptom presentation of these two types of lesions can be very similar so the possibility of an ablative lesion must be ruled out before the diagnosis of a physiological lesion is made.

For example, in *Huntington's disease* (HD) the neurons in the neostriatum degenerate. The degeneration appears to be more pronounced in the output neostriatal neurons of the indirect pathway. This results in the disinhibition of the globus pallidus pars externa (GPe), which in turn results in an overinhibition of the subthalamic nucleus. The functional overinhibition of the subthalamic nucleus results in a situation that resembles an ablative lesion to the subthalamic nucleus and results in a hyperkinetic movement disorder. In this case the lesion is not purely physiological in nature because the neostriatal neurons have actually degenerated but the result is the physiological functional state of overinhibition of a neuron system.

Fundamental Functional Projection Systems

In order to apply the neurophysiological concepts discussed thus far in a clinical setting an understanding of some of the basic fundamental functional projection systems utilized by the cortex to modulate activity in wide-ranging areas of the neuraxis must be gained.

About 90% of the output axons of the cortex are involved in modulation of the neuraxis. About 10% of the cortical output axons of the cortex are involved in motor control and form the corticospinal tracts.

Of the 90% output dedicated to neuraxis modulation about 10% projects bilaterally to the reticular formation of the mesencephalon (MRF) and 90% projects ipsilaterally to the reticular formation of the pons and medulla or pontomedullary reticular formation (PMRF). The cortical projections to both the MRF and the PMRF are excitatory in nature. The neurons in the MRF and some of those in the PMRF project bilaterally to excite

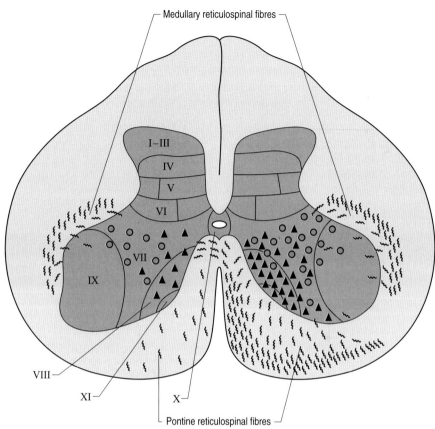

Fig. 1.13 The relative distribution of neuron cell bodies and projection fibre tracts of the pontomedullary reticulospinal tracts (PMRF). Although both the neurons and the projection fibres occur bilaterally, the majority of neurons and projections are ipsilateral in nature.

neurons in the intermediolateral (IML) cell columns located between T1 and L2 spinal cord levels in the grey matter of the spinal cord; however, the majority of the PMRF remain ipsilateral (Fig. 1.13) (Nyberg-Hansen 1965). These neurons in the IML form the presynaptic output neurons of the sympathetic nervous system, and project to inhibit neurons in the sacral spinal cord regions that form the output neurons of the parasympathetic nervous system.

Following the stimulus flow through the functional system it can be seen that high cortical output results in high PMRF output, which results in strong inhibition of the IML, which in turn results in disinhibition of the sacral parasympathetic output. The bilateral excitatory output of the MRF is overshadowed by the powerful stimulus from the cortex to the PMRF (Fig. 1.14).

To further illustrate the impact that an asymmetric cortical output (hemisphericity) could potentially have clinically, consider the affects of an asymmetric cortical output on the activity levels of the sympathetic and parasympathetic systems on each side of the body. Autonomic asymmetries are an important indicator of cortical asymmetry as this reflects on fuel delivery to the brain (sympathetic system) and the integrity of excitatory and inhibitory influences on sympathetic and parasympathetic function throughout the rest of the body.

The PMRF has other modulatory effects in addition to modulation of the IML neurons. All of the modulatory interactions of the PMRF have clinical relevance and include:

1.   Inhibition of pain ipsilaterally;

2.   Inhibition of the inhibitory interneurons which project to ventral horn cells (VHCs) ipsilaterally which acts to facilitate muscle tone—this is another example of inhibition of inhibition in the neuraxis as discussed above; and

3.   Inhibition of the ipsilateral anterior muscles above T6 and the posterior muscles below T6.

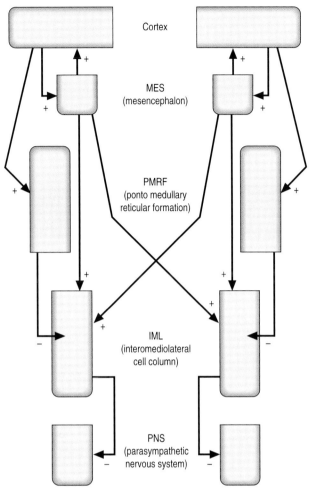

Fig. 1.14 A simplified schematic of the cortical projection system to the sympathetic (SNS) and parasympathetic nervous systems (PNS). All outputs of the cortex in this system are excitatory to both the mesencephalon (MES) and the pontomedullary reticular formation (PMRF); however, 90% of the cortical projections are to the PMRF and 10% to the MES. Bilateral, excitatory projections from the MES to the intermediolateral (IML) cell column neurons result in activation of the sympathetic preganglionic neurons. Ipsilateral inhibitory projections from the PMRF to the IML result in inhibition of the sympathetic preganglionic neurons. Because of the distribution of projection fibres, cortical activation will result in an ipsilateral inhibition of the IML or SNS and an ipsilateral activation of the PNS. These functional loops will be discussed in much more detail later in the text.

A sense of the clinical impact that asymmetric stimulation of the PMRF can produce symptomatically in the patient becomes apparent when it is considered that all of the following can result:

- Increased blood pressure systemically or ipsilaterally to the side of decreased PMRF stimulation, which results in differences in blood pressure between right and left sides of the body;
- Increased vein-to-artery ratio, which is most apparent on examination of the retina;
- Increased sweating globally or ipsilaterally to the side of decreased PMRF stimulation;
- Decreased skin temperature globally or ipsilaterally to the side of decreased PMRF stimulation;
- Arrhythmia if decreased left PMRF stimulation occurs or tachycardia if decreased right PMRF stimulation occurs;
- Large pupil (also due to decreased mesencephalic integration) to the side of decreased PMRF stimulation;
- Ipsilateral pain syndromes to the side of decreased PMRF stimulation;
- Global decrease in muscle tone ipsilaterally to the side of decreased PMRF stimulation;

- Flexor angulation of the upper limb ipsilaterally to the side of decreased PMRF stimulation; and

- Extensor angulation of the lower limb ipsilaterally to the side of decreased PMRF stimulation.

Clinical presentation of ipsilateral flexor angulation of the upper limb and extensor angulation of the lower limb is known as *pyramidal paresis,* and is an important clinical finding in many patients with asymmetric cortical function.

The fundamental projection systems (Fig. 1.14) presented above are simplified for the purposes of introduction and will be discussed more thoroughly throughout the rest of the text.

Longitudinal Level of a Lesion in the Neuraxis

Lesions may occur at one or more points along a nerve pathway. Identifying the level at which the lesion has occurred is usually accomplished by taking a thorough history and performing a thorough physical examination of the patient. A nerve pathway may become dysfunctional at one or more of the following:

- The receptor level;
- The effector organ level;
- In the efferent and afferent nerve axons of the peripheral nerve;
- The spinal cord level;
- The brainstem and cerebellar level;
- The thalamus/basal ganglionic level; or
- The level of the cortex.

Lesions at the receptor level may be ablative, may be caused by states of habituation, or may be due to a decreased environmental stimulus. Often the sensitivity of a receptor is cortically mediated and cortical hyper- or hyposensitivity states may be confused with a receptor lesion. The level of response of a receptor is often measured through the response of an effector organ and this may also result in confusion between a receptor lesion and an effector dysfunction.

Effector or end organ lesions may be hyper- or hypofunctional in nature. In skeletal muscle hypofunctional disorders can be caused by myopathies, neurotransmitter or neuroreceptor dysfunction, oxidative phosphorylation disorders, or lack of use. Hyperfunctional disorders can be caused by metabolic and ionic imbalances. Often, disinhibition of VHCs can result in a hyperfunctional state, such as rigidity and spasms of the end organ. This is actually a spinal cord (corticospinal tract lesion) or supraspinal (upper motor neuron) level of involvement which could be confused with an end organ dysfunction.

Peripheral nerve lesions usually involve both motor and sensory functional disturbances. The distributions of the peripheral nerves have been anatomically and functionally mapped fairly accurately and these distributions can be used to identify the location of a specific peripheral nerve dysfunction. Often the end organs such a muscle will show specific forms of activity (flaccid paralysis) or neurologically induced atrophy (muscle wasting) when a peripheral nerve is involved.

Spinal cord lesions may exhibit disassociation of sensory and motor symptoms depending on the specific areas of involvement of the spinal cord. Specific tract lesions may demonstrate classical symptoms (dorsal column lesions and loss of proprioception) and when specific areas of the cord are involved the patient may exhibit classical symptoms of a well-defined syndrome (posterior lateral medullary infarcts and symptoms of Wallenberg's syndrome).

Lesions of the brainstem and cerebellum often result in widespread seemingly unrelated symptoms (cerebellar degeneration and changes in cognitive function, or dysautonomia with brainstem dysfunction). These can be one of the most challenging levels of lesion to treat, due to the involvement of both upstream and downstream neuronal systems which experience altered function concomitantly.

Basal ganglionic and thalamic levels usually result in movement disorders and disorders of sensory reception including pain disorders. Basal ganglionic disorders have also been implicated in a variety of cognitive function disorders as well.

Lesions at the cortical level can manifest as dysfunction at any other level in the neuraxis and as such are often very difficult to pinpoint. Many of the cortical functions, if not all cortical functions, are highly integrated over diffuse areas of cortex, which once again makes targeting specific neuron circuits difficult.

The Concepts of Direct Linearity and Singularity

The neuraxis utilizes a number of types of synaptic connections including monosynaptic and polysynaptic relays.

Monosynaptic connections between two structures suggest an important functional relationship between the two structures in question. Polysynaptic connections may be important as well but are not as well understood. For example, the existence of monosynaptic connections between the hypothalamus and the preganglionic sympathetic neurons in the IML suggests an important functional relationship between the output of the sympathetic nervous system and the CIS of the hypothalamus.

An area of singularity is a neuronal circuit or system that has one or very few input pathways that can modulate its activities. For example the globus pallidus is a very difficult area of the neuraxis to influence clinically because the area can only be accessed via projections from neurons in the neostriatum, whereas ventral horn neurons in the spinal cord can be influenced by modulating a multitude of different pathways.

The Physiological 'Blind Spot' as a Measure of Cortical Activation

A visual image inverts and reverses as it passes through the lens of the eye and forms an image on the retina. Image from the upper visual field is projected on the lower retina and from the lower visual field on the upper retina. The left visual field is projected to the right hemiretina of each eye in such a fashion that the right nasal hemiretina of the left eye and the temporal hemiretina of the right eye receive the image. The central image or focal point of the visual field falls on the fovea of the retina, which is the portion of the retina with the highest density of retinal cells and as such produces the highest visual acuity. The fovea receives the corresponding image of the central $1°-2°$ of the total visual field but represents about 50% of the axons in the optic nerve and projects to about 50% of the neurons in the visual cortex. The macula comprises the space surrounding the fovea and also has a relatively high visual acuity. The optic disc is located about 15° medially or towards the nose on each retina and is the convergence point for the axons of retinal cells as they leave the retina and form the optic nerve. This area although functionally important has no photoreceptors. This creates a blind spot in each eye about 15° temporally from a central fixation point. When both eyes are functioning, open, and focused on a central fixation point, the blind spots do not overlap so all of the visual field is represented in the cortex and one is not aware of the blind spot in one's visual experience. The area of the visual striate cortex which is the primary visual area of the occipital lobe, representing the blind spot and the monocular crescent which are both in the temporal field, does not contain alternating independent ocular dominance columns. This means that these areas only receive information from one eye. If you close that eye, the area representing the blind spot of the eye that remains open will not be activated due to the lack of receptor activation at the retina.

It would be expected that when one eye is closed the visual field should now have an area not represented by visual input and one should be aware of the absence of vision over the area of the blind spot. However, this does not occur. The cortical neurons responsible for the area of the blind spot must receive stimulus from other neurons that create the illusion that the blind spot is not there. This is indeed the case and is accomplished by a series of horizontal projection neurons located in the visual striate cortex that allow for neighbouring hypercolumns to activate one another. The horizontal connections between these hypercolumns allow for perceptual completion or 'fill in' to occur (Gilbert & Wiesel 1989; McGuire et al 1991).

The blind spot is therefore not strictly monocular, but it is dependent on the FOF of horizontal connections from neighbouring neurons. These may be activated via receptors and pathways from either eye.

Perceptual completion refers to the process whereby the brain fills in the region of the visual field that corresponds to a lack of visual receptors. This explains why one generally is not aware of the blind spot in everyday experience. The size and shape of the blind spots can be mapped utilizing simple procedures as outlined in Chapter 4.

The size and shape of the blind spots is dependent to some extent on the CIS of the horizontal neurons of the cortex that supply the stimulus for the act of completion to occur. The integrative state of the horizontal neurons is determined to some extent by the activity levels of the neurons in the striate cortex in general. Several factors can contribute to the CIS of striate cortical neurons; however, a major source of stimulus results from thalamocortical activation via the reciprocal thalamocortical optic radiation pathways involving the lateral geniculate nucleus (LGN) of the thalamus. Only 10–20% of the projections arriving in the LGN nucleus are derived directly from the retina. The remaining projections arise from the brainstem reticular formation, the pulvinar, and reciprocal projections from the striate cortex.

It is clear from the above that the majority of the projection fibres reaching the LGN are not from retinal cells. This strongly suggests that the LGN acts as a multimodal sensory integration convergence point that in turn activates neurons in the striate cortex appropriately. The level of activation of the LGN is temporally and spatially dependent on the activity levels of all the multimodal projections that it receives.

In 1997, Professor Frederick Carrick discovered that asymmetrically altering the afferent input to the thalamus resulted in an asymmetrical effect on the size of the blind spot in each eye. The blind spot was found to decrease on the side of increased afferent stimulus. This was attributed to an increase in brain function on the contralateral side due to changes in thalamocortical activation that occurred because of multimodal sensory integration in the thalamus.

The stimulus utilized by Professor Carrick in his study was a manipulation of the upper cervical spine which is known to increase the FOF of multimodal neurons in areas of the thalamus and brainstem that project to the visual striate cortex. These reciprocal connections lower the threshold for activation of neurons in the visual cortex. By decreasing the threshold for firing of neurons in the visual cortex the blind spot became smaller because the area surrounding the permanent geometric blind spot zone is more likely to reach threshold and respond to the receptor activation that occurs immediately adjacent to the optic disc on the contralateral side. The size and shape of the blind spot will also be associated with the degree of activation of neurons associated with receptors adjacent to the optic disc. The receptors surrounding the optic disc underlie the neurons that form the optic nerve exiting by way of the optic disc. The amplitude of receptor potentials adjacent to the optic disc may therefore also be decreased due to interference of light transmission through the overlying fibres even though they should have lost their myelin coating during development; otherwise, interference would be even greater. This interference results in a decreased receptor amplitude, which in turn results in decreased FOF of the corresponding primary afferent nerve. This may result in a blind spot physiologically larger than the true anatomical size of the blind spot.

This lead to the understanding that the size and shape of the blind spots could be used as a measure of the CIS of areas of the thalamus and cortex due to the fact that the amplitude of somatosensory receptor potentials received by the thalamus will influence the FOF of cerebellothalamocortical loops that have been shown to maintain a CIS of the cortex.

Therefore, muscle stretch and joint mechanoreceptor potentials will alter the FOF of primary afferents that may have an effect on visual neurons associated with the cortical receptive field of the blind spot when visual afferents are in a steady state of firing. Professor Carrick proposed that 'A change in the frequency of firing of one receptor-based neural system should effect the central integration of neurons that share synaptic relationships between other environmental modalities, resulting in an increase or decrease of cortical neuronal expression that is generally associated with a single modality' (Carrick 1997).

Care should be taken not to base too much clinical significance on the blind spot sizes until any pathological or other underlying cause that may have resulted in the changes in blind spot size are ruled out. The blind spot has been found to increase in size due to the following conditions:

- Multiple evanescent white dot syndrome;
- Acute macular neuroretinopathy;
- Acute idiopathic blind spot enlargement (AIBSE) syndrome;
- Multifocal choroiditis;
- Pseudo presumed ocular histoplasmosis;
- Peripapillary retinal dysfunction; and
- Systemic vascular disease.

An ophthalmoscopical examination is therefore an important component of the functional neurological examination. There are several other valuable ophthalmoscopic findings discussed in Chapter 4 that can assist with estimating the CIS of various neuronal pools.

Upper and Lower Motor Neurons

The concept of a group of upper motor neuron pools versus groups of lower motor neuron pools can be of great value when localizing lesions in the neuraxis in the clinical setting. Upper motor neurons are considered all of the neuron pools which project directly or indirectly to the final common path motor neurons. Lower motor neurons are the neurons that supply the final common projection to the skeletal muscles. Some examples will illustrate the concepts.

The pyramidal neurons in the motor cortex project via the corticospinal tracts to the ventral grey area of the spinal cord where they synapse on the VHCs. The ventral horn neurons are the final common pathway to the skeletal muscles and as such are considered lower motor neurons. The cortical neurons and their projections in the corticospinal tracts are considered the upper motor neurons.

The same concept applies to the cortical neurons that modulate the motor output of cranial nerves. The cortical neurons in the motor strip that project their axons via the corticobulbar tracts to the motor nuclei of the cranial nerves in the brainstem are considered upper motor neurons. The cranial nerve motor neurons in the brainstem are considered the final common pathway to the muscles that they supply and are considered the lower motor neurons of this system.

The functional effects of upper and lower motor neuron dysfunction are distinct and important clinically.

Lower motor neuron lesions will produce flaccid muscle weakness, muscular atrophy, fasciculations, and hyporeflexia. Upper motor neuron lesions will produce spastic muscle weakness, and hyperreflexia. Upper motor neuron dysfunction involving the corticospinal tracts usually produces a classic reflex sign referred to as Babinski's sign or reflex. Under normal conditions stroking the plantar aspect of the foot will produce a reflex flexion of the toes. In cases of corticospinal tract dysfunction stroking the plantar surface of the foot produces an 'up-going' or extended big toe and fanning action of the rest of the toes. This is referred to as a positive or present Babinski sign or up-going plantar reflex. Other reflex signs of upper motor neuron dysfunction will be discussed in Chapter 4. Initially, in the acute stages, the signs of upper motor neuron dysfunction may mimic lower motor neuron dysfunction exhibiting flaccid muscle weakness and hyporeflexia. These signs change progressively over hours or days to the true signs of upper motor neuron dysfunction. In the case of long-standing upper motor neuron dysfunction the involved muscles may atrophy due to disuse and give the appearance of a lower motor neuron involvement.

References

Alberts B, Bray D, Lewis J et al 1994 Energy conversion: mitochondria and chondroplasts in molecular biology of the cell. 3rd edn. Garland, New York.

Brock LG, Coombs JS, Eccles JC 1952 The recording of potential from motor neurones with an intercellular electrode. Journal of Physiology 117:431–460.

Brooks VB 1984 The neural basis of motor control. Oxford University Press, Oxford.

Carrick FR 1997 Changes in brain function after manipulation of the cervical spine. Journal of Manipulative and Physiological Therapeutics 20(8):529–545.

Connor JA, Stevens CF 1971 Prediction of repetitive firing behaviour from voltage clamp data on an isolated neurone soma. Journal of Physiology 23:31–53.

Cragg B 1975 The density of synapses and neurons in normal, mentally defective, and aging human brains. Brain 98:81–90.

Davidson RJ, Hugdahl K 1995 Brain asymmetry. MIT Press, Cambridge, MA/London.

Destexhe A, Sejnowski TJ 2003 Interactions between membrane conductances underlying thalamocortical slow wave oscillations. Physiological Reviews 83:1401–1453.

Eccles JC 1951 Interpretation of action potentials evoked in the cerebral cortex. Journal of Neurophysiology 3:449–464.

Falk D, Hildebolt C, Cheverud J et al 1991 Human cortical asymmetries determined with 3D-MR technology. Journal of Neuroscience Methods 39(2):185–191.

Galaburda AM, LeMay M, Geschwind N 1978 Right-left asymmetries in the brain. Science 199:852–856.

Ganong WF 1983 Excitable tissue: nerve. In: Review of medical physiology. Lange Medical, Los Altos, CA.

Geschwind N, Levitsky W 1968 Human brain: Left-right asymmetries in temporal speech regions. Science 161:186–187.

Getting PA 1989 Emerging principals governing the operation of neuronal circuits. Annual Review of Neuroscience 12:185–204.

Gilbert CD, Wiesel TN 1989 Columnar specificity of intrinsic horizontal and corticocortical connections in the cat visual cortex. Journal of Neuroscience 9:2432–2442.

Huttenlocher PR 1994 Synaptogenesis, synapse elimination, and neural plasticity in human cerebral cortex. In: Nelson CA (ed) Threats to optimal development: integrating biological, psychological, and social risk factors: the Minnesota symposia on child psychology. L Erlbaum, Mahwah, NJ, vol 27, p 35–54.

Jacobson M 1991 Developmental neurobiology, 3rd edn. Plenum Press, New York/London.

LeMay M, Culebras A 1972 Human brain morphological differences in the hemispheres demonstrable by carotid arteriography. New England Journal of Medicine 287:168–170.

McGuire BA, Gilbert CD, Rivlin PK et al 1991 Targets of horizontal connections in macaque primary visual cortex. Journal of Comparative Neurology 305:370–392.

Mitchell PJ, Tjian R 1989 Transcriptional regulation in mammalian cells by sequence specific DNA proteins. Science 245:371–378.

Nyberg-Hansen R 1965 Sites and mode of termination of reticulospinal fibers in the cat. An experimental study with silver impregnation methods. Journal of Comparative Neurology 124:74–100.

Savic I, Pauli S, Thorell JO et al 1994 In vivo demonstration of altered benzodiazepine receptor density in patients with generalized epilepsy. Journal of Neurology, Neurosurgery, and Psychiatry 57:784–797.

Steinmetz H, Volkmann J, Jancke L et al 1991 Anatomical left-right asymmetry of language-related temporal cortex is different in left-handers and right handers. Annals of Neurology 29(3):315–319.

Stevens CF 1979 The neuron. Scientific American (Sept) 241:54.

Williams PL, Warwick R 1980 Some general features of neural organisation. In: Gray's anatomy. Churchill Livingstone, Edinburgh, p 808–810.

Chapter

2

Early Developmental Events

Clinical Cases for Thought

Case 2.1   A young couple have presented to your office with their 3-week-old male child concerned about the possibility of spina bifida. The father reports that when he was born the doctor stated to his parents that he may have spina bifida and that it may be hereditary. The father, aged 23, has had no clinical signs or symptoms to date.

Questions

2.1.1   Describe the different types of spina bifida and the mechanism of development in each case.

2.1.2   Describe the critical period of development when the risk of spina bifida is greatest.

2.1.3   What tests can be done to rule out whether spina bifida is present in the foetus?

Introduction

Clinicians and researchers concerned with the function of the nervous system are focusing increasing attention on brain and nervous system development as a window of insight into both brain functionality and new treatment possibilities directed at nervous system dysfunction. Dysfunctions that may be associated with developmental abnormalities of the brain range from a mild reduction of cortical function to severe psychiatric disorders, such as infantile autism and schizophrenia. In man, the brain and nervous system are the most complex part. In the time span of a few months from conception, a microscopic speck of embryonic neuroblasts will have expanded into an intricate neural network with a few billion interconnections. Perhaps even more amazing is the fact that the entire mass of this fragile structure will fit very nicely into the palm of one's hand! By five years of age the human brain has reached 90% of its adult weight and in the cortex, the maximum density of synaptic connections will have already maximized and started to decline. Although there has been in the past few years an explosion in the knowledge and understanding of some of the mechanisms involved in neural development the story of how these extraordinary events unfold is one of the great mysteries of mankind. It is important to recognize that the development of the brain and nervous system is influenced by the interaction of both endogenous and exogenous mechanisms. Endogenous mechanisms include innate pre-programmed genes and chemical morphogens. Exogenous mechanisms involve the interaction of the developing nervous system with its environment.

Development of the Nervous System

The location of the cells destined to develop into the neuraxis (nervous system) is probably already defined in the late gastrula stage of the embryo, at about 18 postovulatory days. At this point the embryo is about 1.5 mm in length (Huttenlocher 2002).

The development proper of the nervous system can first be identified at approximately 3 weeks (21 days) after conception, with the appearance of the neural plate. Originally the neural plate is roughly the shape of a Ping-Pong paddle, but soon develops a distinct neural groove, flanked by neural folds (Fig. 2.1). This fold is eventually drawn together by contractile tissue deep to the neural groove which pulls the folds together. Initially while the tube is closing, its walls consist of a single layer of neuroepithelial cells. Each of these cells contacts both the internal (luminal) and external (basal) limiting membranes. This fold fuses by the end of the third week to the early fourth week, generally in what will eventually become the cervical region of the spinal cord and then extends zipper-like, rostrally forming the brain proper and caudally forming the thoracic, lumbar, sacral, and coccygeal regions of the spinal cord (Fig. 2.2).

The neural tube is originally open to the amniotic cavity by virtue of the neuropores located both rostrally and caudally, but by the end of the fourth week the neural tube closes at both ends with the closure of the neuropores. At the rostral end of the neural tube the primitive forebrain divides into two cerebral hemispheres and forms the two lateral ventricles and the third ventricle. The embryo is about 7 mm long at this point (day 32) in development (Behrman & Vaughan 1987). Once the neural tube has closed, the ectoderm forming the lips of the neural fold separates and forms the neural crest tissue (Fig. 2.3).

The neural crest cells give rise to several components of the peripheral nervous system, as well as a number of non-neural tissues. Tissues eventually formed by the neural crest cells include pigment cells of the skin; medullary cells of the adrenal gland; calcitonin-secreting cells of the thyroid gland; neurons of the paravertebral ganglia; many of the

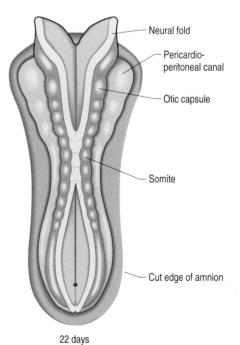

22 days

Fig. 2.2 Dorsal aspect of a human embryo at day 22. Note the initial closure of the neural fold forming the neural tube, which will progress both caudally and dorsally until complete closure. The appearance of the bilateral forked primitive ventricles caudally and the bilateral otic placodes should also be noted.

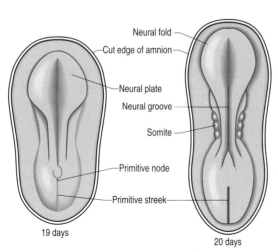

19 days

20 days

Fig. 2.1 Dorsal aspect of a human embryo at day 19 (left) and day 20 (right). Note the rapid progression of somite formation, the appearance of the neural fold, and the deepening of the neural groove from day 19 to day 20 in development.

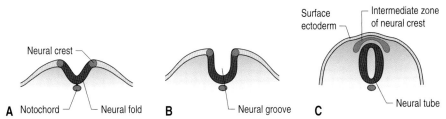

Fig. 2.3 Cross-sectional progression of the formation of the neural tube and the migration of the neural crest tissue. (A) The formation of the neural fold and differentiation of the neural crest tissue. (B) The neural fold deepens to form the neural groove, and the neural crest tissues enlarges and approximates. (C) Closure of the neural groove forms the neural tube. The neural crest tissue separates from the neural tube and is enveloped by surface ectodermal tissue. The neural crest tissue is initially connected by an intermediate zone, which will in turn separate as development progresses. Note the presence of the notochord throughout the sequence which is destined to form the nucleus pulposus of the intervertebral disc.

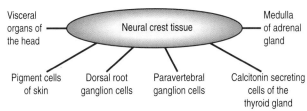

Fig. 2.4 The various structures that arise from the neural crest tissue. The dorsal root ganglion cells form the basis of all sensation received below the head and neck. The paravertebral ganglion cells will form the majority of the post-ganglionic catacholaminergic (noradrenaline) output cells of the sympathetic nervous system. The adrenal medulla cells will form the major catacholaminergic (adrenaline) output of the hypothalamic-pituitary-adrenal axis. Calcitonin is a hormone that lowers the blood calcium concentration in the blood. As we will discover calcium is a major second messenger signalling molecule in neurons. Alterations in melatonin distribution and formation can signal underlying neurological conditions such as neurofibromatosis.

neurons in the ganglia of the cranial nerves V, VII, VIII, IX, and X; and neurons of the dorsal root ganglia (Leikola 1976) (Fig. 2.4). The cells of the neural crest disperse by migrating along well-defined pathways to their destinations. The phenotype of each cell seems to be largely determined by the position that they eventually occupy (Le Douarin 1982). For example, cells destined to migrate to the adenyl medulla (norepinephrine-secreting cells) have been experimentally transplanted to sites that give rise to cholinergic (acetylcholine-secreting) cells. The transplanted cells converted to cholinergic-secreting neurons (Cowan 1992).

The continued growth and expansion of the neural tube leads to the stimulation of overlying ectodermal tissues at various sites called ectodermal placodes. These ectodermal placodes lead to the development and formation of the sensory epithelia and cranial nerve ganglia. The various placodal development sites include the olfactory placode, the trigeminal placode, the auditory/vestibular placode, the facial placode, the vagal placode, and the glossopharyngeal placode.

These early stages of development are largely dependent on the processes of primary embryonic induction, which is largely under genetic control (Williams & Warwick 1980).

Gross Morphological Development

Shortly after the closure of the neural tube, a series of three vesicle-like swellings appear at the rostral apex of the tube. These swellings will eventually form the three primary brain vesicles: the prosencephalic (forebrain), the mesencephalic (midbrain), and the rhombencephalic (hindbrain) areas. Through various folding patterns the three primary vesicles ultimately give rise to the mature brain structures. The development of the three primary vesicles into their representative mature structures results in the following progression: the prosencephalic region develops into the telencephalon and the diencephalon; the mesencephalon remains undifferentiated, giving rise to the mature mesencephalon; and the rhombencephalon develops into the myelencephalon and metencephalon. Each of these secondary brain vesicles further develops into the recognized mature divisions of the human brain (Figs 2.5 and 2.6).

Embryological Development of the Primary Vesicles of the Neuraxis

Forebrain-----------Prosencephalon------------Telencephalon
                                              Diencephalon

Midbrain------------Mesencephalon-------------Mesencephalon

Hindbrain-----------Rhombencephalon----------Myelencephalon
                                             Metencephalon

Embryological Development of the Secondary Vesicles of the Neuraxis

Telencephalon ---------Cerebral cortex
                       Basal ganglia

Diencephalon ----------Pituitary gland
                       Thalamus
                       Hypothalamus

Mesencephalon --------Corpora quadrigemina
                      Red nucleus
                      Substantia nigra

Metencephalon---------Cerebellum
                      Pons

Myelencephalon--------Medulla oblongata

Fig. 2.5 This figure demonstrates the development of primary and secondary brain vesicles.

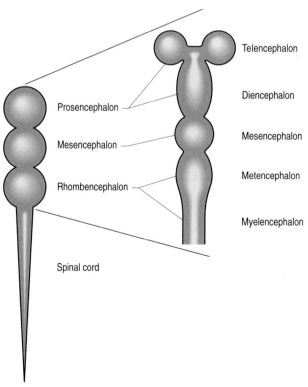

Fig. 2.6 Development of the secondary vesicles from the precursor primary vesicles. The prosencephalon differentiates into the telencephalon and the diencephalon. The mesencephalon remains undifferentiated as the mesencephalon. The rhombencephalon differentiates into the myelencephalon and the metencephalon.

Primary Developmental Processes

The development of the mature nervous system is brought about by a series of steps that include processes both progressive and regressive (Cowan 1978). These steps include cell proliferation, neuronal migration, selective cell aggregation, cytodifferentiation, axonal outgrowth, and synapse formation. The first regressive events occur about the time that neurons in each population begin to form connections within their prospective projection fields. This phase is marked by the selective death of a substantial proportion (50%) of the initial population of prospective neuron cells. Many connections that were initially formed are eliminated and certain axon terminals are withdrawn. A large number of axon collaterals are also removed at this stage (Cowan et al 1985). Each phase is considered in detail below.

Why Study the Development of Neural Structures? QUICK FACTS 1

1. How do neurons arise?

2. How do neurons know where to send their axons?

3. How are neural pools connected?

4. What are the functional relationships between neuron pools?

Can we use our knowledge of embryological and fetal development to better understand and treat developmental and other functional pathology?

Cell Proliferative Phase

The wall of the neural tube is formed initially by pseudostratified columnar epithelium that rests on the external basement membrane. Each cell sends a peripheral process to both the external (basal) lamina and the neural tube internal (luminal) surface. At the luminal surface a complex of junctional connections allows communication with other cells. The nuclei are found at different levels within the neuroepithelium, except those in the later stages of mitosis which are constantly found at the luminal aspect (Cowan 1981). The young neurons constantly migrate from the internal or luminal lamina to the external or basal lamina in a process called interkinetic nuclear migration. Throughout this process the neurons must continually retract and reform their peripheral processes. At this stage of development the neural tube consists of two histological areas of tissues, the ependymal or germinal cell layer found on the luminal aspect of the tube and the ventricular zone or matrix layer which spans the remainder of the tube and is in contact with the basal membrane. Continued cell division leads to growth and expansion of the neural tube in three ways: general expansion of the neural tube surface epithelium, rapid growth of the brain and spinal cord, and differentiation of the different lineages of cell types including glial cells and neurons. This differentiation phase is marked by a migration of some of the cells from the ventricular zone to the newly emerging intermediate or mantle zone, away from the luminal surface. The neurons in the intermediate zone send processes outward towards the basal membrane which eventually develops into the marginal zone. To summarize, at this point (4 weeks or 28 days) the development of the neural tube consists of four histologically identifiable layers: the ependymal or germinal layer, from which all the cells of the central nervous system will develop; the ventricular or matrix layer, which consists of newly formed cells undergoing interkinetic nuclear migration and mitosis; the intermediate or mantle zone, which consists of cells migrating from the intermediate zone; and the marginal zone, which consists of the elongated cytoplasmic processes of the cells in the intermediate zone. Interposed throughout these layers are developing glial cells including the radial glial cells which seem to act as guide cells for the migrating neurons (Fig. 2.7).

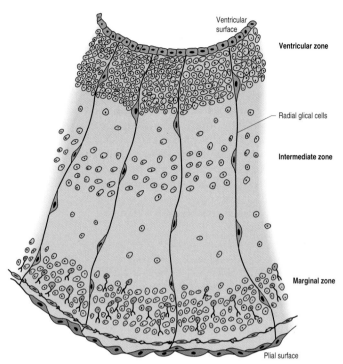

Ventricular surface

Ventricular zone

Radial glical cells

Intermediate zone

Marginal zone

Plial surface

Fig. 2.7 This figure illustrates the migration of neurons from the ventricular surface toward the plial surface of the neural tube. This migration takes part along highly specialized cells called neural glial cells. Note that neural migration appears to occur in cohorts, with neural cells born at or near the same time migrating at the same time.

Each population of neurons is generated during a distinct period of embryonic or foetal life. This period is usually quite short, ranging from a few days to a week. Cells born of the same cohort can be classified as embryological homologues. The relationships that each cohort of neurons forms with other neurons of the same cohort become very important as the system matures. These relationships can be used clinically to gain insight into the function of other related homologous systems by stimulating one system of neurons and measuring the response of a homologous system through a variety of clinical testing procedures (see Embryological Homologous Relationships later in this chapter). The sequence at which the cells withdraw from the proliferative pool is well defined. For example, in the retina the ganglion cells farthest from the original luminal zone are generated first, followed by the inner nuclear layer, which are in turned followed by the photoreceptors. The actual sequence may vary somewhat from region to region; for example, the situation in the motor cortex is completely reversed with the deepest cells forming first (Fig. 2.8).

The process of neurogenesis seems to be highly programmed in both space and time. The process seems to progress largely in a ventral to dorsal, and cervical to sacral gradient (above, down, inside, out). In keeping with this strategy, the motor systems arising from the basal plate located ventrally are generally generated before the sensory systems arising from the alar plate, which is located dorsally (Figs 2.9A and 2.9B).

It is now apparent that neurons and glial cells are generated simultaneously, and not in isolation as was once thought. Glial cells, however, tend to develop and proliferate long after neurons have been generated. This is evident in the formation of myelinated axons by the proliferation of glial cells subsequent to axon formation.

In a vast majority of cases the larger neurons of a system are generated before the smaller neurons of the same general type in the system. A notable exception to this occurs in the motor cortex where the smaller stellate cells of the cortex develop prior to the large pyramidal cells. The extent to which genetic determination plays a role in the fate of individual cells is unknown in mammals but thought likely to play a role.

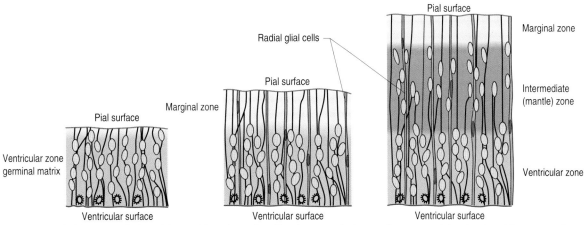

Fig. 2.8 A magnified diagrammatic view of Fig. 2.7. The various cell proliferation zones, the intermediate zone, and the migration of the neurons via the radial glial cells are illustrated.

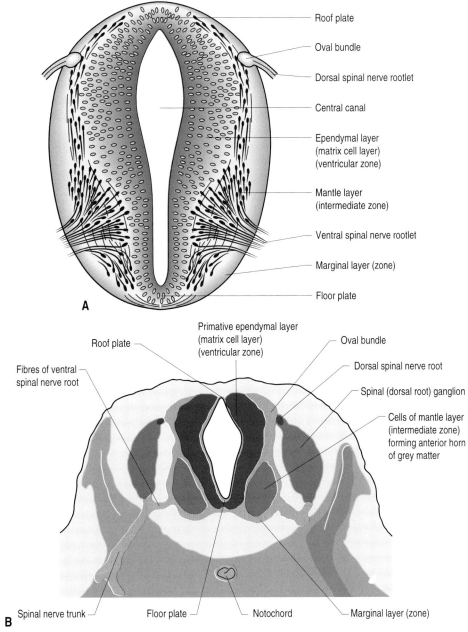

Fig. 2.9 (A) A schematic drawing of the real slide (B). Note the roof or alar plate and the floor or basal plate in (B).

Neuronal Migration

Peripheral Nervous System

Neural crest and placodal precursor cells migrate along predetermined, but as yet molecularly undefined pathways to their various locations in the cranial, spinal, and autonomic ganglia. These cells undergo the majority of their proliferation once they reach their definitive destinations. There is good evidence to suggest that the neural phenotype of most neural crest cells is largely determined by the regions through which they migrate and the location in which they ultimately settle (Sidman & Rakic 1974). Neuropathologies can develop when cells migrate too far or in the wrong direction. This situation results in the condition referred to as neuronal ectopias.

Central Nervous System

In the central nervous system the situation is quite different from the peripheral nervous system in that all cells must undergo at least one migratory phase as a rudimentary neuron or glial cell before locating to their final destination. The cells of the peripheral nervous system are stem cells or immature neurons when they start their migration. The rudimentary cells have a primitive form of differentiation that identifies the cell as either a neuron or a glial cell when they start their migration out of the nuclear zone. The final differentiation of the cell occurs throughout its migratory process through interactions with the various other cells along its determined pathway and is completed when it reaches its final destination through associations with other cells also located there.

Several aspects of the central nervous system migratory process are understood. The initial impetus for the migration of a ventricular zone neuron occurs when it withdraws itself from the cell cycle. The reasons for the withdrawal from the cell cycle are not understood. It appears that by the time a cell withdraws from the cell cycle it has acquired a distinct address for its final destination of both cell body and axonal outgrowths. The cell moves to its final location via ameboid motion guided by a substratum of radial glial cells that extend lengthy processes both the length and depth of the neural tube. It is important to note that some cells migrate in non-radial patterns, which are not consistent with the radial processes of the glial cells, and some neurons migrate beyond the presence of the radial glial cell processes. Clearly other as yet to be identified mechanisms are also involved. Neuronal ectopias can also develop in the central nervous system for the same reasons as previously listed for the peripheral nervous system.

Neuronal Cytodifferentiation

Cells of the potential neuraxis that initiate their migration out of the ventricular or subventricular zones have achieved a rudimentary form of differentiation in that they are destined to become either neurons or glial cells. In the majority of cases, it is only after they have migrated to their desired destination and associated with other cells at their destination that they undergo their major transformation into neurons or glial cells.

Once started, the process of neuronal differentiation proceeds through three major classes of events, including morphological, physiological, and molecular differentiation.

Morphological Differentiation

This process involves the development of a number of different outgrowth processes from the neuron cell body that will eventually become the dendrites and axons of the neuron. The process usually begins with the development of a single axon and one or more dendritic processes. Initially the outgrowths all look remarkably similar and contain the same organelles, including ribosomes that will disappear in the axon processes but remain in the dendritic processes as both structures mature. At this point in their development they are referred to as neurites. The establishment of the dominate axon seems to be dependent on a predetermined polarity thought to be produced by chemical morphogenic gradients produced by guide cells and locator cells in the region of the final destination of the neuron. These morphogenic gradients may act to induce a certain family of genes responsible for the production of growth-associated proteins (GAP). These GAPs are involved with the rapid elongation of the axon at a highly specialized structure referred to as the growth cone of the axon. Growth occurs through continuous addition of cytoplasmic and membrane components supplied by the neuron cell body via anterograde axonal transport to the growth cone. This axonal transport can reach velocities of up to 200 mm/day. The axon itself can reach growth velocities of up to 5 mm/day

(Cowan 1992). Some axons, such as those of the giant pyramidal cells of Betz, can grow to over a metre in length! In such cases it could potentially take proteins and transmitter substance 5–6 days to reach the axon terminal.

The formation of dendrites also occurs at a specialized growth cone structure.

A general genetic plan for the development of the initial dendritic tree seems to determine the original dendritic layout. However, the development and maintenance of dendrites in the neuron seems to maintain plasticity and is quite variable throughout life with a strong dependence on environmental stimulation determining the dendritic layout at any given stage in time.

Physiological and Molecular Differentiation

The cell membrane components necessary for the development of membrane and action potential production, including enzymes, transmembrane proteins, gap junctions, and specific receptors, do not appear simultaneously in the evolving neuron. The development of these specialized membrane structures seems to follow a specific sequential order of appearance and function in most neurons. In the early developmental period when the cells are still in the interkinetic nuclear migration cycle in the ventricular zone they develop electrically coupled (gap) junctions. Just prior to leaving the ventricular zone the cells undergo an uncoupling of their gap junctions. This uncoupling phase is replaced by long-lasting (10–100 ms) action potentials produced by calcium ion fluxes across the membrane. The next phase of development is heralded by the appearance of much shorter (1–2 ms) sodium-produced action potentials superimposed over the long-lasting calcium action potentials. In the final stage of development, in most neurons, the calcium slow potentials disappear, leaving only the sodium action potentials active in the neuron (Spitzer 1981). A complex relationship between calcium and sodium interaction remains in most mature neurons with the permeability of sodium across the neuronal membrane inversely proportional to the concentration of extracellular calcium. It is not clear why this sequence of events occurs in most neurons but it outlines the importance of temporally pre-programmed expression of genes in the development of ion-specific protein channels so important to the establishment of neuron function.

The functional attributes of a neuron begin by the production of at least one group and sometimes several groups of neurotransmitter synthesizing enzymes. Thus a single neuron may produce more than one neurotransmitter. In conjunction with the appearance of these specialized transmitter enzymes, enzymes for the production of neuropeptides, one or several transmitter receptors proteins, pro-oncogenes, growth factor receptor proteins, insertion proteins, and structural maintenance proteins are also produced (Black et al 1984).

Establishment of Neuronal Connections and Axonal Pathfinding

How do the billions of neuronal connections that eventually form come to be? Are they formed randomly? Are they formed due to functional environmental input? Are they genetically predetermined? How do axons know where to go? These are the fundamental questions that investigators have been challenged with in neurobiology. As will be seen the answers to these questions are very complex and probably involve a combination of the above possibilities at various phases of neuron development. Let us address each of these issues individually before considering a holistic view.

Is the formation of the multitude of connections in the nervous system random?

The short answer is probably not. There is insufficient genetic material in any individual neuron to code for all of the neuronal connections that need to develop, breakdown, and reform throughout the life of a neuron in a functional nervous system (Kandel et al 1995). However, there is a good deal of evidence to suggest that neurons have innate predetermined programmes that lay out the basic patterns of connections to be formed initially in their development. Little is known about the mechanism of implementation or of how the information is actually stored in the neurons. Predetermined connection fields develop quite early in some neurons perhaps as early as their positional determination in the neural plate is achieved. This is particularly true in neurons developing as retinal cells. These cells seem to have developed a positional orientation or map of their location in the retina before they start developing their axons which will form the optic nerve. This positional orientation is temporally dependent, although initially maintaining a degree of flexibility, after a certain time period becomes permanently fixed (Cowan & Hunt 1985).

This same pattern seems to apply to other areas of the nervous system also. The initial neurons in any given location seem to be under the influence of a gross general polarity-based guidance system that operates throughout the entire body of the developing embryo. This general positional system is responsible for guiding the initial neurons of a particular local to their destination. Initially this system can be altered or reversed if the conditions in the location are not optimal. Once the original neurons become established they act as guideposts for further infiltration by additional neurons. At a critical point this process becomes irreversible and the destiny of each neuron becomes fixed. How these neurons determine where they need to be from a cellular level is again theoretical, but may be best explained by the chemoaffinity hypothesis first proposed by Sperry in 1963 and further developed by Hunt and Cowan in the 1990s. This theory proposes that the positional address of these cells becomes coded on the cell membrane in the form of a distinct labelling molecule or grouping of molecules that allow neurons to differentiate between areas of attraction and repulsion. The neurons would naturally gravitate to areas of attraction and move away from areas of repulsion, eventually arriving in the most attractive environment (Sperry 1965).

How do axons know where to go?

Developing ganglion cells in the inferior nasal portion of the retina send their axons to the lateral geniculate body of the thalamus, whereas developing ganglion cells of the superior temporal retina send their axons to the superior colliculus of the midbrain (Fig. 2.10).

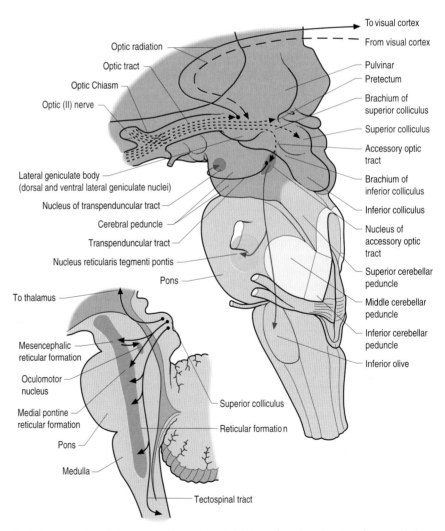

Fig. 2.10 The ganglion cell projections to the midbrain and thalamus from the retina. Note the anatomical relationship between the thalamus and the midbrain.

How do these neurons know where their respective axons are to go? In most developing embryos the paths taken by axons to their respective destinations is very constant and rigidly controlled. Even when axons are experimentally disorientated they still find their way to their target destination. This indicates that axons have some form of homing mechanism that allows them to know when they are going in the right direction and when they have arrived at the right location. Several mechanisms that allow axons to accurately find their way to their target destinations have been identified; these include selective axonal fasciculation; axon substrate interactions; axonal tropisms; and other gradient effects.

Newly formed axons from neighbouring cells often travel together over long distances using some form of axoaxonal connections to communicate. In many cases they follow a previously formed guide axon fibre with which they communicate in a similar axoaxonal fashion. This mechanism is termed axonal fasciculation.

Axons tend to grow in the direction that follows a selective substrate pathway specific for certain axonal membrane receptors contained on the surface of their developing axons. These molecules or receptors include various integrins such as fibronectin and laminin. Tropic influences include substances that promote axon growth along a concentration gradient. One such factor is nerve growth factor (NGF), which has been shown to exert strong grow influences on sympathetic nerve axons to the extent in some cases of causing them to change direction (Gundersen & Barrett 1979).

In light of the above discussion, it must be pointed out that even in fibre systems that seem to show high degrees of topographic order, such as visual systems, individual axons often diverge and follow pathways markedly different from those of neighbouring axons even when the destination is the same.

Synaptogenesis

When the growth cone of an axon comes into close proximity of a postsynaptic cell surface at a potential target destination the terminal portion of the growth cone starts to accumulate vesicles. At the same time morphologic changes occur on the pre- and postsynaptic membranes that allow the presynaptic transmitter to be recognized by the postsynaptic receptors. Functional synaptic integrity has been observed within minutes of the initial contact between an axon growth cone and a target muscle at acetylcholine (ACh) neuromuscular junctions (Kidokoro & Yeh 1982). Initially the effect of the transmitter on the postsynaptic receptors is quite variable but as the functionality of the synaptic connection becomes stabilized, the action of ACh on the postsynaptic receptors results in a progressively shorter opening time of the sodium depolarizing channels until a fairly consistent opening and closing time becomes established.

Initially many more axons form synapses than are present in the mature system. Over time and through a variety of mechanisms a portion of these axons are eliminated.

The mechanisms utilized to remove redundant or inappropriate axons are cell death and selective synaptic elimination.

Most neuronal systems undergo a phase of substantial neuron death at some phase of their development. In most neuron systems about 50% of the initial neurons formed undergo cell death. This process usually occurs temporally at the same time that the axons of the system have formulated contacts with their destination areas. This suggests that a certain amount of the stimulus for neuron death may actually arise or be initiated from the axon destination field through some form of feedback system (Hamburger & Oppenheim 1982). The feedback mechanism may be in the form of tropic growth factors produced at the destination site tissues. Active competition by axons for these growth factors may determine which axons and thus which neurons remain alive. In the case of dorsal root ganglion (DRG) cells one such growth factor that has been isolated is neuron growth factor, without which DRG cells cannot survive (Levi-Montalcini 1982).

Not only is there an overproduction of neurons initially but most neurons establish many more synaptic connections than are necessary or than they can physically maintain. This results in a phase of synaptic elimination in most systems. This was first recognized at the neuromuscular junctions where in the mature system each muscle fibre is innervated by a single axon. Early in development, however, many (6–7) axons may innervate a single muscle fibre (Perves & Lichtmann 1980). This same pattern has been shown to occur in many other systems including the autonomic system and is now thought to be a common strategy in most neuronal systems (Perves 1988). It is important to point out that axon collaterals may be eliminated but the parent axon and other synapses of the parent axon can remain functional and actually multiply in some cases. The most notable example of this occurs in the cortex. Initially all pyramidal cells of lamina V in all cortical areas send axons through the cortical spinal tracts. In the case of the visual and other inappropriate areas of cortex, the inappropriate axons but not the parent cell bodies are eliminated so that only axons from the pyramidal cells of the motor and some areas of sensory cortex remain in the cortical spinal tracts at maturity (O'Leary & Stanfield 1989).

Whether a particular synapse or axon collateral remains and is not eliminated seems to depend on the degree of stimulation generated at the postsynaptic membrane. Synapses that generate a response frequently in the postsynaptic membrane develop a stronger connection with the postsynaptic region which ensures their continued existence. This relationship between stimulation and circuit stability is a form of neural plasticity.

Neural Plasticity

Neural plasticity results when changes in the physiological function of the neuraxis occur in response to changes in the internal or external milieu (Jacobson 1991). Neuroplastic changes are stimulated under two basic conditions.

The first basic condition involves 'normal' physiological change (physiological plasticity) in response to changing afferent sensory stimulation from the environment. The second condition involves injury-related change (injury-related plasticity) in response to damage of areas of the neuraxis through injury or disease.

Physiological plasticity is involved in such processes as learning and is enhanced in situations were the cerebral cortex is still immature such as in early childhood. An excellent example of physiological plasticity is the changes that occur in the geniculo-cortical connections during the development of the visual system. Neurons in the lateral geniculate body of the thalamus project to neurons in the primary visual cortex, and under normal conditions develop equally for both visual fields. However, in the event of a decreased visual input from one eye, most commonly from injury or strabismus, the geniculo-cortical connections from the eye with decreased visual input are weakened and the neural projections from the normal eye are strengthened. This process can develop to the point of complete dominance of the 'normal' eye, which becomes permanent after a critical point in development.

Injury-related plasticity is the response of the normal, remaining tissues to the demands placed on them following injury or disease. Commonly, the remaining tissues will 'take over' some or all of the functions of the damaged tissues over time. This concept is important in a variety of treatment approaches utilized in functional neurology. A striking example of this type of plasticity is the relative normal development of language in young infants who receive damage to their dominant hemisphere. In an adult, damage to the dominant hemisphere usually results in permanent, severe language comprehension and/or articulation problems. This does not occur in infants, even with a complete removal of the dominant hemisphere (hemispherectomy) if the damage occurs before the age of 3, who will, in most cases, develop language skills in a normal fashion. This is the result of other brain areas changing their own response patterns and taking over the responsibilities of the injured areas (Huttenlocher 2002).

The process of neural plasticity appears to occur through the reorganization of synaptic contacts in a neural system in response to changing stimulus in such a way that synapses that receive more stimulation become strengthened and those that receive less stimulation become weakened (Hebb 1949; Lashley 1951). Not all areas of cortex have the same ability to undergo plastic changes. The hard-wired areas of the motor and sensory cortex do not respond to the same extent as certain areas of frontal cortex such as those areas responsible for higher cortical functions like language, mathematics, musical ability, and executive functions. For example, the same left-sided hemispheric injury described above in an infant that did not result in language difficulties will still result in right-sided paralysis or weakness.

Embryological Homological Relationships

In the application of functional neurology the concept of embryological homological relationships between neurons born at the same time frequently needs to be taken into consideration.

The term embryological homologue is used to describe the functional relationships that exist between neurons born at the same time in the cell proliferation phase of development. Cells born at the same time along the length of neuraxial ventricular area develop and retain synaptic contact with each other, many of which remain in the mature functional state. This cohort of cells that remain functionally connected after migration results in groups of neurons that may be unrelated in cell type or location but have an increased probability of firing as a functional group when one member of the group is brought to threshold. The following three examples illustrate the concept.

DRG cells detecting joint motion and muscle contraction maintain synaptic connections with the postsynaptic neurons in the sympathetic ganglia controlling blood flow to the homonymous joints and muscles. This ensures that the appropriate alterations in blood flow occur to support the actions of the muscles and tissues involved in the movement.

Another example includes the motor column of the cranial nerves III, IV, VI, and XII in the brainstem. This mid-line motor column responds functionally as a homologous column, in that alterations in function in one area, eye movement, can also be detected in other areas such as tongue movement.

A third example involves the neurons in the hippocampal formation and parahippocampal gyrus in the medial temporal lobe. During embryological development the neurons that originally were born side by side undergo an elaborate series of folding, resulting in neurons that are physically in different areas (Fig. 2.11). These neurons maintain their original synaptic connections and influence the central integrated state of the others in the functional group (Fig. 2.12). This neural circuit is involved in the development of memory.

Development of the Vertebral Column

During the fourth week of development cells of the sclerotomal tissues surround the spinal cord and the notochord. Areas of mesenchymal tissue embedded in the sclerotomes develop into intersegmental arteries of the spine.

As this development continues, the caudal portion of each sclerotomal segment proliferates extensively and condenses. This proliferation is so extensive that it binds the caudal portion of one sclerotome to the cephalic portion of the subjacent sclerotome.

A portion of mesenchymal tissue does not proliferate, but remains in the space between the sclerotomal development and results in the formation of the intravertebral disc. Embedded still more centrally is the remnant notochordal tissue, which eventually develops into the nucleus pulposus, which is later surrounded by circular fibrous tissue, the annular fibrosis (Sadler 1995) (Fig. 2.13).

A variety of spinal anomalies arise from the abnormal development or closure of the neural tube and/or fusion of the posterior aspects of the vertebral bodies. These anomalies include spina bifida occulta, spina bifida vera, diastematomyelia, and tethered cord (Guebert et al 2005). The term spinal dysraphism refers to a variety of conditions in which the posterior aspects of the first or second sacral segments are involved.

Spina Bifida Occulta

Spina bifida occulta is a defect of the posterior arch of a vertebrae in which one or the other of the developing pedicle segments fails to fuse to form the spinous process. In spina bifida occulta failure of the arch formation does not affect the development of the thecal sac or its contents. The most common areas of the spine involved are the lumbosacral areas. Clinical manifestations of spina bifida occulta usually only become apparent sometime after birth and include back pain, increased incidence of disc herniation, and spondylolisthesis (Fidas et al 1987; Avrahami et al 1994). Although neurological manifestations are rare, a number of conditions have been associated with

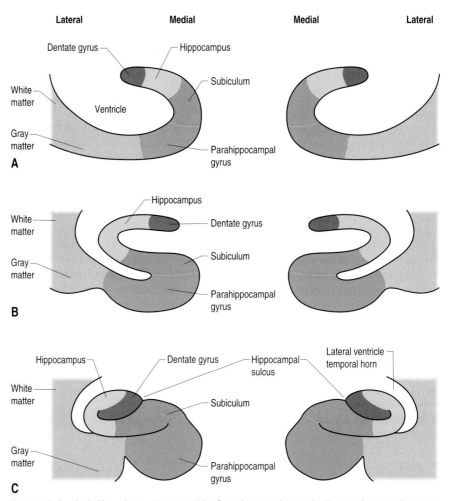

Fig. 2.11 Embryological homologues. Neurons arising from the same tissue maintain synaptic connections even though they may finally come to rest long distances apart. During embryological development of the hippocampal formation the neurons that originally were born side by side undergo an elaborate series of folding resulting in neurons that are located physically in different areas.

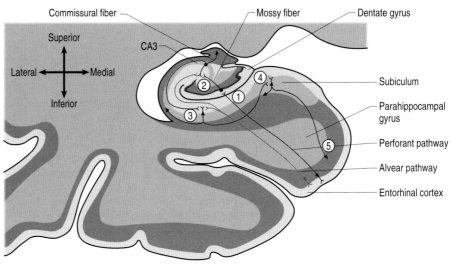

Fig. 2.12 Synaptic connections of the neurons in Fig. 2.11.

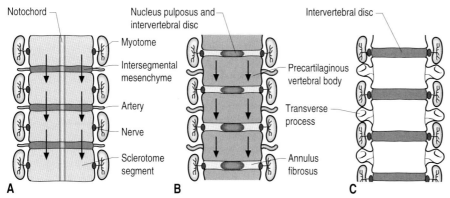

Fig. 2.13 Formation of the vertebral column at various stages of development. (A) At the 4th week of development, sclerotomic segments are separated by less dense intersegmental tissue. Note the position of the myotomes, intersegmental arteries, and segmental nerves. (B) Condensation and proliferation of the caudal half of the subjacent sclerotome. Note the appearance of the intervertebral discs. Note the position of the arrows in (A) and (B). (C) Precartilaginous vertebral bodies are formed by the upper and lower halves of two successive sclerotomes, and the intersegmental tissue. Myotomes bridge the intervertebral discs and, therefore, can move the vertebral column.

spina bifida occulta. These include low termination of the conus medullaris (tethered cord syndrome), syrinx formation, lipoma, nerve root adhesions, and conjoined nerves (Giles 1991; Gregerson 1997).

Spina Bifida Vera

In situations involving spina bifida vera there is a wide bony defect in the posterior arch development of usually more than one vertebrae. The thecal sac and its contents are usually also involved and protrude beyond the confines of the spinal canal. There is some evidence to suggest that an adequate supply of folic acid during this critical period of development can prevent this type of condition. Failure of fusion of the posterior arch to the degree necessary to result in spina bifida vera must take place in the period of the 21st to 29th foetal day. Unfortunately, this is a period in which most women do not realize they are pregnant; thus to be effective supplementation with folic acid must begin prior to conception. Herniation of the fluid-filled sac that contains cerebral spinal fluid is called meningocele. When protrusion includes the meninges, cerebral spinal fluid, and neural elements, it is called a myelomeningocele. When neural elements protrude without thecal covering, it is called a myelocele (Figs 2.14A and 2.14B). Myeloschisis refers to the presence of complete uncovering of the neural elements along a sagittal midline defect that involves bone, thecal sac, and all posterior tissues (Guebert et al 2005) (Fig. 2.15). Failure of closure of the caudal neuropore results in absence of the cranial vault with the cerebral hemispheres either completely missing or reduced to non-functional masses. This condition is referred to as anencephaly (Figs 2.16A and 2.16B).

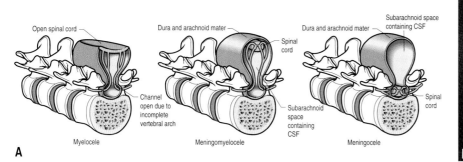

Fig. 2.14 (A) The different variations of spina bifida vera. There is a wide bony defect in the posterior arch development of usually more than one vertebrae. The thecal sac and its contents are usually also involved and protrude beyond the confines of the spinal canal. (B) The appearance of spina bifida vera in an infant.

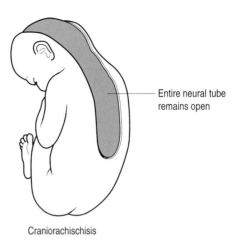

Entire neural tube remains open

Craniorachischisis

Fig. 2.15 Myeloschisis.

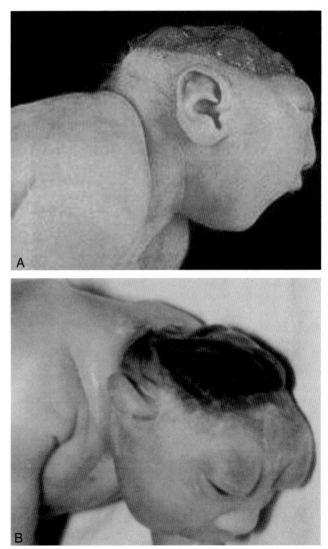

Fig. 2.16 Failure of the caudal neuropore to close. (A, B) This condition results in absence of the cranial vault with the cerebral hemispheres either completely missing or reduced to non-functional masses. This condition is referred to as anencephaly.

References

Avrahami E, Frishman E, Fridman Z et al 1994 Spina bifida occulta is not an innocent finding. Spine 119:12–15.

Behrman RE, Vaughan II 1987 Nelson's textbook of paediatrics. WB Saunders, Philadelphia.

Black JA, Waxman SG, Hildebrand C 1984 Membrane specialization and axo-glial in the rat retinal nerve fibre layer: freeze fracture observations. Journal of Neurocytology 13:417–430.

Cowan WM 1978 Aspects of neural development. In: International review of physiology III. University Park Press, Baltimore, MD, p 149–191.

Cowan WM 1981 The development of the vertebrate central nervous system: an overview. In: Garrod PR, Feldman JD (eds) Development in the nervous system. Cambridge University Press, New York, p 3–33.

Cowan WM 1992 Development of the nervous system. In: Asbury AK, McKhann GM, McDonald WI (eds) Diseases of the nervous system: clinical neurobiology. WB Saunders, Philadelphia/London/Toronto, p 5–24.

Cowan WM, Fawcett JW, O'Leary DD et al 1984 Regressive phenomena in the development of the vertebrate nervous system. Science 225:1258–1265.

Cowan WM, Hunt RK 1985 The development of the retinal-tectal projection: an overview. In: Edelman GM, Gall E, Cowan WM (eds.) Molecular basis of neuronal development. Wiley, New York, p 389–428.

Fidas A, MacDonald HL, Elton RA et al 1987 Prevalence and patterns of spina bifida occulta in 2707 normal adults. Clinical Radiology 38:537–542.

Giles L 1991 Review of tethered cord syndrome with a radiological and anatomical study. Surgical and Radiological Anatomy 13:339–343.

Gregerson DM 1997 Clinical consequences of spina bifida occulta. Journal of Manipulative and Physiological Therapeutics 20:546–550.

Guebert GM, Rowe LJ, et al (2005) Congenital anomalies and normal skeletal variance. In: Yokumw T, Rowe L (eds) Essentials of skeletal radiology. Lippincott Williams and Wilkins, Philadelphia,

Gundersen RW, Barrett JN 1979 Neuronal chemotaxis: Chick dorsal root axons turn toward high concentrations of nerve growth factor. Science 206:1079–1080.

Hamburger V, Oppenheim RW 1982 Naturally occurring neuronal death in vertebrates. Neuroscience Commentaries 1:39–55.

Hebb DO 1949 The organization of behavior. Wiley, New York.

Huttenlocher PR 2002 Neuralanatomical substrates: early developmental events. In: Huttenlocher PR (ed) Neural plasticity: the effects of environment on the development of the cerebral cortex. Harvard University Press, Cambridge, MA/London, p 9–36.

Jacobson M 1991 Developmental neurobiology, 3rd edn. Plenum Press, New York/London.

Kandel ER, Schwartz JH et al 1995 The neuron. In: Kandel ER, Schwartz JH, Jessell TM (eds) Essentials of neural science and behaviour. McGraw-Hill, New York, p 43–69.

Kidokoro Y, Yeh E 1982 Initial synaptic transmission at the growth cone in Xenopus nerve/muscle cultures. Proceedings of the National Academy of Science USA 79:6727–6731.

Lashley KS 1951 Central mechanisms in behavior. Academic Press, New York.

Le Douarin NM 1982 The neural crest. Cambridge University Press, New York.

Leikola A 1976 The neural crest: migrating cells in neurological development. Folia Morphologica 24:155–172.

Levi-Montalcini R 1982 Developmental neurobiology and the natural history of nerve growth factor. Annual Reviews of Neuroscience 5:341–362.

O'Leary DD, Stanfield BB 1989 Selective elimination of axons extended by developing cortical neurons is dependent on regional locale: experiments utilizing fetal cortical transplants. Journal of Neuroscience 9:2230–2246.

Perves D 1988 Body and brain: a trophic theory of neural connections. Harvard University Press, Cambridge, MA.

Perves D, Lichtmann JW 1980 Elimination of synapses in the developing nervous system. Science 210:153–157.

Sadler TW 1995 Vertebral column in Langman's medical embryology. Williams and Wilkins, Baltimore, MD.

Sidman RL, Rakic P 1974 Neuronal migration. In: Berenberg SR, Masse NP (eds) Modern problems in paediatrics, vol 13, p 13–43.

Sperry RW 1965 Embryogenesis of behavioral nerve cells. In: DeHaan RL, Ursprung H (eds) Organogenesis. WB Saunders, Philadelphia, p 161–186.

Spitzer N 1981 Development of membrane properties in vertebrates. Trends in Neuroscience 4:169–172.

Williams PL, Warwick R 1980 Embryology. In: Gray's anatomy. Churchill Livingstone, Edinburgh.

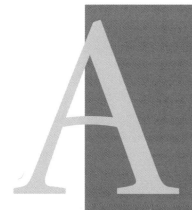

Clinical Case Answers

2.1.1 A variety of spinal anomalies arise from the abnormal development or closure of the neural tube and/or fusion of the posterior aspects of the vertebral bodies. These anomalies include spina bifida occulta, spina bifida vera, diastematomyelia, and tethered cord.

Spina bifida occulta is a defect of the posterior arch of a vertebrae in which one or the other of the developing pedicle segments fails to fuse to form the spinous process. In spina bifida occulta failure of the arch formation does not affect the development of the thecal sac or its contents. The most common areas of the spine involved are the lumbosacral areas. Clinical manifestations of spina bifida occulta usually only become apparent sometime after birth and include back pain, increased incidence of disc herniation, and spondylolisthesis.

In situations involving spina bifida vera there is a wide bony defect in the posterior arch development of usually more than one vertebrae. The thecal sac and its contents are usually also involved and protrude beyond the confines of the spinal canal. There is some evidence to suggest that an adequate supply of folic acid during this critical period of development can prevent this type of condition. Failure of fusion of the posterior arch to the degree necessary to result in spina bifida vera must take place in the period of the 21st to 29th foetal day. Herniation of the fluid-filled sac that contains cerebral spinal fluid is called meningocele. When protrusion includes the meninges, cerebral spinal fluid, and neural elements, it is called a myelomeningocele. When neural elements protrude without thecal covering, it is called a myelocele. Myeloschisis refers to the presence of complete uncovering of the neural elements along a sagittal midline defect that involves bone, thecal sac, and all posture elements. Failure of closure of the caudal neuropore results in absence of the cranial vault with the cerebral hemispheres either completely missing or reduced to non-functional masses. This condition is referred to as anencephaly.

2.1.2 Failure of fusion of the posterior arch to the degree necessary to result in spina bifida vera must take place in the period of the 21st to 29th foetal day. Unfortunately, this is a period in which most women do not realize they are pregnant; thus to be effective supplementation with folic acid must begin prior to conception.

2.1.3 Ultrasound can usually detect the occurrence of spina bifida vera.

Chapter

3

The Biochemistry and Physiology of Receptor Activation

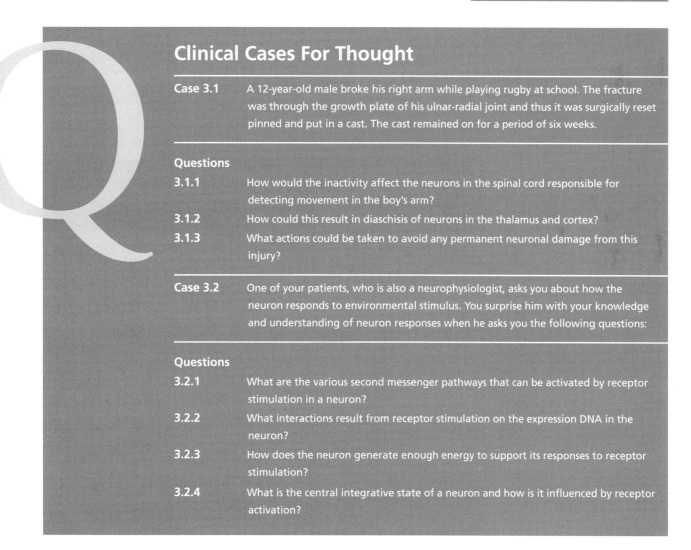

Clinical Cases For Thought

Case 3.1   A 12-year-old male broke his right arm while playing rugby at school. The fracture was through the growth plate of his ulnar-radial joint and thus it was surgically reset pinned and put in a cast. The cast remained on for a period of six weeks.

Questions

3.1.1   How would the inactivity affect the neurons in the spinal cord responsible for detecting movement in the boy's arm?

3.1.2   How could this result in diaschisis of neurons in the thalamus and cortex?

3.1.3   What actions could be taken to avoid any permanent neuronal damage from this injury?

Case 3.2   One of your patients, who is also a neurophysiologist, asks you about how the neuron responds to environmental stimulus. You surprise him with your knowledge and understanding of neuron responses when he asks you the following questions:

Questions

3.2.1   What are the various second messenger pathways that can be activated by receptor stimulation in a neuron?

3.2.2   What interactions result from receptor stimulation on the expression DNA in the neuron?

3.2.3   How does the neuron generate enough energy to support its responses to receptor stimulation?

3.2.4   What is the central integrative state of a neuron and how is it influenced by receptor activation?

Introduction

For neurons, altering gene expression in response to extracellular signals is a fundamental process; thus the biochemical and physiological changes that occur in neurons during the variety of activities experienced in a lifetime are largely a result of gene activation and suppression by signals received via receptor systems from the environment. The receptors are specialized structures present on the surface of the bilaminar neuron plasma membrane that respond in a specific manner when a structurally specific compound or ligand binds to them.

Activation of these receptor systems occurs via a variety of signal-specific chemical transmitters such as hormones, cytokines, neuropeptides, and neurotransmitters. These eventually modulate the activation (increase in transcriptional activity) or the inhibition (decreased transcriptional activity) of specific genes in the neuron through various types of synaptic transmission.

Synaptic transmission has been conceptualized as a set of processes by which neurotransmitters, acting through their receptors, cause changes in the conductance of specific ion into and out of the neuron to produce excitatory or inhibitory postsynaptic potentials. However, it has become evident that neurotransmitters elicit diverse and complicated effects in target neurons. This has led to the development of a much more complex view of synaptic transmission (Huganir & Greengard 1990).

Activation of receptors can also modulate other activities of the neuron such as glucose uptake and consumption rates, oxygen utilization, neurotransmitter production, and enzyme concentrations.

Phenotypic and Functional Development of Neurons is Accomplished through Genetic Lineage and Environmentally Induced Gene Activation

The initial modulation of genetic events by the environment takes place during the differentiation of stem cells into neurons. Neurons are neurons because they produce the proteins and enzymes necessary to carry out the functions of neurons. They can manufacture axons and dendrites because they are rich in tubulin and microtubule-

QUICK FACTS 1	The Five Main Cellular Organelles

Mitochondria
- Metabolize oxygen during cellular respiration to produce ATP for energy.
- Involved in the citric acid cycle and electron transport chain.
- Derived from symbiotic bacteria early in evolution?

Golgi Apparatus
- Involved in protein synthesis and packaging.
- Intracellular and extracellular (secretory) protein packages.

Endoplasmic Reticulum
- Rough (bind with ribosomes) and smooth ER.
- Protein synthesis, lipid metabolism, and calcium storage.

Peroxisomes
- Contain oxidative enzymes, which means that they use oxygen to strip hydrogen from specific molecules to detoxify waste or toxins. This produces H_2O_2 (also a powerful oxidant), which is decomposed by catalase.

Nucleus
- Contains DNA.

associated proteins (Black & Baas 1989). They can maintain a membrane potential that varies within a specific range of values depending on the environmental circumstances because they manufacture gated plasma ion channels (Hess 1990). They can communicate with other neurons because they have neurotransmitter-specific enzymes to produce neurotransmitters (Snyder 1992). In other words, all or most of the necessary functions of a neuron are made possible by the activation of the genes that code for the proteins necessary to subserve those functions and the suppression of those genes that do not.

The gene repertoire available for transcription in a neuron is determined by the lineage of the neuron and the stage of commitment and differentiation that the neuron has achieved (Van den Berg C 1986; Pleasure 1992). There are usually temporally and environmentally dependent branch points in the development of a neuron lineage that can determine a particular course of differentiation or development that the neuron will take (Lillien & Raff 1990). For instance, during one critical phase or branch point in the development of a neuron the type of neurotransmitters that the neuron will be producing is determined by the environment in which the axons have come into contact. The determinant factors encountered by the axons are transported via retrograde axonal flow to the nucleus where the signals are interpreted and the appropriate genes activated to manufacture the enzymes necessary to produce the specific neurotransmitters signalled for.

Environmental Stimulus is Conveyed to the Nucleus of the Neuron via Specialized Receptor Systems on the Membrane

The plasma membrane of a neuron is essential for the survival of the neuron. It encloses the cell and maintains essential differences in composition and ion concentrations between the cytosol of the neuron and the external environment. The plasma membrane is essentially composed of proteins floating in a thin bilayered lipid structure held together by non-covalent interactions. This unique structure forms a relatively impermeable barrier to the passage of most water-soluble compounds. Some of the proteins in the lipid bilayered structure act as structural support, while others act as receptors and transducers that relay information across the membrane about the neuron's environment (Fig. 3.1). Proteins that span the membrane usually assume an α-helical structure as they pass through the lipid portions of the membrane. This configuration is the most thermodynamically stable, due to interactions with the polar peptide bonds of the polypeptide and the hydrophobic nature of the lipid environment. The transmembrane portion of the protein can pass through the membrane only once, resulting in a single-pass transmembrane protein, or multiple times, resulting in the formation of a multipass transmembrane protein (Fig. 3.2). Multipass transmembrane proteins can form channels in the membrane that can be regulated by a variety of mechanisms (Alberts et al 1994). Some channels are intimately associated with specialized proteins that act as receptors. The neuron has specific receptor proteins for a variety of chemical compounds known as transmitters.

All receptors for chemical transmitters have three things in common.

1. They are membrane-spanning proteins in which the external portion of the protein recognizes and binds a specific neurotransmitter. Some common neurotransmitters include acetylcholine (ACh), norepinephrine (NE), epinephrine (E), serotonin or 5-hydroxytryptophan (5-HT), and dopamine (DA).

2. They carry out an effector function within the target cell. This function may include regulation of specific ion channels, release or activation of second messenger compounds, or modulation of activity levels of intracellular enzymes.

3. It is the receptor that determines the action of the transmitter based on the activity it produces inside the cell. This is an important point to remember. Many neurotransmitters are classified as excitatory or inhibitory to certain cellular functions; however, it is the internal wiring of the receptors that determine the response of a transmitter. For example, acetylcholine has an inhibitory or slowing effect on the heart rate but an excitatory effect on skeletal muscle.

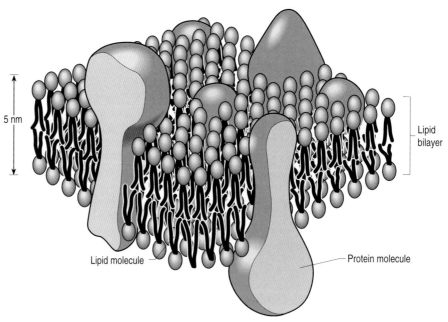

Fig. 3.1 A diagrammatic representation of a cell membrane. This illustration shows the bilaminar nature of the membrane with the phospholipids molecules (red) aligned with the phosphate heads, which are hydrophilic positioned on the external and internal portions of the membrane and the fatty acid portions of the molecules forming the internal area of the membrane. The large proteins (green) float in the phospholipid membrane with some of the proteins transversing the membrane and others only exposed to the inside or the outside of the membrane.

Receptors can be Either Directly or Indirectly Linked to Ion Channels

These two different types of linkage are determined by two different genetic programming families of receptors.

Receptors that gate ion channels directly are called inotropic receptors. Upon binding of a transmitter, the receptor undergoes a conformational change that allows the ion channel to open. The receptor is part of the same molecular structure that composes the channel. The activation of inotropic receptors produces fast synaptic actions (milliseconds in duration), e.g. ACh receptor at the neuromuscular junction (Fig. 3.3).

Receptors that indirectly gate ion channels are called metabotropic receptors. These types of receptors act through a special series of interlinked proteins called G-proteins. G-proteins are so-named because of their ability to bind the guanine nucleotides, guanosine triphosphate (GTP), and guanosine diphosphate (GDP). Four major types of G-proteins are involved in transduction of signals produced by neurotransmitter binding, Gs, Gi/o, Gq, and G12, and multiple subtypes exist for each.

QUICK FACTS 2	The Four Components of a Nerve Cell's Behaviour

1. Input signal

2. Trigger signal (sudden Na⁺ influx)

3. Conducting signal (regenerating)

4. Output signal (releases neurotransmitter)

These behaviours correspond to three types of potentials.

1. Receptor potential

2. Synaptic potential

3. Action potential

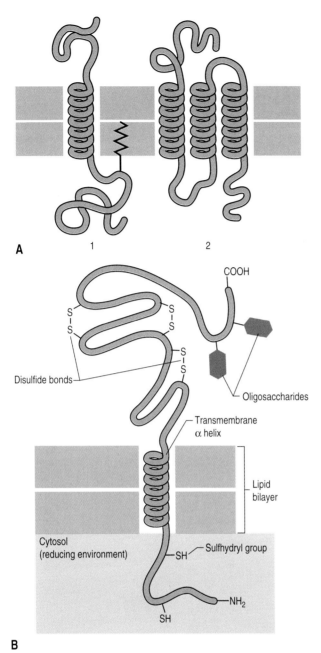

A

B

Fig. 3.2 (A) Proteins that span the membrane usually assume an α-helical structure as they pass through the lipid portions of the membrane. This configuration is the most thermodynamically stable, due to interactions with the polar peptide bonds of the polypeptide and the hydrophobic nature of the lipid environment. The transmembrane portion of the protein can pass through the membrane only once, resulting in a single-pass transmembrane protein, or multiple times, resulting in the formation of a multipass transmembrane protein. (B) A typical single-pass transmembrane protein. Note that the polypeptide chain transverses the lipid bilayer as a right-handed α helix and that the oligosaccharide chains and disulfide bonds are on the noncytosolic surface of the membrane. Disulfide bonds do not form between the sulfhydryl groups in cytoplasmic domain of the protein because the reducing environment in cytosol maintains these groups in their reduced (–SH) form.

Activation of these types of receptors often activates a second messenger such as cyclic AMP (cAMP) or diacylglycerol in the cytoplasm of the neuron. Other prominent second messengers in brain include cyclic GMP (cGMP), calcium, phosphatidylinositol (PI), inositol triphosphate (IP_3), arachidonic acid, and nitric oxide (NO) (Duman & Nestler 2000) (Fig. 3.3).

Many second messengers then act on a variety of intracellular kinases or enzymes to promote or inhibit cellular functions. Such intracellular processes can produce rapid changes in neuronal function such as changes in ionic conductance across the membrane.

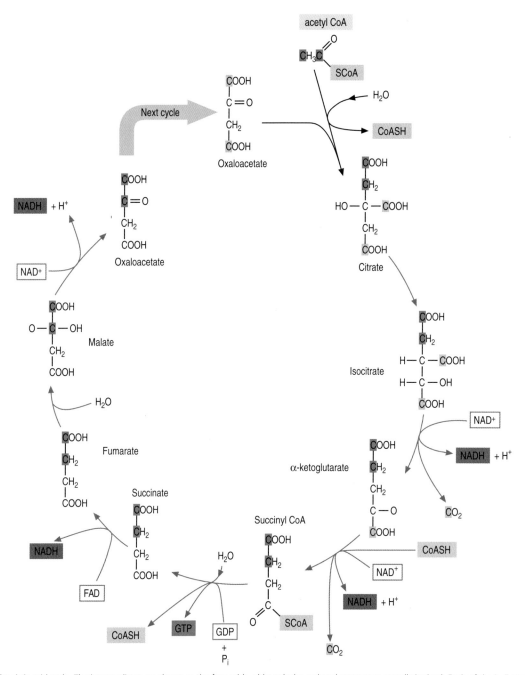

Fig. 3.3 The citric acid cycle. The intermediates are shown as the free acids, although the carboxyl groups are actually ionized. Each of the indicated steps is catalysed by a different enzyme located in the mitochondrial matrix. The two carbons from acetyl CoA that enter this turn of the cycle (shadowed in *red*) will be converted to CO_2 in subsequent turns of the cycle: it is the two carbons shadowed in *blue* that are converted to CO_2 in this cycle. Three molecules of NADH are formed. The GTP molecule produced can be converted to ATP by the exchange reaction GTP + ADP→GDP + ATP. The molecule of $FADH_2$ remains protein-bound as part of the *succinate dehydrogenase complex* in the mitochondrial inner membrane; this complex feeds the electrons acquired by $FADH_2$ directly to ubiquinone.

These second messenger processes can also produce short- to medium-term modulatory effects on neuronal function, such as regulation of the responsiveness of the neuron to the same or different neurotransmitters (transmitter modulation) via changes in receptor sensitivity. Relatively long-term modulatory effects on neuronal function, including changes achieved through the regulation of gene expression, can also be regulated by the actions of second messengers on other intracellular components called third messengers. Such changes can last seconds to minutes and include altered synthesis of receptors, ion channels, and other cellular proteins, or for much longer periods ultimately resulting in forms of learning and memory (Fig. 3.4).

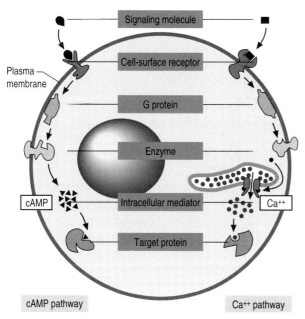

Fig. 3.4 This diagram illustrates two different pathways that are stimulated via receptor activation and also utilize membrane-bound G-proteins to activate their second messengers. The square molecule activates a cascade involving Ca^{++} ions as the second messenger. The teardrop-shaped molecule activates a cascade utilizing cAMP as its second messenger.

Free Levels of Intracellular Ca^{++} can Act as a Potent Second Messenger in a Number of Different Pathways

Under normal conditions the intercellular concentration of free Ca^{++} ions is under strict regulatory control. Receptor activation can result in increases in free intercellular Ca^{++} ion levels in two different ways involving two types of mechanisms that operate to different extents in different cell types. Neurotransmitter receptor activation can alter the flux of extracellular Ca^{++} ions into neurons or can regulate release of Ca^{++} ions from intracellular stores. Once released, Ca^{++} ions can exert multiple actions on neuronal function via intracellular regulatory proteins. Receptors can directly regulate the conductance of specific voltage-gated Ca^{++} channels via coupling with G-proteins. In addition, activation of other second messenger systems can alter Ca^{++} channel conductance. Depolarization of a neuron by any means will activate voltage-gated Ca^{++} channels, which will lead to the flux of Ca^{++} into the cells. Finally, extracellular Ca^{++} can pass through some ligand-gated channels, such as the nicotinic cholinergic and glutamate N-methyl-D-aspartate (NMDA) receptors (Duman & Nestler 2000).

The Structure of Chromatin can Regulate Gene Transcription Induced by Receptor Stimulation

In human neurons, DNA is contained in the nucleus of the cell. The nucleus is also the site of DNA replication and transcription. Chromatin is formed from subunits of nucleosomes, which are chromosomes intimately associated with histone proteins. A chromosome is composed of extremely long molecules of DNA. The DNA not actively involved in transcription processes is stored in supercoiled structures that drastically reduce the space requirements in the nucleus for the storage of DNA. Chromatin is not only structurally important in this storage role but also acts in the regulation of gene expression by inhibiting transcription factors access to binding sites on DNA. Activation of a gene requires that the chromatin or nucleosomal structure be modified to allow the binding of regulatory proteins to the appropriate subset of genes. This is accomplished by a specialized group of proteins referred to as activator proteins that remodel the chromatin and expose core promoter sites on the appropriate genes. This permits the binding of yet another complex of proteins called general transcription factors to the core promoter site on the DNA. This complex of general transcription factors can then recruit and bind with RNA polymerase to enter the transcription initiation phase of the replication process (Workman & Kingston 1998).

The process of transcription can be divided into three steps: initiation, elongation, and termination. Regulation of gene expression can and does occur at each of these steps in the neuron; however, the transcription initiation phase seems to be the most highly regulated step involving extracellular signalling mechanisms.

In humans, three different types of RNA polymerases, I, II, and III, are involved with the transcription of different types of DNA. Polymerase I is involved in the transcription of ribosomal RNAs (rRNA). Polymerase II is involved in the transcription of messenger RNA (mRNA) and another subset of RNAs known as snRNA, which are involved in splicing RNA segments. Polymerase III is involved in the transcription a number of smaller RNA types including transfer RNA (tRNA) (Struhl 1999) (Fig. 3.5).

In humans the expression of highly complex genes requires that additional transcriptional activators are necessary for the transcriptional process to function. These additional transcriptional activation complexes are referred to as functional regulatory elements or transcription factors that bind to specialized sites within the structure of the gene. These functional transcription factors determine the unique pattern of expression for each gene, both in the normal course of development and in response to environmental stimuli. Aspects of gene expression under the control of various transcription factors include the cell type in which the gene is expressed, the time during development when the gene is expressed, and the level to which it will be expressed (Collingwood et al 1999).

Several families of transcription factors as well as several modes of activation or inhibition of these factors have been identified. For example, the cAMP response element binding protein (CREB) family of transcription factors activate transcription of genes to

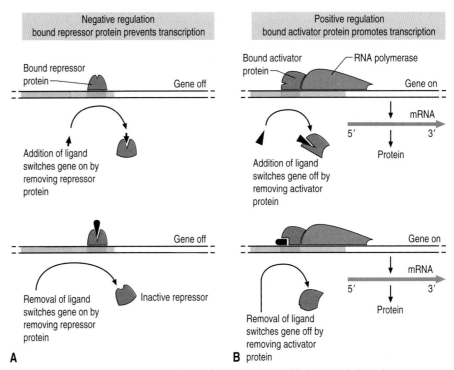

Fig. 3.5 This illustrates the negative and positive regulatory processes modulating transcription polymerase.

which they are linked when they are phosphorylated by cAMP-dependent protein kinase (protein kinase A). Protein kinase A is activated in the presence of cAMP (De Cesare & Sassone-Corsi 2000).

The CREB family of transcription factors can also be activated by other second messengers such as Ca^{++} bound by calmodulin that can activate a variety of protein kinases upon entering the nucleus of the neuron. These kinases can in turn phosphorylate CREB, resulting in the activation of transcription of the specific CREB-linked gene (Nestler & Hyman 2002).

Dissemination of the Receptor Stimulus Throughout the Neuron

The environmental stimulus—whether it be a growth hormone, a neurotransmitter, or a hormone—must get its signal from the receptors on the neuron cell membrane to the transcriptional controlling factors in the nucleus in order for production of the necessary proteins that it calls for.

Some signalling molecules such as hydrophobic hormones (glucocorticoids, oestrogen, and testosterone) can gain direct access to the nuclear apparatus by their lipid-soluble chemical structure that allows them the ability to transverse the highly hydrophobic bilayered lipid plasma membrane dependent mainly on their concentration gradients. These hormones then bind with intracellular hormone receptors that carry them through the cytoplasm and across the nuclear membrane where they bind and alter the conformation of transcriptional factors (Evans & Arriza 1989; Lin et al 1998).

Other signalling molecules such as Ca^{++} ions gain access through specific ion channels present in the neuron plasma membrane (Hess 1990).

Protein hormones, growth factors, peptide neuromodulators, and neurotransmitters must act on their transcription protein targets indirectly by either inducing a change in a transmembrane protein channel related to their receptor proteins (Lester & Jahr 1990) or by inducing a change in linked intramembrane proteins. Changes in these linked intramembranous proteins called G-proteins eventually result in the release of intracellular ions or the generation of intracellular second messenger such as cAMP, diacylglycerol, and inositol triphosphate (Berridge & Irvine 1989; Huang 1989), which then activate directly or through other intermediates the transcription factors in the nucleus such as CREB (Fig. 3.6).

Gene Expression   **QUICK FACTS 3**

- Gene regulatory proteins or transcription factors are activated in the cytosol by second messengers and secondary effectors. This follows the activation of membrane receptors by neurotransmitters and peptides, and changes to intracellular ion concentrations.
- Immediate early gene responses can occur within nanoseconds of cell activation and represent a learned response of the cell. They can lead to protein synthesis or activation, and can also trigger transcription within the nucleus of the cell.
- DNA code is transcribed to produce a single mRNA molecule, which then leaves the nucleus via nuclear pores.
- mRNA passes this code to a ribosome, with the help of rRNA, which reads the base-sequence of the mRNA and translates the code into an amino acid sequence.
- tRNA transfers the appropriate amino acids in the cytosol to their designated site in the sequence being formed by the rRNA.

The number of known second messengers is still relatively small. Response specificity is achieved through one of the following methods:

- Temporally and spatially graded rises in second messenger levels (Berridge & Irvine 1989);
- Recruitment of various combinations of second messengers after a single stimulus (Nishizuka 1988); or
- Regional variations in the intracellular targets on which the second messengers act (Nishizuka 1988; Huang 1989).

Prolonged activity of second messengers can lead to a variety of damaging effects on a neuron, ranging from inappropriate activity to transformation and cell death. This has resulted in the formation of a variety of regulatory mechanisms in the neuron to control the concentration and temporal activity of second messengers. Most commonly, the second messengers are sequestered by intracellular proteins, or degraded by intracellular enzymes within milliseconds of release in the neuron (Boekhoff et al 1990). Because of their size and short span of activity second messengers are limited in their ability to act over the long term and limited in their specificity for precise and effective modulation of protein transcription. These shortcomings have led to the search for a third messenger system within the neuron that can function very specifically and over long periods to modulate gene expression.

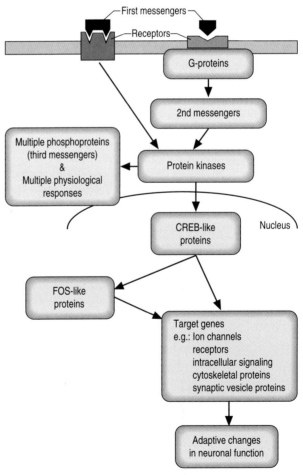

Fig. 3.6 Several families of transcription factors as well as several modes of activation or inhibition of these factors have been identified. For example, the cyclic adenosine monophosphate (cAMP) response element-binding (CREB) protein family of transcription factors activate transcription of genes to which they are linked when they are phosphorylated by cAMP-dependent protein kinase (protein kinase A). Protein kinase A is activated in the presence of cAMP. The CREB family of transcription factors can also be activated by other second messengers such as Ca++ bound by calmodulin that activates a variety of protein kinases upon entering the nucleus of the neuron. These kinases in turn can phosphorylate CREB, resulting in the activation of transcription of the specific CREB-linked gene. The CREB family of transcription factors can act directly on target genes or via fos-like proteins.

Extracellular Signals Result in Activation of a Third Messenger System Coded for by Immediate Early Genes

Third messengers are group of nuclear proteins known as translational factors that are induced by a variety of extracellular signals. These proteins bind to specific nucleotide sequences in the promoter and enhancer regions of genes (Mitchell & Tjian 1989). The third messengers are coded by immediate early genes (IEGs) also referred to as primary response genes or competence genes. The proteins encoded for by immediate early genes in concert with other transcriptional factors exert powerful excitatory or inhibitory effects on the initiation of RNA synthesis (Pleasure 1992). Many of the IEGs were initially recognized because they are the normal nuclear homologues of transforming retroviral oncogenes, which are the class of gene released by viruses immediately upon entering a host cell.

The most fully studied IEG is c-*fos*. The c-*fos* gene has three binding sites for CREB and is activated by neurotransmitters or other stimuli that stimulate the production of cAMP in the neuron (Ahn et al 1998). Changes in the tertiary structure of c-*fos* gene are detectable within one minute after cell stimulation, first appearing in regulatory regions of the gene and then propagating to decoding regions of the gene. The half-life of the c-*fos* gene and the protein it codes for are very short in the range of 20–30 minutes. This time frame of activation is much shorter than other proteins of a structural or enzymatic nature but is many orders of magnitude greater than the half-life of the second messengers.

Fine-tuning of the effects of third messengers is accomplished through a complex network of controls. Since there are now over a hundred IEGs and corresponding proteins composing third messengers a very complex matrix of interactivity which would allow complicated but minor variances in linear and temporal combinations of third messengers for various functions can be developed (Pettersson & Schaffner 1990; Ptashne & Gann 1990) (Table 3.1). For example when *fos* binds to DNA as a heterodimer complex

---

How Are Neurons Stimulated? QUICK FACTS 4

Answer: Receptors
- A receptor converts an impulse of energy into an electrical impulse that travels along the nerve.
- They are derived from mesoderm—therefore, they do not need to be activated in order to stay alive, as is the case with nerve cells.
- The receptor potential is the first representation of an internal or external event to be coded in the nervous system.

Features of Receptor Potentials QUICK FACTS 5

- It is graded (depending on intensity and duration) and unpropagated (amplitude decreases progressively) and needs to be amplified; thus the initial response of a receptor is its greatest.
- Degradation occurs quickly due to Na^+ being drawn out, but the receptor potential may trigger an action potential due to the higher concentration of voltage-gated sodium channels where the axon meets the receptor.
- There is a one-to-one relationship between the environmental stimulus and the receptor potential.

Table 3.1 Diversity of Pro-oncogenes Thus Far Discovered

Class	Proto-oncogene nomenclature	Homologue
Receptor ligand	c-sis	PDGF B chain
	Int-2	Basic-FGF-like
	hst	FGF-like
Transmembrane tyrosine kinases	c-erbB	EGF receptor
	c-fms	CSF -1 receptor
	neu (c-erbB-2)	EGF receptor-like
	trk, trkB, trkC	Neurotrophin receptors
	c-met	Insulin receptor-like
	c-kit	W locus gene
	c-ros	Insulin receptor-like
	c-sea	Insulin receptor-like
Membrane-associated tyrosine kinases	c-src	
	hck	
	c-abl	
	c-yes -1 and -2	
	c-fgr	
	c-lck	
	c-fps/fes	
	fer	
	flk	
	flk	
	c-syn	
	c-lyn	
	c-slk	
	fyn	
Non-tyrosine kinase receptors	mas	Angiotensin receptor
Serine/threonine kinases	c-raf-1	
	c-mos	
	pim-1	
G-protein-like	c-Ha-ras	
	c-Ki-ras	
	c-N-ras	
	rab (1 -4)	
	ypt -1	
	rho	
	smg	
Signal transduction enzymes	crk	Phospholipase c-like
Nuclear proteins	c-ski	
	c-erbA	Thyroid hormone receptor
	snoA and B	
	ets -1 and -2	
	c-myb	Related to NFkB
	mybA and B	
Zinc finger proteins	gli	Related to krueppel
	gr -1 and -2	Related to krueppel
Leucine zipper protein	c-fos	
	fra -1 and -2	AP -1 complexes
	fosB	
	c-jun, -B, -D	
Helix-loop-helix	c-myc	
	N-myc	
	L-myc	

ᵃ Reproduced with permission from *Discussions in Neuroscience*, 7(4) (August 1991), Elsevier Science Publishers B.V.

with another third messenger protein called jun the transcription of the target protein—usually tyrosine hydroxylase, neurotensin, neuromedin, or a proenchephalin—is dramatically increased (Gizang-Ginsberg & Ziff 1990; Kislauskis & Dobner 1990). However when *fos* binds to DNA on its own it inhibits the transcription of *c-fos*, its coding gene (Gius et al 1990).

The *fos* Family of Genes may Act as a Molecular Switch within the Neuron

Under resting conditions the concentration of c-*fos* mRNA and protein in the neuron are extremely low, but c-*fos* expression can be dramatically increased by a variety of stimluli (Correa-Lacarcel et al 2000). For example, experimental induction of a grand mal seizure causes marked increases in c-*fos* mRNA within the brain within 30 minutes and induces the formation of c-*fos* protein within two hours (Sonnenberg et al 1989). The *fos*-like proteins are highly unstable and return to normal values within 4–6 hours. Administration of other substances such as cocaine or amphetamine causes a similar pattern of expression in the striatum (Graybiel et al 1990; Hope et al 1994). With repeated activation, the c-*fos* family of genes become refractory to the stimulus, and other isoforms of the *fos* proteins which express very long half-lives in brain tissue are expressed and accumulate in specific neurons in response to repeated stimulus (Pennypacker et al 1995; Chen et al 1997). The accumulation of these proteins remains in the neurons long after the stimulus has ceased. The prolonged presence of the *fos*-like proteins may act as a molecular switch inside the cell, shutting off or modulating responses to repeated stimulus. The true functional significance of the sustained presence of these *fos*-like proteins in neurons remains unknown but may have a mediating effect on the development of various striatal-based movement disorders (Kelz & Nestler 2000).

We will now look at a variety of receptors and their respective neurotransmitters.

Acetylcholine (Cholinergic) Receptors

Acetylcholine is essential for the communication between nerve and muscle at the neuromuscular junction. ACh is also involved in direct neurotransmission in the autonomic ganglia and is also active in cortical processing, arousal and attention activity in the brain (Karczmar 1993) (Fig. 3.7).

Spatial and Temporal Summation
QUICK FACTS 6

Spatial summation refers to the cumulative effect of inputs from multiple pre-synaptic sources on a single cell occurring at the same time.

Temporal summation refers to the cumulative effect of multiple inputs prior to the degradation of previous inputs. The impulse from a neuron is provided faster than its rate of degradation.

Cholinergic transmission can occur through G-protein coupled mechanisms via muscarinic receptors or through inotropic nicotinic receptors. The activity of ACh is terminated by the enzyme acetylcholinesterase, which is located in the synaptic clefts of cholinergic neurons. To date, seventeen different subtypes of nicotinic receptors and five different subtypes of muscarinic receptors have been identified (Nadler et al 1999; Picciotto et al 2000).

Cholinergic, nicotinic receptors are present on the postsynaptic neurons in the autonomic ganglia of both sympathetic and parasympathetic systems. Cholinergic, muscarinic receptors are present on the end organs of postsynaptic parasympathetic neurons and expressed on a variety of neurons in the brain.

Cholinergic, nicotinic receptors are also present at the neuromuscular junctions of skeletal muscle.

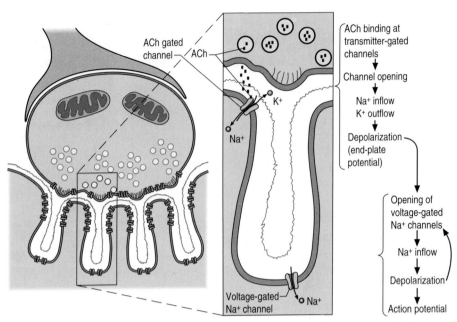

Fig. 3.7 The binding of ACh in a postsynaptic muscle cell opens channels permeable to both Na+ and K+. The flow of these ions into and out of the cell depolarizes the cell membrane, producing the end-plate potential. The depolarization opens neighbouring voltage-gated Na+ channels in the muscle cell. To trigger an action potential, the depolarization produced by the end-plate potential must open a sufficient number of Na+ channels to exceed the cell's threshold.

Adrenergic Receptors

Physiologically, the adrenergic receptors bind the catecholamines norepinephrine (noradrenalin) and epinephrine (adrenalin). These receptors can be divided into two distinct classes, alpha- and beta-adrenergic receptors.

Traditionally, the alpha-adrenergic receptors have been divided into two well-recognized subclasses, alpha-1 and alpha-2 receptors. It is now known that both of these subclasses have as many as three further derivatives.

Alpha-1 receptors have been demonstrated, based on both radioligand and pharmacological data, in the liver, heart, vascular smooth muscle, brain, spleen, and other tissues. All of the derivatives of alpha-1 receptors are related to G-proteins and coupled to distinct second messenger systems controlling intracellular Ca++ levels and are able to mobilize Ca++ from intracellular stores as well as increase extracellular Ca++ entry via voltage-gated Ca++ channels.

Alpha-2 receptors have been demonstrated in wide areas of the central nervous system (CNS) including multiple nuclei of the brainstem and pons, the midbrain, the hypothalamus, the septal region, amygdala, olfactory system, hippocampus, cerebral cortex, spinal cord, and cerebellum and in many neuroendocrine cells (Wang et al 1996). Alpha-2 receptors are mediated by the GTP-binding proteins subfamily and affect three different routes of inhibitory activation:

- Inhibition of adenyl cyclase and thereby inhibit the production of cAMP;
- Suppression of voltage-activated calcium channels, thus reducing the flow of extracellular Ca++ into target cells; and
- Increased conductance of K+ ions through the membranes of target cells.

All three of these activities (inhibition of adenyl cyclase, suppression of voltage-sensitive calcium channels, and stimulation of potassium channels) can contribute to the inhibition of the target cell, and to reduction of neurotransmitter release in neurons or hormone release in neuroendocrine cells (Langer 1974).

The beta-adrenergic receptors have three well-recognized subclasses: beta-1, beta-2, and beta-3 receptors. All three subtypes are coupled to adenyl cyclase activation via stimulatory G-proteins (Barnes 1995).

Beta-1 and -2 receptors have been demonstrated in the lungs, including airway smooth muscle, epithelium, cholinergic and sensory nerves, submucosal glands, and pulmonary vessels, and are also found in the heart; here beta-1 receptors are predominantly in the myocytes, while the beta-2 receptors are on innervating neurons. Beta-2 receptors are also present in saphenous vein, mast cells, macrophages, eosinophils, and T lymphocytes (Ruffolo et al 1995). Beta-3 receptors are primarily expressed in brown and white adipose tissue, although some studies have also reported the presence of beta-3 receptors in oesophagus, stomach, ileum, gallbladder, colon, skeletal muscle, liver, and cardiovascular system (Krief et al 1993; Berlan et al 1995).

Glutamate Receptors

The transmitter L-glutamate or L-glutamic acid (Glu) is the major excitatory transmitter in the brain and spinal cord (Hollmann & Heinemann 1994).

The role of Glu in the function of the nervous system is much more diverse and complex than a simple excitatory neurotransmitter. It also plays a major role in brain development, neuronal migration, differentiation, and axon development and maintenance (Komuro & Rakic 1993; Wilson & Keith 1998). In the mature nervous system, Glu is essential in the processes involving stimulus-dependent modifications of synapses necessary for neural plasticity to occur.

Persistent or overwhelming stimulation of glutamate receptors can result in neuronal degeneration, or in some circumstances neuronal death by necrosis or aptosis. This process is referred to as excitotoxicity and has been linked to the development of a range of disorders including Huntington's disease, Alzheimer's disease, amyotrophic lateral sclerosis, and stroke (Choi 1988; Ankarcrona et al 1995; Olney et al 1997).

NMDA Receptors vs Non-NMDA Receptors—Clinical Considerations   **QUICK FACTS 7**

- They are unique receptors as they depend on membrane potential and activation by glutamate and co-factor glycine. Cell needs to be depolarized first (~20mV) in order for magnesium plug to be expelled, such as:
  - Tinnitus due to overexcitation of NMDA receptors by persistent loud broadband noise, which activates DCN (dorsal cochlear nucleus) output cells of the brainstem; and
  - Fibromyalgia—activation of NMDA receptors in the presence of decreased magnesium. This allows for phosphorylation of the NMDA receptor, therefore allowing continued calcium influx and associated intracellular changes—activation of phospholipases and proteases. NMDA receptors are located on pain fibres.
- Activation of NMDA receptors results in massive influx of calcium, which results in biochemical cascade of events leading to IEG response. NMDA receptors can promote changes in protein production or phosphorylation of intracellular domain of membrane channels.
- NMDA receptor activity promotes synaptogenesis and survivability of the neuron.

Glu is utilized in as many as 40% of all brain synapses and in the spinal cord synapses of dorsal root ganglion cells that detect muscle stretch from muscle spindle fibres in skeletal muscle.

Activation of glutamate receptors results in the opening of both Na and K channels. Glutamate receptors can be either inotropic or metabotropic in nature. There are three major subclasses of glutamate inotropic receptors based on the synthetic agonists that activate them:

- AMPA (α-amino-3-hydroxy-5-methylisoxazole-4-propionic acid);
- Kainate; and
- NMDA.

Because AMPA and Kainate receptors are similar in structure and not voltage-dependent they are sometimes referred to as non-NMDA receptors (Fig. 3.8).

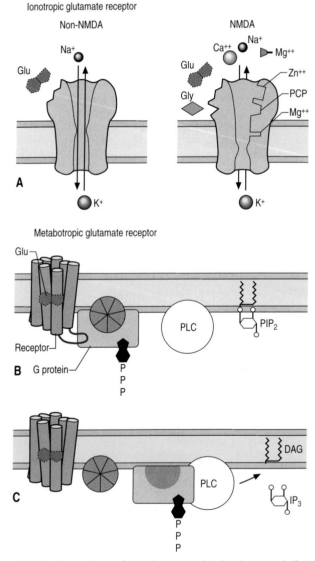

Fig. 3.8 Three classes of glutamate receptors regulate excitatory synaptic actions in neurons in the spinal cord and brain. (A) Two types of inotropic glutamate receptors directly gate ion channels. Two subtypes of non-NMDA receptors bind the glutamate agonists kainate or AMPA and regulate a channel permeable to Na$^+$ and K$^+$. The NMDA (N-methyl-D-aspartate) receptor regulates a channel permeable to Ca^{++}, K$^+$, and Na$^+$ and has binding sites for glycine, Zn^{++}, phencyclidine (PCP, or 'angel dust'), MK801 (an experimental drug), and Mg^{++}, which regulates the functioning of this channel in different ways. (B) The metabotropic glutamate receptors indirectly gate ion channels by activating a second messenger. The binding of glutamate to certain types of metabotropic glutamate receptors stimulates the activity of the enzyme phospholipase C (PLC), leading to the formation of two second messengers derived from phosphatidylinositol 4,5-bisphosophates (PIP$_2$): inositol 1,4,5-triphosphate (IP$_3$) and diacylglycerol (DAG).

Glutamate NMDA Receptors

The NMDA receptor is a complex receptor that has three exceptional qualities:

1. The receptor controls a gated channel permeable to Na, K, and Ca (non-NMDA receptors are not permeable to Ca).

2. The channel will only function if glycine is also present as a co-factor.

3. The function of the channel is dependent on a specific membrane voltage being reached as well as the presence of a chemical transmitter.

A magnesium (Mg) plug blocks the channel pore at the resting membrane potential. As the membrane is depolarized the Mg plug is expelled from the channel. This receptor is inhibited by phencyclidine (angel dust). The hallucinations produced by this inhibition resemble the symptoms of schizophrenia.

Glutamate NMDA Receptor Activation Can Modulate Genetic Expression in the Neuron via Ca^{++}-Induced Second Messenger Systems

When glutamate Kainate and AMPA receptors are activated by glutamate binding, the result is an influx of Na$^+$ ions into the neuron, which depolarizes the neuron, bringing its membrane potential towards threshold. Simultaneously, glutamate will also bind to the NMDA receptors on the neuron membrane. Recall that in order to activate NMDA receptors, which allow Ca^{++} to move into the neuron, the membrane potential must meet certain criteria. The membrane potential necessary to activate NMDA receptors is usually sufficient to bring the postsynaptic neuron to threshold so that an action potential is initiated. Thus glutamate-induced Ca^{++} influx is associated with action potential initiation in the postsynaptic neuron. Ca^{++} influx into the postsynaptic neuron results in the activation of a variety of second and third messenger systems that result in modulation of mRNA and protein production in the neuron (see below).

Ionotropic vs Metabotropic Receptors QUICK FACTS 8

Ionotropic
- Fast
- Short-lived
- GABA-A (gates Cl channel)

Metabotropic
- Slow
- Long-lasting
- Can ↑ or ↓ channel opening
- Can change RMP, Ri, length and time constants, threshold potentials, AP duration, and repetitive firing
- Modulates pre-synaptic (Ca^{++}/K$^+$), postsynaptic (ionotropic), and electrical properties
- GABA-B (gates K$^+$ channel)

Overstimulation or prolonged stimulation of glutamate NMDA receptors can result in excitotoxcity in the neuron, which results in damage or death of the neuron.

GABA Receptors

GABA, γ-aminobutyric acid, is the major inhibitory neurotransmitter in the brain and spinal cord. It acts on two receptor types, GABA-A and GABA-B. GABA-A is an inotropic channel that gates Cl ions. When GABA binds to A-type receptors the activation of proteins that open selective channels for Cl ions results, the Cl ions flow down their concentration gradient into the neuron, resulting in a hyperpolarization or movement away from the threshold potential of the neuron. This results in a decreased probability that the neuron will produce an action potential per unit stimulus and is referred to as inhibition of the neuron.

GABA-B is a metabotropic receptor that activates a second messenger that gates K channels. When GABA binds to B-type receptors activation of proteins that cause gates selective for K^+ takes place and K^+ flows down its concentration gradient out of the cell. The movement of the positively charged ions out of the cell results in a hyperpolarization state. This decreases the probability that the neuron will produce an action potential per unit stimulus and is referred to as inhibition of the neuron.

Glycine Receptors

Glycine is a less common inhibitory transmitter that acts on inotropic channels that gate Cl. The inhibition that these receptors produce is due to the increased conductance of Cl ions. Since the concentration of Cl outside the cell is much greater than that inside the cell Cl flows down its concentration gradient into the cell, making the inside more negative and hyperpolarizing the cell. This results in a decreased probability that the neuron will produce an action potential per unit stimulus and is referred to as inhibition of the neuron.

Serotonin or 5-Hydroxy-Tryptophan (5-HT) Receptors

Serotonin has been implicated in a staggering array of physiological and behavioural activities including affect, aggression, appetite, cognition, emesis, gastrointestinal function, perception, sensory function sex, and sleep (Bloom & Kupfer 1995).

To date, five different subtypes of 5-HT receptor have been isolated. All members of the 5-HT type-1 receptor family tend to modulate inhibitory effects through either presynaptic or postsynaptic action. All members of the 5-HT type 2 subgroup modulate excitatory activity (Aghajanian & Sanders-Bush 2002).

Dense concentrations of 5-HT receptors are found in the dorsal raphe nucleus, hippocampus, and cerebral cortex. The facial nerve and other cranial motor nuclei also have high densities of 5-HT receptors (Chalmers & Watson 1991).

Dopamine Receptors

There are five types of dopamine (DA) receptors that are classified into two major categories. The five receptor types are D1–D5. These receptors fall into two class categories, the D1-like receptor class and the D2-like receptor class (Spano et al 1978; Su et al 1996). The D1-like receptor class includes D1 and D5 receptor types. The D2-like receptor class includes D2, D3, and D4 receptor types (Sunahara et al 1990; Sumiyoshi et al 1995).

Dopamine receptors are present in most parts of the CNS but in particular they are found in three main projection systems: the nigrostriatal pathway, comprising the neurons of the substantia nigra pars compacta, which project to neurons of the neostriatum; the mesolimbic pathway comprising neurons of the ventral tegmental area of the mesencephalon, which project to wide-spread areas of the limbic system; and the mesocortical pathways, which involve neurons in the substantia nigra and the ventral tegmental areas of the mesencephalon that project to the prefrontal cortical areas of the brain (Bjorklund & Lindvall 1964; Blumenfeld 2002).

Attempts to understand the actions of the different DA receptors are often stymied by the complex array of activities that these receptors can produce. DA receptors have been shown to interact via both inotropic and G-protein coupled mechanisms. DA has also been shown to have a modulatory affect on other transmitters in the region of its activity and to alter the actions of groups of neurons through modulation of gap junction activities between the neurons (Grace 2002). DA can also regulate its own levels of interaction by activating autoreceptors sensitive to local DA concentrations. These autoreceptors have been found on the soma of dopaminergic neurons as well as at the dopaminergic nerve terminal synapses.

Several studies have shown the presence of dopaminergic neurons in the substantia nigral and ventral tegmental areas of the mesencephalon. The majority of these neurons seem to exhibit spontaneous action potential generation driven by an endogenous pacemaker conductance activity (Grace & Bunney 1984). The rate of this pacemaker generation is normally closely regulated by feedback from autoreceptors located on the soma and synaptic areas of the neurons (Harden & Grace 1995).

The activity of dopamine is probably best described as a neuromodulator rather than an excitatory or inhibitory transmitter. For example in combination with glutamate activation DA seems to act as a facilitator of rapid alterations to neuron function as well as an attenuator of long-term changes that have occurred in the neuron. It also acts at the neuron gap junctions to facilitate the formation of reversible hardwiring networks that may be involved in enhancing performance of previously learned tasks.

The complexity of the interactions involving dopaminergic receptors can be illustrated in the following example. D1 receptor activation in dorsal striatum neurons results in further inhibition of previously hyperpolarized neurons. However, with repeated stimulation of D1 receptors in previously hyperpolarized neurons excitation can occur. When D1 and D2 receptors are stimulated simultaneously the result is a synergistic inhibition of the neuron. However, the D1-mediated inhibition previously described can be reversed by subsequent stimulation of D2 receptors on the neuron (Cepeda et al 1995; Hernandez-Lopez et al 1997; Onn et al 2000).

Receptor Modulation of Neuron Bioenergetic Processes Require ATP for Energy

Bioenergetics describes the transfer and utilization of energy in biological systems. Essential processes like transferring ions across a membrane against their concentration gradients to maintain a membrane potential require energy to operate. In the neuron most energy-requiring processes are made possible by either direct or indirect coupling with an energy-releasing mechanism involving the hydrolysis of adenosine triphosphate (ATP).

Energy Transfer in the Neuron   QUICK FACTS 9

- Energy in the electrons of the free hydrogen atoms is carried by NAD and FAD into the electron transport chain—a series of electron carrier molecules on the inner mitochondrial membrane lining the cristae. The electrons fall to successively lower energy levels along the chain as they synthesize more ATP via ATP synthetase.
- Complexes I and II collect electrons from the catabolism of fats, proteins, and carbohydrates and transfer them to ubiquinone (CoQ10). The electrons are then transferred successively to complexes III and IV and to oxygen, which is the final electron acceptor. Three sites along the electron transport chain (complexes I, III, and IV) use the energy released from the transfer of electrons to transport hydrogen ions across the inner mitochondrial membrane to the intermembrane space—thus driving a proton gradient.
- The [H^+] is higher in the intermembrane space so it travels back to the matrix via channels that contain ATP synthetase, which is activated by H^+ flow.
- ADP + Pi (ATP synthetase) → ATP (32 more molecules per glucose molecule).

The ATP molecule is composed of an adenosine base segment to which three phosphate groups attach. The two terminal phosphate groups release a relatively high amount of energy (7.3 kcal/mol) when they are chemically broken down; these are referred to as high-energy phosphate bonds. The monophosphate bond adjacent to the adenosine base releases about 4.0 kcal/mol when broken down and is referred to as a low-energy phosphate bond. Other compounds such as phosphoenolpyruvate and phosphocreatine contain phosphate bonds which release energy approaching 10 kcal/mol when they are broken down and are referred to as very-high-energy phosphate bonds (Champe & Harvey 1994). These compounds can convert ADP to ATP over short time periods in situations when ATP demands are higher then ATP production. Glucose-6-phosphate and glycerol 3-phosphate both have phosphate bonds that release about 4.0 kcal/mol and are referred to as low-energy phosphate bonds. Thus, ATP is placed in the middle ground between very-high- and low-energy phosphate bonds and acts as a middleman in the transfer of energy between molecules that regulate processes.

ATP is synthesized in the mitochondria of the neuron via the processes of electron transfer and oxidative phosphorylation and in the cytoplasm via glycolysis.

Energy-rich compounds such as glucose can be oxidized through a series of reactions in the mitochondrial matrix to produce reduced coenzymes such as nicotinamide adenine dinucleotide (NADH) and flavin adenine dinucleotide (FADH) that in-turn transfer their electrons down the electron transfer chain of specialized enzymes to form water from hydrogen and oxygen. This process produces energy at various points in the enzyme chain as the electrons lose much of their energy as they move down the chain of reactions. This energy is utilized to convert ADP and a phosphate group to ATP.

When large molecules such as proteins, sugars, or fats are broken down to their component parts to produce ATP the process is referred to as catabolic. When ATP is converted to ADP and the energy used to build up complex molecules from component parts the process is referred to as anabolic.

Glycolysis (Embden-Meyerhof pathway) is the metabolism of glucose to pyruvate and lactate. This process results in the net production of only 2 mol of ATP/mol of glucose (Fig. 3.9). On the other hand, pyruvate can pass into the tricarboxylic acid cycle (Krebs

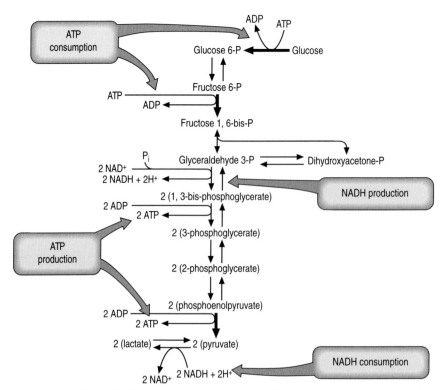

Fig. 3.9 Summary of anaerobic glycolysis. Reactions involving the production or consumption of ATP or NADH as indicated. The irreversible reactions of glycolysis are shown with thick arrows.

cycle) in the mitochondria and via the oxidative phosphorylation cascade produce 30 mol of ATP/mol of glucose (see Fig. 3.3). The energetic benefit of utilizing the oxidative phosphorylation route over the glycolytic route is obvious from an energetic perspective (Magistretti et al 2000).

The glycolytic route may not always be utilized for the production of ATP in neurons because of saturation of enzymes in the Krebs pathway or the oxidative phosphorylation cascades pathways in the mitochondria. Several studies have shown that the ATP production capability of the neuron operating at a basal rate is operating at near maximal capacity. When the neuron undergoes activation it needs to utilize the glycolytic pathway for ATP production, thus producing lactate, which converts to lactic acid under certain conditions (Fox & Raichle 1986; Van den Berg 1986; Fox et al 1988).

Metabolic Demands of the Brain Require Glucose as a Substrate for ATP Synthesis

The brain, which represents about 2% of the total body weight in humans, consumes 15% of the cardiac output blood flow, 20% of the total body oxygen consumption, and 25% of total body glucose utilization (Kety & Schmidt 1948). Glucose utilization calculations need to take into account the fact that glucose can have metabolic fates other than that of ATP production. Glucose can produce metabolic intermediates such as lactate and pyruvate, which when released do not necessarily enter the tricarboxylic acid cycle but can be removed by the circulation. Glucose can also be incorporated into lipids, proteins, and glycogen and can also be utilized in the formation of a variety of neurotransmitters including GABA, glutamate, and acetylcholine. It is estimated that about 17% of the glucose in neurons is utilized in metabolic processes other than that of ATP production (Magistretti et al 2000).

QUICK FACTS 10

Pathway	Rate	Capacity	ATP/glucose
Creatine phosphate	Very fast	Very limited	0
Anaerobic glycolysis	Fast	Limited	2–3
Oxidative phosphorylation	Slow	Unlimited	36

Numerous studies have tried to identify molecules other than glucose that could substitute for glucose in brain energy metabolic processes. To date, no other physiologically available substrate has been identified that can substitute for glucose under normal basal conditions. Under a certain set of conditions such as starvation, diabetes, or in breast-fed neonates, acetoacetate and D-3-hydroxybutyrate can be used by the brain as a metabolic substrate for glucose (Owen et al 1967).

Other Cells such as Vascular Endothelial Cells and Astrocytes also Participate in Neural Activation Processes

Brain metabolism studies in the past have assumed that energy metabolism at the cellular level represented predominantly neuronal activity. However, it is now clear that other types of cells such as neuroglia and vascular endothelial cells not only consume energy but also play a part in the neural activation process and in maintenance of neuron function. In studies spanning a variety of species, the ratio of non-neural to neural substrate is about 50% (Kimelberg & Norenberg 1989). In addition there is very good evidence to suggest that the astrocyte to neuron ratio increases with increasing brain size.

Two well-established functions of astrocytes include the maintenance of extracellular K[+] ion levels within a narrow range and to ensure the reuptake of neurotransmitters. Activation of neurons results in increases of extracellular K[+] ion concentrations and increases in concentrations of the synaptic-specific neurotransmitters released by the neuron. For example, at excitatory synapses where glutamate is the activating neurotransmitter, it not only depolarizes the postsynaptic neuron but also stimulates the uptake of K[+] ions into the surrounding astrocytes (Barres 1991).

Astrocytes may also play a role in supplying the neuron an adequate energy substrate during the initial periods of activation when the neuron may be unable to produce adequate amounts of ATP via oxidative phosphorylation pathways.

Recent studies have also shown that the metabolic activity of astrocytes can be mediated by norepinephrine and other vasoactive substances and that activation of the locus coeruleus in the brainstem prior to activation of neurons may indicate that the metabolic priming of astrocytes is preset prior to neuron activation by the nervous system and is not solely dependent on the generation of local metabolites for activation (Magistretti et al 1981, 1993; Magistretti & Morrison 1988).

Clinical Signs and Symptoms of Altered Brain Metabolism can be Demonstrated with Positron Emission Tomography (PET) Studies

Under normal conditions neurons are dependent on glucose for their supply of ATP (see above). Since as much as 75% of ATP produced is utilized by neurons to produce and maintain action potentials and membrane potentials the rate of glucose metabolism can be used as a reliable measure of synaptic activity in neurons. Positron emission tomography (PET) utilizes this concept by assessing the amount glucose consumed in neurons or the amount of oxygen consumed by the neuron and relating these data to the activity of the neurons in question.

Glucose consumption is measured by infusion of a radioactive tracer (F-fluorodeoxyglucose) utilized at the same rate as glucose by the metabolic enzymes of the neuron. The regional concentration of the tracer is measured by receptors that detect the positron emissions from the tracer compound. Since glucose can be used for other purposes in the neuron besides ATP production the oxygen utilization rate of the neuron can result in a somewhat more accurate measure of synaptic activity in the neuron.

The value of PET scans in the development of our understanding of the function of the nervous system is becoming more apparent with each successive study. The following studies outline some of the recent applications of PET scans.

PET studies of patients with Huntington's disease without hyperactive behaviour have shown normal frontal lobe metabolism in the presence of decreased caudate and putamen metabolism (Kuhl et al 1982; Young et al 1986).

PET scans in patients with Parkinson's disease have shown decreased cortical glucose consumption in the frontal cortex in conjunction with decreased D2 receptor uptake ratios in the nigrostriatal (substantia nigra) regions (Brooks 1994).

Similar findings have been found in children with ADHD or childhood hyperkinetic disorder, where researchers found that after receiving Ritalin previously normal subjects showed decreased activity in the basal ganglia and those previously diagnosed with ADHD (originally decreased basal ganglionic activity compared to normal levels) showed and increased activity of basal ganglial areas (Young et al 1986; Rogers 1998).

Mitochondrial Activation and Interactions in the Neuron

Mitochondria are membrane-bound cytoplasmic organelles that vary in size, number, and location between the various cell types found in humans. They have many functions including maintaining and housing most of the enzymes necessary for the citric acid and fatty acid oxidation pathways in their cellular matrix substance, active regulation of Ca[++]

concentrations within cells, and production of ATP via oxidative phosphorylation complexes contained in their inner membranes.

The most likely theory explaining the presence of mitochondria in eukaryotic cells involves the development of a symbiotic relationship between a previously independent aerobic bacteria and ancient eukaryotic cells. The relationship has evolved to the point that although the mitochondria still maintain the majority of their own DNA and RNA and still reproduce via fission, some of the genes necessary for the survival of the mitochondria in the eukaryotic cell have moved into the nucleus of the host cell.

The mitochondria are bounded by two highly specialized membranes that create two separate mitochondrial compartments, the inner membrane space and the matrix space. The matrix contains a highly concentrated mixture of hundreds of enzymes, including those required for oxidation of pyruvate, the citric acid cycle, and the oxidation of fatty acids. The mitochondrial DNA, mitochondrial ribosomes, and mitochondrial transfer RNAs are also contained in the matrix space.

The inner membrane is impermeable to virtually all metabolites and small ions contained in the mitochondria. The inner membrane contains specialized proteins that carry out three main functions including oxidative reactions of the respiratory chain, the conversion of ADP to ATP (ATP synthase), and the transport of specific metabolites and ions in and out of the mitochondrial matrix. The inner membrane space contains several enzymes required for the passage of ATP out of the matrix space and into the cytoplasm of the host cell (Alberts et al 1994) (Fig. 3.10).

Mitochondrial dysfunction through genetic mutation, free radical production, and aging mechanisms can result in a variety of neurological consequences. Neurons are heavily dependent on the mitochondria for ATP production in order to survive. This coupled with the non-replication state of most neurons makes them exceptionally vulnerable to diseases or malfunction of the mitochondria.

Genetic mutation of mitochondrial DNA can be maternally inherited, congenital, or due to genetic mutations or defects obtained through physiological activities throughout the life span of the individual.

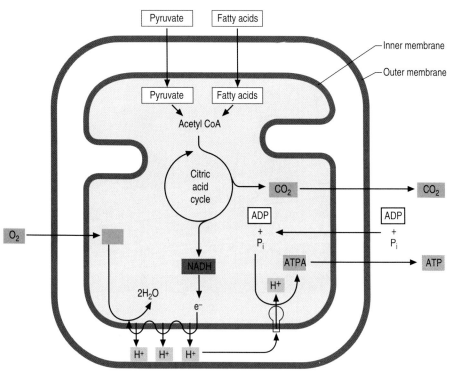

Fig. 3.10 Different compartments of the mitochondria. A large concentration of H^+ ions builds up in the intramembranous space between the inner and the outer membrane, which then flows through the transmembrane enzyme, which phosphorylates ADP to ATP. Note that the citric acid cycle occurs in the matrix of the mitochondria within the bounds of the internal membrane.

Mitochondrial Oxidative Phosphorylation (OxPhos) Disorders

As previous discussed the mitochondria play a key role in energy production in the neuron. The energy produced is largely in the form of ATP produced in the process of respiration by the oxidative phosphorylation enzymes contained in the mitochondrial matrix.

The respiratory chain is composed of five multienzyme complexes, which include flavin and quinoid compounds, transition metals such as iron–sulphur clusters, hemes, and protein-bound copper compounds. The respiratory chain can be grouped into five complexes that in addition to two small carrier molecules, coenzyme Q and cytochrome c, can be grouped into the following complexes (Mendell & Griggs 1994):

- Complex I—contains NADH and the coenzyme Q oxidoreductase;
- Complex II—contains succinate and the coenzyme Q oxidoreductase;
- Complex III—contains coenzyme Q and cytochrome c oxidoreductase;
- Complex IV—contains cytochrome c oxidase; and
- Complex V—composed of ATP synthase.

Complexes I and II collect electrons from the catabolism of fat, protein, and carbohydrates and transfer these electrons to ubiquinone (CoQ_{10}), and then pass them on through to complexes III and IV before the electrons react with oxygen, which is the final electron receptor in the pathway (Smeitink & Van den Heuvel 1999).

Complexes I, III, and IV use the energy from electron transfer to pump protons across the inner mitochondrial membrane, thus setting up a proton gradient. Complex V then uses the energy generated by the proton gradient to form ATP from ADP and inorganic phosphate (Pi) (Nelson & Cox 2000) (Fig. 3.11). During this process, about 90–95% of the oxygen delivered to the neuron is reduced to H_2O; however, about 1–2% is converted to oxygen radicals by the direct transfer of reduced quinoids and flavins. This activity produces superoxide radicals at the rate of 10^7 molecules per mitochondria per day. Superoxide radicals are part of a chemical family called reactive oxygen species or free

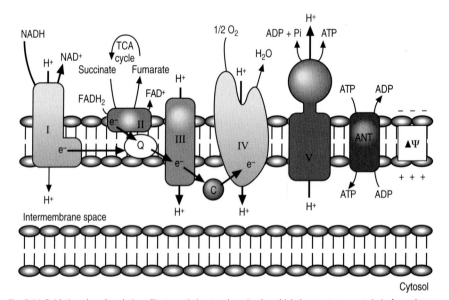

Fig. 3.11 Oxidative phosphorylation. Electrons (e⁻) enter the mitochondrial electron transport chain from donors such as reduced nicotinamide adenine dinucleotide (NADH) and reduced flavin adenine dinucleotide ($FADH_2$). The electron donors leave as their oxidized forms, NAD⁺ and FAD⁺. Electrons move from complex I (I), complex II (II), and other donors to coenzyme Q_{10} (Q). Coenzyme Q_{10} transfers electrons to complex III (III). Cytochrome c (c) transfers electrons from complex III to complex IV (IV). Complexes I, III, and IV use the energy from electron transfer to pump protons (H⁺) out of the mitochondrial matrix, creating a chemical and electrical ($\Delta\psi$) gradient across the mitochondrial inner membrane. Complex V (V) uses this gradient to add a phosphate (P_i) to adenosine diphosphate (ADP), making adenosine triphosphate (ATP). Adenosine nucleotide transferase (ANT) moves ATP out of the matrix. *From D. Wolf, with permission.*

radicals. They are extremely reactive molecules because they contain an oxygen molecule with an unpaired electron (Del Maestro 1980). Although production of free radicals can occur during specialized cellular process such as in lysozyme production in neutrophils the vast majority of all free radical production occurs in the mitochondria.

Excessive free radical production can damage or slow the enzyme activity of the oxidative phosphorylation (OxPhos) chain. This in turn decreases the ability of the OxPhos system to operate. Severe defects in any of the OxPhos components can result in decreased ATP synthesis. The inability to sustain ATP production profoundly affects the homeostatic function of the neuron and will eventually result in necrotic neuron death.

Oxygen free radicals can also bind to iron–sulphur-containing proteins, releasing ferrous iron moieties that react with hydrogen peroxides to form an extremely reactive and damaging hydroxyl radical that can overwhelm the neuron's normal biochemical supplies of antioxidants and result in oxidative stress (Jacobson 1996).

Free radicals can also attack the phospholipids membranes of the mitochondria and the neuron. As much as 80% of the mitochondrial membrane is composed of the phospholipids phosphatidylcholine and phosphatidylethanolamine, which are particularly susceptible to free radical attack. Free radicals can also react with proteins and alter their conformation and functional capabilities. Many proteins that undergo conformational changes are attracted to other proteins and form aggregates that build up in the neurons. The presence of protein aggregates in neurons is a common pathological hallmark in many movement disorders.

A unique characteristic of the genetics of the respiratory chain enzyme complexes is that the genes that code for each enzyme complex are composed of some from the mitochondrial DNA (mtDNA) and some from the host neuron DNA (Hatefi 1985; Birky 2001). Another fact that complicates the genetics of mitochondria is that the vast majority of the mtDNA comes directly from the mother. This is because very little mtDNA is carried or transferred by the sperm at fertilization (Giles et al 1980; Sutovsky et al 1999).

MtDNA is susceptible to damage by oxygen radicals due to the lack of protective histones, which leaves mtDNA exposed to the free radicals. The physical location of the mtDNA, which is very close to the area in the mitochondria where the free radical formation occurs, also increases its susceptibility to damage. MtDNA also has very 'primitive' DNA repair mechanisms that results in damage remaining for long periods on the mtDNA, which results in ongoing mutation accumulation during protein synthesis. This is extremely important in neurons that have a very slow rate of replication because they tend to accumulate large amounts of mutated mtDNA proteins over time, which eventually starts to interfere with the function of the neuron.

The Substantia Nigra, Caudate Nucleus, and Putamen Are at Increased Risk of Damage from Oxidative Radicals

Oxidative deamination of dopamine by monoamine oxidase-B (MAO-B) at the outer mitochondrial membrane results in H_2O_2 production as well as high rates of production of other radical moieties. The auto-oxidation of dopamine to form neuromelanin, which is a dopamine-lipofuscin polymer, also results in high rates of oxidative radical formation in dopaminergic neurons. This means that the substantia nigra, the caudate nucleus, and the putamen, all nuclei with large concentrations of dopaminergic involvement and all of which are involved in motor function, are at increased risk for mitochondrial OxPhos disorders.

Particular Mutations in mtDNA Are Responsible for Specific Patient Presentations

MtDNA mutations cause a range of movement disorders including ataxias, dystonias, myoclonic epilepsy with lactic acidosis and stroke-like episodes (MELAS), and Kearn's-Sayer (KS) syndrome, and more and more evidence points to their involvement in Parkinson's disease. MELAS and KS syndrome will be briefly discussed here, while ataxias, dystonias, and Parkinson's disease are covered in Chapter 11.

MELAS can occur at any age but is particularly prevalent in youth. The presentation usually involves some form of epileptic movement disorder, cerebellar ataxia, ragged red fibres in muscle, which increase with age as the OxPhos capability decreases, and stroke-like episodes. Ataxic episodes may proceed the other symptoms by a number of years.

KS syndrome consists of variable but often significant organic dysfunction such as proximal tubule dysfunction of the kidneys, with associated aminoaciduria and increased levels of lactate, pyruvate, and alanine in the blood, urine, and cerebral spinal fluid (CSF). Involvement of the extrinsic ocular muscles of the eye, with ptosis and extraocular weakness, often present as the first clinical sign of this syndrome.

Diagnosis of OxPhos Disorders

The clinical presentation and histories will most often suggest a mitochondrial involvement. However, the following findings are essential in establishing the definitive diagnosis:

- Elevated levels of lactate, pyruvate, and alanine in urine, blood, and CSF;
- Positive OxPhos enzymology;
- Positive microscopy findings with muscle biopsy; and
- Confirmation by genetic and mitochondrial analysis of the specific mutation.

Conservative Treatment of OxPhos Disorders

CoQ_{10} supplementation given at 2–4 mg/kg/day has been effective for improving symptoms in patients with OxPhos disorders. The same treatment has been effective for increasing the mitochondrial respiration rate, which declines with age naturally by approximately 1% per year after the age of 40 (Bresolin et al 1988; Ihara et al 1989).

Young males can increase their mitochondrial volume by 100% with exercise training while older adults can increase volumes by around 20% by increasing the size of their existing mitochondria.

Apoptosis is a Controlled, Preprogrammed, Process of Neuron Death

Apoptosis, which differs from necrotic cell death, involves a complex set of specific preprogrammed activities that result in the death of the neuron. This type of activity is actually an important part of normal embryological development of the nervous system which has been linked to the absence or lack of appropriate concentrations of nerve growth factors. The involvement of the mitochondria in apoptosis is well documented (Green & Reed 1998; Desagher & Martinou 2000). When activated by cellular damage or other proapoptotic signals, apoptogenic molecules that normally remain dormant in the membrane of the mitochondria become activated. These molecules then activate aspartate-specific cysteine protease (caspase), a major effector in apoptosis in neurons (Schulz et al 1999). The caspase pathway is also activated by other cellular insults such as DNA damage and anoxia. The processes involved in apoptosis result in neuron shrinkage, condensation of chromatin, cellular fragmentation, and eventual phagocytosis of cellular remnants.

QUICK FACTS 11	Two Factors That Influence the Survivability of a Neuron

- Frequency of firing (FOF)—neuron activation.
- Fuel delivery—O_2 and glucose.

The Central Integrative State of the Neuron is Determined by Receptor Activation and Production Levels of ATP

A single neuron may receive synaptic input from as many as 80,000 different neurons. Some of the synapses are excitatory, some inhibitory and modulatory as described above. Integration of the input received occurs in the neuron or neuron system, and the output response of the neuron or neuron system is determined mostly by modulation of the

When the FOF of Presynaptic Neurons Is Decreased, as Would Occur Because of Subluxation, the Following Events May Take Place: QUICK FACTS 12

- ↓ CIEGr (cellular Immediate Early Gene responses)
- ↓ Protein production
- ↓ Cellular respiration (via mitochondrial electron transport chain)
- ↓ ATP synthesis
- ↑ Resting membrane potential (RMP)
- ↑ Free radical formation
- Further inhibition of cellular respiration (electron transport chain) in the mitochondria
- Transneuronal degeneration (TND) and diaschisis

FOF—Frequency of firing (action potential generation)

Presynaptic—Events occurring prior to activation

Postsynaptic—Events occurring during and after activation

membrane potential of the neurons. The decision of whether to fire an action potential is finally determined in an area of the neuron known as the axon hillock, where large populations of voltage-gated channels specific for Na$^+$ ions are located.

This implies that the position of a synapse on the host neuron is an important determinant in the probability of firing an action potential. Synapses closer to the axon hillock will have more influence than those farther away.

The number of synapses firing at any one time (spatial summation) and the frequency of firing of any one synapse (temporal summation) are integral in determining the *central integrative state* of the neuron at any given moment.

As discussed previously in this chapter a variety of neuronal intracellular and intercellular functions are determined by the frequency of action potential generation or frequency of firing (FOF) in the neuron, as well as the synaptic activity experienced by the neuron. Numerous second messenger systems and genetic regulatory systems are dependent on the synaptic stimulation received by the neuron. Ultimately the ability of the neuron to respond with the appropriate reactions to the environmental stimulus it receives is dependent upon the expression of the appropriate genes at the appropriate time in the appropriate amount. The neuron's ability to perform these functions is summarized in the expression 'the central integrative state of the neuron'.

Transneural Degeneration

Intimately related to the concept of central integrative state of the neuron is the concept of transneural degeneration. Neurons that have been subject to a lack of synaptic activity, low glucose supplies, low oxygen supplies, decreased ATP supplies, etc., may not be able to respond to a sudden synaptic barrage in the appropriate manner and the overfunctional integrity of the system becomes less than optimal. In neurons that have been exposed to a decreased frequency of synaptic activation a number of responses can be found in the neurons including:

- Decreases in cellular immediate early gene responses (CIEGr);
- Decreases in protein production;
- Decreases in cellular respiration (via mitochondrial electron transport chain);
- Decreases in ATP synthesis;
- Increases in resting membrane potential (RMP) in initial stages;
- Hyperpolarization of membrane potential in the late stages of degeneration;

- Increased free radical formation; and
- Further inhibition of cellular respiration (electron transport chain) in the mitochondria.

All of these processes will contribute to the development of transneural degeneration (TND), which refers to a state of instability of the nerve cell as a result of changes in FOF and/or fuel delivery to the cell. It also represents a state of decline that will proceed to cell death if fuel delivery, activation, and FOF are not restored.

Diaschisis refers to the decrease in FOF of neurons that are postsynaptic to an area of damage and is one example of how TND can occur in a neuronal system. For example, Broca's aphasia due to ischaemia in the left inferior frontal cortex can lead to diaschisis in the right hemisphere of the cerebellum due to a decrease in FOF of cerebropontocerebellar projections.

Changes in the FOF and fuel delivery can have a deleterious effect on the central integrated state (CIS) of a neuronal pool. The CIS determines the integrity of a neuronal pool and its associated functions and dictates the presence of neurological signs and symptoms.

References

Aghajanian GK, Sanders-Bush E 2002 Serotonin. In: Davis K, Charney D, Coyle J, Nemeroff C (eds) Neuropsychopharmacology: the fifth generation of progress. Lippincott Williams and Wilkins, New York, p 15–25.

Ahn S, Olive M, Aggarwal S et al 1998 A dominant-negative inhibitor of CREB reveals that it is a general mediator of stimulus-dependent transcription of c-fos. Molecular and Cellular Biology 18:967–977.

Alberts B, Bray D, Lewis J et al 1994 Energy conversion: mitochondria and chondroplasts in molecular biology of the cell. Garland, New York.

Ankarcrona M, Dypgukt JM, Bonfoco E et al 1995 Glutamate induced neuronal death: a succession of necrosis or apoptosis depending on mitochondrial function. Neuron 15:961–973.

Barnes PJ 1995 β-Adrenergic receptors and their regulation. American Journal of Respiratory and Critical Care of Medicine 152:838–860.

Barres BA 1991 New roles for glia. Journal of Neuroscience 11:3685–3694.

Berlan M, Galitzky J, Monastruc JL 1995 Beta 3-adrenoceptors in the cardiovascular system. Fundamental and Clinical Pharmacology 9:234–239.

Berridge MJ, Irvine RF 1989 Inositol phosphates and cell signalling. Nature 341:197–205.

Birky CW 2001 The inheritance of genes in mitochondria and chloroplasts: Laws, mechanisms, and models. Annual Review of Genetics 35:125–148.

Black MM, Baas PW 1989 The basis of polarity in neurons. Trends in Neuroscience 12:211–214.

Bloom FE, Kupfer DJ (eds) 1995 In: Psychopharmacology: the fourth generation of progress. Raven Press, New York, p 407–471.

Blumenfeld H 2002 Brainstem III: internal structures and vascular supply. In: Neuroanatomy through clinical cases. Sinauer Associates, Sunderland, MA, p 575–651.

Boekhoff I, Tareilus E, Strotmann J 1990 Rapid activation of alternative second messenger pathways in olfactory cilia from rats by different odorants. The EMBO Journal 9:2453–2458.

Borklund A, Lindvall O 1974 Acta Physiologica Scandinavica, Supplementum 412:1–48.

Bresolin N, Bet L, Binda A et al 1988 Clinical and biochemical correlations in mitochondrial myopathies treated with coenzyme Q10. Neurology 38:892–899.

Brooks VB 1984 The neural basis for motor control. Oxford University Press, Oxford.

Cepeda C, Chandler SH, Shumate LW et al 1995 Persistent Na$^+$ conductance in medium-sized neostriatal neurons: characterization using infrared videomicroscopy and whole cell patch-clamp recordings. Journal of Neurophysiology 74:1343–1348.

Chalmers DT, Watson SJ 1991 Comparative anatomical distribution of 5-HT$_{1A}$ receptor mRNA and 5-HT$_{1A}$ binding in rat brain—a combined in situ hybridization/in vitro receptor autoradiographic study. Brain Research 561:51–60.

Champe P, Harvey R 1994 Bioenergetics and oxidative phosphorylation. In Lippincott's illustrated reviews: biochemistry, 2nd edn. Lippincott, Philadelphia, p 61–74.

Chen J, Kelz MB, Hope BT et al 1997 Chronic FRAs: stable variants of δFosB induced in brain by chronic treatments. Journal of Neuroscience 17:4933–4941.

Choi DW 1988 Glutamate neurotoxicity and diseases of the nervous system. Neuron 1:623–634.

Collingwood TN, Urnov FD, Wolffe AP 1999 Nuclear receptors: coactivators, corepressors and chromatic remodeling in the control of transcription. Journal of Molecular Endocrinology 23:255–275.

Correa-Lacarcel J, Pujante M, Terol F et al 2000 Stimulus frequency affects c-fos expression in the rat visual system. Journal of Chemical Neuroanatomy 18:135–146.

De Cesare D, Sassone-Corsi P 2000 Transcriptional regulation by cyclic AMP-responsive factores. Progress in Nucleic Acid Research and Molecular Biology 64:343–369.

Del Maestro RF 1980 An approach to free radicals in medicine and biology. Acta Physiologica Scandinavica Supplementum 492:153–168.

Desagher S, Martinou JC 2000 Mitochondria as the central control point of apoptosis. Trends in Cellular Biology 10:369–377.

Duman RS, Nestler EJ 2000 Signal transduction pathways for catecholamine receptors. In: Bloom FE, Kupfer DJ (eds) Psychopharmacology: the fourth generation of progress. American College of Neuropsychopharmacology.

Evans RM, Arriza JL (1989) A molecular framework for the actions of glucocorticoid hormones in the nervous system. Neuron 2:1105–1112.

Fox PT, Raichle ME 1986 Focal physiological uncoupling of cerebral blood flow and oxidative metabolism during somatosensory stimulation in human subjects. Proceedings of the National Academy of Science USA 83:1140–1144.

Fox PT, Raichle ME, Mintun MA et al 1988 Nonoxidative glucose consumption during focal physiologic neural activity. Science 241:462–464.

Giles RE, Blanc H, Cann HM et al 1980 Maternal inheritance of human mitochondrial DNA. Proceedings of the National Academy of Science USA 77:6715–6719.

Gius D, Cao X, Rauscher FJ III et al 1990 Transcriptional activation and repression by fos are independent functions: the C-terminus represses immediate early gene expression via CArG elements. Molecular and Cellular Biology 10:4243–4255.

Gizang-Ginsberg E, Ziff EB 1990 Nerve growth factor regulates tyrosine hydroxylase gene transcription through a nucleoprotein complex that contains c-fos. Genes and Development 4:447–491.

Grace A 2002 Dopamine. In: Davis KL, Charney D, Coyle JT et al (eds) Neuropsychopharmacology: the fifth generation of progress. Lippincott Williams and Wilkins, New York, p 119–132.

Grace AA, Bunney BS 1984 The control of firing pattern in nigral dopamine neurons: single spike firing. Journal of Neuroscience 4:2866–2876.

Graybiel AM, Moratalla R, Robertson HA 1990 Amphetamine and cocaine induce drug specific activation of the c-fos gene in striosome-matrix compartments and limbic subdivisions of the striatum. Proceedings of the National Academy of Science USA 87:6912–6916.

Green DR, Reed JC 1998 Mitochondria and apoptosis. Science 281:1309–1312.

Harden DG, Grace AA 1995 Activation of dopamine cell firing by repeated L-DOPA administration to dopamine-depleted rats: its potential role in mediating the therapeutic response to L-DOPA treatment. Journal of Neuroscience 15:6157–6166.

Hatefi Y 1985 The mitochondrial electron transport and oxidative phosphorylation system. Annual Reviews of Biochemistry 54:1015–1069.

Hernandez-Lopez S, Bargas J, Surmeier DJ et al 1997 D1 receptor activation enhances evoked discharge in neostriatal medium spiny neurons by modulating an L-type Ca^{2+} conductance. Journal of Neuroscience 17:3334–3342.

Hess P 1990 Calcium channels in vertebrate cells. Annual Reviews of Neuroscience 13:337–356.

Hollmann M, Heinemann S 1994 Cloned glutamate receptors. Annual Reviews of Neuroscience 17:31–108.

Hope BT, Nye HE, Kelz MB et al 1994 Induction of a long lasting AP-1 Complex composed of altered Fos-like proteins in brain by chronic cocaine and other chronic treatments. Neuron 13:1235–1244.

Huang KP 1989 The mechanism of protein kinase C activation. Trends in Neuroscience 12:425–432.

Huganir RL, Greengard P (1990) Regulation of neurotransmitter receptor desensitization by protein phosphorylation. Neuron 5:555–567.

Ihara Y, Namba R, Kuroda S et al 1989 Mitochondrial encephamyopathy (MELAS): Pathological study and successful therapy with coenzyme Q10 and idebenone. Journal of Neurological Science 90:262–263.

Jacobson MD 1996 Reactive oxygen species and programmed cell death. Trends in Biochemical Science 21:83–86.

Karczmar AG 1993 Brief presentation of the story and present status of studies of the vertebrate cholinergic system. Neuropsychopharmacology 9:181–199.

Kelz MB, Nestler EJ 2000 δFosB: a molecular switch underlying long-term neural plasticity. Current Opinions in Neurology 13:715–720.

Kety SS, Schmidt F 1948 The nitrous oxide method for the quantitative determination of cerebral blood flow in man: theory, procedure, and normal values. Journal of Clinical Investigation 27:476–483.

Kimelberg HK, Norenberg MD 1989 Astrocytes. Scientific American 260:44–52.

Kislauskis E, Dobner PR 1990 Mutually dependent response elements in the cis- regulatory region of neurotensin/neuromedin N gene integrate environmental stimuli in PC12 cells. Neuron 4:783–795.

Komuro H, Rakic P 1993 Modulation of neuronal migration by NMDA receptors. Science 260:95–97.

Krief S, Lonnqvist F, Raimbault S et al 1993 Tissue distribution of beta 3-adrenergic receptor mRNA in man. Journal of Clinical Investigation 91:344–349.

Kuhl DE, Phelps ME, Markham CH et al 1982 Cerebral metabolism and atrophy in Huntington's disease determined by 18 FDG, and computed tomographic scan. Annals of Neurology 12:425–434.

Langer SZ 1974 Presynaptic regulation of catecholamine release. British Journal of Pharmacology 60:481–497.

Lester RAJ, Jahr CE 1990 Quisqualate receptor-mediated depression of calcium currents in hippocampal neurons. Neuron 4:741–749.

Lillien LE, Raff MC 1990 Differentiation signals in the CNS: type-2 astrocyte development in vitro as a model system. Neuron 5:111–119.

Lin RJ, Kao HY, Ordentlich P et al 1998 The transcriptional basis of steroid physiology. Cold Spring Harbor Symposia on Quantitative Biology 63:577–585.

Magistretti PJ, Morrison JH, Shoemaker WJ et al 1981 Vasoactive intestinal polypeptide induces glycogenolysis in mouse cortical slices: a possible regulatory mechanism for the local control of energy metabolism. Proceedings of the National Academy of Science USA 78:6535–6539.

Magistretti PJ, Morrison JH 1988 Noradrenaline- and vasoactive intestinal peptide-containing neuronal systems in neocortex: functional convergence with contrasting morphology. Neuroscience 24:367–378.

Magistretti PJ, Sorg O, Martin JL 1993 Regulation of glycogen metabolism in astrocytes: physiological, pharmacological, and pathological aspects. In: Murphy S (ed) Astrocytes: pharmacology and function. Academic Press, San Diego, p 243.

Magistretti P, Pellerin L, Martin J 2000 Brain energy metabolism: an integrated cellular perspective. In: Bloom FE, and Kupfer DJ (eds) Psychopharmacology: the fourth generation of progress. American College of Neuropsychopharmacology.

Mendell JR, Griggs RC 1994 Inherited, metabolic, endocrine and toxic myopathies. In: Isselbacher K, Braunwald E, Martin JB (eds) Harrison's principles of internal medicine, 13th edn. McGraw-Hill, New York, vol. 2.

Mitchell PJ, Tjian R 1989 Transcriptional regulation in mammalian cells by sequence specific DNA proteins. Science 245:371–378.

Nadler LS, Rosoff ML, Hamilton SE et al 1999 Molecular analysis of the regulation of muscarinic receptor expression and function. Life Science 64:375–379.

Nelson DL, Cox MM 2000 Lelninger principles of biochemistry. Worth, New York.

Nestler E, Hyman S 2002 Regulation of gene expression. In: Davis KL, Charney D, Coyle JT, Nemeroff C (eds) Neuropsychopharmacology: the fifth generation of progress. Lippincott Williams and Wilkins, New York, p 217–228.

Nishizuka Y 1988 The molecular hydrogeneity of protein kinase C and its implications for cellular recognition. Nature 334:661–665.

Olney JW, Wozniak DF, Farber NB 1997 Excitotoxic neuro-degeneration in Alzheimer disease. New hypothesis and new therapeutic strategies. Archives of Neurology 54:1234–1240.

Onn SP, West AR, Grace AA 2000 Dopamine regulation of neuronal and network interactions within the striatum. Trends in Neuroscience 23:S48–S56.

Owen OE, Morgan AP, Kemp HG et al 1967 Brain metabolism during fasting. Journal of Clinical Investigation 46:1589–1595.

Pennypacker KR, Hong JS, McMillian MK 1995 Implications of prolonged expression of Fos-related antigens. Trends in Pharmacological Science 16:317–321.

Pettersson M, Schaffner W 1990 Synergistic activation of transcription by multiple binding sites for NF-kB even in absence of cooperative factor binding to DNA. Journal of Molecular Biology 214:373–380.

Picciotto M, Caldarone BJ, King SL et al 2000 Nicotinic receptors in the brain: links between molecular biology and behaviour. Neuropsychopharmacology 22:451–465.

Pleasure D 1992 Third messengers that regulate neural gene transcription. In: Asbury AK, McKhann GM, McDonald WI (eds) Diseases of the nervous system. WB Saunders, Philadelphia, p 56–62

Ptashne M, Gann AAF 1990 Activators and targets. Nature 346:329–331.

Rogers A 1998 Thinking differently. Brain scans give new hope for diagnosing ADHD. Newsweek 132:(23):60.

Ruffolo RR Jr, Bondinell W, Hieble JP 1995 α- and β-adrenoceptors: from the gene to the clinic. 2. Structure-activity relationships and therapeutic applications. Journal of Medicinal Chemistry 38:3681–3716.

Schulz JB, Weller M, Moskowitz MA 1999 Caspases as treatment targets in stroke and neurodegenerative diseases. Annals of Neurology 45:421–429.

Smeitink J, Van den Heuvel L 1999 Human mitochondrial complex I in health and disease. American Journal of Human Genetics 64:1505–1510.

Snyder SH 1992 Neurotransmitters. In: Asbury AK, McKhann GM, McDonald WI (eds) Diseases of the nervous system. WB Saunders, Philadelphia, p 47–55.

Sonnenberg JL, Macgregor-Leon PF, Curran T et al 1989 Dynamic alterations occur in the levels and composition of transcription factor AP-1 complexes after seizure. Neuron 3:359–365.

Spano PF, Govoni S, Trabucchi M 1978 Studies on the pharmacological properties of dopamine receptors in various areas of the central nervous system. Advances in Biochemical Psychopharmacology 19:155–165.

Struhl K 1999 Fundamentally different logic of gene regulation in eukaryotes and prokaryotes. Cell 98:1–4.

Su T-P, Breier A, Coppola R et al 1996 D2 receptor occupancy during risperidone and clozapine treatment in chronic schizophrenia: Relationship to blood level, efficacy and EPS. Society of Neuroscience Abstracts 22:265.

Sumiyoshi T, Stockmeier CA, Overholser JC et al 1995 Dopamine D4 receptors and effects of guanine nucleotides on [^{3}H]raclopride binding in postmortem caudate nucleus of subjects with schizophrenia or major depression. Brain Research 681:109–116.

Sunahara RK, Niznik HB, Weiner DM et al 1990 Human dopamine D1 receptor encoded by an intronless gene on chromosome 5. Nature 347:80–83.

Sutovsky P, Moreno RJ, Ramalho-Santos J et al 1999 Ubiquitin tag for sperm mitochondria. Nature 402:371–372.

Van den Berg C 1986 On the relation between energy transformations in the brain and mental activities. In: Hockey GRJ, Gaillard AWK, Coles MGH (eds) Energetics and human information processing. Nijhoff, Boston, p 131–135.

Wang R, Macmillan LB, Fremeau Jr RT 1996 Expression of alpha 2-adrenergic receptor subtypes in the mouse brain: evaluation of spatial and temporal information imparted by 3kb of 5' regulatory sequence for the alpha 2A AR-receptor gene in transgenic animals. Neuroscience 174:199–218.

Wilson MT, Keith CH 1998 Glutamate modulation of dendrite outgrowth: alterations in the distribution of dendritic microtu-bules. Journal of Neuroscience Research 52:599–611.

Workman JL, Kingston RE 1998 Alteration of nucleosome structure as a mechanism of transcriptional regulation. Annual Review of Biochemistry 67:545–579.

Young AB, Penney JB, Starosta-Rubinstein S et al 1986 PET scan investigations of Huntington's disease: cerebral metabolic correlates of metabolic features and functional decline. Annals of Neurology 20:296–303.

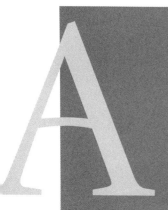

Clinical Case Answers

Case 3.1

3.1.1 The reduced activation of the movement receptors in the joints of his arm will result in a decreased afferent input or reduced synaptic activity of the dorsal root ganglion cells responsible for detection of proprioception in his arm. The number of synapses firing at any one time (spatial summation) and the frequency of firing of any one synapse (temporal summation) are integral in determining the *central integrative state* of a neuron at any given moment. When a neuron is exposed to a decrease in synaptic activity over a period of time it may undergo a change in central integrative state that results in transneuron degeneration. Once normal activity is attempted in the arm the neurons that have been subject to a lack of synaptic activity, low glucose supplies, low oxygen supplies, decreased adenosine triphosphate (ATP) supplies, etc., may not be able to respond to a sudden synaptic barrage of restored movement in the appropriate manner and the overfunctional integrity of the system becomes less than optimal. In neurons that have been exposed to a decreased frequency of synaptic activation a number of responses can be found in the neurons including:

- Decreases in cellular immediate early gene responses;
- Decreases in protein production;
- Decreases in cellular respiration (via mitochondrial electron transport chain);
- Decreases in ATP synthesis;
- Increases in resting membrane potential in initial stages;
- Hyperpolarization of membrane potential in the late stages of degeneration;
- Increased free radical formation; and
- Further inhibition of cellular respiration (electron transport chain) in the mitochondria.

All of these processes will contribute to the development of transneural degeneration, which refers to a state of instability of the nerve cell as a result of changes in frequency of firing (FOF) and/or fuel delivery to the cell. It also represents a state of decline that will proceed to cell death if fuel delivery, activation, and FOF are not restored. The sudden return of attempted movement in his arm may severely damage some of the neurons in the spinal cord that have undergone TND as a result of decreased movement over time.

3.1.2 Diaschisis refers to the decrease in FOF of neurons that are postsynaptic to an area of damage and is one example of how TND can occur in a neuronal system. The neurons in the spinal cord project to neurons of the thalamus and cerebellum. Diaschisis could cause TND in these neuronal pools downstream from the neurons involved through a resulting decrease in activation at the neuronal pools.

3.1.3   A variety of things could be done to prevent any serious damage from occurring:

1. The arm could be gently moved several times per day to stimulate proprioceptors.
2. Transepithelial electrical nerve stimulation (TENS) could be applied on a daily basis to maintain action potential frequency in the system.
3. Appropriate rehabilitation needs to be carried out before return to full activity.

Case 3.2

3.2.1   The environmental stimulus whether it be a growth hormone, a neurotransmitter, or a hormone must get its signal from the receptors on the neuron cell membrane to the transcriptional controlling factors in the nucleus in order for production of the necessary proteins that it calls for.

Some signalling molecules such as hydrophobic hormones (glucocorticoids, oestrogen, and testosterone) can gain direct access to the nuclear apparatus by their lipid soluble chemical structure that allows them the ability to transverse the highly hydrophobic bilayered lipid plasma membrane dependent mainly on their concentration gradients. Other signalling molecules such as Ca^{++} ions gain access through specific ion channels present in the neuron plasma membrane.

Protein hormones, growth factors, peptide neuromodulators, and neurotransmitters must act on their transcription protein targets indirectly by either inducing a change in a transmembrane protein channel related to their receptor proteins or by inducing a change in linked intramembrane proteins. Changes in these linked intramembranous proteins called G-proteins eventually result in the release of intracellular ions or the generation of intracellular second messenger such as cyclic adenosine monophosphate (cAMP), diacylglycerol, and inositol triphosphate, which then activate directly or through other intermediates the transcription factors in the nucleus such as cAMP response element binding protein (CREB).

The number of known second messengers is still relatively small. Response specificity is achieved through one of the following methods:

- Temporally and spatially graded rises in second messenger levels;
- Recruitment of various combinations of second messengers after a single stimulus; and
- Regional variations in the intracellular targets on which the second messengers act.

3.2.2   Third messengers are groups of nuclear proteins known as translational factors induced by a variety of extracellular signals. These proteins bind to specific nucleotide sequences in the promoter and enhancer regions of genes. Fine-tuning of the effects of third messengers is accomplished through a complex network of controls. Since there are now over a hundred IEGs and corresponding proteins composing third messengers a very complex matrix of interactivity which would allow complicated but minor variances in linear and temporal combinations of third messengers for various functions can be developed. Activation of a gene requires that the chromatin or nucleosomal structure be modified to allow the binding of regulatory proteins to the appropriate subset of genes. This is accomplished by a specialized group of proteins referred to as activator proteins that remodel the chromatin and expose core promoter sites on the appropriate genes. This permits the binding of yet another complex of proteins called general transcription factors to the core promoter site on the DNA. This complex of general transcription factors can then recruit and bind with RNA polymerase to enter the transcription initiation phase of the replication process. Several families of transcription factors have been identified as well as several modes of activation or inhibition of these factors. For example, the CREB family of transcription factors activate transcription of genes to which they are linked when they are phosphorylated by cAMP-dependent protein kinase (protein kinase A). Protein kinase A is activated in the presence of cAMP.

The CREB family of transcription factors can also be activated by other second messengers such as Ca^{++} bound by calmodulin that can activate a variety of protein kinases upon entering the nucleus of the neuron. These kinases can in turn phosphorylate CREB, resulting in the activation of transcription of the specific CREB-linked gene.

3.2.3   In the neuron most energy-requiring processes are made possible by either direct or indirect coupling with an energy-releasing mechanism involving the hydrolysis of ATP. ATP is synthesized in the mitochondria of the neuron via the processes of electron transfer and oxidative phosphorylation and in the cytoplasm via glycolysis. Glycolysis (Embden-Meyerhof pathway) is the metabolism of glucose to pyruvate and lactate. This process results in the net production of only 2 mol of ATP/mol of glucose. On the other hand, pyruvate can pass into the tricarboxylic acid cycle (Krebs cycle) in the mitochondria and via the oxidative phosphorylation cascade produce 30 mol of ATP/mol of glucose. The energetic benefit of utilizing the oxidative phosphorylation route over glycolytic route is obvious from an energetic perspective.

3.2.4   The number of synapses firing at any one time (spatial summation) and the frequency of firing of any one synapse (temporal summation) are integral in determining the *central integrative state* of the neuron at any given moment.

As discussed previously in this chapter a variety of neuronal intracellular and intercellular functions are determined by the frequency of action potential generation or frequency of firing (FOF) in the neuron, as well as the synaptic activity experienced by the neuron. Numerous second messenger systems and genetic regulatory systems are dependent on the synaptic stimulation received by the neuron. Ultimately the ability of the neuron to respond with the appropriate reactions to the environmental stimulus it receives is dependent upon the expression of the appropriate genes at the appropriate time in the appropriate amount. The neuron's ability to perform these functions is summarized in the expression 'the central integrative state of the neuron'.

Chapter

4

The Fundamentals of Functional Neurological History and Examination

Clinical Cases for Thought

Case 4.1   A 54-year-old woman present to your office via referral from her cardiologist. She has a spectrum of complaints ranging from irregular heart beat, dizziness on standing, feelings of hot and cold in her arms and feet, and stomach upset including irregular bowel movements through the day. She has had a complete cardiac work-up done by her cardiologist in which all findings were normal. The cardiologist feels that this patient may be suffering from a form of dysautonomia.

Questions

4.1.1   Which cranial nerves can you examine that will give you information about the level of function of her parasympathetic nervous system? Which tests would you perform?

4.1.2   What examinations would you perform to evaluate the level of function of her sympathetic nervous system?

4.1.3   What is dermatographia and in what situations would you expect to find it?

Case 4.2   A 23-year-old male presents to your office with double vision and headaches. On examination you discover that he has an exophoria of the right pupil.

Questions

4.2.1   What are the causes of exophoria? What is exotropia?

4.2.2   How would you differentiate between a weak medial rectus muscle and an overactive lateral rectus muscle?

Introduction

The neurological examination is traditionally taught using a disease or ablative lesion-orientated model. While this approach may help to detect the presence of both serious and benign disorders, it is less helpful for the practitioner who wishes to investigate and estimate the physiological functional integrity of the nervous system. A more functional approach to the neurological examination heightens the examiner's sensitivity to physiological aberrations responsible for the vast majority of neurological symptoms. At the same time, a practitioner using this approach is more likely to detect subtle signs of pathology.

The practitioner who intends to utilize the functional approach of examination must be concerned with the identification of ablative lesions and the presence of disease processes, but must also attempt to identify any physiological lesions manifesting themselves as physical symptoms.

For example, if a patient presents with a recent history of an inner ear infection complicated by hearing loss and balance disturbances, one might assume the possibility of potential damage to the vestibular and/or cochlear hair cells, which are the receptors responsible for balance and hearing. At follow-up after a course of antibiotics, a commonly occurring scenario is that the patient states that their hearing has returned and their balance is no longer a concern to them but they are starting to experience migraines, which they have not experienced before. The vestibular system can have a profound influence on peripheral resistance due to disynaptic or polysynaptic connections between vestibular neurons and the tonic vasomotor neurons of the rostral ventrolateral medulla. The purpose of these connections is for protection against orthostatic stress. Should a comprehensive examination focused on the functional state of the vestibular-cerebellar and medullary areas show dysfunction or asymmetry of function in this patient, it would be of great value to the patient for you to address the central consequences of the inner ear infection and attempt to reduce the vasomotor dysregulation that has no doubt developed during the course of their illness. Treatment, involving appropriate afferent stimulation and exercises aimed at restoring symmetry and integrity to the vestibular system and associated brainstem nuclei, should be a primary consideration in this patient's management in addition to any pharmaceutical approach also applied.

In learning the traditional approach to the neurological examination a student or inexperienced practitioner may be less interested in minor asymmetries of cranial nerve function or motor and sensory signs, especially when the history does not alert to serious pathology. This is not the case in the functional examination were minor asymmetries or altered functional output are of great significance in the analysis of the physiological lesion. Each test must be performed with alert observational skills and meticulous care, comparing the results bilaterally when possible.

The functional neurological examination aims to elicit information about mental, sensory, and motor functions. Sensory functions are analysed by observing the patient's mental or motor response to stimulation of the various sensory receptors in the head and body. Motor functions are analysed by observing the patient's requested or spontaneous volitional actions. Sensory and motor functions can also be analysed by observing both muscle and glandular responses to sensory stimulation. The muscles and glands are the final common effector systems of the body. Their responses are normally dependent on the output from complex neuronal integration, and as such, can be utilized in assessment of the functional state of the neuron pools that control their output.

The Five Parameters of Effector Response are Important Clues in Gauging the CIS of Upstream Neuron Systems

The response of an effector (e.g., muscle) to a stimulus or command is largely dependent on the central integrative state (CIS) of the presynaptic neuronal pool projecting to the motor neuron of the effector. Therefore, the CIS of a neuronal pool can be predicted or estimated by observing the characteristics of the motor response of the downstream motor neuron to a unit stimulus. The parameters of the effector response observed can be summarized under the following observational findings:

QUICK FACTS 1	Central Integrative State (CIS) Is Dependent on the Following

1. Fuel delivery
2. FOF of presynaptic pools

Energy Production in the Cell	QUICK FACTS 2

1. Glycolysis
2. Citric acid cycle
3. Electron transport chain

1. Latency and velocity of the response;
2. Amplitude of the response;
3. Smoothness of movement of the response;
4. Fatigability of the response; and
5. Direction of the response.

All of the responses observed during the functional examinations performed on a patient, should be evaluated with the above parameters in mind. It is also important to visualize the pathways actively involved in producing the actions that one is examining. This allows the practitioner the advantage of performing additional or more detailed tests directed at the same pathways throughout the examination should disparities in the patient's responses become apparent.

Latency and Velocity of a Response

The latency refers to the time between the presentation of a stimulus and the motor, sensory, autonomic, or behavioural response of the patient. This provides information concerning conduction time along nerve axons and spatial and temporal summation occurring in the neurons involved in the functional action chain of the response. The velocity of the response is another window of spatial and temporal summation and conduction time.

Diagnostic Approach	QUICK FACTS 3

1. Serious disorders
2. Common disorders
3. Underlying issues
4. Masquerades
5. Level of the lesion
6. Frequency of firing (FOF)
7. Fuel delivery

The time to summation (TTS) and time to peak summation (TTSp) are abbreviations that describe, respectively, the latency and average velocity of effector responses. The pupillary action observed in response to a light stimulus offers a good illustration of these concepts. Under normal conditions, the pupils will respond with a relatively equal TTS and TTSp in both eyes when stimulated with an equal light stimulus. However, in the situation where the central integrative state of the neurons in the right Edinger-Westphal nucleus or mesencephalic reticular formation is further away from threshold, the TTS of the right eye would be expected to be increased from that of the left. The same result may be expected when measuring the velocity of the response, or an increased time to maximal pupil constriction (increased TTSp). The same result, that is increased TTS and TTSp in the right eye, may be found with an afferent pupil defect such as would occur if the right eye end organ was impeded by a photoreceptor or axonal conduction deficit such as in retinal or optic nerve dysfunction. Thus there is the need for a complete fundoscopic and visual acuity exam when unequal pupil responses are present.

Amplitude of a Response

The amplitude of the response refers to the maximum change in the parameters being assessed. This can be a useful indicator of the relative frequency of firing in a neuronal pool. For example, the degree of excursion of the eye during the smooth phase of pursuit movement during optokinetic testing of eye movements. Or, in keeping with our first example, the maximum change in pupil size when testing the pupil light reflex.

Smoothness of a Response

Smoothness of any movement is dependent on complex interactions between multiple neuronal pools. An example is the smoothness of visual tracking in the horizontal plane. This requires complex interactions between the cerebellum, vestibular system, neural integrator, and occipital, parietal, and frontal lobes. A poor central integrative state in any of these areas may affect the quality of visual tracking in one or more directions. Specific features of the visual tracking deficit may alert to greater involvement of one area over another. Uncoordinated or jerky movements are referred to as dysmetric.

Fatigability of a Response

This refers to the ability to maintain a response during continued or repeated presentation of a stimulus. A progressive reduction in ocular roll and skew deviation between successive head tilts is an example of increasing fatigue of the ocular tilt reaction (OTR). Poor maintenance of a response reflects increased fatigability. The fatigability coefficient is an arbitrary descriptor of the fatigability of a neuronal pool.

Direction of a Response

The direction of response elicited is compared to the expected normal response to provide further information about the integrity of a neuronal pool. For example, the direction of change of pupil size when shining a light in the eye, the direction of nystagmus during caloric irrigation of the ear, and the direction of change of skin temperature in response to a cognitive task or vestibular stimulation all have an expected normal response direction. If the direction of response is different to the expected outcome, this may indicate the presence of pathology, fatigue, or plastic alterations in neural circuitry.

QUICK FACTS 4	Five Components of Effector Response

1. Latency and Velocity
2. Amplitude
3. Smoothness
4. Fatigability
5. Direction

The Longitudinal Level of the Lesion

When examining a patient, the practitioner needs to consider that dysfunction at any level of the pathway, from the sensory receptor to the effector, may result in aberrant findings during an examination of body function. The usually considered longitudinal levels that may be involved in a dysfunctional output response include the following: the receptor or effector, the afferent or efferent pathways of the peripheral nerve, the spinal cord, the brainstem or cerebellum, the thalamus or basal ganglia, the cortex. It is important to remember that a dysfunction at one longitudinal level of the neuraxis may result in dysfunction at other levels also.

The following example illustrates the concept. A patient presents with unilateral ptosis. The cause of the ptosis might be occurring at the effector level involving the ACh receptors of the orbicularis oculi muscle as in myasthenia gravis. The cause of the ptosis might be occurring at the peripheral nerve level as could occur in a partial third nerve compression palsy. The cause of the ptosis may involve disruption of the sympathetic fibres to the levator palpebrae superiorus muscle at any point along the sympathetic projections from the hypothalamus, through the spinal cord, the superior cervical ganglia, and postsynaptic projections that follow the oculomotor nerve to the muscle as in Horner's syndrome. Alternatively, it may be caused by asymmetric cortical output resulting in overstimulation of the pontomedullary reticular formation (PMRF), which has inhibited sympathetic output to the eyelid.

A complete history and examination of the patient would enable the correct diagnosis without too much difficulty in this case.

Approaches to Developing a Differential Diagnosis

Before discussing the history and physical examination procedures in general, it is necessary to give some thought to the reason for performing these activities in the first place. The history and physical examination are procedures that allow the practitioner to develop a clinical impression of the state of health or disease of the patient. Based on the clinical impression, the practitioner then arrives at a working diagnosis of the patient's condition and develops the most appropriate approach to treatment of the patient.

The Basic Functional Neurological Examination   QUICK FACTS 5

- Blind spots and visual fields;
- Pupil size and PLRs (pupil light reflexes);
- Motor and sensory examination of the head;
- Motor and sensory examination of the trunk and limbs;
- Skin and tympanic temperature patterns;
- Ophthalmoscopic/otoscopic examination;
- Vestibular, cerebellar, and spatial awareness tests; and
- Specific cortical tests.

The process of arriving at a diagnosis usually first involves the development of a differential diagnosis, which is the consideration of a number of alternative diagnostic possibilities in light of the history. The list of differential diagnoses is then systematically reduced by the results obtained from further tests performed on the patient. The most common tests utilized clinically include the examination procedures that compose the physical examination, laboratory blood or body fluid analysis, diagnostic imaging such as plain film X-rays, MRI, fMRI, or PET scans, and electrophysiological evaluations such as qEEG, EEG, and EMG.

Space limitations only allow for a brief overview and suggested approach to differential diagnosis at this time, but several excellent texts on the subject can be found in the additional reading section at the end of the chapter.

One approach to developing a differential diagnosis is to consider the possible causes of the patient's presenting symptom picture with respect to a list of major classifications of pathological processes. The major classifications include vascular disorders, infectious conditions, neoplastic disorders, neurological disorders, degenerative disorders, inflammatory disorders, congenital disorders, connective tissue disorders, autoimmune disorders, trauma, endocrine disorders, and soft tissue disorders. The pneumonic VINDICATES can be used to remember the major classifications for this approach.

Once a clear history has been taken from the patient, possibilities from each category can be considered and analysed in light of the symptom picture that the patient has presented with. The following example should illustrate the approach: A 54-year-old male presents with a history of low back pain that radiates into his left leg. The patient works as a construction worker and has a 30-year history of smoking. Diagnostic possibilities based on the VINDICATES approach should be considered (see Table 4.1).

Table 4.1 Diagnostic Possibilities Utilizing the VINDICATE Pneumonic

V= Vascular	Deep vein thrombus, varicose veins, Burger's disease, heart failure, myocardial infarction (atypical presentation), abdominal aortic aneurysm, arthrosclerosis
I = Infection	Meningitis, HIV, osteomyelitis
N = Neoplastic, Neurological	All carcinomas including emphasis on prostate carcinoma, lung carcinoma—Pancoast tumour, tumours of spinal cord and brain—Schwannomas, glioma, MM, Mets, osteosarcoma, Ewings sarcoma. Herniated or prolapsed vertebral disc, sciatic neuralgia, cervical spondylitic myelopathy, piriformis syndrome, cauda equine syndrome, neurogenic claudication
D = Degenerative	Spondylosis of IVF, osteoarthritis, DISH
I = Inflammatory	Osteomyelitis, RA, AS, EA, more arthropathie, gout
C = Cartilagenous, Congenital, Connective tissue	Pagets (as 'bone softening' disease), osteoporosis, scoliosis, spondylolisthesis Duchenne muscular dystrophy and Becker's, congenital MD Systemic lupus erythematosus
A = Autoimmune	RA, Sjogrens , MS, SLE, AIDS
T = Trauma	Fracture, → complete, stress, compression. Whiplash syndrome. Muscle strain, ligament sprain, e.g., lumbosacral strain-sprain Haematoma, fibromyalgia
E = Endocrine	Hyperthyroidism, hypothyroidism, hypercalcaemia, hypocalcaemia Hyperparathroidism, hypoparathyroidism. Diabetes mellitus (ID and NIDDM), diabetes insipidus. Cushings, Addisons
S = Soft tissue (involvement)	Muscle strain, ligament sprain, e.g., lumbosacral strain-sprain. Haematoma , fibromyalgia, piriformis syndrome, facet syndrome, SI syndrome, torticollis, VSC, TMJ syndrome, tension/cervicogenic

Order of the History and Examination Process

Any healthcare practitioner with training in clinical and neural science has the ability to perform the neurological history and examination in a proficient manner. The key is to develop a routine that can easily be remembered, that can be performed in logical sequential order, and that can be easily improvised for different patient presentations. Two systematic approaches to the neurological examination include the anatomical and functional approaches. The anatomical approach requires examination of the nervous system in a rostrocaudal order (i.e., brain, brainstem/cranial nerves, spinal cord, spinal nerves, receptors etc.), while the functional approach requires examination of related functions in groups (i.e., mental, motor, sensory, visceral etc.). A combination of these two approaches is likely to be more efficient, less repetitive, and more appropriate for both the history-taking process and examination as well.

Greater efficiency may be achieved by limiting movement of the patient and using each tool or each type of test only once throughout the examination. If possible, the patient should be assessed in the sitting, standing, and lying positions once and should be assessed in a rostrocaudal order for each function tested. This will reduce the frequency of switching between tools and patient positions. Each instrument used in the examination should be laid out in order of use and within easy reach of the practitioner. With this orderly approach, the practitioner will be less likely to miss any component of the examination (DeMyer 1994). For example, it might be more efficient for the practitioner to determine sensitivity to pain at all levels from the ophthalmic division of the trigeminal nerve to sacral innervated regions, rather than switching between motor and sensory tests at each level.

Details gathered from the neurological history and examination may only provide information concerning the type and location of aberrant neuronal function. A thorough physical and orthopaedic examination and laboratory or ancillary neuro-diagnostic tests may be more useful in establishing the aetiology in some cases.

The following lists provide an overview of the breadth of information concerning the neurological history and examination. This should serve as a useful reference and template.

The Neurological History

1. Initial History

Onset and Character of Health Complaints

What and where are the symptoms and when did they first occur?

Was there any illness, trauma, or significant event prior to or during the onset?

What is the nature of the sensations, disabilities, or problems that have arisen?

Pain/Headaches/Fever/Energy or Weight Change

Has the patient experienced any pain, headaches, fever, energy, or weight change?

If weight change has occurred, was it expected from a diet or exercise programme?

Duration and Frequency

How long do the symptoms last and how often do they occur? Are they recurrent in nature?

Course

Has the patient's condition or the symptoms changed since the onset of their condition?

Aggravating Factors

Is there anything that makes their symptoms worse?

Relieving Factors

Is there anything that makes their symptoms better?

Timing of Symptoms

Do the symptoms occur at a particular time of day, month, or year?

Treatment

Has the patient received any treatment? If so, what did it involve?

Sneeze/Cough/Valsalva One

Are the symptoms aggravated by pressure changes in the thorax or abdomen?

Are the symptoms affected by changes in position such as rising from a sitting or lying position?

2. General Health History

Family History

Have any immediate or extended family members suffered from a major or hereditary illness or expressed symptoms similar to the patient's symptoms?

Accidents/Trauma

Past trauma such as motor vehicle accidents, falls, concussions, fractures, etc.

Medications/Supplements

Past (long-term prescriptions, etc.) or present medications.

Is the patient exposed to any other chemicals at work or home?

Is the patient taking any vitamins, remedies, or supplements?

Illnesses

Are there any current or past illnesses that the patient has experienced?

Tests and Imaging

Have any laboratory, imaging, or electrodiagnostic procedures been performed?

Operations/Hospitalization

Has the patient had any surgery or admissions to hospital in the past?

Nutrition

What is the patient's diet like?

3. **Social History**

Family Life

What is the patient's marital status?

Do they have any dependants?

Do they feel much stress at home?

Recreation

Does the patient partake in recreational activities and exercise?

Education

What is their level of education?

Occupation

What is their job description and have there been any recent changes at work?

Social Drugs

Does the patient smoke or drink alcohol? If yes, how much?

4. **Systems History (special senses, motor, sensory, autonomic, mental)**

Smell and Taste

Have there been any changes to smell or taste?

Has the patient noticed any spontaneous smells or tastes?

Vision

Has the patient noticed any cloudiness, haziness, blurring, or double vision?

Does the patient have difficulty in stabilizing their focus?

Does the patient ever experience movement of their visual environment?

Does the patient experience any pain in or around their eyes?

Is the patient more sensitive to light in one or both eyes?

Hearing

Has the patient ever noticed any changes to their hearing in either ear?

Does the patient find it difficult to listen when there is background noise?

Does the patient experience any ringing or whooshing noises in either ear?

Does the patient experience any pain or itchiness in or around their ears?

Does the patient experience a 'fullness' or 'blocked' sensation in either ear?

Balance

Does the patient find it harder to walk in a straight line?

Does the patient tend to deviate more to the left or right when walking?

Does the patient ever feel as though they are falling or leaning to one side?

Does the patient feel as though they are spinning or moving when they are still?

Does the patient ever experience any movement of their visual environment?

Has the patient experienced any nausea or vomiting?

Does the patient feel dizzy or light-headed when looking at moving objects?

Does the patient feel dizzy or light-headed when they change their posture?

Motor

Does the patient have any difficulty with chewing or swallowing their food?

Has the patient noticed any difficulties with speech (e.g. slurring or stuttering)?

Has the patient noticed any clumsiness (e.g. using tools and utensils, or tripping)?

Has the patient noticed any tremors or uncontrollable movements?

Has the patient noticed any stiffness, cramping, or twitching anywhere?

Has the patient noticed any weakness or wasting of muscles?

Sensory

Has the patient noticed any changes in skin sensitivity anywhere?

Has the patient noticed any unusual sensations anywhere (e.g. tingling, coldness)?

Autonomic

Has the patient noticed any changes with salivation or tearing?

Has the patient noticed any changes in sweating on either side of the body?

Has the patient noticed any coldness or puffiness in their extremities?

Does the patient feel dizzy or light-headed when they change their posture?

Does the patient experience arrhythmia or rapid changes in heart rate?

Does the patient experience any breathing difficulties?

Does the patient have any problems with digestion or bowel movements?

Does the patient suffer from ulcers or irritability in the GI tract?

Does the patient have any difficulties with initiating or controlling urination?

Has the patient experienced any signs of sexual dysfunction?

Mental

Have there been any changes in decision making, planning, or organization skills?

Have there been any changes in attention levels or concentration?

Have there been any changes in behaviour, mood, or personality?

Have there been any changes in the ability to express thoughts or words?

Have there been any changes in the comprehension of speech or the written word?

Have there been any problems with the recognition of people or objects?

Have there been any changes with regard to orientation or spatial awareness?

Have there been any changes in short- or long-term memory?

Has the patient experienced any seizures, anxiety, or panic attacks?

Learning these questions as a basis for taking a neurological history can help the practitioner to gain experience by learning more about classic and unusual symptom patterns.

The Neurological Examination

There are numerous excellent texts that cover neurological examination techniques and these have been outlined in the Further Reading section. What will be attempted here is a description of examination techniques or procedures that either differ from the norm or are not covered in traditional texts. As each technique is encountered in the text it will be expanded on to explain in detail the approach necessary. First, some neurodiagnostic testing equipment often utilized in functional neurology will be discussed.

Neurodiagnostic Tests

A variety of neurodiagnostic testing equipment can be utilized to investigate or objectively quantify dysfunction. These include:

1. *Video nystagmography* (VNG)—for objective analysis and documentation of visual tracking, saccade, and optokinetic dysfunction, spontaneous nystagmus with and without visual fixation, unilateral weakness (canal paresis) and directional preponderance (central asymmetry) via caloric irrigation, positional tests, and others.

2. *Vestibular evoked myogenic potentials* (VEMPs)—for objective analysis of certain components of the vestibulocollic reflex. Latency and amplitude of motor signals to the Sternocleidomastoid (SCM) muscle are measured following stimulation of the saccule with loud auditory stimuli.

3. *Balance platform*—Objective analysis of postural sway in various conditions using a force platform.

4. *Electrocochleography*—Objective analysis of short latency responses from the cochlear apparatus and nerve.

5. *Auditory brainstem responses*—Objective analysis of brainstem responses to auditory stimuli to complement VEMPs.

6. *Electroencephalography* (EEG) and qEEG—the neuron electrical activity is measured over the scalp by very powerful receptors and then amplified to produce wave patterns that can be used to give objective projections of the state of brain function. This technique has become very powerful with the addition of source localization software such as that offered by the Key institute which can combine low-resolution tomographic analysis (LORETA) and MRI anatomical library data to give very accurate localization of EEG data.

7. *Advanced imaging*—MRI, CT, Doppler ultrasound if history and examination suggests ablative lesion of sinister aetiology or if patient is not responding to care. To be discussed further.

8. *Audiometry*—also useful and it is important that copies of all reports concerning hearing, vision, balance, and imaging are requested.

The Examination Process
Observation

1. Note the general appearance of the patient and their body morphology.
2. Note the patient's manner and disposition.
3. Look for postural angulations of the head, trunk, and limbs.
4. Note the condition of the skin, nails, and hair.
5. Note skin lesions, pigmentary differences, nevi, oedema, and vascularity.
6. Note any asymmetries of pupil size or position, and observe for ptosis and lid lag.
7. Note any asymmetries of facial muscles and structure and observe the hairline.

Vital signs

1. Determine the heart and respiratory rate and rhythm. These signs can give an indication of the tone of the sympathetic and parasympathetic systems.
2. Determine respiratory dynamics including depth and inspiration/expiration ratio. This can give an indication of the ventilation patterns and thus the pH or acid/base state of the patient.
3. Determine blood pressure bilaterally and record even minor differences as these along with other findings can be important in determining the state of the sympathetic nervous system. Blood pressure should always be measured on both arms. Blood pressure is dependent in part on the peripheral resistance, which can be different on either side of the head and body due to asymmetrical control of vasomotor tone. Increased vasomotor tone can occur because of decreased integrity or CIS of the ipsilateral PMRF, or because of excitatory vestibulosympathetic reflexes.
4. Measure the core temperature. This may give you an indication of the basal metabolic rate of the patient, which is elevated in hyperthyroidism and some cases of infection.
5. Measure the skin and tympanic temperature bilaterally, again recording any differences as these seemingly small variations may be of great clinical importance in determining the blood flow and thus activity levels in each frontal cortex.
6. Determine oxygen saturation if the technology is available.

Visual Fields and Pupil Responses

1. Check the upper and lower temporal and nasal visual fields. This is best done using confrontational testing procedures with a red tipped pointer.
2. Check the patient's pupil sizes and response to light. Both consensual and direct reflexes need to be tested and recorded.

Examination of the Pupils
Pupil size reflects a balance in tone between the sympathetic and parasympathetic nervous systems. You can get a reasonable measure of the actual sympathetic tone in the patient by measuring the resting pupil size in darkness. The sympathetic tone represents the degree of dilation of the pupil but the degree of resting vascular constriction in vascular smooth muscle in most parts of the body. Vestibular, cerebellar, and cortical influences on both sympathetic and parasympathetic tone should also be considered.

Various components of the pupil light reflex are subserved by each component of the autonomic nervous system. The TTA, amplitude of constriction, smoothness and maintenance of constriction, TTF, and time to redilation of the pupil response need to be measured and recorded in each pupil. These are all aspects of the pupil light reflex that have been researched and correlated with central integrative state of the various contributing components of the nervous system.

Pupil Constriction Pathways

Accommodation is the constriction of the pupil that occurs during convergence of the eyes for close focusing. The Edinger-Westphal nucleus is activated by the adjacent oculomotor nucleus, which activates the medial rectus muscle more powerful than the light reflex. There is also contraction of the ciliary muscle to aid close focusing which is referred to as the 'near response'. Parasympathetic fibres lie superficially on the oculomotor nerve and they relay in the ciliary ganglion of the orbit, which lies on the branch to the inferior oblique muscle. They begin in dorsal position and rotate to a medial and then inferior position as they enter the orbit. Blood supply to the pupil fibres is different to the main trunk of the nerve. The pupil fibres receive their blood supply from the overlying pia mater; therefore, the pupil fibres are usually spared in an oculomotor nerve trunk infarction.

An 'afferent pathway lesion' results in a *Marcus-Gunn pupil*. The swinging light test will reveal that the affected pupil will not react to light as well as the other pupil, but it may constrict normally in response to stimulation of the opposite pupil during testing of the consensual light reflex. This occurs in multiple sclerosis, and diabetes conditions that affect the optic nerve because of demyelination or vascular lesions. One might also expect this to occur when there is an increase in sympathetic tone to the pupil on the side of relative 'afferent' defect. This could distinguish a high firing IML column from TND in the mesencephalon.

The *'Wernicke' pupil* reaction refers to differential summation depending on whether you are shining the light into the nasal or temporal aspects of the retina (i.e. intact or ablated fields). This may be observed in an optic tract lesion. Supposedly, the resting size of the pupil is uninterrupted because of the consensual light reflex. The nasal half of the retina is significantly more sensitive to light than the temporal half of the retina and the direct responses are significantly larger than the consensual response. Direct and consensual pupil reactions when stimulating the temporal retina are nearly equal. This may suggest an input of temporal retina to both sides of the pretectum. Such a crossing of temporal fibres may take place in the chiasm. The net effect of the pupillary light reaction, which involves shining light into the monocular zone from the temporal hemi-field of one eye, leads to greater constriction of the pupil on that side (Schmid et al 2000).

Parinaud syndrome results when damage to decussating fibres of the light reflex at the level of the superior colliculus is present. This results in semi-dilated pupils fixed to light, plus loss of upward gaze.

Argyll Robertson pupil is most commonly seen in neurosyphilis: bilateral ptosis, increased frontalis tone, pupil that is irregular, small, and fixed to light, but constricts with accommodation. The pupil can not be dilated by atropine. Differential diagnosis of this particular pupillary dysfunction includes senile miosis, pilocarpine, or β-blocker drops for glaucoma. This pattern of findings is reversed in encephalitis lethargica.

Holmes-Adie pupil or 'tonic' pupil occurs because of degeneration of the nerve fibres in the ciliary ganglion and is thought to be produced by a combination of slow inhibition of the sympathetic and partial reinnervation by parasympathetic fibres. This condition can also be associated with loss of patella reflex, decreased sweating, blurred vision for near work, and eye pain in bright light.

Horner's Syndrome

Disruption of the sympathetic chain at any point from the hypothalamic or supraspinal projections to the oculomotor nerve can result in a spectrum of symptoms referred to as Horner's syndrome. The classic findings in this syndrome include ptosis, miosis, and anhidrosis but a number of other abnormalities may also be present. Ptosis or drooping of the upper eyelid is caused by the interruption of the sympathetic nerve supply to the muscles of the upper eyelid. Miosis or decreased pupil size is a result of the decreased action of the dilator muscles of the iris due to decreased sympathetic input. This results in the constrictor muscles acting in a relatively unopposed fashion, resulting in pupil constriction. A Horner's pupil will still constrict when light is shined on the pupil although careful observation is sometimes required to detect the reduced amount of constriction that occurs. Innervation to superior and inferior tarsus muscles is carried in CN III. Vasomotor fibres are carried in the nasociliary branch of CN V and make no synapses in the ciliary ganglion after branching off from the carotid tree. Pupillodilator fibres are carried in the long ciliary branches of the nasociliary nerve.

This syndrome is characterized by the following signs and symptoms;

- Ptosis/apparent enophthalmos;
- Small pupil;
- Anhydrosis (forehead or forequarter of body);
- Bloodshot eye (loss of vasoconstrictor activity);
- Heterochromia; and

Horner's syndrome can occur because of lesions at various peripheral and central sites: hemispheric lesions, brainstem, spinal cord especially in central syringomyelia, nerve root lesions, carotid artery, jugular foramen, orbit, and cavernous sinus. Depending on the location, other cranial nerves may be involved such as III, IV, VI, and Vi near the cavernous sinus or superior orbital fissure and IX, X, and XII at the base of the skull. In the spinal cord, the mixed signs associated with syringomyelia may be present because of widening of the central canal. This would include loss of segmental reflexes, descending hypothalamospinal fibres, spinothalamic sensation (segmentally ipsilaterally and then descending contralaterally or bilaterally), ventral horn cell function, and atypical pain patterns.

With T1 nerve root involvement, Horner's syndrome may be present with weakness of finger abduction and adduction, wasting of the intrinsic hand muscles, loss of pain sensation in the medial aspect of the arm and armpit, and deep pain in the armpit. This is rarely due to spinal degeneration, and serious causes such as Pancoast's tumour should be considered. Referral for MRI, chest X-rays, and/or CT scan should then be considered.

Different lesion levels affect sweating differently. Central lesions may affect sweating over the entire forequarter due to involvement of the descending pathways from the hypothalamus. Lower neck lesions may affect sweating over the face only because of involvement of sympathetic efferents in the arterial plexus (carotid/vertebral). Lesions above the superior cervical ganglion may not affect sweating at all, or it may be restricted to the forehead.

Blind Spots and Ophthalmoscopy
What are Blind Spots?
The area of the retina occupied by the nerves and blood vessels is not populated with visual receptor cells. Normally the cells of the retinal project to the thalamus and then to the occipital cortex where their projections form ocular dominance columns, or hypercolumns. Hypercolumns represent all the possible visual characteristics of a specific point in the visual field including binocular interaction (independent ocular dominance columns), angle of perceived stimulus (orientation columns), blobs, and interblobs (colour perception units). There are a series of horizontal projecting neurons located in the visual striate cortex that allow for neighbouring hypercolumns to activate one another. The horizontal connections between these hypercolumns allow for perceptual completion to occur.

The area of the visual striate cortex (occipital lobe) representing the blind spot and the monocular crescent (both in the temporal field) does not contain the alternating independent ocular dominance columns. This means that these areas only receive information from one eye. If one closes that eye, the area representing the blind spot of the eye remaining open (on the contralateral side) will not be activated because of the lack of receptor activation at the retina.

The blind spot is therefore not strictly monocular, but it is dependent on the FOF of horizontal connections from neighbouring neurons. These may be activated via receptors and pathways from either eye. Perceptual completion refers to the process whereby the brain fills-in the region of the visual field that corresponds to a lack of visual receptors; therefore, we generally are not aware of the blind spot.

The size of the blind spot has been linked to the CIS of the cortex (Carrick 1997).

The Parts of Two Commonly Used Ophthalmoscopes QUICK FACTS 6

Figure 4.1 The parts of two commonly used ophthalmoscopes.

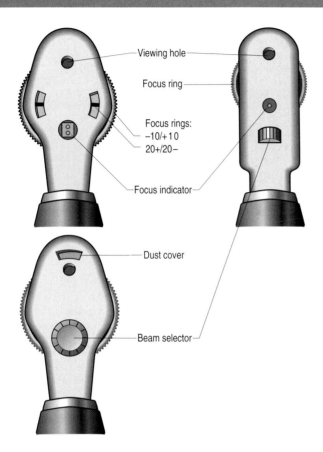

1. Measure the size of the patient's blind spots using perimetry techniques (Figs. 4.3 and 4.4).

   a) Use a white-backed business card with a red circle drawn in one corner.

   b) Stick a piece of A4 white paper on the wall or desk in landscape orientation and place a black dot in the centre that the patient can focus on.

What Does it Mean? QUICK FACTS 7

Exotropia—permanent outward deviation of one eye

Exophoria—outward deviation of one eye that corrects when the eye focuses on an object

Anisocoria—pupils of unequal size

Corectasia—dilation of the pupil

Cormyosis—constriction of the pupil

Intorsion—rotation of the eyeball towards the nose

Extorsion—rotation of the eyeball away from the nose

QUICK FACTS 8   **Anisocoria with Right Corectasia**

Figure 4.2 Anisocoria with right corectasia.

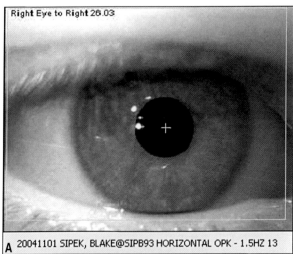

A 20041101 SIPEK, BLAKE@SIPB93 HORIZONTAL OPK - 1.5HZ 13

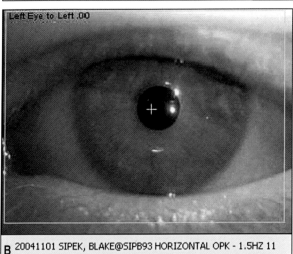

B 20041101 SIPEK, BLAKE@SIPB93 HORIZONTAL OPK - 1.5HZ 11

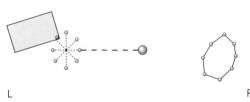

L   R

Fig. 4.3 The procedure for manual determination of blind spots.

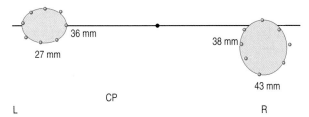

Fig. 4.4 A blind spot map generated by a blind spot mapping computer program. The deviation of one blind spot either above or below the centre line by a significant amount can indicate a dysfunction in the optic radiations as they pass through the parietal or temporal pathways. A similar effect can be seen when the patient has tilted their head or has ocular skew when measuring the blind spots. In these cases the deviation of the blind spots will be equidistant from the centre line. This figure demonstrates the appearance of the blind spots with a right parietal radiation dysfunction.

c) Cover one of the patient's eyes and place the patient 28cm from the paper, ensuring that there is no head tilt present. The head should not move for the duration of the testing.

d) Move the red circle outwards from the centre and instruct the patient to inform you when the red circle disappears. Then move the circle back towards the centre until the patient informs you that the circle has returned.

e) Move the dot outwards again and repeat for eight separate points in the horizontal (2), vertical (2), and diagonal (4) planes.

f) Repeat for the other eye ensuring that the patient has not altered the position of their head.

g) Connect the dots and measure the perimetry or horizontal and vertical dimensions.

Blind spots can also be mapped using the Microsoft Paint program or using the computerized physiological blind spot mapper (Fig. 4.5).

2. Observe the anterior to posterior and nasal to temporal structures of the eye.

a) Observe the condition of the retinal vessels and determine the vein-to-artery (V:A) ratio utilizing ophthalmoscopy (Fig. 4.7). *Ophthalmoscopy* is useful for assessing the vascularity of the optic disc and retina. This should accompany measurement of the blind spot size as changes in the morphology of the optic disc and peripapillary region of the retina could explain the shape or size of the blind spot. Changes that occur before and after an adjustment or other activity are functional in nature.

The V:A ratio refers to the difference in diameter of the veins and arteries that branch from the central retinal artery. A large difference may be due to increased sympathetic output, which causes greater peripheral resistance and constriction of arteries. The condition of blood vessels can also be helpful as an indicator of cerebrovascular integrity. Look through the ophthalmoscope and locate the vessels of the fundus. Identify a vein, which is normally larger than an artery, and an artery and then compare the sizes. The ratio of vein diameter to artery diameter can then be recorded. This is a useful procedure to perform following any intervention that may affect the sympathetic/parasympathetic activity ratio in the neuraxis.

Physiologic blind spot evaluation

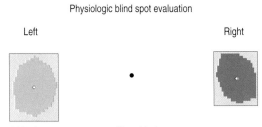

Fig. 4.5 A relatively normal blind spot map generated by a blind spot map computer program. Note the volume calculations listed at the top of the figure for each blind spot. This blind spot map shows centre points that are roughly equidistant from the centre line and are thus not the result of ocular skew or head tilt.

Figure 4.6 A lateral (top) and a superior (bottom) view of the correct angle of approach to start the ophthalmoscopic examination. If the patient is looking straight ahead, it also demonstrates the area of the retina that this approach should expose in the eye field of the ophthalmoscope as a point of reference for the examination. Note your viewing eye and the eye being examined in the patient should be the same, and both of your eyes should remain open during the examination.

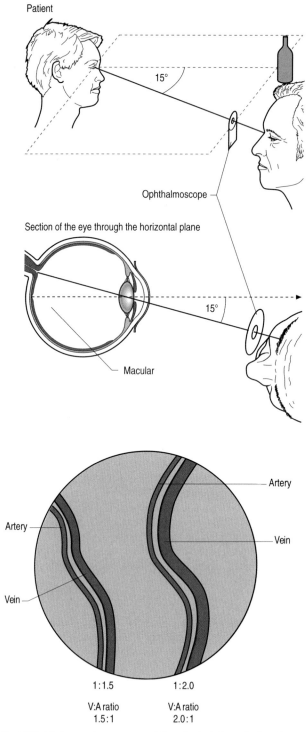

Patient

15°

Ophthalmoscope

Section of the eye through the horizontal plane

15°

Macular

Artery

Artery

Vein

Vein

1:1.5   1:2.0

V:A ratio   V:A ratio
1.5:1   2.0:1

Fig. 4.7 Ophthalmoscopic appearance of the retinal arteries and veins when attempting to determine the vein-to-artery (V:A) ratio. The V:A ratio on the left is normal and on the right is increased, indicating an overactive sympathetic input to the retinal artery.

b) Observe *the fundus* and look for normal appearance or any normal variants that may be present (Fig. 4.8). Observe the fundus for any pathology that may be present including vein/artery nipping, clouding or discolouration, optic nerve head swelling, subhyaloid haemorrhages, papilloedema, scarring, or melanomas (Fuller 2004) (Figs 4.9 and 4.10).

c) *Nystagmus*, which is a slow drift of the pupil in one direction followed by a fast correction in the opposite direction, can also be detected very easily utilizing the magnification of the scope. When recording the nystagmus, it is convention to describe the direction of the fast phase as the direction of the nystagmus. For example if the pupil is seen to move slowly to the left than correct with a fast phase to the right this would be described as a right nystagmus. Nystagmus can be *physiological* as seen when the head is rotated or in people looking out the window of a car, *peripheral*, due to abnormalities of the vestibular system, *central*, due to cerebellar dysfunction, or *retinal*, due to the inability to fixate the retina on a target. *Opticokinetic reflexes* (OR) can be used to test visual tracking and nystagmus. *Optokinetic testing* can be extremely useful for determining the

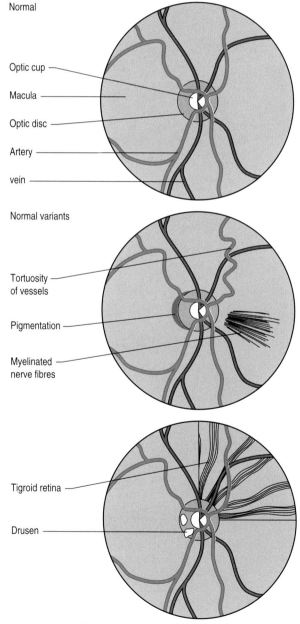

Normal

Optic cup

Macula

Optic disc

Artery

vein

Normal variants

Tortuosity of vessels

Pigmentation

Myelinated nerve fibres

Tigroid retina

Drusen

Fig. 4.8 A normal fundus (top) and normal variants (middle and bottom) that may be observed during examination.

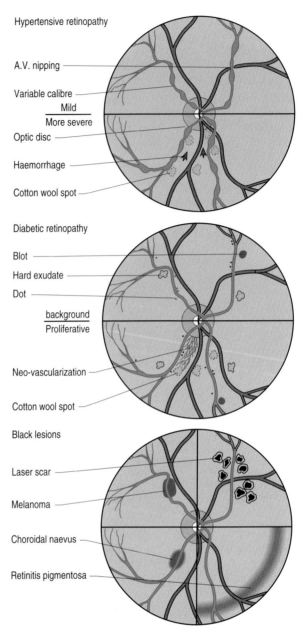

Hypertensive retinopathy

A.V. nipping

Variable calibre

Mild

More severe

Optic disc

Haemorrhage

Cotton wool spot

Diabetic retinopathy

Blot

Hard exudate

Dot

background

Proliferative

Neo-vascularization

Cotton wool spot

Black lesions

Laser scar

Melanoma

Choroidal naevus

Retinitis pigmentosa

Fig. 4.9 The retina in a variety of retinopathies as it may be observed during examination of the fundus. These conditions, unlike the normal variants in Fig. 4.7, warrant significant medical follow-up.

presence of vestibulocerebellar dysfunction and cortical hemisphericity. There is a high expectation of abnormal reflexes in patients who suffer from learning or behavioural disorders, balance problems, dizziness, vertigo, migraine, spondylosis, whiplash syndrome, anxiety, or symptoms known to be associated with cortical dysfunction (e.g. stroke).

OR can be tested by passing a opticokinetic tape in front of the patient's eyes, first in one direction and then in the other, and observing the motion of the eyes as the tape is passed. The motion of the eyes should be observed keeping in mind the latency and velocity of the response, the amplitude of the response, smoothness of movement of the response, the fatigability of the response, and the direction of the response, all of which should be recorded (Fig. 4.11). The opticokinetic tape can be made using a piece of white cloth about 5 cm wide and 1m long, onto which red pieces of cloth about 5 × 5 cm^2 have been stitched at regular 5-cm intervals.

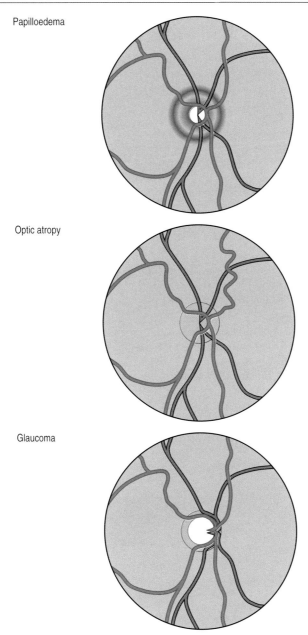

Papilloedema

Optic atropy

Glaucoma

Fig. 4.10 Pathologies that may be observed during examination of the fundus. These conditions, similar to those in Fig. 4.9, warrant significant medical follow-up.

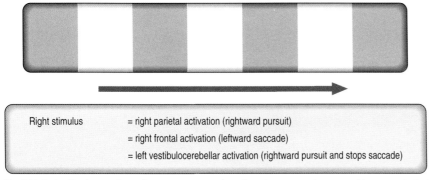

Right stimulus	= right parietal activation (rightward pursuit)
	= right frontal activation (leftward saccade)
	= left vestibulocerebellar activation (rightward pursuit and stops saccade)

Fig. 4.11 Opticokinetic tape. Saccadic eye movements, also referred to as saccades, are rapid movements that move the eye from one object to the next. The saccadic reflexes can be tested by holding an opticokinetic tape about 14 in. from the eyes and moving the tape slowly and steadily first in one direction and then the other direction. Observation of the amplitude, frequency, direction, and smoothness of the saccades generated can give a clue as to the area of the neuraxis that is dysfunctional. The areas of the neuraxis largely responsible for the various phases of the slow pursuit and saccades of the eyes are highlighted in pink.

Perception of self-motion or vertigo can occur because vision-related neurons project to the medial vestibular nucleus via the nucleus of the optic tract in the pretectum.

A cortical *smooth pursuit* system is involved when one tries to maintain fixation of gaze on a moving object. This can be tested by slowly moving a finger from left to right in front of the patient and asking the patient to watch your finger only moving their eyes, and not their head.

Saccadic eye movements, which are also referred to as saccades, are rapid movements that move the eye from one object to the next. These can be tested by holding up fingers about 1m apart in front of the patient and asking the patient to look from one finger to the other.

Motor Examination of the Head

1. Observe the orientation of the pupils and the corneal reflections. This test utilizes the reflection of light off the cornea of the eyes when the patient is looking off into the distance. The reflections should be equal in size and position if the eyes are equally deviated.

2. Test the six positions of gaze and look for conjugate movements and nystagmus (Fig. 4.12). Relate the movement of the eyes to the anatomy of the eye muscles and note that the muscles of the eye will have different actions when the eye is in different positions (Fig. 4.13).

3. Observe the quality of smooth pursuit in the planes of the semicircular canals. These eye movements require activation of the cerebellum without the activation of the vestibular system and can be used to differentiate between a cerebellar and vestibular dysfunction (Fig. 4.14).

4. Palpate the jaw muscles, observe for jaw deviation, and check the jaw jerk reflex. This reflex tests the motor and sensory divisions of the mandibular division of the trigeminal nerve.

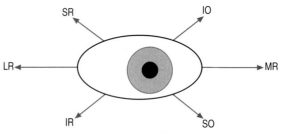

Fig. 4.12 Movement directions produced by contractions of the extraocular muscles. The directions outlined represent the primary direction of movement of each muscle when the eyeball is facing forward in a neutral gaze and with no synergic activity of other extraocular muscles involved. SR = superior rectus, IR = inferior rectus, IO = inferior oblique, SO = superior oblique, LR = lateral rectus, MR = medial rectus.

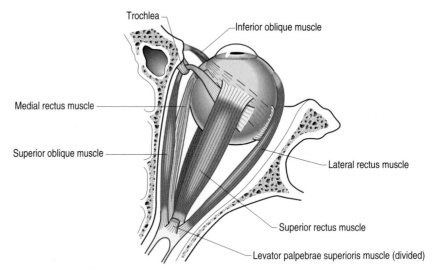

Fig. 4.13 Superior view of the extraocular muscles of the eye. Note the origin and insertion of the muscles with respect to the midline of the eyeball.

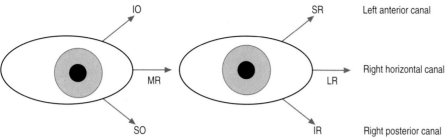

Fig. 4.14 Eye movements and their related vestibular canals stimulated when these eye movements are accompanied by a rotation of the head in order to focus on a moving object or keep an object in focus while the head is moving.

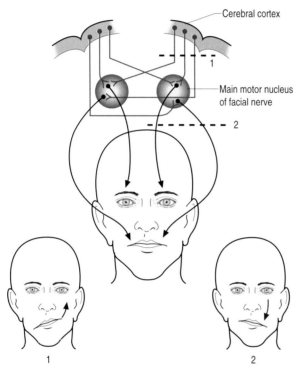

Fig. 4.15 Innervation of the facial muscles by the facial nerve (CN VII). The corticobulbar projections (1) arise from the cortical facial areas and project to the facial nerve nuclei. These projections are bilateral from the cortex to the areas of the facial nucleus supplying the upper eyelid and forehead and ipsilateral to the nuclei supplying the lower face. The projections of the cranial nerve nuclear neurons form the facial nerve (CN VII) proper and project ipsilateral to the upper and lower face (2). Thus, a facial nerve (CN VII) lesion, also referred to as a lower motor neuron lesion, will result in paralysis of the ipsilateral facial muscles of both the upper and lower face. A lesion to the cortical areas or the corticobulbar projection pathways, also referred to as an upper motor neuron lesion, will result in a contralateral facial paralysis of the upper face (forehead and upper eyelid region) only.

5. Observe for asymmetries in facial muscle contraction, both voluntary and involuntary actions and both upper and lower face need to be tested. The CN VII nucleus is innervated bilaterally by upper motor cortico bulbar neurons. The CN VII nerve itself is ipsilateral in projection to the face. This results in a situation where damage to the CN VII nerve (lower motor neuron) results in ipsilateral paralysis involving the whole side of the face. When supranuclear damage (upper motor neuron) is present, the paralysis is limited to the contralateral forehead area (Fig. 4.15).

6. Observe for asymmetry in palate elevation (Fig. 4.16).

7. Observe for fasciculations, atrophy, and deviation of the tongue.

8. Observe and feel the tone of the SCM and trapezius muscles during head turning.

9. Observe the quality of the ocular tilt reaction. The OTR is a reflex movement of the eyeball when the head is tilted from one side to the other. When the head tilts to

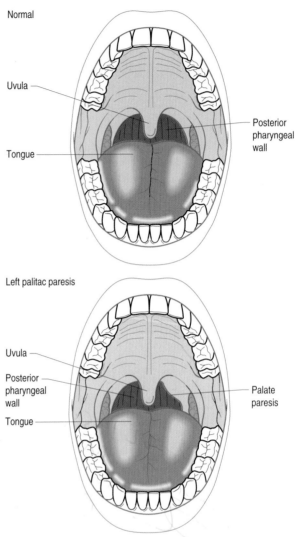

Normal

Uvula

Posterior
pharyngeal
wall

Tongue

Left palitac paresis

Uvula

Posterior
pharyngeal
wall

Palate
paresis

Tongue

Fig. 4.16 View of the mouth and palate during examination. (Top) Normal palatal elevation and (bottom); left palatal paresis. The latter may be due to a number of reasons including muscular weakness, glossopharyngeal nuclear dysfunction, and decreased neural stimulus from the ipsilateral corticobulbar neurons. Note the uvula rarely deviates in this condition as opposed to the complete paralysis of the glossopharyngeal nerve where it deviates away from the side of the lesion.

the right the right eye should intort (roll towards the nose) and the left eye should extort (roll away from the nose). This is a vestibular ocular reflex.

10. Observe the patient's optokinetic reflexes (see above).

11. Observe the patient's saccades and anti-saccades (see above).

Sensory Examination of the Head

1. Check sensation to pinprick (or pinwheel) in trigeminal and cervical zones (Fig. 4.17).

2. Check sensation to light touch if indicated.

3. Check for quality and asymmetry of the *corneal reflex*. Many students and practitioners get false results from this reflex because of faulty technique. Several common mistakes include touching the conjunctiva instead of the cornea, approaching the eye too quickly which is perceived as menacing and results in a blink reflex, testing over a contact lens, all of which result in inaccurate findings. The area of the eye touched to trigger this reflex correctly is shown in Fig. 4.18. The reflex is performed by asking the patient to look up and away and slowly bring a piece of cotton wool twisted to a point in contact with the cornea. Watch for the reaction of both eyes, and the ocular muscles surrounding the eye. The normal response is a bilateral blink and contracture of the muscles of the eyebrows bilaterally. If there is

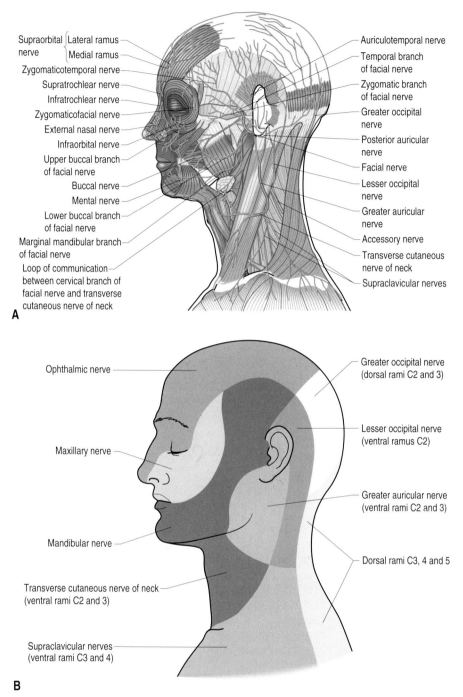

Supraorbital { Lateral ramus
nerve { Medial ramus
Zygomaticotemporal nerve
Supratrochlear nerve
Infratrochlear nerve
Zygomaticofacial nerve
External nasal nerve
Infraorbital nerve
Upper buccal branch of facial nerve
Buccal nerve
Mental nerve
Lower buccal branch of facial nerve
Marginal mandibular branch of facial nerve
Loop of communication between cervical branch of facial nerve and transverse cutaneous nerve of neck

Auriculotemporal nerve
Temporal branch of facial nerve
Zygomatic branch of facial nerve
Greater occipital nerve
Posterior auricular nerve
Facial nerve
Lesser occipital nerve
Greater auricular nerve
Accessory nerve
Transverse cutaneous nerve of neck
Supraclavicular nerves

A

Ophthalmic nerve
Maxillary nerve
Mandibular nerve
Transverse cutaneous nerve of neck (ventral rami C2 and 3)
Supraclavicular nerves (ventral rami C3 and 4)

Greater occipital nerve (dorsal rami C2 and 3)
Lesser occipital nerve (ventral ramus C2)
Greater auricular nerve (ventral rami C2 and 3)
Dorsal rami C3, 4 and 5

B

Fig. 4.17 (A) Actual nerve pathways of the face and head. (B) Dermatomal distribution of the receptive fields of the nerves of the head and face. Note that the trigeminal nerve's occipital division has a dermatomal distribution that projects from the tip of the nose to well past the ears on the top of the head and the mandibular division projects anterior to the ear to cover the temporal area.

failure of either side to blink you can suspect an ipsilateral trigeminal nerve (CN V) V1 lesion on the side you are testing. If only one side fails to respond you could expect a facial (CN VII) lesion on the side that fails to contract.

4. Perform gag reflex if indicated.

Taste, Smell, Hearing, and Otoscopic Inspection

1. Check taste sensation on each side of the tongue.
2. Test for smell sensation in each nostril.
3. Check hearing with Weber's, Rinne's, and other tests if necessary.

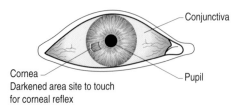

Fig. 4.18 The corneal reflex.

4. Perform otoscopic inspection. This is useful for observing the integrity of the tympanic membrane and investigating the presence of middle and outer ear abnormalities including wax accumulation. History of ear infection may provide an insight into the aetiology of vestibular and auditory symptoms.

Cranial Nerve Screening

The majority of signs and symptoms associated with brainstem dysfunction can be revealed by performing a thorough history and examination of the cranial nerves and their effects on sensory, motor, autonomic, and mental functions. The list below includes motor, sensory, and autonomic signs observed at both cranial and spinal levels that may be mediated by the various cranial nerves and neighbouring reticular formation.

QUICK FACTS 10 **Commonly Presenting Movement Disorders**

- Essential tremor
- Parkinson's disease
- Dystonia
- Spasmodic torticollis
- Writer's cramp
- Primary dystonia of essential tremor
- Restless leg syndrome
- Spasmodic dysphonia
- Meige's syndrome

CN I	Olfactory

1. Smell in independent nostrils

CN II	Optic

1. Pupil size
2. Pupil light reflexes
3. Light sensitivity—vestibular-induced increase contralaterally
4. Blind spot size and orientation
5. Acuity
6. Visual fields

A upper temporal field deficit may be found in the contralateral eye to an optic nerve lesion because of looping of the contralateral lower nasal retinal fibres back along the optic nerve. Incongruous field defects can occur because of involvement of the optic tracts between the optic chiasm and the lateral geniculate nucleus (LGN) (thalamus) and midbrain. This is due to the 90° inward rotation of the tracts so that both sets of lower field fibres lie medially, and both sets of upper field fibres from each eye lie laterally.

CN III: Oculomotor

1. Corneal reflection abnormalities
2. Weakness on gaze
3. Nystagmus—vestibular-induced slow phase contralaterally
4. Opticokinetic reflexes (OPK)—slower contralateral to deficit
5. Saccades/pursuits—dysmetric contralaterally
6. OTR
7. Blepharospasm—vestibular-induced enhancement of blink reflex

CN IV Trochlear

1. Corneal reflection abnormalities
2. Weakness on gaze
3. Nystagmus
4. OKN
5. Saccades/pursuits
6. OTR

CN V Trigeminal

1. Masticator tone—vestibular-induced increase (esp. contralaterally)
   Sensation—vestibular-induced disinhibition of pain
2. Ear pain
3. Corneal reflex (afferent limb)—vestibular/anxiety-induced enhancement

CN VI Abducens

1. Corneal reflection abnormalities
2. Weakness on gaze
3. Nystagmus
4. OKN
5. Saccades/pursuits

CN VII Facial

1. Facial tics—peripheral or basal ganglionic mechanisms
2. Ear pain
3. Salivation—vestibular-induced increase due to PMRF integration (superior salivatory nucleus)

CN VIII Vestibular and Cochlear

1. OTR
   a. Skew deviation
   b. Ocular torsion
   c. Head tilt
   d. Subjective visual vertical (SVV)—cortical consequences
2. Corneal reflection abnormalities
3. Weakness on gaze—contralateral to deficit
4. Nystagmus—vestibular-induced slow phase contralaterally
5. OKN
   a. Slower pursuit contralateral to deficit
   b. Dysmetric pursuit contralateral to hyper- or hypofunction
6. Saccades/pursuits—as above
7. Vestibulo-ocular reflexes (VORs)—decreased gain with rotation to side of deficit
8. Vestibulo-autonomic reflexes as above and below (heart, lungs, gut, head)
9. Neck muscle tension and pain—vestibular-induced increase
10. Extensor muscle tone—vestibular-induced increase
11. Somatic sensation—vestibular-induced pain, 'numbness', tingling, etc.
12. Motor and sensory trigeminal signs as above (5)
13. Light sensitivity—vestibular-induced increase contralaterally
14. Postural head tilt—most commonly to side of deficit
15. Deviation on Romberg's test or walking—most commonly to side of deficit

16. Increased postural sway in sagittal or coronal planes
17. Rotation or side-stepping on Fukuda's test (marching on the spot with eyes closed for 30 s)—most commonly to side of deficit
18. Accompanying hearing deficits and tinnitus—peripheral mechanisms
19. Hearing deficits and/or tinnitus—altered autonomic and/or dorsal cochlear nucleus integration
20. Aural fullness—sensation of fullness or pain in the ear or surrounding head
21. Frequent headaches (occipital to frontal)—aggravated by fatigue, visual work, light, oversleeping

CN IX   Glossopharyngeal

1. Baroreceptor reflexes—interaction with vestibulosympathetic reflexes
2. Ear pain
3. Salivation—vestibular-induced increase due to PMRF integration (inferior salivatory nucleus)

CN X   Vagus

1. Difficulty or tightness swallowing—vestibular-induced anxiety syndrome
2. Increased or decreased bowel movements/sounds (auscultation)—vestibular-induced activation of DMN X
3. Bradycardia—depending on interaction with vestibulosympathetic reflexes (vestibular-induced activation of nucleus ambiguus)
4. Nausea—activation of NTS, DMN X, and emetic centres
5. Ear pain

CN XI   Spinal Accessory

1. Postural deviations of head—most commonly tilted to side of deficit (there are other important factors such as increased posterior muscle tone)

CN XII   Hypoglossal

1. Tongue muscle tone—vestibular-induced increase

QUICK FACTS 11 | **Frequently Observed in Patients with Chronic Vestibulocerebellar Disorders**

General Dystonias
- Writer's cramp
- Causalgic-dystonia (reflex sympathetic dystrophy (RSD), repetitive strain, chronic pain, etc)

Facial Tics
- Peripheral nerve lesion (see slides on blepharospasm)
- Vestibular disorders
- Mood disorders—anxiety, panic, and obsessive-compulsive disorder (OCD)
- Dystonic

Restless Leg Syndrome
- Akathisia

Essential Tremor
- Vestibular and cerebellar dysfunction (inner ear disease)

Parkinsonism
- Mood disorders
- Medications

Motor Examination of the Trunk and Limbs

1. Check upper and lower limb muscles for segmental or suprasegmental weakness (see muscle testing diagrams in Appendix 1 at the end of this chapter).

2. Check upper and lower limb reflexes (see reflex diagrams in Appendix 1 at the end of this chapter). Reflexes should be tested by applying repeated equal strikes of the reflex hammer to the tendon until fatigue occurs or until six or seven strikes have been performed. If the muscle maintains equal responses throughout the six or seven repeated stimuli then the area supplying that reflex can be thought of as expressing a healthy CIS.

3. Check the resistance in muscles to joint motion (muscle tone).

4. Assess for percussion irritability and myotonia.

5. Check flexor reflex afferent reflexes, which include the superficial abdominal and plantar reflexes. The superficial abdominal reflex is performed by scratching the abdominal wall as shown in Fig. 4.19 and observing the reaction of the abdominal muscles, which should contract on the same side. The afferent supply for this reflex is thought to be the segmental sensory nerves and the efferent supply the segmental motor nerves. The roots tested when striking above the umbilicus are T8–T9 and below the umbilicus T10 and T11. No reaction of the abdominal muscles is a positive response and is thought to indicate an upper motor neuron lesion at the level being tested, but may also present if the lower motor neuron is involved. However, this test is not accurate in a large number of individuals because of the presence of large amounts of abdominal fat or scar tissue formation, or in women who have experienced multiple pregnancies.

6. The plantar reflex or response (Fig. 4.20) is performed by stroking the plantar aspect of the foot making sure to curve under the area where the toes join the foot. A normal response involves the toes curling downwards and a mild jerk of the foot

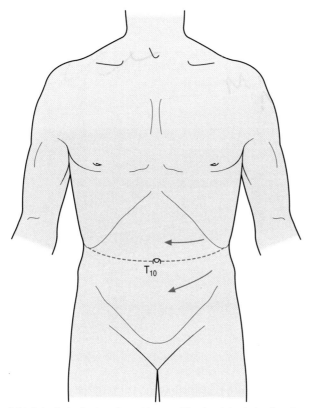

Fig. 4.19 The superficial abdominal reflex is performed by scratching the abdominal wall as shown and observing the reaction of the abdominal muscles, which should contract on the same side.

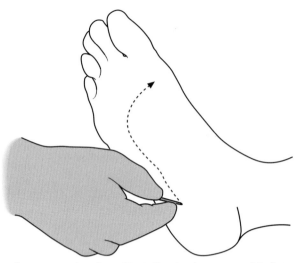

Fig. 4.20 The plantar reflex or response is performed by stroking the plantar aspect of the foot with a blunted sharp edge such as the pointed end of the reflex hammer.

away from the stimulus. A positive response, also known as a Babinski response, involves the upward movement of the toes, and in some cases only the big toe moves upwards, which is referred to as an up-going toe. A positive response indicates a lesion to the corticospinal tract on the ipsilateral side below the decussation of the fibres in the medulla, or a contralateral lesion of the corticospinal tracts above the decussation. Commonly this type of neuron injury is referred to as an upper motor neuron lesion.

Sensory Examination of the Trunk and Limbs

1. Check spinothalamic sensation, which includes pain and temperature in upper and lower limbs. A common mistake made when performing this test is to be too gentle and not actually cause pain. The patient may respond that they felt the stimulus but the stimulus they felt was not pain but pressure. If you are testing pain then it must cause pain to test it.

2. Check dorsal column sensation, which includes two-point discrimination and vibration sense, in upper and lower limbs. A good way to check vibration sense is to use a low C tuning fork, set it ringing, and apply the single pronged end to a distal point on the fingers or toes.

QUICK FACTS 12

The Following Points Are Central to the Initial Assessment of a Movement Disorder

1. Determine the characteristics of the movement.
2. Determine the likelihood of heredity.
3. Enquire about inciting events and exposures to drugs/toxins, etc.
4. Determine the time course of the disorder.
5. Investigate for coexisting medical or neurological disease.

---

3. Determine presence of:
   a. Astereognosis, which is the inability to identify a common object when placed in the hand with eyes closed;
   b. Atopognosia, which is the inability to correctly localize a sensation; and
   c. Graphanaesthesia which is the failure to recognize a number drawn on the patient's palm which is not in view of the patient.

Cerebellar (and Further Vestibular) Examination

1. Observe for the presence of a resting, postural, or kinetic tremor.

   a. Check all limbs for past pointing/overshooting, by asking the patient to extend their arms out to each side with their first finger extended and touch the fingers in alternating fashion to their nose. Do this first with eyes open and then with eyes closed. To test the lower limbs have them run the heel of one foot down the shin of the opposite leg to the toes.

Testing for Cerebellar Dysfunction *CELLS OF* **QUICK FACTS 13**

- Walk in tandem, on heels, on toes, and backwards
- Accentuate dysmetria by increasing inertial load of limb (overshooting and undershooting)
- Finger opposition, pronation, and supination of the elbow, heel/toe floor tapping (disdiadochokinesia)
- Finger to nose, toe to finger, heel to shin, figure of 8 (kinetic tremor and dysmetria)
- Rotated postures of the head

Not to be Missed Tests in All Cases of Suspected Vestibular and Auditory Dysfunction *CELLS OF* **QUICK FACTS 14**

1. Cranial nerve screen
2. Corneal reflexes
3. Trigeminal sensation (especially 1st division)
4. Plantar reflexes
5. Basic motor and sensory examination
6. Cerebellar screening

---

   b. Dysmetria—check all movements for smoothness and accuracy of performance.

   c. Disdiadochokinesia is present if the patient cannot perform rapid alternating movements in a consistent, symmetrical, and coordinated fashion. A good test is to ask the patient to rapidly turn both of their hands from palm up to palm down as rapidly as they can and compare the actions of each hand.

2. Instruct the patient to walk on their toes and heels and perform tandem gait.

3. Perform:

   a. *Romberg's test*, which is testing the posterior columns and cerebellum. Ask the patient to stand with their feet close together or touching. Then ask them to raise their arms to shoulder height and keep them extended in space at the same height. Observe the degree to which they sway. If the sway is not to such an extent that they may fall, ask them to close their eyes and again observe the sway. Watch very closely for the direction of movement or any preferences in direction that they like to move into. Have them maintain this posture for approximately 30 s. Then ask them to open their eyes and tell you what they felt. Patients will usually fall to the side of decreased cortical muscle tone or the side of increased cerebellar activation.

b. *Fukuda's marching in place test,* which is performed by asking the patient to march on the spot, lifting their right arm and leg in unison and likewise for the left arm and leg. Have them complete the cycle a few times and then ask them to close their eyes. Keep them marching for about 30 s and note any deviation from the spot that they started on.

Orthopaedic Examination

Check both passive and active range of motion of all joints including the extremities. Check muscle strength (see muscle testing diagrams at the end of this chapter). Observe the patient's gait and posture.

Physical (Visceral) Examination

1. Chest—not covered in this text.

    a. Heart: Tachycardia or arrhythmia—due to IML escape (especially on the right and left respectively as the right IML has greater control of the sinoatrial node, while the left IML has greater control of the atrioventricular node). This may occur because of decreased integrity of the PMRF or increased expression of vestibulosympathetic reflexes. Arrhythmias and changes in heart sounds can occur due to altered CIS of the PMRF.

    b. Lungs—not covered in this text

2. Abdominal exam—not covered in this text

Examination of Mental State

The patient should be tested for orientation to person: Do they know who they are?; place—Do they know where they are?; and time—Do they know what day, month, and year it is? One should also test for both short- and medium-term memory by asking the patient to remember a six-digit number and repeat it back immediately and then again after a few minutes have past and they have been distracted by other testing.

We have now covered some background information about neuron theory, functional neuroanatomy, and the objectives of performing a functional neurological examination. The focus in the following will now be on determining the presence of dysfunction and asymmetry as part of the wider functional neurological examination.

1. Vestibulocerebellar system

2. Autonomic system

3. Cerebral neuronal activity—hemisphericity

Vestibulocerebellar Dysfunction and Asymmetry

The SEE Principle (Spine, Ears, and Eyes)

There is substantial integration of spine, ear, and eye afferents at numerous levels of the neuraxis. The four major areas involved in this multimodal integration include the following.

1. Vestibulocerebellar system;

2. Mesencephalon;

3. Pulvinar and posterior thalamic nuclei; and

4. Parietotemporal association cortex.

Integration in all regions may affect the CIS of the IML column and autonomic nuclei in the brainstem. However, convergence of spine, ear, and eye afferents in the vestibulocerebellar system and mesencephalon will have a more direct affect and the

Frontal Lobe Testing CELLS OF   **QUICK FACTS 15**

- Clinical tests
- Digit span (forwards and backwards)
- Motor strength and tone
- Limb control
- Blink rates
- Glabellar tap test (e.g. depression, mania, Parkinson's, dementia)
- Other release phenomena
- Spontaneous lateral eye movements
- Saccade accuracy
- Anti-saccades
- Remembered saccades
- Forehead skin temperature
- Tympanic temperature

relationship between dysfunction in these areas and autonomic asymmetry can be readily observed.

Signs and symptoms of vestibulocerebellar dysfunction may be associated with increased or decreased vestibular output, referred to below as 'vestibular-induced' and 'deficit-induced', respectively. Despite these delineations, a vestibular-induced symptom may in fact be due to vestibular hypofunction on the contralateral side and vice versa. Dysmetric eye movements and some signs associated with autonomic function are not classed as being due to hypo- or hyperfunction as individual bedside tests may not be adequate to confirm this relationship. All clinical signs and symptoms help to establish the diagnosis or clinical impression.

The following aspects need to be considered when determining the presence of vestibulocerebellar dysfunction.

- Vestibulosympathetic reflexes;
- Vestibular/fastigial connections to the PMRF;
- Motor consequences;
- Sensory consequences; and
- Mental consequences.

Extraocular Movements

1. Dorsal vermis

   Saccadic dysmetria (hypermetric) and macrosaccadic oscillations

   Pursuit

   Saccadic lateropulsion

2. Flocculus and paraflocculus

   Gaze-evoked nystagmus

   Rebound nystagmus

   Downbeat nystagmus

   Smooth tracking

   Glissadic, postsaccadic drift

   Disturbance in adjusting the gain of the VOR

3. Nodulus

   Increase in duration of vestibular response

   Periodic alternating nystagmus

Autonomic Dysfunction and Asymmetry

What components of the neurological, physical, or orthopaedic examinations allows one to gain some information about autonomic function?

1. Width of palpebral fissure (ptosis)—This is dependent on both sympathetic and oculomotor innervation. Therefore, one needs to differentiate between a Horner's syndrome, oculomotor nerve lesion, or physiological changes in the CIS of the mesencephalic reticular formation.

2. Skin condition—Increased peripheral resistance may result in decreased integrity of skin, particularly at the extremities.

3. Ophthalmoscopy—V:A ratio and vessel integrity

4. Heart auscultation—Arrhythmias and changes in heart sounds can occur because of altered CIS of the PMRF.

5. Bowel auscultation—This can be particularly useful during some treatment procedures to monitor the effect of stimulation on vagal function (e.g., caloric irrigation—further instruction required, adjustments and visual stimulation or exercises, etc).

6. Skin and tympanic temperature and blood flow—This is particularly useful as a pre- and post-adjustment check. Profound changes in skin temperature asymmetry can occur following an adjustment. These changes are side dependent. An adjustment on the side of decreased forehead skin temperature will commonly result in greater symmetry or reversed asymmetry. Conflicting results are likely to be dependent on a number of factors, which are currently being investigated further. Remember that forehead skin temperature depends on fuel requirements of the brain, and vestibular and cortical influences on autonomic function among other things.

7. Dermatographia—The red response is often observed in patients who suffer from sympathetically mediated pain.

8. Lung expansion, respiratory rate and ratio, etc.—An inspiration:expiration ratio of 1:2 is considered to represent approximately normal sympathovagal balance. This means that expiration should take twice as long as inspiration. This is difficult to achieve for some patients at first and requires some training.

    Shallow and rapid breathing can result in respiratory alkalosis, which leads to hypersensitivity in the nervous system. CO_2 is blown off at a higher rate, resulting in decreased $[H^+]$ ions in the blood. Lower $[Ca^{++}]$ follows, causing $[Na^+]$ to rise in extracellular fluid. This can be seen clinically by the presence of percussion myotonia, which is also often seen in various metabolic and hormonal disorders.

9. Forehead skin temperature—Measurement of skin temperature above the browline may provide useful information concerning sympathetic control of blood vessels to the eye, as sympathetic supply to the vessels of the forehead are branches of the sympathetic supply to the retinal vessels.

    Activation of cervical afferents has been found to have an antagonistic effect on the excitatory vestibulosympathetic reflexes. It is therefore proposed that a cervical spine adjustment may enhance cervical inhibition of the vestibulosympathetic reflex, resulting in increased blood flow to the eye and brain (Sexton 2006).

Appendix 1

Motor Examination of the Trunk and Limbs

Table 4.2 Muscle Innervation Listed by Individual Nerves

Upper Extremity		Lower Extremity	
Suprascapular nerve	**Radial nerve**	**Superior gluteal nerve**	Leg
Shoulder girdle	Arm	Buttock	Tibialis posterior
Supraspinatus	Triceps (long head,	Gluteus medius	Flexor digitorum
Infraspinatus	lateral head,	Gluteus minimus	longus
Long thoracic nerve	medial head)	Tensor fasciae	Flexor hallucis
Shoulder girdle	Anconeus	latae	longus
Serratus anterior	Brachioradialis		Foot
	Extensor carpi radialis	**Inferior gluteal nerve**	Abductor hallucis
Axillary nerve	longus	Buttock	Abductor digiti
Shoulder girdle	Forearm	Gluteus maximus	minimi
Teres minor	Extensor carpi		Dorsal interossei
Deltoid	radialis brevis	**Femoral nerve**	
	Supinator longus	Thigh	**Sciatic nerve, peroneal**
Musculocutaneous	Extensor digitorum	Pectineus	**division**
nerve	communis	Sartorius	Thigh
Arm	Extensor digit quinti	Quadriceps	Biceps (short head)
Biceps brachii	Extensor carpi ulnaris	femoris (rectus	Leg (deep peroneal
Coracobrachialis	Abductor pollicis	femoris, vastus	nerve)
Brachialis	longus	lateralis, vastus	Tibialis anterior
	Extensor pollicis brevis	intermedius,	Extensor hallucis
Median nerve	Extensor indicis	vastus medialis)	longus
Forearm	proprius		Extensor digitorum
Pronator teres		**Obturator nerve**	longus
Flexor carpi radialis	**Ulnar nerve**	Thigh	Peroneus tertius
Palmaris longus	Forearm	Adductor longus	Foot
Flexor digitorum	Flexor carpi ulnaris	Gracilis	Extensor digitorum
sublimes	Flexor digitorum	Adductor brevis	brevis
Flexor pollicis	profundus	Obturator	Leg (superficial
longus	(medial half)	externus	peroneal nerve)
Pronator	Hand	Adductor magnus	Peroneus longus
quadratus	Flexor digiti quinti		Peroneus brevis
Hand	brevis	**Sciatic nerve, tibial**	
Abductor pollicis	Abductor digiti quinti	**division**	
brevis	Oppenens digiti	Thigh	
Opponens pollicis	quinti	Semitendinosus	
Flexor pollicis	Interossei	Biceps (long	
brevis	Lumbricales III	head)	
Lumbricales I	and IV	Semimembranosus	
and II	Adductor pollicis	Popliteal space	
	Flexor pollicis brevis	(tibial nerve)	
	(deep part)	Gastrocnemius	
		Plantaris	
		Popliteus	
		Soleus	

From Chusid 1964 with permission.

Table 4.3 Motor Function Chart

Action to be Tested	Muscles	Cord Segment	Nerves	Plexus
Shoulder Girdle and Upper Extremity				
Flexion of neck Extension of neck Rotation of neck Lateral bending of neck	Deep neck muscles (sternomastoid and trapezius also participate)	C1–4	Cervical	Cervical
Elevation of upper thorax	Scaleni	C3–5	Phrenic	
Inspiration	Diaphragm			
Adduction of arm from behind to front	Pectoralis major and minor	C5–8, T1	Thoracic anterior (from medial and lateral cords of plexus)	Brachial
Forward thrust of shoulder	Serratus anterior	C5–7	Long thoracic	
Elevation of scapula	Levator scapulae	C5 (3, 4)	Dorsal scapular	
Medial adduction and elevation of scapula	Rhomboids	C4, 5		
Abduction of arm	Supraspinatus	C4–6	Suprascapular	
Lateral rotation of arm	Infraspinatus	C4–6		
Medial rotation of arm Adduction of arm from front to back	Latissimus dorsi, teres major and subscapularis	C5–8	Subscapular (from posterior cord of plexus)	
Abduction of arm	Deltoid	C5, 6	Axillary (from posterior cord of plexus)	
Lateral rotation of arm	Teres minor	C4, 5		
Flexion of forearm Supination of forearm Adduction of arm	Biceps brachii Coracobrachialis	C5, 6 C5–7	Musculocutaneous (from lateral cord of plexus)	
Flexion of forearm				
Flexion of forearm	Brachialis	C5, 6		
Ulnar flexion of hand	Flexor carpi ulnaris	C7, 8, T1	Ulnar (from medial cord of plexus)	
Flexion of terminal phalanx of Ring finger Little finger	Flexor digitorum profundus (ulnar portion)	C7, 8, T1		
Flexion of hand				
Adduction of metacarpal of thumb	Adductor pollicis	C8, T1		
Abduction of little finger	Abductor digiti quinti	C8, T1		
Opposition of little finger	Opponens digiti quinti	C7, 8, T1		
Flexion of little finger	Flexor digiti quinti brevis	C7, 8, T1		
Flexion of proximal phalanx, extension of 2 distal phalanges, adduction and abduction of fingers	Interossei	C8, T1		

Action to be Tested	Muscles	Cord Segment	Nerves	Plexus
Pronation of forearm	Pronator teres	C6, 7	Median (C6, 7 from lateral cord of plexus; C8, T1 from medial cord of plexus)	
Radial flexion of hand	Flexor carpi radialis	C6, 7		
Flexion of hand	Palmaris longus	C7, 8, T1		
Flexion of middle phalanx of { Index finger / Middle finger / Ring finger / Little finger }	Flexor digitorum sublimes	C7, 8, T1		
Flexion of hand				
Flexion of terminal phalanx of thumb	Flexor pollicis longus	C7, 8, T1		
Flexion of terminal phalanx of { Index finger / Middle finger }	Flexor digitorum profundus (radial portion)	C7, 8, T1		
Flexion of hand				
Abduction of metacarpal of thumb	Abductor pollicis brevis	C7, 8, T1	Median (C6, 7 from lateral cord of plexus; C8, T1 from medial cord of plexus)	
Flexion of proximal phalanx of thumb	Flexor pollicis brevis	C7, 8, T1		
Opposition of metacarpal of thumb	Opponens pollicis	C8, T1		
Flexion of proximal phalanx and extension of the 2 distal phalanges of { Index finger / Middle finger / Ring finger / Little finger }	Lumbricals (the 2 lateral)	C8, T1		
	Lumbricals (the 2 medial)	C8, T1	Ulnar	
Extension of forearm	Triceps brachii and anconeus	C6–8	Radial (from posterior cord of plexus)	
Flexion of forearm	Brachioradialis	C5, 6		
Radial extension of hand	Extensor carpi radialis	C6–8		
Extension of phalanges of { Index finger / Middle finger / Ring finger / Little finger }	Extensor digitorum communis	C6–8		
Extension of hand				

(Continued)

107

Table 4.3 Motor Function Chart—Cont'd

Action to be Tested	Muscles	Cord Segment	Nerves	Plexus
Extension of phalanges of little finger	Extensor digiti quinti pro-prius	C6–8		
Extension of hand				
Ulnar extension of hand	Extensor carpi ulnaris	C8–8		
Supination of forearm	Supinator	C5–7	Radial (from posterior cord of plexus)	Brachial
Abduction of metacarpal of thumb	Abductor pollicis longus	C7, 8		
Radial extension of hand				
Extension of thumb	Extensor pollicis brevis and longus	C7, 8		
Radial extension of hand		C6–8		
Extension of index finger	Extensor indicis proprius	C6–8		
Extension of hand				
Trunk and Thorax				
Elevation of ribs	Thoracic, abdominal and back		Thoracic and posterior lumbo-sacral branches	Brachial
Depression of ribs				
Contraction of abdomen				
Anteroflexion of trunk				
Lateral flexion of trunk				
Hip Girdle and Lower Extremity				
Flexion of hip	Iliopsoas	L1–3	Femoral	Lumbar
Flexion of hip (and eversion of thigh)	Sartorius	L2, 3		
Extension of leg	Quadriceps femoris	L2–4		
Adduction of thigh	Pectiwneus	L2, 3	Obturator	
	Adductor longus	L2, 3		
	Adductor brevis	L2–4		
	Adductor magnus	L3, 4		
	Gracilis	L2–4		
Adduction of thigh	Obturator externus	L3, 4		
Lateral rotation of thigh				
Abduction of thigh	Gluteus medius and minimus	L4, 5, S1	Superior gluteal	Sacral
Medial rotation of thigh				
Flexion of thigh	Tensor Fasciae latae	L4, 5		
Lateral rotation of thigh	Piriformis	S1, S2		

Action to be Tested	Muscles	Cord Segment	Nerves	Plexus
Abduction of thigh	Gluteus maximus	L4, 5, S1, 2	Inferior gluteal	
Lateral rotation of thigh	Obturator internus	L5, S1	Muscular branches from sacral plexus	
	Gemelli	L4, 5, S1		
	Quadratus femoris	L4, 5, S1		
Flexion of leg (assist in extension of thigh)	Biceps femoris	L4, 5, S1, 2	Sciatic (trunk)	
	Semitendinosus	L4, 5, S1		
	Semimembranosus	L4, 5, S1		
Dorsal flexion of foot	Tibialis anterior	L4, 5	Deep peroneal	
Supination of foot				
Extension of toes II – V	Extensor digitorum longus	L4, 5, S1		
Dorsal flexion of foot				
Extension of great toe	Extensor hallucis longus	L4, 5, S1		
Dorsal flexion of foot				
Extension of great toe and the 3 medial toes	Extensor digitorum brevis	L4, 5, S1		
Plantar flexion of foot in pronation	Peronei	L5, S1	Superficial peroneal	
Plantar flexion of foot in supination	Tibialis posterior and triceps surae	L5, S1, 2	Tibial	
Plantar flexion of foot in supination	Flexor digitorum longus	L5, S1, 2		
Flexion of terminal phalanx of toes II–V				
Plantar flexion of foot in supination	Flexor hallucis longus	L5, S1, 2		
Flexion of terminal phalanx of great toe				
Flexion of middle phalanx of toes II–V	Flexor digitorum brevis	L5, S1		
Flexion of proximal phalanx of great toe	Flexor hallucis brevis	L5, S1, 2		
Spreading and closing of toes	Small muscles of foot	S1, 2		
Flexion of proximal phalanx of toes				
Voluntary control of pelvic floor	Perineal and sphincters	S2–4	Pudendal	

Modified from JC McKinley, reproduced with permission.

Muscle Testing of the Upper Limbs

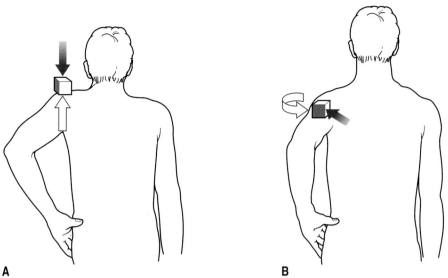

Fig. 4.21 (A) Trapezius, upper portion (C3, 4; spinal accessory nerve). The shoulder is elevated against resistance. (B) Trapezius, upper portion (C3, 4; spinal accessory nerve). The shoulder is thrust backward against resistance. From Chusid 1964 with permission.

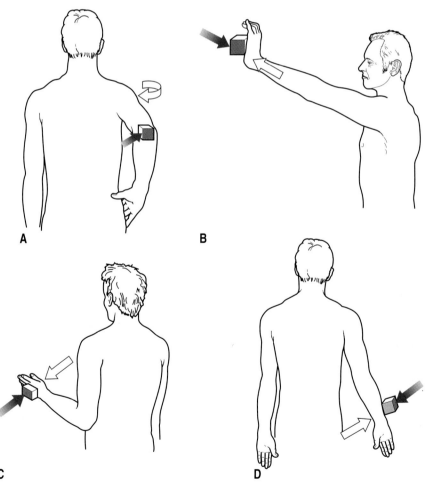

Fig. 4.22 (A) Rhomboids (C4, 5; dorsal scapulary nerve). The shoulder is thrust backward against resistance. (B) Serratus anterior (C5–7; long thoracic nerve). The subject pushes hard with outstretched arms; the inner edge of the scapula remains against the thoracic wall. (If the trapezius is weak, the inner edge may move from chest wall.) (C) Infraspinatus (C4–6; suprascapular nerve). With the elbow flexed at the side, the arm is externally rotated against resistance on the forearm. (D) Supraspinatus (C4–6; suprascapular nerve). The arm is abducted from the side of the body against resistance. From Chusid 1964 with permission.

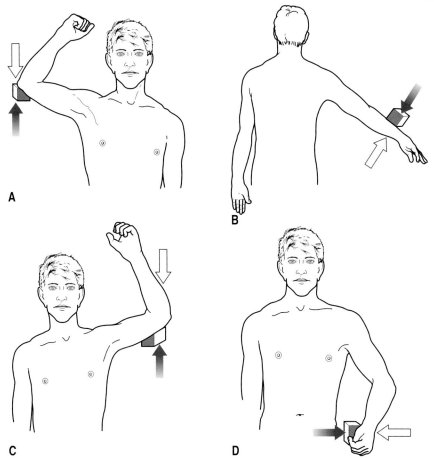

Fig. 4.23 (A) Latissimus dorsi (C6–8; subscapular nerve). The arm is abducted from a horizontal and lateral position against resistance. (B) Deltoid (C5, 6; axillary nerve). Abduction of laterally raised arm (30°–75° from body) against resistance. (C) Pectoralis major, upper portion (C5–8; lateral and medial pectoral nerves). The arm is abducted from an elevated or horizontal and forward position against resistance. (D) Pectoralis major, lower portion (C5–8, T1; lateral and medial pectoral nerves). The arm is abducted from forward position below horizontal against resistance. From Chusid 1964 with permission.

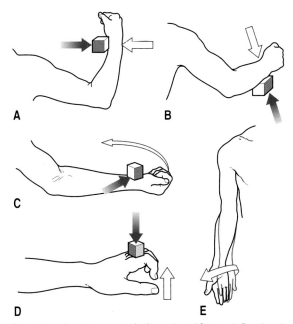

Fig. 4.24 (A) Biceps (C5, 6; musculocutaneous nerve). The supinated forearm is flexed against resistance. (B) Triceps (C6–8; radial nerve). The forearm, flexed at the elbow, is extended against resistance. (C) Brachioradialis (C5, 6; radial nerve). The forearm is flexed against resistance while it is in 'neutral' position (neither pronated nor supinated). (D) Extensor digitorum (C7, 8; radial nerve). The fingers are extended at the metacarpophalangeal joints against resistance. (E) Supinator (C5, 6; radial nerve). The hand is supinated against resistance, with arms extended at the side. Resistance is applied by the grip of the examiner's hand on patient's forearm near the wrist. From Chusid 1964 with permission.

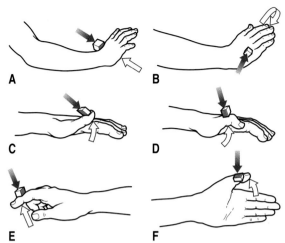

Fig. 4.25 (A) Extensor carpi radialis longus (C6–8; radial nerve). The wrist is extended to the radial side against resistance; fingers extended. (B) Extensor carpi ulnaris (C6–8; radial nerve). The wrist joint is extended to the ulnar side against resistance. (C) Extensor pollicis longus (C7, 8; radial nerve). The thumb is extended against resistance. (D) Extensor pollicis brevis (C7, 8; radial nerve). The thumb is extended at the metacarpophalangeal joint against resistance. (E) Extensor indicis proprius (C6–8; radial nerve). The index finger is extended against resistance placed on the dorsal aspect of the finger. (F) Abductor pollicis longus (C7, 8, T1; radial nerve). The thumb is abducted against resistance in a plane at right angle to the palmar surface. From Chusid 1964 with permission.

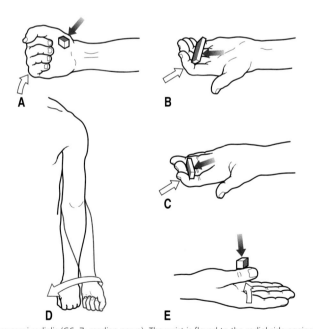

Fig. 4.26 (A) Flexor carpi radialis (C6, 7; median nerve). The wrist is flexed to the radial side against resistance. (B) Flexor digitorum sublimis (C7, 8, T1; median nerve). Fingers are flexed at first interphalangeal against resistance; proximal phalanges fixed. (C) Flexor digitorum profundus I and II (C7, 8, T1; median nerve). The terminal phalanges of the index and middle fingers are flexed against resistance, the second phalanges being held in extension. (D) Pronator teres (C6, 7; median nerve). The extended arm is pronated against resistance. Resistance is applied by grip of examiner's hand on patient's forearm near the wrist. (E) Abductor pollicis brevis (C7, 8, T1; median nerve). The thumb is abducted against resistance in a plane at a right angle to the palmar surface. From Chusid 1964 with permission.

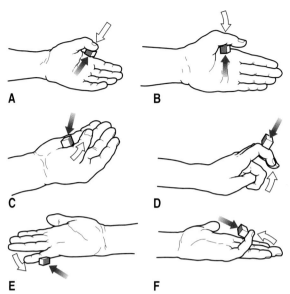

Fig. 4.27 (A) Flexor pollicis longus (C7, 8, T1; median nerve). The terminal phalanx of the thumb is flexed against resistance as the proximal phalanx is held in extension. (B) Flexor pollicis brevis (C7, 8, T1; median nerve). The proximal phalanx of the thumb is flexed against resistance placed on its palmar surface. (C) Opponens pollicis (C8, T1; median nerve). The thumb is crossed over the palm against resistance to touch the top of the little finger with the thumbnail held parallel to the palm. (D) Lumbricalis-interossei (radial half) (C8, T1; median and ulnar nerves). The second and third phalanges are extended against resistance; the first phalanx is in full extension. The ulnar has the same innervation and can be tested in the same manner. (E) Flexor carpi ulnaris (C7, 8, T1; ulnar nerve). The little finger is abducted *strongly* against resistance as the supinated hand lies with fingers extended on table. (F) Flexor digiti quinti (C7, 8, T1; ulnar nerve). The proximal phalanx of the little finger is flexed against resistance. From Chusid 1964 with permission.

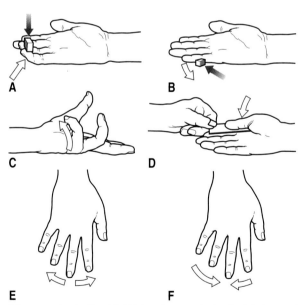

Fig. 4.28 (A) Flexor digitorum profundus III and IV (C8, T1; ulnar nerve). The distal phalanges of the little and ring fingers are flexed against resistance; the second phalanges are held in extension. (B) Abductor digiti quinti (C8, T1; ulnar nerve). The little finger is abducted against resistance as the supinated hand with fingers extended lies on table. (C) Opponens digiti quinti (C7, 8, T1; median nerve). With fingers extended, the little finger is moved across the palm to the base of the thumb. (D) Abductor pollicis (C8, T1; ulnar nerve). A piece of paper grasped between the palm and the thumb is held against resistance with the thumbnail kept at a right angle to the palm. (E) Dorsal interossei (C8, T1; ulnar nerve). The index and ring fingers are abducted from midline against resistance as the palm of the hand lies flat on the table. (F) Palmer interossei (C8, T1; ulnar nerve). The abducted index, ring, and little fingers are adducted to midline against resistance as the palm of the hand lies flat on the table. From Chusid 1964 with permission.

Muscle Testing of the Lower Limbs

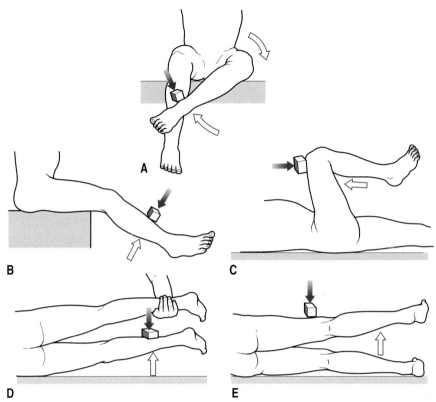

Fig. 4.29 (A) Sartorius (L2, 3; femoral nerve). With the subject sitting and the knee flexed, the thigh is rotated outward against resistance on the leg. (B) Quadriceps femoris (L2–4; femoral nerve). The knee is extended against resistance on the leg. (C) Iliopsoas (L1–3; femoral nerve). The subject lies supine with knee flexed. The flexed thigh (at about 90°) is further flexed against resistance. (D) Adductors (L2–4; obturator nerve). With the subject on one side with knees extended, the lower extremity is adducted against resistance; the upper leg is supported by the examiner. (E) Gluteus medius and minimus; tensor fasciae latae (L4, 5, S1; superior gluteal nerve). Testing abduction: With the subject lying on one side and the thigh and leg extended, the uppermost lower extremity is abducted against resistance. From Chusid 1964 with permission.

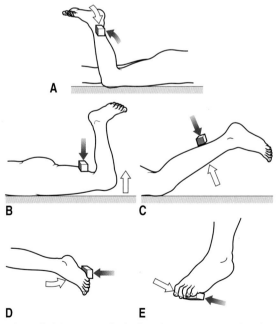

Fig. 4.30 (A) Gluteus medius and minimus; tensor fasciae latae (L4, 5, S1; superior gluteal nerve). Testing internal rotation: With the subject prone and the knee flexed, the foot is moved laterally against resistance. (B) Gluteus maximus (L4, 5, S1, 2; inferior gluteal nerve). With the subject prone, the knee is lifted off the table against resistance. (C) 'Hamstring' group (L4, 5, S1, 2; sciatic nerve). With the subject prone, the knee is flexed against resistance. (D) Gastrocnemius (L5, S1, 2; tibial nerve). With the subject prone, the foot is plantar-flexed against resistance. (E) Flexor digitorum longus (S1, 2; tibial nerve). The toe joints are plantar-flexed against resistance. From Chusid 1964 with permission.

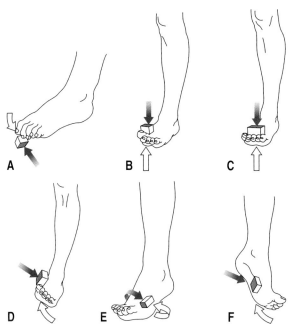

Fig. 4.31 (A) Flexor hallucis longus (L5, S1, 2; tibial nerve). The great toe is plantar-flexed against resistance. The second and third toes are also flexed. (B) Extensor hallucis longus (L4, 5, S1; deep peroneal nerve). The large toe is dorsiflexed against resistance. (C) Extensor digitorum longus (L4, 5, S1; deep peroneal nerve). The toes are dorsiflexed against resistance. (D) Tibialis anterior (L4, 5; deep peroneal nerve). The foot is dorsiflexed and inverted against resistance applied by gripping the foot with the examiner's hand. (E) Peroneus longus and brevis (L5, S1; superficial peroneal nerve). The foot is everted against resistance applied by gripping the foot with the examiner's hand. (F) Tibialis posterior (L5, S1; tibial nerve). The plantar-flexed foot is inverted against resistance applied by gripping the foot with the examiner's hand.
From Chusid 1964 with permission.

Testing Reflexes

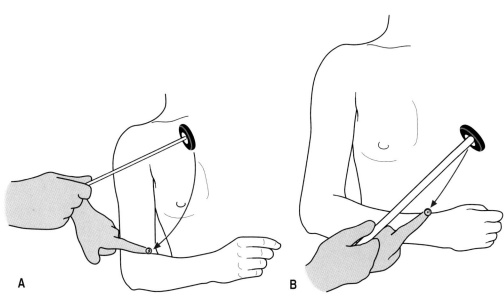

Fig. 4.32 (A) Testing the biceps reflex; (B) testing the supinator reflex;

(continued)

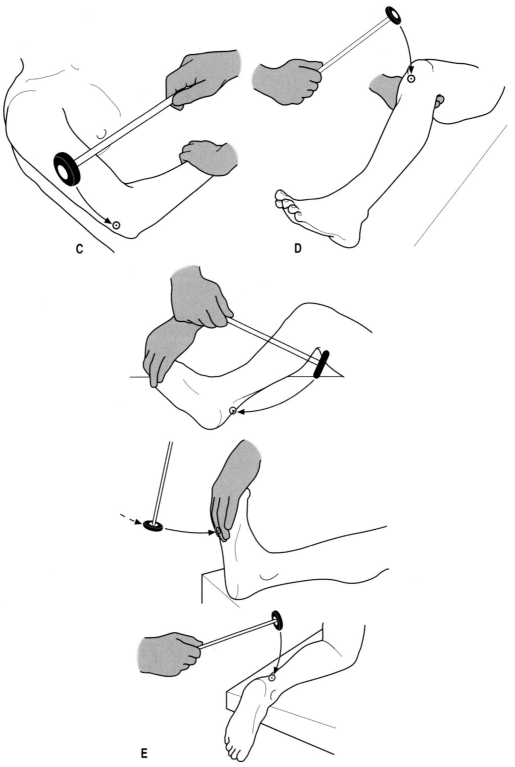

Fig. 4.32 Cont'd (C) testing the triceps reflex; (D) testing the knee reflex; (E) the ankle reflex and three ways to get it. From Chusid 1964 with permission.

References

Carrick FR 1997 Changes in brain function after manipulation of the cervical spine. Journal of Manipulative and Physiological Therapeutics 20:529–545.

Chusid JG 1964 Correlative neuroanatomy and functional neurology. Lange Medical Publishers, Los Altos, California.

DeMyer WE 1994 Technique of the neurologic examination: a programmed text, 4th edn. McGraw-Hill, New York.

Fuller G 2004 Neurological examination made easy, 3rd edn. Churchill Livingston, New York.

Schmid R, Wilhelm B, Wilhelm H 2000 Naso-temporal asymmetry and contraction aniscoria in the pupillomotor system. Graefe's Archive for Clinical and Experimental Ophthalmology 238(2)123–128.

Sexton SG 2006 Forehead temperature asymmetry: A potential correlate of hemisphericity. (Personal communication)

Further Reading

Bickley L, Hoekelman R 1999 Bates' guide to physical examination and history taking, 7th edn. Lippincott Wilkins and Williams, Philadelphia.

Blumenfeld H 2002 Neuroanatomy from clinical cases. Sinauer Associates, Sunderland, MA.

DeMyer WE 1994 Technique of the neurologic examination: a programmed text, 4th edn. McGraw-Hill, New York.

Fuller G 2004 Neurological examination made easy, 3rd edn. Churchill Livingston, New York.

Patten J 2004 Neurological differential diagnosis, 2nd edn. Springer, New York.

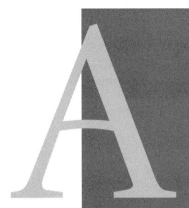

Clinical Case Answers

Case 4.1

4.1.1   You would need to examine CN III, V, VII, IX, and X. The examinations one would perform are;

1. Width of palpebral fissure (ptosis)—This is dependent on both sympathetic and oculomotor innervation. Therefore, one needs to differentiate between a Horner's syndrome, oculomotor nerve lesion, or physiological changes in the CIS of the mesencephalic reticular formation.

2. Skin condition—Increased peripheral resistance may result in decreased integrity of skin, particularly at the extremities.

3. Ophthalmoscopy—V:A ratio and vessel integrity

4. Heart auscultation—Arrhythmias and changes in heart sounds can occur because of altered CIS of the PMRF.

5. Bowel auscultation—This can be particularly useful during some treatment procedures to monitor the effect of stimulation on vagal function (e.g. caloric irrigation—further instruction required, adjustments and visual stimulation or exercises, etc).

6. Skin and tympanic temperature and blood flow—This is particularly useful as a pre- and post-adjustment check. Profound changes in skin temperature asymmetry can occur following an adjustment. These changes are side dependent. An adjustment on the side of decreased forehead skin temperature will commonly result in greater symmetry or reversed asymmetry. Conflicting results are likely to be dependent on a number of factors, which are currently being investigated further. Remember that forehead skin temperature depends on fuel requirements of the brain, and vestibular and cortical influences on autonomic function among other things.

7. Dermatographia—The red response is often observed in patients who suffer from sympathetically mediated pain.

8. Lung expansion, respiratory rate and ratio, etc.—An inspiration: expiration ratio of 1:2 is considered to represent approximately normal sympathovagal balance. This means that expiration should take twice as long as inspiration. This is difficult to achieve for some patients at first and requires some training.

    Shallow and rapid breathing can result in respiratory alkalosis, which leads to hypersensitivity in the nervous system. CO_2 is blown off at a higher rate, resulting in decreased $[H^+]$ ions in the blood. Lower $[Ca^{++}]$ follows, causing $[Na^+]$ to rise in extracellular fluid. This can be seen clinically by the presence of percussion myotonia, which is also often seen in various metabolic and hormonal disorders.

9. Forehead skin temperature—Measurement of skin temperature above the browline may provide useful information concerning sympathetic control of blood vessels to the eye, as sympathetic supply to the vessels of the forehead are branches of the sympathetic supply to the retinal vessels.

Activation of cervical afferents has been found to have an antagonistic effect on the excitatory vestibulosympathetic reflexes. It is therefore proposed that a cervical spine adjustment may enhance cervical inhibition of the vestibulosympathetic reflex, resulting in increased blood flow to the eye and brain.

4.1.2
1. Pupil size and reactivity
2. Retinal artery V:A ratios
3. Bilateral blood pressure
4. Skin temperature and sweat production
5. Presence of dermatographia
6. Heart rate

4.1.3 Dermatographia is an exaggerated wheal and flare response to lines drawn on the skin with a pointed but blunt instrument. It is also referred to as the red response. The red response is often observed in patients who suffer from an overactive sympathetic nervous system or sympathetically mediated pain.

Case 4.2

4.2.1 Exotropia is the deviation of the eye away from the nose when the eye is stationary but the degree of deviation usually remains no matter how the eye is moved. It is a form of strabismus (see Fig. 4.2.1). Exophoria is a mild deviation of the eye towards the nose during movement of the eye that is normally not detected by the individual because integration in the brain can accommodate the minor variance. Both may be caused by a weak medial rectus muscle or an overactive lateral rectus muscle.

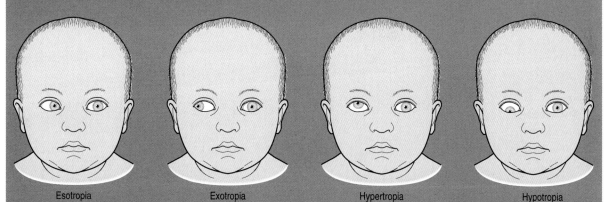

Esotropia   Exotropia   Hypertropia   Hypotropia

Fig. 4.2.1 Esotropia is a deviation of the eye towards the nose when at rest. Exotropia is the deviation of the eye away from the nose when at rest. Hypertropia is the deviation of the eye upwards when at rest. Hypotropia is the deviation of the eye downward when at rest.

4.2.2 The activity level of both the involved muscles may be due to the activity in the respective innervating neuron pools. Testing of the mesencephalon (Oculomotor) activity and the pontine (Abducens) activity may give an indication which of overactivity or underactivity may be occurring.

Chapter

5

Neurology of Sensory and Receptor Systems

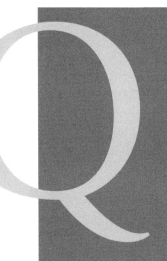

Clinical Cases for Thought

Case 5.1   A 36-year-old male presents with severe buttock pain radiating down his right leg to the outside of his foot. He first noticed the pain while helping his brother shift house 3 days ago. Coughing and straining seem to aggravate the pain. On physical examination a straight leg raise limited to 20° by pain and a positive Bowstring's sign are found. His low back area is inflamed and sensitive to palpation at the L5–S1 area. His right gastrocnemius tendon reflex is diminished and he has no sensation of vibration in his lateral foot.

Questions

5.1.1   Explain the suspected mechanism of injury in this case.

5.1.2   Explain the loss of reflex activity in his gastrocnemius muscle.

5.1.3   Explain the loss of vibration sensation in his lateral foot.

5.1.4   What imaging studies might you request to confirm your diagnosis above?

Case 5.2   A 68-year-old woman presents with mild low back pain and a severe left-sided limp of 3 months duration. On examination a moderate deformation of her left knee joint when compared to the right is noted. She denies any pain or discomfort arising from the knee but only from the back. On examination a loss of deep tendon reflexes and sensation below her knee are found. Radiographs of her back were unremarkable. Radiographs of her knee revealed joint debris, dislocation, disorganization, and bony destruction of the tibial plateau. On further questioning, she admits that she is an uncontrolled diabetic.

Questions

5.2.1   Outline the top five differential diagnoses for this patient.

5.2.2   How would one test for sensation of her lower legs?

5.2.3   Explain the absent reflexes and sensation.

5.2.4   Explain the mechanism of joint damage in this unfortunate woman.

Introduction

The conversion of external stimuli to neuron activity occurs in specialized structures called receptors. Each different type of receptor has a specialized ability to detect a specific modality or type of stimulus. Light receptors are most sensitive to light, pressure receptors are most sensitive to pressure, etc. However, each type of receptor may be excited by other modalities of stimulation if the stimulus is of sufficient amplitude. Try closing your eyes and rubbing with gentle pressure over your eyelids. Some of you will perceive flashes of light floating across your visual field. This sensation is caused by the light sensitive cells in your retina depolarizing due to the pressure that you have exerted on your eyeball. The pressure causes the cells to depolarize but you do not perceive pressure but flashes of light! This is due to the hard wiring of these cells to your visual cortex which normally receive action potential activity for light stimulation. The cells in your visual cortex quite naturally 'believe' that the reason they have received an increase in action potential activity is due to light stimulus so you perceive light! We will see that we often do not construct a true representation of the outside world in our minds. Our mind's interpretation of the stimulus becomes our perception and thus our reality.

The common modalities consciously perceived by humans include light, pain, pressure, vibration, taste, touch, smell, hearing, and temperature. Some modalities such as muscle length, joint position sense, and internal organ function are not always consciously perceived but are none the less essential for normal function. With very few exceptions, each of these different modalities is detected by the receptors of a distinct set of dorsal root ganglion or primary afferent neurons.

Sensory information is essential for a variety of reasons such as to construct a perception of ourselves in the universe, muscle movement control, internal organ and blood flow functionality, maintaining arousal, and developing and maintaining survival and plasticity in neural networks.

Clinically, we can utilize the various modalities and how they are perceived by our minds to test the functionality of various pathways, to localize dysfunction in the system, and identify intact pathways for utilization in treatment of dysfunction. It is important to remember that malfunction at any level in the system from receptor to perception may be the cause of a patient's symptoms or dysfunction.

In this chapter we will examine the different types of receptors and the characteristic modalities that they detect and outline where and how this information is integrated in the brain to form a perception.

Reception and Sensation of Afferent Stimulation

The physical properties of the stimuli detected by our receptors often differs dramatically from the perceptions that we form from these stimuli. For example, our retinal cells detect electromagnetic radiation patterns but we perceive the Mona Lisa. Our ears detect sound wave variations and patterns but we perceive a Mozart symphony. Our nociceptors detect chemical imbalances but we perceive pain. This amazing ability of our brain to process this information in an individually unique but universally characteristic fashion is one of the fundamental attributes that determines our humanism. Colours, sounds, feelings, pain, and all other human perceptions do not exist outside of the human mind. Thus our perception of our universe is not a true representation of our physical universe but a mental construct composed by our mind's interpretation of all of the integrated nervous input available to it at any given moment (Martin & Jessell 1995). It is important to remember this when a patient presents with symptoms that cannot be explained by our traditional understanding of neuroscience or neuroanatomy. The patient's perception is their reality. For example, in people with fibromyalgia, the detection of movement by their joint receptors is perceived as pain in their mind. To this patient this perception of pain is very real.

The Sensory Neurons

Virtually all of the afferent or sensory information that reaches the spinal cord arrives via the dorsal root ganglion or primary afferent cells. All other afferent information reaches

Somatic Sensation | **QUICK FACTS 1**

Somatic sensibility has four major types of modalities:

1. Discriminative touch—Discrimination of size, shape, texture, and movement across the skin.

2. Proprioception—The sense of static and kinetic position of the limbs and body without visual input.

3. Nociception—The signalling of tissue damage or chemical irritation, typically perceived as pain or an itch.

4. Temperature sense—Warmth and cold perception.

the central nervous system via embryological homologues of the dorsal root ganglion cells, the cranial nerve nuclei, located throughout the brainstem.

The cell bodies of the primary afferent neurons of the spinal cord live in the dorsal root ganglia situated adjacent to the spinal cord in the immediate vicinity of the intervertebral foramen from which they enter the spinal canal (Schwartz 1995). The primary afferent neurons are classified as pseudounipolar cells because they give rise to only one axon that transmits information from the periphery to the spinal cord. The segment of the axon that transmits information from the peripheral receptor towards the cell body is called the peripheral axon branch, and the portion of the axon transmitting information away from the cell body towards the spinal cord is called the central axon branch. The dorsal root neurons do not form dendrites as most other neurons do; thus any modulatory activity occurring at these neurons must occur at the cell body or presynaptically on the central process as it enters the grey matter spinal cord. Most of the central processes of the primary afferent develop collateral axon branches as they enter the spinal cord (Fig. 5.1). These collateral branches synapse with a variety of other neurons depending on the type of modality that the primary afferent cell is relying. The collateral branching and synapse formation of each type of primary afferent will be described in detail as each individual modality is described below.

The axons of the various primary afferents display a variety of different diameters and myelination densities. Functionally, these morphological differences result in axons that transmit impulses at different rates of speed or conduction velocities. Table 5.1 outlines the various conduction velocities and diameters of different primary afferent axons.

Because of different growth rate patterns between the spinal cord and the vertebral column the dorsal root ganglion cells below T3 are located at increasingly further

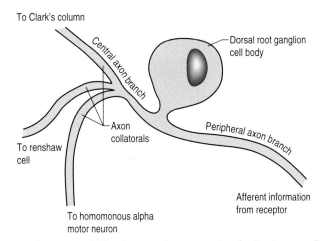

Fig. 5.1 Dorsal root ganglion neuron. This is a diagrammatic representation of a dorsal root ganglion cell illustrating the unique properties associated with this type of neuron. Note the axon is both afferent (peripheral axon branch) and efferent (central axon branch) in nature. The central axon branch has a number of collateral axon branches that project to a variety of other neurons, both segmentally and suprasegmentally. This illustrates the principal of divergence of receptor information in the neuraxis.

Table 5.1 Nerve Fibre Types in Mammalian Nerve

Fibre Type		Function	Fibre Diameter (μm)	Conduction Velocity (m/s)	Spike Duration (ms)	Absolute Refractory Period (ms)
A	α	Proprioception; somatic motor	12–20	70–120	0.4–0.5	0.4–1
	β	Touch, pressure	5–12	30–70		
	γ	Motor to muscle spindles	3–6	15–20		
	ς	Pain, temperature, touch	2–5	12–30		
B		Preganglionic autonomic	<3	3–15	1.2	1.2
C	Dorsal root	Pain, reflex responses	0.4–1.2	0.5–2	2	2
	Sympathetic	Postganglionic sympathetics	0.3–1.3	0.7–2.3	2	2

distances from the segmental spinal cord levels that they supply. This results in the progressive lengthening of the central processes of the primary afferents and in the formation of the cauda equina after the spinal cord ends at the level of L1–L2 in most people. It is these central processes that may experience compression from a posterior central or posterior lateral vertebral disc herniation (Figs. 5.2 and 5.3).

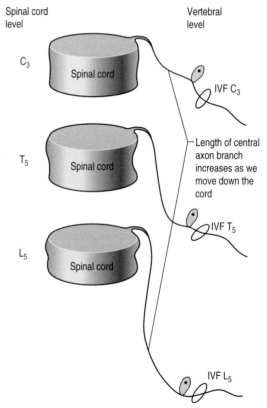

Fig. 5.2 Length of central axons of dorsal root ganglion neurons. This figure demonstrates the fact that the spinal vertebra continue to grow after the spinal neurons have established their connections to the dorsal root ganglion neurons. The central axon projections of the dorsal root ganglion neurons must elongate to keep pace with the growing vertebral column. This results in a physical separation of the spinal cord level neurons with the dorsal root ganglion neurons, which remain at their original location in the vertebral foramina of the spinal column. Thus spinal root level and spinal cord level functional units are located at different physical locations.

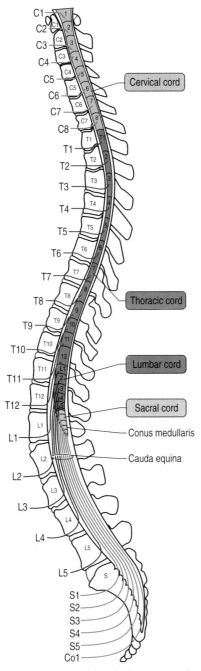

Fig. 5.3 Cauda equina The relationship between the spinal cord and spinal vertebral levels is shown a lateral view. Also illustrated is the cauda equina, which is formed by the elongated central processes of the dorsal root ganglion neurons from the lumbar, sacral, and coccygeal vertebral spinal levels and the efferent motor projection of the ventral horn cells of the lumbar, sacral, and coccygeal spinal cord levels. Note as the spinal column grows the efferent fibres arising from the ventral horn neurons must also elongate to exit the vertebral column at the appropriate foraminal level.

Receptors of Primary Afferent Input

Structurally, receptors can be classified into three basic morphological forms: neuroepithelial receptors, visual receptors, and primary afferent receptors. In the case of the neuroepithelial receptor, the sensory sensitive detection apparatus is contained in the neuron cell body itself. These types of neurons are situated near the sensory surface with their axons projecting back towards the central nervous system. The unique quality of these receptors is that the neuron cell body has derived from epithelial tissue and remains in that tissue as a receptor organ. In humans the only known example of this type of sensory reception can be found in the

QUICK FACTS 2 — **Somatosensory Information Pathways**

Regardless of modality all somatosensory information from the limbs and trunk is conveyed to the CNS via dorsal root ganglion (DRG) cells.

Somatosensory information from the cranial structures (face, lips, oral cavity, conjunctiva, and dura mater) is transmitted via trigeminal sensory neurons, which are structurally and morphologically equivalent to DRG neurons.

sensory cells of the olfactory epithelium. Here the axons of these neurons which form the olfactory nerve or 1st cranial nerve (CN I) traverse the cribriform plate of the ethmoid bone to synapse in the glomeruli of the olfactory bulb (Williams & Warwick 1984) (Fig. 5.4).

The second type of receptor can be classed as visual receptors. These receptors are similar to the neuroepithelial receptors in that the receptive apparatus is in their cell bodies; however, in this case, their cell bodies are derived from neuroectoderm of the foetal ventricles which form the foetal brain and migrate to the retinal areas (Fig. 5.5).

In the third type of receptor, which may be classified as a primary afferent receptor, the cell body is located near to or in the central nervous system. Long peripheral processes extend to the receptive area and form the specialized receptive structures that act as the receptors. All cutaneous and most proprioceptors are composed of this type of receptor (Williams & Warwick 1984) (Fig. 5.1).

A variety of different receptor types and axonal and neuronal specialization give rise to a vast array of sensory information reaching the spinal cord via the primary afferent neurons. The primary modality types are outlined below.

The Muscle Spindle

Muscle spindles provide the nervous system with information concerning the instantaneous static length of a muscle at any given moment and the rate of change of muscle length during any movement. The output of the muscle spindle is simultaneously transmitted to a variety of interneuron networks in the spinal cord. This information is then relayed to areas in the brainstem, cerebellum, and basal ganglia. The axons of the primary afferent neurons that relay muscle spindle information to the spinal cord form many collateral branches as they enter the spinal cord. Some of these collaterals proceed without synapsing on an interneuron to synapse directly (monosynaptic connection) on the alpha motor neuron pools of the muscle fibres from which they are relaying information (homonymous muscle), resulting in an excitatory stimulus (Fleshman et al 1981). Other collaterals first synapse (polysynaptic connection) on interneurons in lamina VIII of the grey matter of the spinal cord referred to as Clark's column. These interneurons then project to the brainstem reticular formation nuclei, various cortical areas of the cerebellum via mossy fibres, and the basal ganglia (Cram & Kasman 1998). The spinocerebellar tracts are formed from the axons of these interneurons in Clark's columns. The anterior spinocerebellar tracts receive axons from both ipsilateral and contralateral lamina VIII neurons. The posterior spinocerebellar tracts receive axons from only ipsilateral lamina VIII neurons. This is an example of reciprocal innervation that occurs when vital information transfer is required (Fig. 5.6). All regions other than the segmental interneurons and their associated alpha motor neurons receiving input from the primary afferents at that level are referred to as suprasegmental to the input. Most suprasegmental integration is involved with modulation of movement, or in feedback control of the accuracy of the movement generated. Some controversy exists as to whether the receptive input of muscle spindles can be consciously perceived. Since muscle spindles do not project directly to the somatosensory cortex, their activity was thought not to be consciously perceived. However, some research has indicated that conscious perception is possible (Williams & Warwick 1984).

The specialized receptors on the muscle spindle afferent axons are associated with the intrafugal fibres of the muscle. These intrafugal fibres are interposed between the major contractile tissues referred to as the extrafugal fibres of the muscle. The intrafugal fibres

Olfactory receptors

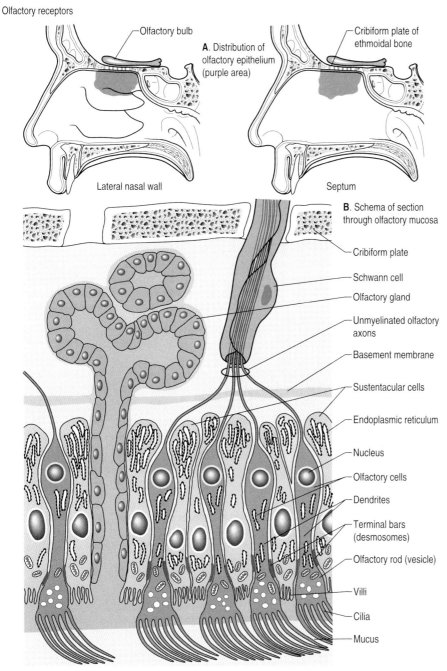

Fig. 5.4 Formation of the olfactory nerves from the olfactory cells. Note the passage of the myelinated axon complex through the cribriform plate.

are surrounded by a sheath that separates them from the extrafugal fibres, which is filled with a fluid rich in hyaluronic acid. The intrafugal fibres can be classified into nuclear bag and nuclear chain fibres. Nuclear bag fibres have their nuclei clustered in the central area of the fibre, giving them a fusiform appearance. Within the nuclear bag fibres a further distinction between static and dynamic fibre types can also be made. The nuclear bag fibres are much longer then the nuclear chain fibres and extend beyond the capsule of the spindle to attach to the endomysium of the surrounding extrafugal fibres. The nuclear chain fibres have their nuclei lined up centrally along the midline of the length of the fibre and are attached to the nuclear bag fibres at their poles. Sensory endings in the muscle spindles give rise to two types of afferent axons emerging from a muscle fibre. The large myelinated, type Ia afferent fibres—also known as annulospiral endings—innervate all types of primary sensory endings in an intrafugal muscle fibre and are rapidly adapting and extremely sensitive to changes in muscle fibre length (Banks et al 1981).

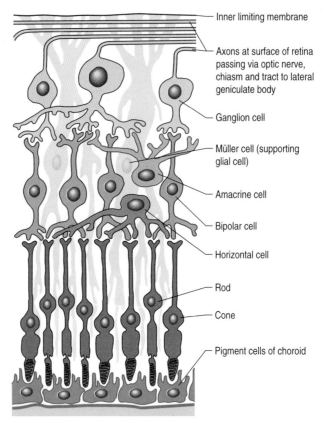

Fig. 5.5 The complex array of neurons and other cells that form the retina of the eye. Note the formation of the optic nerve from the axons of the ganglion cells.

- Inner limiting membrane
- Axons at surface of retina passing via optic nerve, chiasm and tract to lateral geniculate body
- Ganglion cell
- Müller cell (supporting glial cell)
- Amacrine cell
- Bipolar cell
- Horizontal cell
- Rod
- Cone
- Pigment cells of choroid

The type II afferent fibres—also known as flower spray endings—emerge from the sensory endings of nuclear chain and static nuclear bag fibre types and are slow adapting and highly sensitive to static muscle length (Cooper & Daniel 1963; Boyd 1980) (Fig. 5.7). Human muscle spindle sensory endings also respond to tendon percussive stimulation, vibration, and other forms of rhythmic stretch (Burke 1981). Most types of human muscle tissue have one nuclear bag dynamic fibre, one nuclear bag static fibre, and a number of nuclear chain fibres per muscle spindle (Ghez & Gorden 1995). When the intrafugal fibres become stretched, the nerve endings depolarize and an increase in action potential firing occurs. This process is known as 'loading' the spindle. 'Unloading' the spindle occurs when the intrafugal fibre returns toward its normal length. This results in a decrease in the action potential frequency of firing in the afferent nerve fibres.

Gamma Motor Fibres Can Change the Sensitivity and Gain of the Muscle Spindle
The intrafugal fibres contain specialized areas of contractibility innervated by efferent motor fibres referred to as gamma motor fibres (Matthews 1981). Each intrafugal fibre receives motor innervation from more than one gamma motor axon. This is termed polyneuronal innervation and is peculiar for the most part to the intrafugal fibres of muscle. (Polyneuronal innervation does occur in extrafugal fibres in neonates before functional maturation has occurred and occasionally in the early stages of reinnervation of muscle tissue following injury (Burke & Lance 1992).) These gamma motor fibres release acetylcholine at their synapses and arise from gamma motor neurons that live in lamina IX of the anterior grey matter of the spinal cord of the same segmental level as the alpha motor neurons supplying the extrafugal fibres from the homonymous muscle (Hunt 1974). The contractile elements of the nuclear bag fibres are rich in mitochondria and oxidative enzymes, whereas the nuclear chain fibres have more extensive sarcoplasmic reticulum and T-fibre development but fewer mitochondria and oxidative enzymes. This results in a slower contraction of nuclear bag fibres than nuclear chain fibres when the spindle is stimulated (Williams & Warwick 1984).

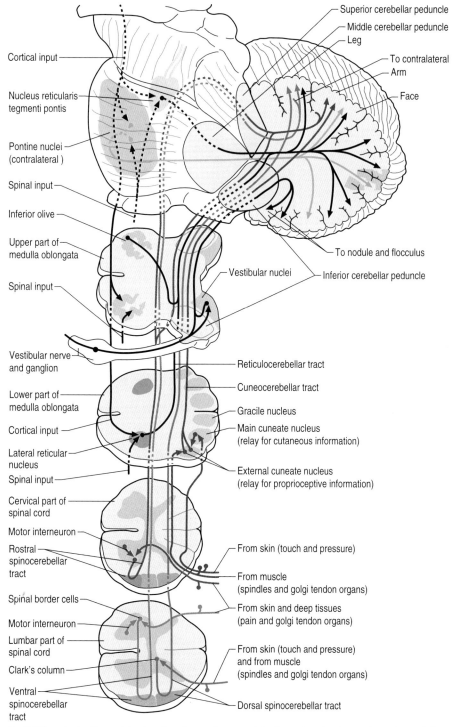

Fig. 5.6 The spinal pathways taken by afferent axons from a variety of proprioceptors in muscles to the cerebellum. Note the axons that form the ventral and dorsal spinocerebellar tracts and the cuneocerebellar tracts, and the afferent axons that form the inferior, middle, and superior cerebellar peduncles.

The gamma motor input to the intrafugal fibres is involved with adjusting the appropriate length of intrafugal fibres in order to maintain an accurate measure of the degree of contraction of the muscle. If the length of the intrafugal fibre was not constantly adjusted as the extrafugal fibres contracted, it would become slack and fail to accurately record further contraction or the static state of the muscle at that instant. Loading of the intrafugal fibres may occur by increasing the stretch on the extrafugal fibres or by increasing the activity of the contractile elements of the intrafugal fibres by increasing the gamma motor activity. Increasing the gamma motor activity results in

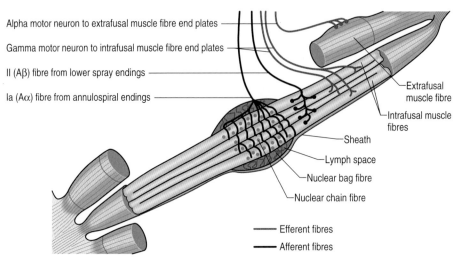

Alpha motor neuron to extrafusal muscle fibre end plates
Gamma motor neuron to intrafusal muscle fibre end plates
II (Aβ) fibre from lower spray endings
Ia (Aα) fibre from annulospiral endings

Extrafusal muscle fibre
Intrafusal muscle fibres
Sheath
Lymph space
Nuclear bag fibre
Nuclear chain fibre

—— Efferent fibres
—— Afferent fibres

Fig. 5.7 The afferent and efferent innervation of extrafusal and intrafusal muscles. The alpha motor neuron axons form the efferent supply to the extrafusal muscle fibres. The gamma motor neuron axons form the efferent projections to the intrafusal motor fibres. The afferent sensory information from the annulospiral endings of the intrafusal fibres is transmitted to the neuraxis via the type Ia fibres and the afferent information from the flower spray endings of the intrafusal fibres is transmitted to the neuraxis via the type II fibres.

QUICK FACTS 3	Two Classes of Somatic Sensation can be Distinguished Neurologically

1. Epicritic sensation—Involves fine aspects of touch and is mediated by encapsulated receptors; for example:
   a. Topognosis (gentle touch, localizing position of touch)
   b. Vibration sense (frequency and amplitude)
   c. Two-point discrimination
   d. Stereognosis (recognize the shape of objects held in the hand)
2. Protopathic sensations—Involve pain, temperature, itch, and tickle sensations and are mediated by receptors with bare nerve endings.

a high specificity of muscle activity with a small amplitude of sway variation in maintaining extrafugal to intrafugal muscle length within a tight oscillating pattern. The degree of oscillation occurring in a muscle is referred to as gain. Thus with increasing gamma activation the specificity of movement or sensitivity increases and the gain decreases. This interaction provides for the occurrence of a reflex compensation for small irregularities of movement that may occur between the suprasegmental programming and the performance of the actual movement (Burke & Lance 1992). This modulation circuit is referred to as the motor servo mechanism (see Chapter 6). In order to ensure that this system performs properly there is an interactive connection between the alpha and gamma motor neurons that results in a co-activation of both systems simultaneously. So important is knowing the moment to moment state of our muscle position to the nervous system that nearly 30% of all descending efferent motor control systems are associated with the gamma motor modulation of spindle fibres and the feedback information from these fibres is transmitted from the spinal cord to the suprasegmental areas via redundant pathways. As a general rule only information crucial to the nervous system is transmitted by more than one pathway. As previously mentioned, when information is transmitted through more than one pathway it is referred to as redundant transmission. To exemplify this point the information from the muscle spindles below vertebral level of T1 travels up the spinal cord via the ipsilateral dorsal or posterior spinocerebellar tract and bilaterally in the ventral or anterior spinocerebellar tracts to the cerebellum. The axons of the posterior spinocerebellar tracts and the ipsilateral anterior spinocerebellar tracts pass through the ipsilateral inferior cerebellar peduncles to reach the ipsilateral cerebellum. The axons of the contralateral anterior spinocerebellar tracts cross back to the side of their origin in the superior cerebellar peduncles and thus maintain the rule that cerebellar input from muscle spindles occurs ipsilaterally. The paravertebral muscles of the spine have one of the highest concentrations of spindle receptors in the body and the upper cervical region of the spinal cord has the highest density of muscle spindle receptors in the spine (Kulkarni et al 2001).

The muscle spindles of humans are usually well developed at birth. The development of the spindles in the foetus depends solely on the presence of the primary afferent axon. After the spindles have formed they can tolerate periods of denervation; however, they often undergo marked changes in function and reactivity even when reinnervation occurs by the original axon (Milburn 1973). The altered functional activity in muscle spindles following injury can contribute to asymmetries in cortical afferent input, resulting in hemispheric asymmetry. This presents one of the clinical challenges facing a patient following axon injuries or demyelination conditions.

Free Nerve Endings	**QUICK FACTS 4**

- C-fibres (group IV)
- Unmyelinated
- Slow conducting (0.25–0.35 m/s)
- Pain
- Temperature
- Itch
- Tickle

Golgi Tendon Organs

These specialized receptors are found extensively in the collagen fibres of the muscle tendon junction. These receptors align themselves in series with the muscle fibres in such a way that stretching the tendon results in depolarization of the receptors (Barker 1974). Some tendon organs are activated with even the weakest of contractions. The total discharge frequency of the organ increases with the strength of contraction of the homonymous muscle. The tendon organs are generally silent in relaxed muscle. There is some controversy as to when the tendon organs actually become activated. It has been the prevailing view that tendon organs become active whenever the muscle is stretched either by active contraction or by passive stretch (Matthews 1972). However, another opinion which states that tendon organs usually will not activate even if the muscle is stretched unless the muscle contracts during the stretch has recently arisen. Thus, the newest theory is that these organs monitor muscle contraction in conjunction with tendon tension and not just tendon tension in isolation (Houk & Crago 1980). One of the actions of stimulating the tendon organs of a muscle is a reflex inhibitory feedback stimulus on the alpha motor neurons controlling the homonymous muscle (Fig. 5.8).

The sensory organs of Golgi tendon organs give rise to type Ib afferent fibres, which are myelinated but slightly smaller in diameter than the type Ia fibres of the muscle spindles. The fibres intertwine between the collagenous fibres of the tendon muscle junction where they are unmyelinated and highly branching. As they emerge from the collagen fibre network they bundle together and form a single myelinated axon. Usually, each individual tendon organ gives rise to one type Ib axon (Schoultz & Swett 1974; Ghez & Gorden 1995). Although the receptor information from the Golgi tendon organs does not reach the somatosensory cortex directly, and thus is not consciously perceived, the information supplied by the Golgi tendon organs is very important in the integration of inhibition of motor activity. This is especially apparent when learning how to perform a new motor function. For example, when learning how to hit a tennis ball, the player learns after many attempts not only how to perform the coordinated actions of the muscles involved in the correct swing, but also the 'feel' of the muscle tensions involved in the correct swing (see Chapter 6).

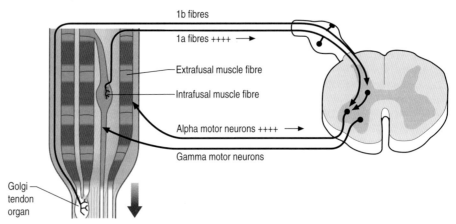

1b fibres

1a fibres ++++ →

Extrafusal muscle fibre

Intrafusal muscle fibre

Alpha motor neurons ++++ →

Gamma motor neurons

Golgi tendon organ

Fig. 5.8 Segmental reflex activity. Both intrafusal and extrafusal muscle fibres stretched; spindles activated. Reflex via la fibres and alpha motor neurons causes secondary contraction (basis of stretch reflexes, same as knee jerk). Stretch is too weak to activate Golgi tendon organs.

Tactile (Meissner's) Corpuscles

These receptors are present on all parts of the hands and feet, on the forearm, the lips, and the tip of the tongue. The corpuscles consist of a capsule and a core portion. The capsule is formed by layers or lamellae between which substantial amounts of collagen have been laid down. The core consists of epidermally derived cells and nerve fibres. Each corpuscle is supplied by several large, heavily myelinated nerve (Aα) fibres and a few small unmyelinated (C) fibres. These receptors are low threshold, rapidly adapting and thus provide information concerning the change of mechanical pressure on the overlying skin. Interestingly these receptors are formed in abundance at birth and over our lifetimes reduce in number by some 80% unless constantly maintained by stimulation (Cauna 1966) (Fig. 5.9).

QUICK FACTS 5	Merkel Discs

- Slow adapting mechanoreceptor
- Deformation of the skin surface
- Large to medium diameter axon
- Aa/group I, Ab/group II
- 30–120 m/s
- One afferent fibre forms from branches of several Merkel discs
- Touch
- Pressure

QUICK FACTS 6	Meissner Corpuscles

- Rapidly adapting, large diameter fibre
- Aa/group I and Ab/group II
- 30–120 m/s
- Stroking
- Fluttering

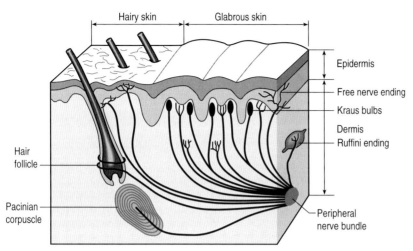

Fig. 5.9 Receptors of the skin. A variety of peripheral receptors including Ruffini endings, Pacinian corpuscles, free nerve endings, Merkle discs are shown. Note the axons of all of these receptors contribute to the formation of a peripheral nerve fibre.

Pacinian Corpuscles

These receptors are sensitive to changes in pressure in a variety of tissues in the body. Pacinian corpuscles are found on the palmer aspects of the hands and feet, the genital organs of both sexes, and buried deep in most muscle tissues. These receptors are extremely sensitive to mechanical disturbances and are particularly sensitive to vibration (Gray & Sato 1953). In muscle tissue they give feedback on the internal pressure changes inside the muscle fibres during both stretch and contraction.

Each corpuscle consists of a capsule and a central core containing a nerve fibre. The capsule is lamellar in nature, with the lamellae separated by layers of collagen. The amounts of collagen deposited between the lamellae increases with age, decreasing the sensitivity of the receptors. Each corpuscle is supplied by one thickly myelinated nerve fibre of the Aα type (Williams & Warwick 1984) (Fig. 5.9).

Merkel Cell Endings

These receptors are found immediately under the epidermis or around the base of certain hair follicles. The nerve fibres expand at their periphery into flattened disc-like structures that come into close association with a non-neural type cell called the Merkel cell. The Merkel cells have a number of interdigitating processes that contact other neighbouring cells. The nerve/Merkel cell units together are called Merkel discs and are sensitive to vertical pressure. The receptors are slow adapting and transmit information via large, myelinated (Aα) afferent fibres (English 1977) (Fig. 5.9).

Krause End Bulbs   CELLS OF   **QUICK FACTS 7**

- Thermal receptors
- Ag/group III
- 10–30 m/s
- Ruffini endings
- Aa, Ab fibres, rapidly conducting
- Skin stretch

Ruffini Endings

The Ruffini system of receptors including the Ruffini endings and Ruffini nuclei are found in each and every joint complex and in the dermis of hairy skin. These receptors respond to changes in stress levels in collagen. In joint capsules they are very sensitive to capsular deformation and may be activated by changes in the degree of arc about a joint. In most cases involving peripheral joints they can detect a 1° change of arc about the joint. In the case of certain types of receptors in the upper cervical spine as little as a 0.4° change of arc has been shown to cause activation. This is probably due to the high concentration of joint receptors in the upper cervical spine region which has been shown to contain the highest concentration of joint receptors in the spine (Vele 1970). These receptors are slowly adapting and utilize large, myelinated (Aα) afferent fibres for transmission (Chambers et al 1972) (Fig. 5.9).

Joint Receptors

A complex system of specialized receptors that supply feedback concerning the static and dynamic position of joints has been described by Wyke (1966). His description involves a classification of four types of joint receptors, which are described as follows.

Type I or tonic receptors have a low threshold and are slow adapting. These receptors are active both at rest and during changes of joint arc. Thus when the joint arc changes, these receptors show an initial burst of activity and continue to fire at a reduced but specific frequency until another change in joint angle occurs. These types of receptors are multibranched, encapsulated Ruffini ending type receptors. These receptors appear to be the most abundant type of joint receptor and are most highly concentrated in the weight-bearing joints where static postural information is crucial. It is thought that the information transferred by these receptors may reach conscious perception (Skoglung 1973).

Type II joint receptors are similar to Pacinian corpuscles but much smaller in size and have a low threshold but are rapidly adapting. Their activity increases at both the initiation and cessation of movement. They are highly sensitive to movement and pressure changes in the capsule and are thought to detect duration of movement. The information from these receptors is thought not to reach conscious awareness (Skoglung 1973).

Type III receptors have a high threshold and are slowly adapting to stimuli. They are inactive in non-moving joints and fire only at extremes of joint motion. They are similar in structure to the Golgi tendon organs of tendons and cause a reflex inhibition of the homonymous muscle when highly stimulated (Williams & Warwick 1984) (Fig. 5.10).

Type IV receptors are nociceptive in function and have a high threshold and do not adapt. These types of receptors are free nerve endings that invade the synovial layers, blood vessels, and fat pads surrounding the joint and are normally inactive. They seem to be most sensitive to excessive joint movement and all causes of damaging stimuli that result in the perception of joint pain (Wyke 1966; Newton 1982; Fitz-Ritzon 1988; McLain & Picker 1998; Eriksen 2004).

This diverse variety of receptors in the joint capsule allows these receptors to supply the nervous system with a continuous input stream regarding joint position at any given moment in time. Some of the input from this system of receptors can be volitionally perceived although most of the time we are not consciously aware of the position of each of our joints (Fitz-Ritzon 1988).

Free Nerve Endings

Free nerve endings are found in all types of connective tissue including dermis, fascia, ligaments, tendon sheaths of blood vessels, meninges, joint capsules, periosteum,

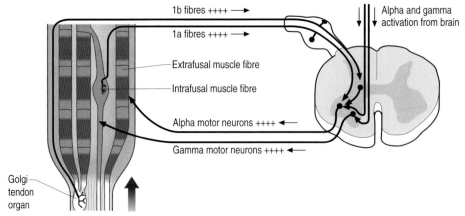

Fig. 5.10 Supraspinal modulation of reflex control. Intrafusal as well as extrafusal fibres contract; spindles activated, reinforcing contraction stimulus via Ia in accord with resistance. Tendon organ activated, causing relaxation if load is too great.

perichondrium, Haversian systems of bone, and endomysial tissue of all muscles. Nociceptive fibres may be depolarized by a number of different modalities termed nociceptive stimuli such as alterations in pH (acid or base environment), the presence of chemicals or collagenous deformation such as those associated with swelling and inflammation, heat, physical damage, and some chemicals normally contained inside of cells.

Three different types of nociceptors can be distinguished by the various stimuli to which they respond. These are mechanical, thermal, and polymodal receptor types (Gardner et al 2000). Mechanical receptors are responsive to sharp penetration of objects into the skin or tissues. They are also sensitive to pinching or squeezing actions. The axons are mechanical nociceptors, are myelinated, and thus are the fastest conducting fibres of the nociceptors receptors. Thermal receptors are excited by extremes of temperature. The two different types of thermal receptors respond to cold and heat. Polymodal receptors respond to a variety of stimuli including mechanical, chemical, and temperature extremes. These receptors evoke the sensation of deep burning pain when their activation becomes perceived consciously.

Some of the nociceptive input may reach the somatosensory cortex where it is consciously perceived most commonly as pain (Cauna 1966). Nociceptive information is conveyed from the spinal cord to the thalamus and then to the sensory cortex. The spinal tracts that convey this information to the thalamus or hypothalamus include the spinothalamic, spinoreticular, spinomesencephalic, cervicothalamic, and spinohypothalamic tracts. The most prominent nociceptive tract is the spinothalamic tract of which both anterior and lateral divisions participate in nociceptive signal transmission (Basbaum & Jessell 2000).

A good illustration of the chemical activation of nociceptors involves the build-up of lactic acid inside a working muscle. When a muscle contracts in an anaerobic environment, lactic acid is produced as a bi-product. When this substance builds to a threshold value usually due to a lack of circulation caused by sustained muscle contraction, the nociceptors fibres depolarize and fire a series of action potentials along the peripheral branch of the primary nociceptive afferent neuron's axon which arrive eventually in the dorsal horn of the spinal cord. Here the fibre synapses with a variety of cells in the interneuron pools of the substantia gelatinosa. Some of these neurons send inhibitory stimuli back to the muscle while others project via the contralateral lateral spinothalamic pathways to the ventral posterior lateral nucleus of the thalamus. Here depending on the central integrative state of the thalamus further stimuli may or may not be relayed to the somatosensory cortex where perception of the pain may occur.

Integration of Receptor Input

Natural movement is accomplished by active and passive changes in the length of muscles surrounding a joint which act to cause the desired change of arc and appropriate stabilization to allow the desired motion to occur. While this motion is occurring other changes to the joint and its surroundings are also occurring such as deformation of the joint capsule, and deformation of the skin around the joint and tensions and lengths of the homonymous and stabilizing muscles and tendons of the joint. All of these changes in collagen tension, deformation, and movement are being detected and transmitted to the spinal cord and central nervous system by the various receptors previously discussed. All of this afferent information acts to modulate the excitability of the alpha and gamma motor neurons either via segmental or suprasegmental integration.

How do We Begin to Understand the Complexity of the Integration that Must be Occurring for Even the Most Primitive Type of Movement?

At this point we will start to investigate this marvelous feat of integration with two relatively simple spinal reflexes, the deep tendon or muscle stretch reflex and the Golgi tendon inhibition reflex.

The muscle stretch reflex occurs because the group Ia (primary afferent) fibres from the muscle spindles have an overall excitatory effect on the motor neuron pools of the homonymous and heteronymous (synergistic) muscles and an overall inhibitory effect on the antagonistic motor neuron pools. The excitatory effects are produced through a number of pathways including monosynaptic and polysynaptic connections (Jankowska et al 1981). The spindle afferent fibres branch to form collateral fibres on entering the grey area of the spinal cord. Some of these fibres proceed to synapse directly on the homonymous and heteronymous alpha motor neuron pools, forming an excitatory monosynaptic connection. Other collaterals synapse on interneurons called Ia inhibitory interneurons. The spindle collaterals excite the Ia inhibitory interneuron pools that in turn cause an inhibitory stimulus to be received by the antagonist motor neuron pools. A collateral axon from the alpha motor neuron also synapses with another interneuron called a Renshaw cell that in turn inhibits both the original alpha motor neuron and the Ia interneuron. Thus the inhibitory pathway from the agonist to the antagonist is momentarily opened and that from the antagonist to the agonist is momentarily closed until the activity of the Renshaw cell returns the cycle to neutral (Crone et al 1987) (Fig. 5.10). The overall response produced by this activity of stretching the spindle fibres is an increase in the probability of both a contraction of the agonist and inhibition of the antagonist muscles surrounding the joint in question. This is the response normally observed when we strike the tendon of a muscle with a reflex hammer. The impact of the hammer results in a momentary lengthening of the spindle fibres, which sets in motion the events previously described. This sequence of events can be modulated by input from other neurons in either segmental or suprasegmental pools via presynaptic modulation at the primary afferent central process, modulation of interneuron pool central integrative states, and modulation of the alpha and gamma motor neurons directly (Pearson & Gorden 1991).

Activation of the Golgi tendon organs leads to an inhibitory stimulus at the homonymous muscle. This inhibition is accomplished through the excitation of an interneuron called a Ib inhibitory interneuron. When the afferent fibre of the Golgi tendon organ enters the grey area of the spinal cord it synapses on a Ib interneuron, which then in turn synapses on the homonymous alpha motor neuron, increasing the probability of the cell not reaching threshold. The integration of this reflex is complicated because the Ib interneuron pool also receives modulatory input from other interneuron pools that receive their stimulus from joint receptors, muscle spindles, and cutaneous skin receptors and from descending supraspinal neurons (Fig. 5.8).

Clinical Application

Activation of both of the above reflex mechanisms may be lost because of a neuropathy or dysfunction affecting the large afferent fibres. Any situations in which the motor neurons are deprived of the primary afferent loops results in abolishment of the myotactic (stretch and Golgi) reflexes (Sherrington 1906). Muscle stretch reflexes may be absent even in the presence of upper motor neuron disease, which usually manifests as a hyperactive reflex, if afferent dysfunction coexists. Examples of conditions that afferent dysfunction and upper motor neuron lesions may coexist include subacute combined degeneration and Friedreich's ataxia (Williams & Warwick 1984). Posterior root compression by extruded disc material or tumour may impair the conduction of large-diameter fibres before affecting the smaller, slower fibres. Thus stretch reflexes or vibration sense may be lost before loss of pain and temperature sensation. Other compressive or traumatic lesions of the spinal cord may abolish these reflexes by interrupting the reflex arc at the segmental root level, thus identifying the level of the lesion (Nakashima et al 1989).

References

Banks R, Barker D, Stacey MJ 1981 Structural aspects of fusimotor effects on spindle sensitivity. In: Taylor A, Prochazka A (eds) Muscle receptors and movement. Macmillian, London, p 5–16.

Basbaum A, Jessell T 2000 The perception of pain. In: Kandel E, Schwartz J, Jessell T (eds) Essentials of neural science. McGraw-Hill, New York, p 472–491.

Boyd I 1980 The isolated mammillian muscle spindle. Trends in Neuroscience 3:258–265.

Burke D 1981 The activity of human muscle spindle endings in normal motor activity. International Review of Physiology 25:91–126.

Burke D, Lance J 1992 The myotactic unit and its disorders. In: Asbury A, McKhaun, McDonald W (eds) Diseases of the nervous system: clinical neurobiology. WB Saunders, Philadelphia, p 270–284.

Cauna N 1966 Fine structure of the receptor organs and its probable functional significance. In: deReuck A, Knight J (eds) Ciba Foundation: touch, heat and pain. Churchill, London, p 117–127.

Chambers M, Andres K, von Duering M et al 1972 The structure function of the slowly adapting type II receptors in hairy skin. Quarterly Journal of Experimental Physiology and Cognate Medical Sciences 57:417–445.

Cooper S, Daniel P 1963 Muscle spindles in man: Their morphology in the lubricals and deep muscles of the neck. Brain 86:563–587.

Cram JR, Kasman GS 1998 Anatomy and physiology. In: Cram JR, Kasman GS (eds) Introduction to surface electromyography. Aspen Publishers, p 9–38.

Crone C, Hultborn H, Jespersen B et al 1987 Reciprocal Ia inhibition between the ankle flexors and extensors in man. Journal of Physiology 389:163–185.

English K 1977 The ultrastructure of cutaneous type 1 mechano-receptors in cats following denervation. Journal of Comparative Neurology 172:137–164.

Eriksen K 2004 Upper cervical neurology. In: Eriksen K (ed) Upper cervical subluxation complex: a review of the chiropractic and medical literature. Williams and Wilkins, Baltimore, p 59–74.

Fitz-Ritzon D 1988 Neuroanatomy and neurophysiology of the upper cervical spine. In: Vernon H (ed) Upper cervical sydrome. Williams and Wilkins, Baltimore, p 48–54.

Fleshman J, Munson J, Sypert GW et al 1981 Rheobase, input resistance, and motor unit type in medial gastrocnemius motor neurons of the cat. Journal of Neurophysiology 46:1326–1338.

Gardner E, Martin J, Jessell TM 2000 The bodily senses. In: Kandel E, Schwartz J, Jessell T (eds) Principles of neural science. McGraw-Hill, New York, p 430–449.

Ghez C, Gorden J 1995 Muscle and muscle receptors. In: Kandel E, Schwartz J, Jessell T (eds) Essentials of neural science and behavior. McGraw-Hill, New York, p 501–514.

Gray J, Sato M 1953 Properties of receptor potentials in Pacinian corpuscles. Journal of Physiology 122:610–636.

Houk JC, Crago PE, Rymer WZ 1991 Functional properties of Golgi tendon organs. In: Desmedt IE (ed) Progress in clinical neurophysiology. Karger, Basel, vol 8, p 33–43.

Hunt C 1974 The physiology of muscle receptors. In: Hunt C (ed) Handbook of sensory physiology. Springer-Verlag, Berlin, vol 3, p 191–234.

Jankowska E, McCrea D, Mackel R 1981 Oligosynaptic excitation of motor neurons by impulses in group Ia muscle spindle afferents in the cat. Journal of Physiology 316:411–425.

Kulkarni V, Chandy M, Babu KS 2001 Quantitative study of the muscle spindles in suboccipital muscles of human foetuses. Neurology India 49(4):355–359.

McLain R, Picker J 1998 Mechanoreceptor endings in human thoracic and lumbar facet joints. Spine 23(2):168–173.

Martin J, Jessell T (1995) The sensory systems. In: Kandel E, Schwartz J, Jessell T (eds) Essentials of neural science and behaviour. McGraw-Hill, New York, p 369–387.

Matthews P 1972 Mammillian muscle receptors and their control actions. Arnold, London.

Matthews P 1981 Evolving views on the internal operation and functional role of the muscle spindle. Journal of Physiology 320:1–30.

Milburn A 1973 The early development of muscle spindles in the rat. Journal of Cellular Science 12:175–195.

Nakashima K, Rothwell J, Day BL et al 1989 Reciprocal inhibition between forearm muscles in patients with writers cramp and other occupational cramps, symptomatic hemidystonia and hemipareis due to stroke. Brain 112:681–697.

Newton RA 1982 Joint receptor contributions to reflexive and kinesthetic response. Physical Therapy 62:22–29.

Pearson K, Gorden J 1991 Spinal reflexes. In: Kandel E, Schwartz J, Jessell T (eds) Principles of neural science. McGraw-Hill, New York.

Schoultz T, Swett J 1974 Ultrastructural organisation of the sensory fibres innervating the Golgi tendon organs. The Anatomical Record 179:147–162.

Schwartz J 1995 The neuron. In: Kandel E, Schwartz J, Jessell T (eds) Essentials of neural science and behavior. McGraw-Hill, New York, p 45–55.

Sherrington C 1906 Integrative actions of the nervous system. Yale University Press, New Haven, CT.

Skoglung S 1973 Joint receptors and kinaesthesis. In: Iggo A (ed) Handbook of sensory physiology. Springer-Verlag, Berlin.

Vele F 1970 The origin of proprioceptive information in the Zygapophyseal joints and the processing of their afferences. In: Wolff H (ed) Manual medicine. McGraw-Hill, New York, p 78–83.

Williams PL, Warwick R 1984 Sensory receptors. In: Gray's anatomy. Churchill-Livingston, Edinburgh, p 849–860.

Wyke B 1966 The neurology of joints. Proceedings of the Royal College of Surgeons of England.

Yochum T, Rowe L 1996 Neurotropic arthropathies. In: Yochum T, Rowe L (eds) Essentials of skeletal radiology. . Williams and Wilkins, Baltimore, vol 2, p 842–850.

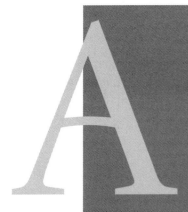

Clinical Cases Answers

Case 5.1

5.1.1 This man has most probably suffered an intervertebral disc protrusion or herniation at the L5 disc. Damage to the disc such as this commonly occurs when twisting or bending occurs while lifting an object. This protrusion has resulted in an increased pressure on the S1 nerve root as it exits the spinal cord, resulting in local inflammation and muscle guarding as well as dysfunction of the nerve itself.

5.1.2 The loss of reflex activity is most probably due to a reduction or loss of the afferent portion of the reflex arc mainly arising from the muscle spindles of the gastrocnemius muscle due to damage to the S1 nerve afferent fibres. When any portion of the reflex loop is lost or dysfunctional the reflex will be diminished or lost.

5.1.3 The large-diameter fast conduction fibres are the most greatly affected by increasing pressure on a nerve. These are the same type of fibres that transmit vibration stimulus. Remember that most encapsulated receptors are sensitive to vibration but the Pacinian corpuscles are particularly sensitive to vibration. This also explains how a patient can have a loss of vibration sense but still feel pain, which is transmitted via the small, unmyelinated, C fibres, which are not as sensitive to pressure as the large, myelinated fibres.

5.1.4 The standard imaging requested for this patient should include anterior to posterior (AP), lateral (LAT) lumbosacral radiographs followed by lumbosacral MRI. While it is true that disc protrusions rarely manifest on plain film radiographs they are useful in ruling out other causes such as fracture, dislocation, or unexpected pathologies.

Case 5.2

5.2.1 Neurotrophic arthropathy, osteoarthritis, fracture/dislocation/sprain, infection, vascular pathology.

5.2.2 Each individual modality must be tested separately: dermatomal distribution of pain, light touch, temperature. Vibration and proprioception of the joints below the knee must also be evaluated.

5.2.3 In diabetic patients a neurotrophic cause to their symptoms must always be considered. In this case the neurotrophic degeneration of the afferent nerve fibres from the muscle spindles and joint receptors of the knee has resulted in a loss of the deep tendon reflex and all other sensations including pain and proprioception.

5.2.4 Loss of proprioception, pain, and other modalities from the knee joint has resulted in a continued dysfunction of motion in the joint, resulting in excessive destruction of the joint's structure. Neurological signs such as altered gait, loss of deep tendon reflexes, and loss of pain sensation should alert you to the possibility of a neurotrophic or Charcot's joint (Yochum & Rowe 1996).

Neuronal Integration and Movement

Clinical Cases for Thought

Case 6.1   A 46-year-old male presents with chronic low back pain. He has had this chronic pain for the past 5 years following a motorcycle crash. Recently he has found that his activity level has been slowly decreasing because of the pain and discomfort of his injury. He has also noticed a definite decline in his motivation to take part in activities that he once greatly enjoyed.

Questions

6.1.1   What neurological structures are involved in the creation of motivation to move?

6.1.2   How is this thought process transformed into mechanical movement of muscles?

6.1.3   Based on neural pathways and integrative circuits what theory can be formed connecting his declining activity level and his lack of motivation?

Case 6.2   A 78-year-old woman presents following a stroke involving a branch of her anterior spinal artery. What clinical findings would you expect to find in each of the following?

Questions

6.2.1   The stroke involved the inhibitory interneurons of the ventral horn.

6.2.2   The stroke involved the alpha motor neurons of the ventral horn.

Case 6.3   What clinical picture would one expect to find in a patient with each of the following?

Questions

6.3.1   A dysfunction of the corticopontocerebellar thalamic loop.

6.3.2   A dysfunction of the corticostriatal thalamic loop.

Introduction

Human motion is a miraculously complex interaction of a multitude of neuronal circuits. The control and integration of these complex interactions are investigated in this chapter by breaking down and analysing the components of a simple human movement, that of reaching for and pinch-grasping an object between the thumb and first finger.

Many questions immediately spring to mind such as what motivated him or her to reach out and grasp the object in the first place. Was it hunger? Was it curiosity? Was it habit? How did the message of wanting to grasp the object find its way to producing the muscular contractions, co-contractions, and inhibition necessary to actually performing the function? These are perplexing questions and indeed the answers to these questions for the most part remain cloaked in mystery and complexity of the human nervous system. However, this mysterious cloak of secrecy is slowly but surely being unravelled and maybe one day someone will be able to answer these questions without the slightest hesitancy or uncertainty that his/her story is the right one. Until then we tell the story of our time and understanding which has almost as many endings as storytellers. Our story begins with the limbic system and motivation, travels through the hierarchies of the cortex, thalamus, cerebellum, and brainstem and ends with the final common pathways of the alpha motor neurons of the spinal cord.

Postures and Movements are Controlled by a Hierarchy of Systems

Postures and movements are controlled simultaneously by different levels of nervous organization including the cortex (cognitive control), the sensory system (sensory control), and the emotional system (emotive control). These levels of the organization first suggested by Jackson are classified into a vague three-tier system.

The highest levels of cognition are concerned with the relevance and importance of the task to the present situation. This analysis seems to occur prior to communicating with the lower levels of the hierarchy. The 'cognitive 'component is composed of sensory, motor, and associative systems and the 'emotive' component is largely composed of limbic circuits (Fig. 6.1).

Limbic and Hypothalamic Involvement in Movement

The limbic system has been traditionally described as involving a complex network of neural circuitry composed of the parahippocampal gyrus, the cingulated gyrus, the subcallosal gyrus (which is the anterior and inferior continuation of the cingulate gyrus),

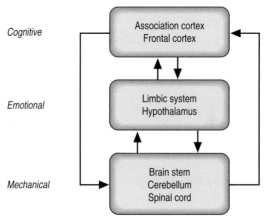

Fig. 6.1 Jackson's hierarchy of movement. The relationships of the emotional, cognitive, and mechanical components of Jackson's hierarchy of movement to the physical locations of the neuraxis thought to be involved are outlined. Note that although the different parts of the system are diagrammatically segregated into components, all components of the system are interconnected, and functionally act as a unit.

the hippocampal formation (which includes the hippocampus proper, the dentate gyrus, and the subiculum), various nuclei of the septal region, the nucleus accumbens (which is an extension of the caudate nucleus), neocortical areas such as the orbital frontal cortex, subcortical structures such as the amygdala, and various nuclei of the hypothalamus (Iversen et al 2000) (Fig. 6.2).

The hypothalamus contributes to limbic system function primarily through controlling influences on the pituitary gland. Neurons in the medial basal region of the hypothalamus release peptide neurohormones that act as stimulators or releasing factors that act on the cells of the anterior pituitary gland or adenohypophysis. The pituitary cells then release a variety of hormones including luteinizing hormone (LH), the growth hormone (GH) somatotrophin, adrenocorticotrophic hormone (ACTH), thyroid stimulating hormone (TSH), follicle-stimulating hormone (FSH), and prolactin. Axons of neurons in the supraoptic and paraventricular nuclei release the neurohormone oxytocin and the antidiuretic hormone vasopressin (Fig. 6.3).

The hypothalamus also functions as a communication relay by funnelling information from the cortex via the cingulate gyrus, to the hippocampal formation, where the information is processed and reciprocally fed back to the cingulate gyrus via the mammillary bodies and anterior thalamic nuclei.

Neurons in a variety of hypothalamic nuclei also project to the intramedial lateral (IML) cell columns of the spinal cord grey regions where they modulate the activity of the pre-ganglionic neurons of the sympathetic nervous system, which control a variety of functions including blood flow to virtually all areas of the body. This pathway is important in modulating blood flow to various muscle groups and organs including the brain, prior to and during movement. The control of the blood flow to the hypothalamus arises from post-ganglionic sympathetic neurons located in the superior cervical ganglion, which are under the influence of the hypothalamus itself (Fig. 6.4).

The Development of Motivational Drives

The limbic system is deeply involved in the creation of motivational states or drives that modulate the central integrative states of neurons in wide-ranging areas of the central nervous system (CNS) that produce a variety of behavioural responses such as movement, temperature regulation, active procurement of food, sexual drive, emotional context, and curiosity (Swanson & Mogenson 1981; Brooks 1984; Kupfermann et al 2000).

Motivational drives produced in the limbic system appear to be the products of integrated sensory and emotional cues, which have been triaged into some order of importance that result in the activation of the appropriate areas of cortex to a readiness or activation mode. Thus, through motivational activation from the limbic system the appropriate areas of cortex increase their central integrative state to a state of awareness

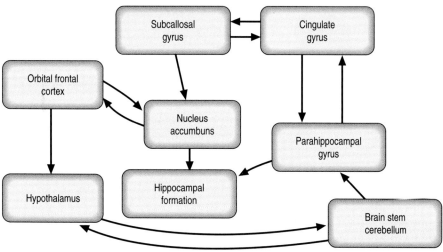

Fig. 6.2 Traditional limbic structures. The traditional components of the limbic system and the projections thought to exist between the anatomical components are illustrated. The projections shown are probably incomplete as the limbic system, like most other functional neural circuits, functions as a unit, utilizing a variety of components simultaneously or independently as necessary.

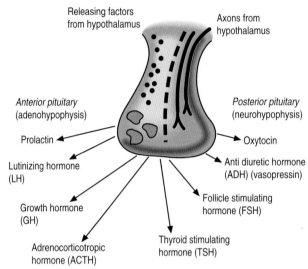

Fig. 6.3 Hormones of the pituitary gland. The relationship between the hypothalamus, the pituitary gland, and the hormones secreted from the pituitary gland is illustrated. The pituitary gland is often referred to as the 'master gland' of the endocrine system because it coordinates many functions of the other glands. The endocrine system itself consists of a group of organs whose main function is to produce and secrete hormones directly into the blood that act to control a variety of functions all over the body. The major organs of the endocrine system are the hypothalamus, the pituitary gland, the thyroid gland, the parathyroid glands, the islets cells (Beta cells) of the pancreas, the adrenal glands, the testes, and the ovaries. The hypothalamus releases messengers that act as releasing or stimulating agents on the pituitary as well as inhibiting factors that inhibit the activation or release of certain hormones of the pituitary. Not all endocrine glands are under the sole control of the pituitary. Some glands such as the insulin-secreting (Beta) cells of the pancreas also respond to local levels of glucose and fatty acids; the parathyroid glands also respond to local concentrations of calcium and phosphate in the blood; and the adrenal medulla or the adrenaline-producing cells of the adrenal glands also respond to direct stimulation from the sympathetic nervous system.

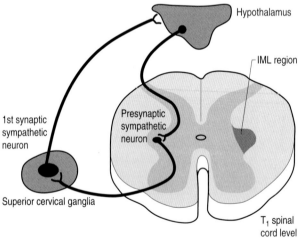

Fig. 6.4 Control of blood flow to the hypothalamus. The cells of the hypothalamus project directly to the presynaptic sympathetic neurons in the intermediolateral (IML) cell column of the spinal cord. These neurons project to the postsynaptic cells of the sympathetic system located in the superior cervical ganglia. The axons of these neurons follow a variety of blood vessels into the skull and innervate the blood vessels supplying the hypothalamus.

looking for something about to happen such as a change in posture or a change of emotional state.

The transition from motivation to the initiation of movement involves pathways from multiple premotor regions of the cortex to the motor regions of cortex.

The majority of the neurons in the inferior and posterior regions of the intraparietal sulcus (Brodmann area 7) show an early response to sensory cues that relate to the execution of movement (Mountcastle et al 1975). Smaller numbers of neurons in area 7 exhibited more complex response patterns, where activation only occurred in specific

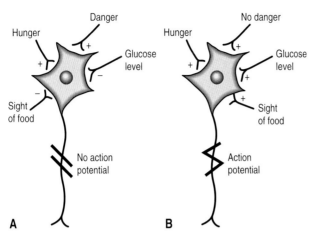

Fig. 6.5 Complex stimulus firing patterns demanded by some neurons before firing. (A) Although hunger stimulus is firing on this neuron, either other inputs are not sufficient to stimulate an action potential or they are inhibitory to the formation of an action potential threshold stimulus. No action potential is generated. (B) All conditions are met in this neuron and an action potential fires.

situations where a number of variables were met simultaneously, e.g. sight of food and the presence of hunger (Fig. 6.5).

This type of processing suggests that motivational drives received from the limbic system are not blindly obeyed but are first presented to the association areas of premotor and parietal cortex, where a rudimentary form of judgment as to the appropriateness of the behaviour required is made.

Corticoneostriatal and Corticopontine Projections

The judgment system seems to consist of a series of complex gate systems of 'and' or 'or' gates that are both involved directly in gating inputs and are indirectly gated themselves by being involved in the more complex array of interactions involved in the complete execution command required. This complex array of gated pathways in the association cortex projects directly to the motor cortex via association fibres as well as to the striatum and pontine nuclei. These projections to the striatum and pontine nuclei further project to other areas of the nervous system and form indirect pathway projection loops from the association cortex to the motor cortex (Rolls 1983; deZeeuw et al 1997).

The first indirect projection loop involves the striatum (caudate nucleus and putamen), whose output nuclei the globus pallidus pars interna projects through the anterior division of the thalamic fasciculus to the pars oralis area of the ventral lateral and ventral anterior thalamic nuclei. Neurons of the ventral lateral thalamic nuclei project their axons to the ipsilateral motor, premotor, and parietal cortical areas (Fig. 6.6).

The second indirect projection loop involves projections to the ipsilateral pontine nuclei via the corticopontine projection fibres, which in turn project to two output nuclei of the contralateral cerebellum via the pontocerebellar fibre system. These deep cerebellar nuclei, the dentate, and the interposed nuclei (emboliform and globose nuclei) then project to the contralateral pars caudalis area of the ventrolateral thalamic nuclei via the posterior division of the thalamic fasciculus. Neurons of the ventrolateral thalamic nuclei project their axons to the ipsilateral motor, premotor, and parietal cortical areas (Fig. 6.7).

To further complicate matters, the major indirect pathways from the premotor to the motor cortex involving the basal ganglionic and pontine-cerebellar loops are not equivalent in the cerebral cortical areas from which they receive inputs nor the projections to the cortex that arise from them.

The Basal Ganglionic Loops

The basal ganglionic loops involve two distinct pathways. The first involves input pathways to the caudate nucleus (Fig. 6.6); the second involves input pathways through the putamen (Fig. 6.7). For instance, the caudate nuclei receive inputs from many areas of

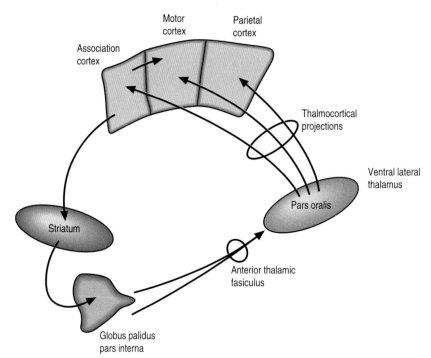

Fig. 6.6 The first indirect corticostriatal–thalamocortical loop.

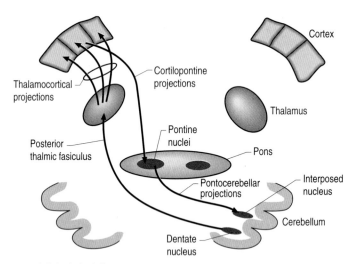

Fig. 6.7 Corticopontocerebellulo-thalamic loop.

cortex including the association regions of the frontal, parietal, and temporal lobes. Most of the afferent or return projections from this loop arise from the globus pallidus pars interna of the basal ganglia and project to the ventral anterior nuclei of the thalamus. Neurons in the ventral anterior nuclei of the thalamus project to the premotor cortex (Brodmann area 6).

The second pathway of the basal ganglionic loop involving the putamen receives the majority of its input from the sensorimotor cortex (Brodmann areas 3, 2, 1, and 5) and projects via the globus pallidus pars interna to the ventrolateral nuclear group of the thalamus. The ventrolateral group of thalamic neurons then project to premotor areas including Brodmann area 6 (Delong et al 1983). This projection loop is very important for basal ganglionic modulation of motor cortical output since the basal ganglia do not possess direct projections from the thalamus to primary motor cortex (Schell & Strick 1984).

The pontine and cerebellar loops receive the majority of their inputs from the primary motor (area 5), somatosensory areas (areas 4, 3, 2, and 1), and some input from association and visual areas (areas 17 and 18). Very little input to the pontine and cerebellar loops comes from high-level association areas (Rolls 1983).

The Thalamocortical Projections

All of the indirect loops described above contain reciprocal innervation pathways above the thalamus (thalamus to cortex, cortex to thalamus) and only unidirectional pathways below the thalamus (basal ganglia to thalamus, pontine nuclei to thalamus) (Sherman & Guillery 2001) (Fig. 6.8). In fact, the thalmocortical projections form a loop in which the 'feedforward' portion is part of the classic pathway relaying sensory information to the cortex and the 'feedback' portion is composed of cortical control or modulation over thalamic operation. This feedback control can be either excitatory or inhibitory depending on the central integrative state of the cortex and is modulated itself by sensory input from the thalamus (Llinas 1991; Destexhe 2000). This results in a variety of intrinsic thalamocortical and corticothalamic oscillations that can be observed via electroencephalograph (EEG) and qualitative electroencephalograph (qEEG) recordings over the cortex (Destexhe & Sejnowski 2003).

A Brief Summary Thus Far

To summarize thus far using our example of a pinch grasp of an object between the finger and thumb, the neural activity involved depends on the motivation for the movement in the first place. Is the object food and is the subject hungry? Is the subject just curious as to what the object is? The pathways through which movement is initiated depend on a number of variables such as prelearning of movement components, the relevance and importance of the movement at the time, and whether a variety of movement choices must be considered. Once initiated the plastic nature of the system provides a multitract system (basal ganglionic and pontine/cerebellar) which can consider a multitude of physical variables as well as the initial motivation in order to complete the desired movement.

Once the 'what am I going to do' instructions have been established, integrated, and weighed with respect to relevance and appropriateness by the limbic system and high-level association cortex, the high-level areas of the hierarchy, the neural information is transferred to the middle layers of the hierarchy which involves the creation of the 'how am I going to do it' outflow.

Formulation of the 'how to' instructions involves the premotor cortex (area 6), which acts as an organizer for the principal output area, the primary motor cortex (area 4) (Brooks & Thach 1981).

Instructions for acts of different complexity enter the middle-level areas via separate routes. For example, motor programmes for complex movement patterns enter from the

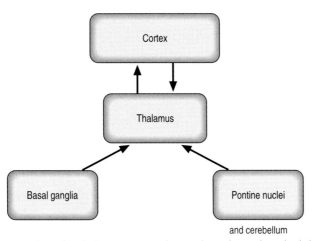

Fig. 6.8 All of the indirect loops described contain reciprocal innervation pathways above the thalamus (thalamus to cortex, cortex to thalamus) and only unidirectional pathways below the thalamus (basal ganglia to thalamus, pontine nuclei to thalamus).

caudate circuit of the basal ganglia, whereas instructions for less complex actions enter the premotor area via the putamen circuit of the basal ganglia as well as the lateral cerebellum pontine nuclei circuit (Brooks 1984).

Changes in neuron potentials have been recorded over the motor cortex 800 ms before the onset of voluntary movement (Krakauer & Ghez 2000). In this period before the onset of movement the higher centres seem to be presetting the neuron response patterns in relation to the specific preset programmes that specify the intended movement. The set of preset programmes that describe a specific movement are referred to as a motor set.

Thus, the various levels of instruction from the basal ganglia, the cerebellum, and transcortical input from association areas integrate to prepare the motor cortex prior to the initiation of movement to ensure the correct motor sets will be initiated at the right time and in the right sequence.

Output Commands from the Motor Cortex

The output instructions from the motor cortex are relayed through two different component systems. The first component arises from the postcentral cortical areas and projects through the pyramidal and extrapyramidal pathways to areas in the dorsal grey matter of the spinal cord where modulation of the central integrative state of spinal dorsal horn cells takes place. The second component is the slower precentral system, which modulates the central integrative state of alpha motor neurons in the anterior horn of the grey matter via the axons of the corticospinal tracts (Brooks 1984).

The organization of the neurons in the cortex of area 4 is somatotopic due to the extensive and specific synapses formed on the spinal motor neurons via the corticospinal tracts. This somatotopic representation is known as the motor homunculus of man (Fig. 6.9). Neurons in the somatosensory cortex receive information in a somatotopic array called the sensory homunculus of man (Fig. 6.10).

The neurons of the motor cortex are grouped into arrays of perpendicular columns called cortical efferent zones or motor columns. Axons from the thalamus and other cortical areas terminate in the superficial layers of the cortical efferent zones by synapsing with dendrites of the pyramidal neurons and on a wide variety of cortical interneurons. These interneurons then send impulses in a cascading fashion to other interneurons

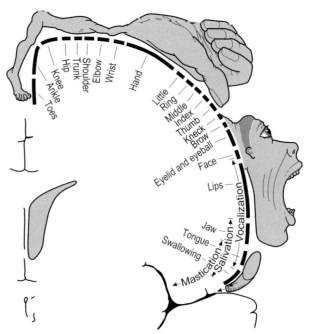

Fig. 6.9 The motor homunculus. The *motor homunculus* showing proportional somatotopical representation in the main cortical area. (After W. Penfield and T. Rasmussen, *The Cerebral Cortex of Man*, Macmillan, 1950.)

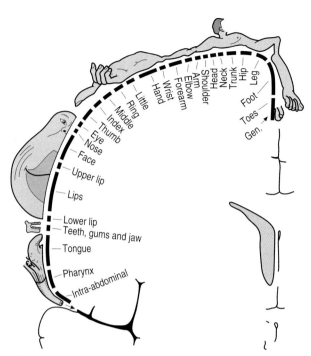

Fig. 6.10 The sensory homunculus. The *sensory homunculus* showing proportional somatotopical representation in the somesthetic cortex. (After W. Penfield and T. Rasmussen, *The Cerebral Cortex of Man*, Macmillan, 1950.)

radially down the cortical columns where they finally reach the pyramidal and large pyramidal neurons. The pyramidal neurons have different adaptation patterns which seem to depend on the diameter of their axons. Pyramidal neurons with larger diameter axons tend to fire when transient high frequency input is received and adapt very quickly to this stimulus, whereas smaller diameter axons respond to low frequency input and adapt slowly (Krakauer & Ghez 2000).

How Do Pyramid Cells Fire to Produce Complex Movements Such as a Pinch Grasp?

Most probably, cortical motor columns are directionally oriented so that increasing the central integrative state (CIS) results in an increased probability that the preferential direction represented by the column will be reproduced by the somatotopic corticospinal projections to the appropriate motor neurons. When a particular movement direction is desired, the firing frequency in the appropriate cortical column which represents the desired direction increases. Interneurons contained within the desired cortical column that project to antagonist motor columns are also brought to threshold and fire inhibitory barrages. Individual neurons do not seem to encode direction individually but require a population of neurons firing in a coordinated fashion to generate a desired directional movement. The end result of this activity is that the alpha motor neurons in the spinal cord that represent the desired direction have an increased probability of reaching activation threshold and those representing the opposite direction have a decreased probability of reaching activation threshold. The corticospinal tract is only one of several tracts that synaptically modulate the alpha motor neurons to determine their CIS. It may be recalled that dorsal root ganglion cells arising from the tendons and the muscle spindles also project either directly or indirectly to modulate the CIS of the alpha motor neurons, as do neurons in the reticular formation and vestibular areas. It has been estimated that approximately 10,000 synapses, some inhibitory and some excitatory, converge onto each alpha motor neuron. The cumulative effect of all of this synaptic activity largely determines the CIS of the neuron at any given moment. Other factors influencing the CIS include the nutritional, biochemical, and oxygen status of the neuron.

The timing and the pattern of activation of the desired muscles during movement are largely controlled by the cerebellum.

Timing and Pattern Control of Movement Involves the Cerebellum

The cerebellum receives input from all areas of motor and association cortex via corticoponto and corticoolivary tract projections. The inferior olivary nucleus receives input from the midbrain reticular neurons and the cortex as well as feedback information from the muscle spindle organs. This type of input information allows the cerebellum to act as a comparator centre where comparisons between commands sent and action produced by the muscles can be evaluated and corrected while still in motion if necessary. The cerebellum also contributes in the control of the initiation, trajectory correction following perturbation, and the stopping or braking of movement.

The Fine Tuning of Motor Control and the Basal Ganglia

The basal ganglia are a group of nuclei situated deep in the brain at the junction of telencephalic and diencephalic functional areas. These nuclei include the caudate and putamen, which are composed of similar cell types and fused anteriorly, the globus pallidus, the subthalamic nuclei, and the substantia nigra (Anderson et al 2003). All input to the basal ganglia projects onto either the caudate nucleus or the putamen. The input arises from four main areas which include wide areas of motor and association cortex, the midline intralaminar thalamic nuclei, the zona compacta of the substantia nigra, and the raphe nuclei of the midbrain. The basal ganglia do not project directly to neurons that would allow them to effect control of motor activity but seems to act in a coordination role between the cortex and the thalamus by filtering or gating the information stream that the thalamus receives from the periphery (Fig. 6.11). The basal ganglia are also involved in the coordination of movement necessary in the maintenance of static postures and the initiation of controlled or detailed movements (Martin 1967; Kornhuber 1971).

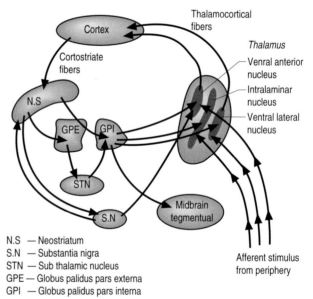

N.S — Neostriatum
S.N — Substantia nigra
STN — Sub thalamic nucleus
GPE — Globus palidus pars externa
GPI — Globus palidus pars interna

Fig. 6.11 Diagram outlining the gating action of the basal ganglia on the thalamus. There are two predominant pathways (direct and indirect) from the neostriatum to the output nuclei of the basal ganglia, the globus pallidus pars internus (GPi) and the substantia nigra pars reticulate (SN). The direct pathway involves the neostriatal projections to the GPi, which in turn projects to the thalamic nuclei. The indirect pathway involves the neostriatal projections to the globus pallidus pars externus (GPe). The GPe then projects to the subthalamic nuclei, which in turn projects to the GPi. The GPi then completes the loop to the thalamus. Because of the different neurotransmitters released through the loops they each result in a different modulatory activity on the thalamus (see Chapter 11).

The Final Common Pathway and Supraspinal Modulation

All of the processing, integration, and complex decision making involved in movement generation and control by the higher centres is finally conveyed to the final common pathway known as the alpha motor neurons.

Supraspinal pathways descend in two major groups, the ventromedial group of axons and the lateral group of axons. The ventromedial group arises from nuclei in the brainstem and descends in the ipsilateral ventral funiculi of the spinal cord and mainly terminates on the medial motor neurons, the interneurons, and propriospinal neurons of the intermediate zone of the spinal cord grey matter. These pathways express the general characteristic of functional divergence of their nerve terminals, giving off many collateral axons and innervating wide-ranging areas. This type of distribution is best suited for the control of a variety of synergistic muscular activities like those involved in postural or strut stabilization roles rather than finely controlled movements. These pathways involve the tectospinal, pontoreticulospinal, medullary reticulospinal, and the lateral and medial vestibulospinal tracts.

The second group of pathways arises from neurons in the cortex and the red nucleus and descends in the contralateral lateral funiculi of the white matter. These axons terminate in the intermediate zone of grey matter and on the motor neurons innervating the more distal muscles. The tracts of this group include the lateral corticospinal tract and the rubrospinal tract. The corticospinal tracts arise from the pyramidal neurons of the sensory–motor cortex and are characteristically focused on a small number of muscle groups and are thus suited for delicate fine movement control. Another pathway that arises from the pyramidal neurons in the motor cortex descends ipsilaterally in the ventromedial area and is called the ventral corticospinal tract. This tract is mostly involved in intricate control of postural muscles of the spinal column (Fig. 6.12).

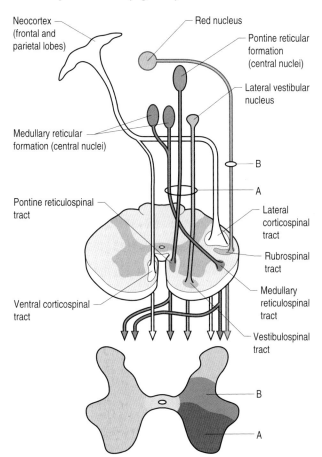

Fig. 6.12 Major brainstem descending pathways concerned with the control of movement in the human (groups A and B) and their spinal terminations.

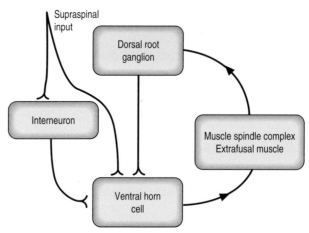

Fig. 6.13 Feedback loop of the motor servo.

In order for meaningful supraspinal coordination of movement to occur the intention command and the actual movement performed must be compared and evaluated for accuracy. This is accomplished via feedforward activation, collateral activation, and feedback mechanisms. This requires that both output information and feedback information are accurate and quickly corrected when they are not accurate. Correction of variances between the command and the actual performance is initially evaluated by a mechanism referred to as the motor servo loop. This loop involves feedback from the muscle spindle via the dorsal root ganglion cell to the alpha motor neuron innervating the same muscle. The muscle servo loop is usually self-correcting but is under the modulatory control of supraspinal neurons, which can alter the balance of the servo loop in either direction (Fig. 6.13).

Another influence of supraspinal control of movement is the coordination of alpha–gamma co-activation of muscle groups whose actions oppose one another and to muscle groups providing supportive roles in the movement. This requires instructions to both the agonist and antagonist muscles as well as to the appropriate strut stabilizing muscles that will act to provide a stable foundation from which the desired contractions can occur.

Summary

Movement involves the enlistment and activation of an amazingly complex sequence of events.

The motivation to move is established by internal interpretations of external stimuli that may involve accessing memory areas to recall the outcome of past performance in similar situations and a decision whether to move is determined. Next the plan or strategy which specifies the 'when', 'where', and 'how' of the movement is conceived. The necessary information is then integrated into packages of motor sets that will result in the completion of the desired movement and these cascades of neural activation alter the CIS of the alpha motor neurons in such a way that the neurons are activated or inhibited in the appropriate sequences that cause the movement to be accomplished. The spinal servomechanisms as well as the supraspinal motor centres monitor the progress of the movement based on the feedback received from a vast array of peripheral receptors, making corrections in the CIS of the appropriate ventral horn cells if necessary. Throughout the entire process the nutritional and oxygen demands of the neurons involved must also be monitored, adapted, and maintained to ensure adequate adenosine triphosphate (ATP) supplies are available to fuel the process.

References

Anderson ME, Postupna N, Ruffo M 2003 Effects of high-frequency stimulation in the internal globus pallidus on the activity of thalamic neurons in the awake monkey. Journal of Neurophysiology 89:1150–1160.

Brooks VB 1984 The neural basis of motor control. Oxford University Press, Oxford.

Brooks VB, Thach WT 1981 Cerebellar control of posture and movement. In: Brooks VB (ed) The handbook of physiology, section 1: the nervous system, vol ii: motor control, part 2. American Physiological Society, Bethesda, MD, p 877–946.

DeLong MR, Georgopoulos AP, Crutcher MD 1983 Cortico-basal ganglia relations and coding of motor performance. In: Massion J, Paillard J, Schultz W (eds) Neural coding of motor performance, Experimental Brain Research Supplement. Springer, Berlin, vol 7, p 30–40.

Destexhe A 2000 Modeling corticothalmic feedback and gating of the thalamus by the cerebral cortex. Journal of Physiology 94:391–410.

Destexhe A, Sejnowski TJ 2003 Interactions between membrane conductances underlying thalamocortical slow wave oscillations. Physiological Reviews 83:1401–1453.

deZeeuw CI, Strata P, Voogd J (eds)1997 The cerebellum: from structure to control. Progress in Brain Research, Elsevier, New York.

Iversen S, Kupferman I, Kandel E 2000 Emotional states and feelings. In: Kandel E, Schwartz J, Jessell T (eds) Principles of neural science, 4th edn. McGraw-Hill, New York.

Kornhuber H 1971 Motor functions of the cerebellum and basal ganglia; the cerebellocortical saccadic ballistic clock, and the basal ganglia as a ramp generator. Kybernetic 8:157–162.

Krakauer J, Ghez C 2000 Voluntary movement. In: Kandel E, Schwartz J, Jessell T (eds) Principles of neural science, 4th edn. McGraw-Hill, New York.

Kupfermann I, Kandel E, Iversen S 2000 Motivational and addictive states. In: Kandel E, Schwartz J, Jessell T (eds) Principles of neural science. McGraw-Hill, New York.

Llinas RR 1991 Of dreaming and wakefulness. Neuroscience 44:521–535.

Martin JP 1967 The basal ganglia and posture. Pitman Medical, London, p 1–152.

Mountcastle VB, Lynch JC, Georgopoulos A et al 1975 Posterior parietal association cortex of the monkey: command functions for operating in extra space. Journal of Neurophysiology 38:871–908.

Rolls ET 1983 The initiation of movements. In: Massion J, Paillard J, Schultz W et al (eds) Neural coding of motor performance, Experimental Brain Research Supplement. Springer, Berlin, vol 7, p 97–113.

Schell GR, Strick PL 1984 The origin of thalamic inputs to the arcuate premotor and supplementary motor area. Journal of Neurological Science 4:539–560.

Sherman SM, Guillery RW 2001 Exploring the thalamus. Academic Press, New York.

Swanson LW, Mogenson GJ 1981 Neural mechanisms for the functional coupling of autonomic, endocrine and somatomotor responses in adaptive behavior. Brain Research 3:1–34.

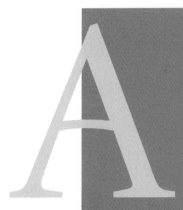

Clinical Case Answers

Case 6.1

6.1.1　The limbic system is deeply involved in the creation of motivational states or drives that modulate the central integrative states of neurons in wide-ranging areas of the CNS that produce a variety of behavioural responses such as movement, temperature regulation, active procurement of food, sexual drive, emotional context, and curiosity.

　　Motivational drives produced in the limbic system appear to be the products of integrated sensory and emotional cues, which have been triaged into some order of importance that result in the activation of the appropriate areas of cortex to a readiness or activation mode. Thus, through motivational activation from the limbic system the appropriate areas of cortex increase their central integrative state to a state of awareness looking for something about to happen such as a change in posture or a change of emotional state.

6.1.2　The transition from motivation to the initiation of movement involves pathways from multiple premotor regions of the cortex to the motor regions of cortex. All of the processing, integration, and complex decision making involved in movement generation and control by the higher centres is finally conveyed to the final common pathway known as the alpha motor neurons.

　　Supraspinal pathways descend in two major groups, the ventromedial group of axons and the lateral group of axon. The ventromedial group arises from nuclei in the brainstem and descends in the ipsilateral ventral funiculi of the spinal cord and mainly terminates on the medial motor neurons, the interneurons, and propriospinal neurons of the intermediate zone of the spinal cord grey matter. The second group of pathways arises from neurons in the cortex and the red nucleus and descends in the contralateral lateral funiculi of the white matter. These axons terminate in the intermediate zone of grey matter and on the motor neurons innervating the more distal muscles. The tracts of this group include the lateral corticospinal tract and the rubrospinal tract. In order for meaningful supraspinal coordination of movement to occur the intention command and the actual movement performed must be compared and evaluated for accuracy. This is accomplished via feedforward activation, collateral activation, and feedback mechanisms. This requires that both output information and feedback information are accurate and quickly corrected when they are not accurate. Correction of variances between the command and the actual performance is initially evaluated by a mechanism referred to as the motor servo loop. This loop involves feedback from the muscle spindle via the dorsal root ganglion cell to the alpha motor neuron innervating the same muscle. The muscle servo loop is usually self-correcting but is under the modulatory control of supraspinal neurons, which can alter the balance of the servo loop in either direction.

6.1.3　Activation levels in one area of the cortex may influence activity levels in other areas of the cortex. Depression may result from a decreased activation of frontal cortical areas that result in a decreased activation of the motor cortex and association cortex of the frontal lobes. Further to this theory a decrease in limbic activation may decrease the drive to move which would also decrease the activation level in the motor cortical circuits.

Case 6.2

6.2.1   A stroke involving the inhibitory interneurons of the ventral horn would most likely result in overactivation of the ventral motor neurons and a hyperkinetic or hypertonic disorder.

6.2.2   A stroke involving the ventral horn motor neurons would most probably result in a decrease in motor activity or hypotonia.

Case 6.3

6.3.1   A person with disruption of the corticopontocerebello-thalamic circuit would most probably display uncoordinated motor activity characterized by dysmetria due to a decrease in cerebellar input to movement commands.

6.3.2   A dysfunction of the corticostriatal thalamic loop would most likely result in a movement disorder similar to Parkinson's or Huntington's disease, depending on what type of dysfunction was present.

Chapter

7

The Spinal Cord and Peripheral Nerves

Clinical Cases for Thought

Case 7.1   An 8-year-old girl presents with right leg pain following a softball game where she received a line drive to the shin 4 months previous to presentation. The child now complains of shin and ankle pain and will not bear weight on the right leg. The leg is cold to the touch and demonstrates marked dermatographia on examination. Previously taken radiographs of the knee, shin, and ankle are negative.

Questions

7.1.1   Describe the neural pathways involved in transmitting this girl's pain from her leg to her brain.

7.1.2   Suggest a list of at least five differential diagnostic possibilities for this girl's presentation.

7.1.3   Describe the presentation of CRPS and discuss the similarities and differences with this case.

Case 7.2   A 19-year-old male presents with incoordination of his right hand. He was previously involved in a motorcycle accident that resulted in a cervical spine fracture at C5. His recovery was uneventful until he noticed that his coordination was failing in his right hand.

Questions

7.2.1   Describe the neural pathways that transmit proprioceptive information from the hand to the brain.

7.2.2   Suggest a list of at least five differential diagnostic possibilities for this young man's presentation.

Introduction

The spinal cord used to be thought of as simply a conduit for nerve pathways to and from the brain. The most elaborate neural integration thought to occur in the spinal cord was limited to simple reflex muscle servo loops. It is now known that the spinal cord is a complex neural integration system contiguous with the neural structures of the brain and is an essential component of the neuraxis in humans. Long-term plasticity of both excitatory and inhibitory transmission, postsynaptic trafficking and recycling of various receptors, activation of immediate early genes in neurons, and constant changes in synaptic structure and connections are all active processes occurring in the spinal cord.

The spinal cord is the first site of sensory modulation and the last site of motor modulation that influences perception and movement of the body parts.

The brain and brainstem also play a part in modulating other sensory systems that influence motor output via the spinal cord.

The peripheral nerves transmit receptor information to neurons in the spinal cord. The peripheral nerves can vary in transmission speeds, size, and modalities that they transmit. The peripheral nerves are also very sensitive to injury, but have specific healing strategies to recover.

The spinal cord also contributes to the integration and modulation of pain. A variety of peripheral and central processes influence pain processing including receptor mechanisms, peripheral sensitization, central sensitization, neural plasticity, and the sympathetic nervous system.

In this chapter we consider all of the above processes.

Anatomy of the Spinal Cord

The spinal cord develops as a contiguous structure with the rest of the neuraxis, arising from the ventricular layer of ependymal cells and maintains the basic dorsal and ventral segregation of sensory and motor function as the brainstem (see Chapter 2). The result of this is that most afferent (sensory) information arrives in the dorsal aspects of the cord and the efferent (motor) information exits from the ventral aspects of the cord (Fig. 7.1). As the spinal cord matures during embryonic development the dorsal/ventral segregation becomes more defined and by about 3 months post-conception two discrete cellular areas can be determined, the alar lamina, which is located dorsally and contains the neurons that will receive the afferent (sensory) information, and the basal lamina, which is located ventrally and contains the neurons that will supply the efferent (motor) outflow from the spinal cord (Fig. 7.2).

QUICK FACTS 1	The Spinal Cord has the Following Functions

1. Is the final common pathway for the somatomotor system.
2. Conveys somatosensory information from the body to higher centres.
3. Contains preganglionic ANS neurons under segmental/suprasegmental control.
4. Mediates spinal and segmental reflexes.
5. Contains central pattern generators for rhythmic movement gait and posture maintenance.

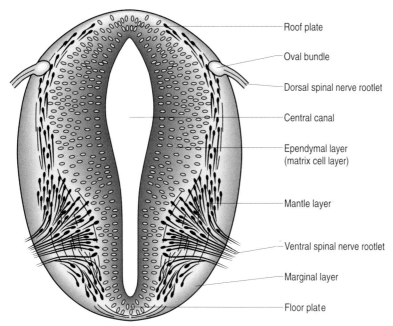

Roof plate
Oval bundle
Dorsal spinal nerve rootlet
Central canal
Ependymal layer (matrix cell layer)
Mantle layer
Ventral spinal nerve rootlet
Marginal layer
Floor plate

Fig. 7.1 A transverse section through the developing spinal cord of a human embryo 4 weeks old.

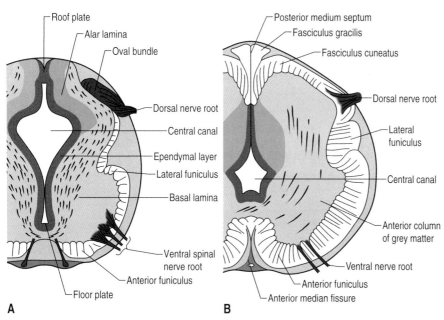

Roof plate
Alar lamina
Oval bundle
Dorsal nerve root
Central canal
Ependymal layer
Lateral funiculus
Basal lamina
Ventral spinal nerve root
Anterior funiculus
Floor plate

A

Posterior medium septum
Fasciculus gracilis
Fasciculus cuneatus
Dorsal nerve root
Lateral funiculus
Central canal
Anterior column of grey matter
Ventral nerve root
Anterior funiculus
Anterior median fissure

B

Fig. 7.2 Transverse sections through the developing spinal cord of human embryos. (A) About 6 weeks old. (B) About 3 months old.

The spinal cord is composed of two major types of matter, one consisting of mainly neurons and neuropil, the grey matter, and the other consisting of mainly axons and supporting glial cells, the white matter. The grey matter forms the central regions of the cord and is surrounded by white matter for its entire course in the spinal cord. The spinal cord proper (medulla spinalis) begins at the superior border of the atlas or first cervical vertebra, and extends to the upper border of the second lumbar vertebra.

For the first 3 months of embryonic development the spinal cord and the vertebral column develop at the same pace and are roughly equal in length. During the rest of embryonic development the vertebra column grows in size faster than the spinal cord, resulting in the spinal cord terminating about two-thirds of the way down the vertebral column (Chusid 1982). The length of the spinal cord, which is usually between 42 and

45 cm, can show significant variation between individuals with the end result affecting the level of termination of the spinal cord (Barson 1970). The variation in the termination of the spinal cord can range from the lower third of the twelfth vertebra to the disc between the second and third lumbar vertebra (Jit & Charnalia 1959). The spinal cord terminates by converging into a cylindrical funnel-shaped structure referred to as the conus medullaris, from the distal end of which extends a thin filament, the filum terminale, to its attachment on the first coccygeal segment. The spinal nerve roots radiating from the spinal cord and the dorsal root ganglion neuron's central projections form a structure referred to as the cauda equina as they traverse the distance, through the spinal canal, between the spinal cord termination point and their exit vertebral foramina in the spinal column (Fig. 7.3).

The volume of the spinal cord is dependent on the number of neurons and axons that it contains at any one point. Because of the increase in afferent input and efferent output that occurs at the level of the cervical and lumbar cord levels, due to the innervation of the arms and legs, the spinal cord expands in circumference, resulting in the cervical and lumbar enlargements.

On cross-sectional views of the spinal cord, the dorsal or posterior median sulcus, which is continuous with a projection of connective tissue that penetrates the posterior aspect of the cord, the dorsal median septum, symmetrically divides the dorsal cord into two halves. Ventrally, the ventral median fissure performs a similar function so that a line connecting it and the dorsal median sulcus effectively divides the spinal cord into left and right symmetrical halves. It is convenient to divide the white matter of the spinal cord into regions referred to as funiculi, so that each half of the spinal cord contains a dorsal or posterior funiculus, a posterior lateral and anterior lateral funiculus, and a ventral or anterior funiculus (Fig. 7.4). In the mature spinal cord the embryonic alar and basal plates, with a few exceptions, maintain their distribution of sensory and motor segregation. These areas can be outlined quite accurately by the funicular divisions just described (Fig. 7.5).

The Grey Matter of the Spinal Cord Is Composed of a High Proportion of Neurons, Neuroglia, and Blood Vessels

Centrally the butterfly-shaped grey matter of the cord is divided in the midline by the central canal. The grey matter passing dorsally to the central canal is referred to as the posterior grey commissure and the grey matter passing ventrally to the central canal is referred to as the anterior grey commissure. Arising from the area of the ventral lateral sulci

QUICK FACTS 2	Spinal Cord Development

- Medulla spinalis extends from the upper border of atlas to the conus medullaris opposite the L1–L2 disc.
- Filum terminale extends to the tip of the coccyx.
- Cord shows cervical and lumbar enlargements.
- In early embryonic development the cord is as long as the vertebral canal but as development proceeds it lags behind the vertebral column.

QUICK FACTS 3	Internal Structure of the Spinal Cord

- Spinal cord consists of a core of neuropil (grey matter) surrounded by an outer axon fibre layer, the white matter.
- The white matter decreases in proportion as the spinal cord lengthens except at the cervical and lumbar enlargements.
- Grey matter is composed of neuron cell bodies, dendrites, and efferent and afferent axons of the neurons.

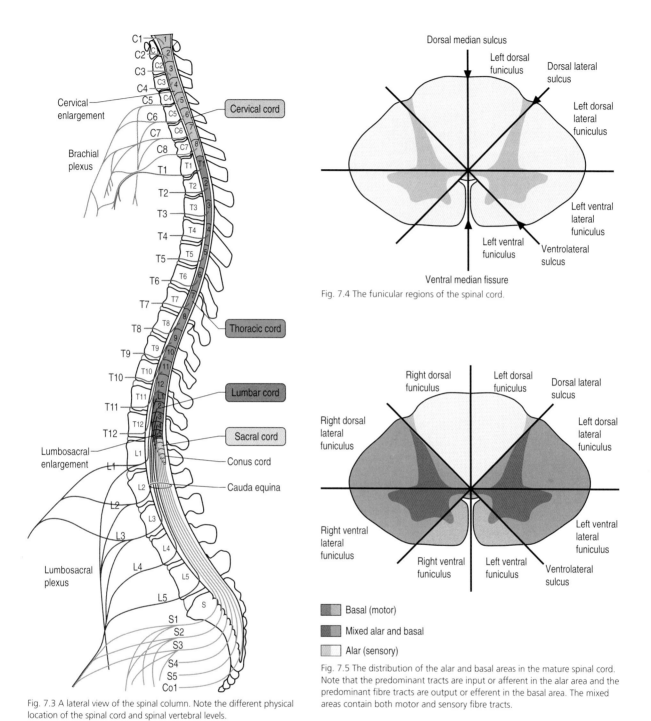

Fig. 7.3 A lateral view of the spinal column. Note the different physical location of the spinal cord and spinal vertebral levels.

Fig. 7.4 The funicular regions of the spinal cord.

■ Basal (motor)

■ Mixed alar and basal

□ Alar (sensory)

Fig. 7.5 The distribution of the alar and basal areas in the mature spinal cord. Note that the predominant tracts are input or afferent in the alar area and the predominant fibre tracts are output or efferent in the basal area. The mixed areas contain both motor and sensory fibre tracts.

are the ventral roots of the spinal cord, which just as they exit the vertebral foramina combine with the afferent axons of the dorsal root ganglion neurons as they enter the vertebral foramina to form the root of the spinal nerve. Entering the spinal cord at the dorsal lateral sulcus are the sensory dorsal roots, completing their journey to the cord from the dorsal root ganglion cells (Fig. 7.6). The areas of grey matter that give rise to or receive the afferent and efferent input resemble the shape of a horn and are thus termed the anterior and posterior horns The anterior horn does not extend through the anterior funiculus and reach the surface of the cord. The posterior horn projects much more deeply into the dorsal funiculus and except for a small band of translucent neurons, the substantia gelatinosa, it would extend to the posterior surface of the cord. A small angular projection from the intermediate areas of the cord forms the lateral horn of grey matter that only occurs between

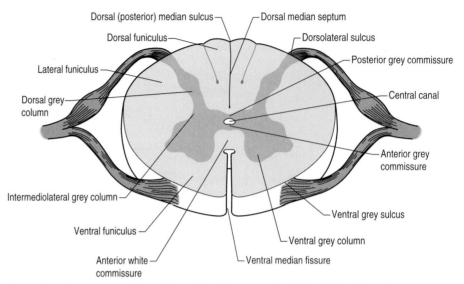

Fig. 7.6 The various structures and nerve fibre pathways in a cross-sectional view of the spinal cord.

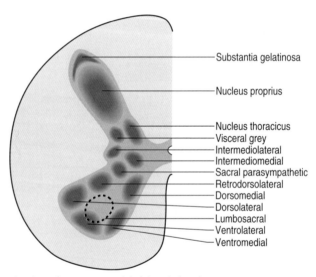

Fig. 7.7 The various locations of grey matter nuclei of the spinal cord.

the levels of the first thoracic to the second lumbar segment. This lateral outgrowth of grey matter houses many of the presynaptic neurons of the sympathetic nervous system.

The neurons of the grey matter form a complex intermingled array involving multiple synaptic connections with many of the axons crossing the midline via the anterior and posterior commissures. Some of the neurons are intrasegmental and their axons and dendrites remain within the same segment of the spinal cord as the neuron soma. Other neurons are intersegmental and their axons and dendrites spread over many segments both rostrally and caudally. In many parts of the neuraxis groups of neurons, usually with a related functional activity, cluster together into nuclei or when large enough ganglia. Several nuclei have been identified in the grey matter of the spinal cord. The most predominant neurons in the ventral grey areas are the large multipolar neurons whose axons emerge from the spinal cord to form the anterior horn, and contribute to the spinal nerves, to ultimately innervate the skeletal muscles of the body. These neurons are also referred to as alpha-efferents or alpha motor neurons. Also present in large numbers in the anterior horn are slightly smaller neurons whose axons supply the intrafusal fibres of the muscle spindle called gamma-efferents or gamma motor neurons (Fig. 7.7).

The neuron groupings in the posterior horns involve four main nuclei, two of which extend through the length of the cord and two that are present only at selective levels of the cord. The substantia gelatinosa of Rolando extends throughout the cord and composes the extreme tip of the dorsal horn. These neurons are involved with signal processing of afferent information from the dorsal root ganglion neurons and are thought to play an essential role in the initial processing of pain due to extensive connections with incoming axons destined to form the spinothalamic tracts (Fig. 7.7).

A second nuclear group that extends throughout the spinal cord is located ventral to the substantia gelatinosa and is referred to as the dorsal funicular group or the nucleus proprius (Fig. 7.7). Lying ventral to the nucleus proprius in the basal region of the dorsal horn and extending from the eighth cervical region of the cord to the fourth lumbar region of the cord is the nucleus dorsalis or Clark's nucleus (Fig. 7.7). Finally, a small group of nuclei known as the visceral grey area, or nucleus centrobasalis, is present only in the lower cervical and lumbosacral segments of the cord.

The intermediate region of the grey matter is composed of relatively small neurons that function as the presynaptic sympathetic neurons of the autonomic nervous system. Two regions are usually identified, the intermediolateral group (IML), which houses the presynaptic sympathetic neurons and the intermediomedial group (IMM), where similar small neurons to the IML reside and probably act as multimodal integrators for the output IML neurons. Neurons from both the IML and IMM send axons via the white rami communicants to the paravertebral ganglia that extend from T1 to L2 vertebral levels.

Rexed's Laminae Can Be Used to Classify Functional Aspects of Grey Matter

In the 1950s and early 1960s an architectural scheme was developed to classify the structure of the spinal cord, based on the cytological features of the neurons in different regions of the grey substance. It consists of nine laminae (I–IX) that extend throughout the cord, roughly paralleling the dorsal and ventral columns of the grey substance, and a tenth region (lamina X) that surrounds the central canal (Rexed 1964) (Fig. 7.9).

A brief description of the functional characteristics of these laminae follows.

Alar and Basal Plate Development   **QUICK FACTS 4**

Fig. 7.8 During embryonic development the alar or roof plate of the spinal cord develops into the neurons that receive afferent information from the dorsal root ganglion cells. The basal or floor plate develops into the motor output neurons of the spinal cord.

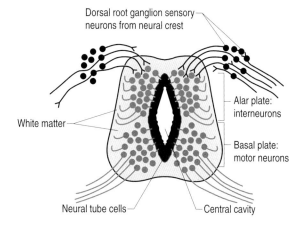

Laminae I–IV

These areas are considered the main receiving junctions for primary afferent information. This region is characterized by complex multisynaptic networks of both intra- and intersegmental neurons. Many of the pathways cross the midline of the cord and ascend or descend in contralateral tracts (Fig. 7.10).

Laminae V and VI

These areas receive proprioceptive primary afferent information as well as descending collateral input from axons of the corticospinal and reticulospinal tracts. This area is probably very involved in multimodal integration and regulation of movement (Fig. 7.10).

Laminae	Names
I	Lamina marginalis
	Layer of Waldeyer
II and III	Substantia gelatinosa
III and IV	Nucleus proprius
V	Deiter's nucleus
VII	Clark's column
	Thoracic nucleus
X	Substantia gelatinosa centralis

Lamina VII

The lateral aspect of this area receives extensive efferent and afferent connections from the cerebellum, spinocerebellar, spinotectal, spinoreticular, and rubrospinal tracts and is involved in the multimodal integration of posture and movement.

The medial aspect of this area contains numerous complex networks of connections between propriospinal neurons. This area is probably involved in the integration of the complex propriospinal reflex network of the spinal cord concerned with both movement and autonomic function (Fig. 7.10).

Lamina VIII

This area receives collateral projections from adjacent laminae, medial longitudinal fasciculus, and vestibulospinal and reticulospinal tracts and profuse projections from the contralateral lamina VIII region. Output of this area influences both ipsilateral and contralateral neuron pools through both direct projections to the alpha motor neurons and projections to the gamma motor neuron pools (Fig. 7.10).

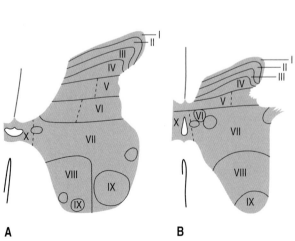

A **B**

Fig. 7.9 The laminar divisions of the spinal grey matter as per Rexed.

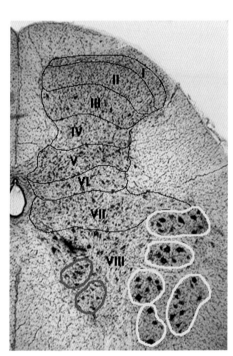

Fig. 7.10 Another view of the grey matter laminae which illustrates the groupings of neurons forming small nuclear units.

Lamina IX
This area is populated with both alpha and gamma motor neurons as well as interneurons.

Lamina X
This area comprises the grey matter in close approximation to and surrounding the central canal. This area also consists of the dorsal and ventral commissures and the central gelatinous substance.

The White Matter of the Spinal Cord is Composed of Axon Fibre Tracts

The spinal cord itself consists of columns of cells and axon fibre tracts that allow communication throughout the length of the spinal cord and with supraspinal levels of the neuraxis. It is convenient to describe the axon fibre tracts of the spinal cord with respect to the funiculus in which they are located.

Axon Fibre Tracts of the Dorsal Funiculus
The *dorsal columns* are composed of the medially located fasciculus gracilis and the more laterally located fasciculus cuneatus (Figs 7.11, 7.12, 7.13). These pathways transport information from receptors in the periphery about fine and discriminative touch, conscious proprioception, pressure, two-point discrimination, and vibration sense. The primary afferent axons enter the spinal cord grey matter through the dorsal horn and synapse on the neurons in laminae V and VI. The secondary afferents ascend in the ipsilateral dorsal columns. Information from the lower limb and trunk is carried in the gracile funiculus and information from the upper limb and hand by the cuneate funiculus and synapse ipsilaterally in the gracile and cuneate nuclei of the caudal medulla.

Neurons then decussate in the caudal medulla as the internal arcuate fibres and ascend to the contralateral thalamus via the medial lemniscus of the brainstem. Some fibres contained in the cuneate fasciculus arising from proprioceptive afferents project to the cerebellum. These projection fibres form the external arcuate fibres and form the cuneocerebellar tract.

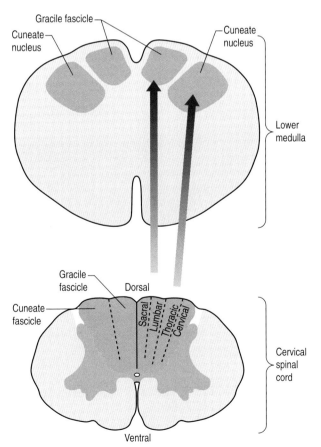

Fig. 7.11 The projections of the dorsal columns to the neurons in the cuneate and gracile nuclei in the caudal medulla region of the neuraxis.

163

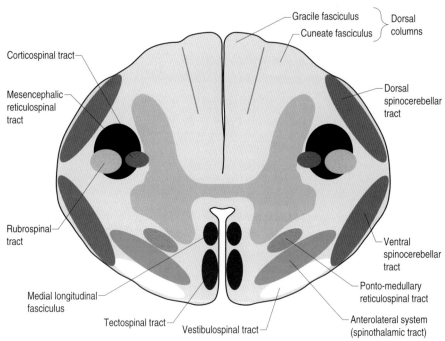

Fig. 7.12 The fibre tracts in a cross-sectional view of the spinal cord.

Axon Fibre Tracts of the Lateral Funiculus

The *anterolateral system* contains the fibre tracts of the spinothalamic tract and some of the fibres comprising the spinoreticular and spinomesencephalic tracts. These last two pathways provide the afferent limb for neuroendocrine and limbic responses to nociception (Figs 7.12 and 7.14).

The *spinothalamic* pathway, from a clinical standpoint, carries pain and temperature sensation from the entire body, excluding trigeminal distributions, to the thalamus. Primary afferent fibres have cell bodies located in the dorsal root ganglion (DRG) and their central processes synapse in the dorsal horn laminae I, II, and V predominately. Secondary afferents, which form the spinothalamic tract proper, decussate (cross the spinal cord) about 2–3 levels higher in the spinal cord and ascend in the anterolateral funiculus to the ventral posterior lateral (VPL) nucleus of the thalamus. Sensory modulation can occur in the brain, thalamus, or spinal cord, especially in lamina II, and is also influenced by visceral afferents in lamina V where convergence of afferent information can result in referred pain phenomena.

The *spinocerebellar* pathways include the ipsilateral dorsal and the contralateral ventral pathways. These pathways convey unconscious proprioception mainly from the joint receptors and muscle spindle fibres of the muscles and joints of the body and integrated data from multimodal neuron systems in the spinal grey matter to the cerebellum.

The *ventral spinocerebellar* pathway conveys information about the ongoing status of interneuronal pools in the spinal cord to the cerebellum. It therefore provides continuous monitoring of ascending and descending information concerning locomotion and posture. The neurons of this tract originate in laminae V–VII between L2 and S3. Their projection axons decussate to the other side so that they ascend in the contralateral anterolateral funiculus. These fibres then decussate again via the superior cerebellar peduncle to synapse on neurons in the anterior part of the ipsilateral cerebellum (Fig. 7.12).

The *dorsal spinocerebellar* tract neurons originate medially to the IML column of the spinal cord between C8 and L2/3.

The primary afferent cell bodies are located in the DRG and their central processes synapse with the above-mentioned neurons near the entry level or after ascending for a short distance in the dorsal columns. Secondary afferents ascend in the ipsilateral dorsolateral funiculus, lateral to the corticospinal tracts, and enter the ipsilateral cerebellum via the inferior cerebellar peduncle. Via this pathway, the cerebellum is provided with ongoing information about joint and muscle activity in the trunk and

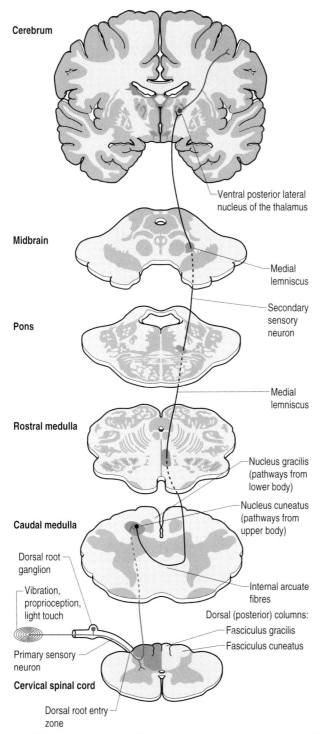

Cerebrum

Ventral posterior lateral
nucleus of the thalamus

Midbrain

Medial
lemniscus

Secondary
sensory
neuron

Pons

Medial
lemniscus

Rostral medulla

Nucleus gracilis
(pathways from
lower body)

Nucleus cuneatus
(pathways from
upper body)

Caudal medulla

Dorsal root
ganglion

Internal arcuate
fibres

Vibration,
proprioception,
light touch

Dorsal (posterior) columns:
Fasciculus gracilis
Fasciculus cuneatus

Primary sensory
neuron

Cervical spinal cord

Dorsal root entry
zone

Fig. 7.13 The pathway of the dorsal column/medial lemniscal system through the various levels of the neuraxis.

limbs. The cuneocerebellar pathway carries the same type of information from the upper limb and cervical spine via the cuneate fasciculus of the dorsal columns (Fig. 7.12).

Motor Pathways

The anterior and lateral corticospinal tracts are important spinal tracts in the control of volitional movement. The fibre tracts are composed of axons from many different areas of the cortex as well as about 50% of their axons from unidentified areas. These tracts

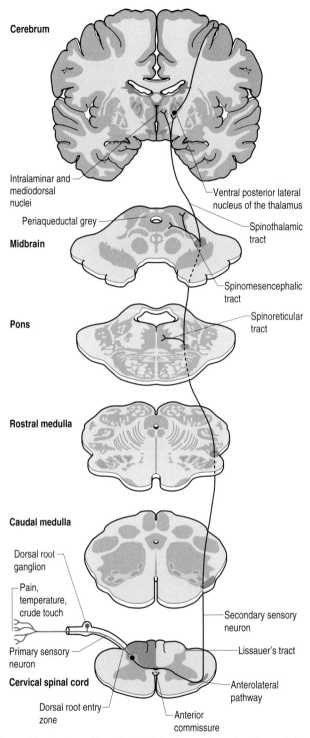

Fig. 7.14 The pathway of the anterior and lateral spinal thalamic tracts (anterolateral system) through the various levels of the neuraxis.

contain about 50% of their axon projections from the large pyramidal neurons of the primary motor cortex and association motor cortex. The *lateral corticospinal tract* descends in the spinal cord anterolateral to the posterior horn of grey matter and medial to the posterior spinocerebellar tract (Figs 7.12 and 7.15). It contains a large number of motor axon projections from cortical areas 1–4 and 6 to the hands, arms, legs, and feet. Its defining role is to convey motor signals to the ventral horn cells (VHCs) at the lower aspect of the cervical and lumbosacral enlargements of the spinal cord, thus controlling distal limb movements and coordinating distal and proximal muscles to

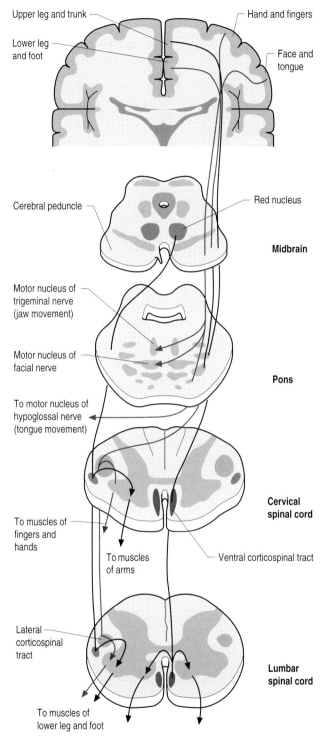

Fig. 7.15 The pathway of the anterior (ventral) and lateral corticospinal tracts through the various levels of the neuraxis.

achieve specific trajectories in space. Each corticomotoneuronal cell can achieve these complex goals by synapsing on interneuronal cells that communicate with whole groups of VHCs.

Axons from the projection neurons in the cortex descend in the internal capsule of the cerebrum through the cerebral peduncle of the mesencephalon and continue through the ventral areas of the pons until they enter the pyramids of the medulla oblongata. As the fibres descend in the medulla about 68% of the fibres cross to form the lateral corticospinal tracts in the lateral funiculus of the contralateral side of the spinal cord;

about 30% of the fibres do not cross and form the *anterior corticospinal tracts* in the ventral funiculus of the ipsilateral side of the spinal cord. The remaining fibres continue as uncrossed fibres of the lateral corticospinal tracts (Fulton & Sheenan 1935).

The anterior corticospinal tract runs adjacent to the anterior median fissure and descends to about the middle of the thoracic region. It contains most of the uncrossed motor projection fibres from the cortex and is thought to modulate axial musculature involved in strut stabilization and postural control.

Traditionally, the anterior and lateral corticospinal tracts were referred to as the pyramidal tracts. These tracts have the distinction among motor pathways of forming a continuous non-interrupted pathway from the cortex to the grey matter of the spinal cord. A number of other tracts also involved in motor control, including the rubrospinal, vestibulospinal, and other tracts that form intermediate synaptic connections in the brainstem, are referred to as the *extrapyramidal tracts*.

Most of the axons of both the anterior and lateral corticospinal tracts synapse on interneurons located in laminae IV to VII of the grey matter of the spinal cord (Nyberg-Hansen 1969). Most physiological evidence suggests that the majority of the corticospinal fibres of both tracts act to facilitate flexor groups of muscles and inhibit extensor groups of muscles, which is the opposite effect observed by projections of the vestibulospinal tracts. Injuries involving the corticospinal tracts affect the motor control of the peripheral muscles differently at different levels of the neuraxis. Injuries above the medulla decussation affect the contralateral peripheral muscles. Injuries below the decussation affect the peripheral muscles ipsilateral to the lesion. It must be remembered that not all of the corticospinal fibres cross the midline so that a lesion to a motor cortical area on one side of the corticospinal tract above the decussation will affect the motor control on both sides of the body to a certain extent. This contributes to the understanding of the ipsilateral pyramidal paresis observed when a decreased cortical function (hemisphericity) occurs.

Vestibulospinal Tract

The vestibulospinal tracts, lateral and medial, descend in the ventral funiculus, and mediate reflexes (vestibulospinal) that enable an individual to maintain balance and posture despite the effect of gravity and changes in the centre of mass due to movement of the trunk, head, and limbs. The lateral segments, the lateral vestibulospinal tract, descend from the lateral vestibular nucleus uncrossed and exert modulatory effects on the ipsilateral anterior column neurons in the grey matter through the length of the cord. The medial segments of this pathway, the medial vestibulospinal tracts, arise from the medial and inferior vestibular nuclei and descend first in the medial longitudinal fasciculus before entering the vestibulospinal tracts of the cord. This pathway is both crossed and uncrossed and only projects to the cervical and thoracic levels of the cord and as such is probably only involved with upper limb and neck movements (Figs 7.12 and 7.16).

QUICK FACTS 6	Spinal Nerve Roots

- There are 31 pairs of spinal nerves:
  - 8 cervical;
  - 12 thoracic;
  - 5 lumbar;
  - 5 sacral; and
  - 1 coccygeal.
- Each root level possesses an oval enlargement of neurons, the dorsal root ganglion.
- Nerve roots of the lower spinal cord exit the cord and form the cauda equina before exiting through their vertebral foramina.

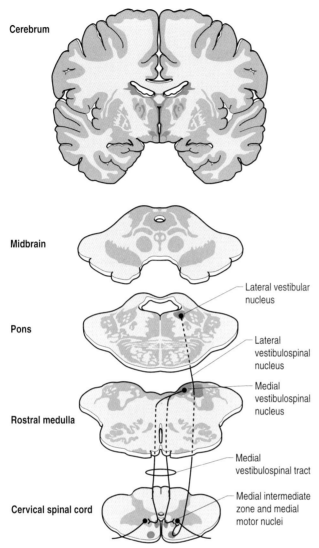

Fig. 7.16 The pathway of the vestibulospinal tracts through the various levels of the neuraxis.

The vestibulospinal tracts transport afferent information from the vestibular apparatus of the inner ear and descending efferent information from the inferior and lateral vestibular nuclei. The pathway descends in the ipsilateral ventral funiculus of the spinal cord, dorsal to the tectospinal tract and immediately adjacent to the anterior median fissure. The axon projections of both pathways synapse predominately on alpha and gamma VHCs of laminae VII and VIII. The physiological evidence to date suggests that this pathway has a facilitory effect on extensor muscles and an inhibitory effect on flexor groups.

Tectospinal Tract

The fibres of this tract originate from the deep layers of the contralateral superior colliculus in the dorsal midbrain (mesencephalon). The tectospinal tract crosses in the dorsal tegmental decussation of the midbrain, which is ventral to the oculomotor nucleus and the medial longitudinal fasciculus (MLF). It maintains a close relationship with the MLF until it reaches the level of the internal arcuate fibres at the decussation of the medial lemniscus. At this point it passes laterally so that it comes to lie in the ventral lateral white matter of the spinal cord. It then descends in the contralateral medial ventral funiculus of the spinal cord, synapsing on interneurons in laminae VI to VIII that communicate with the alpha and gamma motor neurons of the cervical spine (Szentagothai 1948) (Fig. 7.17).

The superior colliculus is a remnant of the optic lobe in primitive animals and is involved in visual reflexes in addition to integration of somatic (especially neck and

169

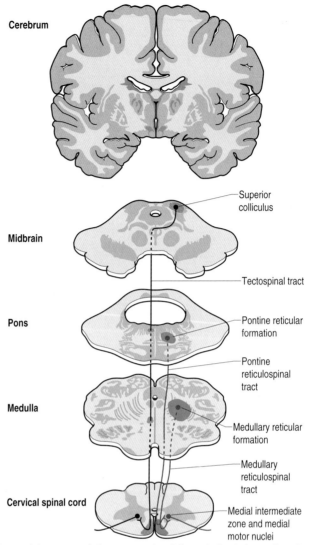

Fig. 7.17 The pathways of the mesencephalic, ponto, and medullary reticulospinal tracts (green) and the tectospinal tract (blue) through the various levels of the neuraxis.

head), auditory, and visual afferents for spatial orientation of incoming stimuli and associated reflex head and eye movements. It facilitates accurate head and eye movements in response to sound and light stimuli.

Rubrospinal Tract

The rubrospinal pathway has been rumoured to be vestigial in humans because of the evolutionary advancement of the corticospinal pathways; however, its presence in primates probably indicates it will eventually be found in humans as well and an open mind needs to prevail. It originates mainly from the large (magnocellular) neurons of the red nucleus in the rostral mesencephalon, decussates slightly more caudally, and descends just ventrally to the corticospinal fibres in the dorsolateral funiculus of the spinal cord contralaterally (Fig. 7.18).

Neurons of the red nucleus share extensive interaction with the cerebellum and basal ganglia and partly mediate their control over spinal motor output. The red nucleus is composed of a magnocellular or large cell and parvicellular or small cell components. Magnocellular components are homologous to the large diameter neurons of the primary motor cortex, while the parvicellular components are homologous to the premotor and supplementary motor areas of the cerebral cortex. The latter component acts as a relay and modulatory centre for feedforward connections between the cerebellum and the cortex.

The anterior spinal nerve roots contain only motor fibres and posterior roots only sensory fibres.

- Charles Bell's work of 1811 contains the first reference to experimental work on the motor functions of the ventral spinal nerve without, however, establishing the sensory functions of the dorsal roots. In 1822 François Magendie definitively discovered that the anterior root is motor and that the dorsal root is sensory.
- Magendie announced that 'section of the dorsal root abolishes sensation, section of ventral roots abolishes motor activity, and section of both roots abolishes both sensation and motor activity.'
- This discovery has been called 'the most momentous single discovery in physiology after Harvey'. In the same volume of *Journal de physiologie expérimentale et de pathologie*, Magendie gave experimental proof of the Bell–Magendie Law.
- Magendie proved Bell's Law by severing the anterior and posterior roots of spinal nerves in a litter of puppies. Stimulation of the posterior roots caused pain. Magendie sums it up: 'Charles Bell had had, before me, but unknown to me, the idea of separately cutting the spinal roots; he likewise discovered that the anterior influences muscular contractility more than the posterior does. This is a question of priority in which I have, from the beginning, honored him. Now, as for having established that these roots have distinct properties, distinct functions, that the anterior ones control movement, and the posterior ones sensation, this discovery belongs to me' (F. Magendie (1847) *Comptes rendus hebdomadaires des séances de l'Académie des sciences*, **24**: 3).

The rubrospinal tract acts much like the corticospinal tracts in that it affects enhancement flexor tone and inhibition of extensor tone, especially in the proximal limb muscles.

Reticulospinal Tract

The reticulospinal pathways can be divided into the medial or pontoreticular and lateral or medulloreticular spinal tracts. The *pontoreticular* neuron projections comprise the *medial reticulospinal pathways* and are predominately ipsilateral. They project to interneurons of laminae VII and VIII where they act to excite VHCs on the same side of origin. Some fibres do cross one or two spinal segments above their target destinations but the main modulating effects remain ipsilateral to the neurons of origin. The *lateral reticulospinal pathways* arise from the neurons in the medullary areas of the reticular formation and in particular from the nucleus reticularis gigantocellularis region. The projections have been found in a variety of fibre tracts in the white matter of the cord, but for the most part travel medial to the corticospinal tracts with a small tract occasionally travelling lateral to the corticospinal tracts in the lateral funiculus. In contrast with the medial reticulospinal tracts, the projections of the lateral tract are largely crossed with some ipsilateral representation (Fig. 7.17). Projections from each half of the medullary reticular formation exert inhibitory effect on spinal cord neurons bilaterally, probably through the activities of inhibitory interneurons (Renshaw cells) of lamina VII of the spinal cord. These projections also modulate the effects of afferent impulses arriving in these areas of the cord (Nyberg Hansen 1965). The loss of inhibitory projections to the spinal cord from the cortex has been thought to play an important role in spasticity observed in lesions of the cord, brainstem, or cortex. However, extrapyramidal, reticulospinal inhibitory dysfunction is also thought to be an important contributing factor. The differential activation of VHC groups by reticulospinal projections

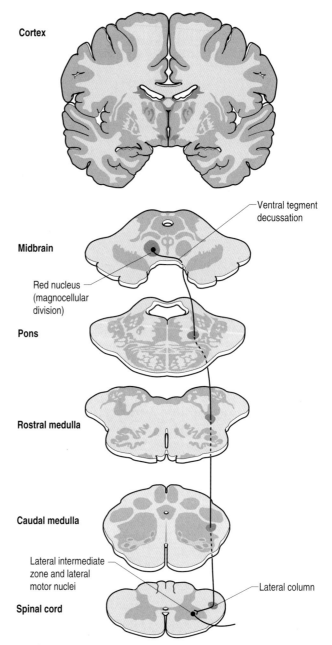

Fig. 7.18 The pathway of the rubrospinal tract through the various levels of the neuraxis.

(e.g. locomotor and inhibitory systems) in combination with the effects of lesions of the corticospinal projections as previously discussed leads to a characteristic weakness or 'soft' weakness pattern in the limbs in response to spinal cord lesions, brain damage, or hemisphericity.

Interstitiospinal Tract
The fibres of this tract arise from the interstitial nucleus and descend in the medial longitudinal fasciculus. They extend into the spinal cord from the MLF into the ipsilateral fasciculus proprius, which terminates on a network of interneurons located in the dorsal horn. These interneurons are thought to participate in intersegmental coordination of various muscles.

Descending Autonomic Modulatory Projections

Autonomic modulatory projection fibres from supraspinal centres to the preganglionic neurons of the autonomic nervous system are known to exist but have been very difficult to isolate as a solid tract of fibres probably because they are composed of polysynaptic columns of neurons and interneurons that range throughout wide areas of the white matter. The best indications are that most of these projections are located in the lateral fasciculus with a smaller number also located in the anterior funiculus. Some findings suggest that some of the pyramidal neurons in the frontal cortex that form the corticospinal tracts are actually autonomic modulatory neurons. Other projections are undoubtedly from various hypothalamic and reticular nuclei.

Spinal Cord Reflexes

Local spinal cord reflex circuits are also important in volitional movement in that descending motor pathways converge on interneurons to allow complex movement patterns to occur— i.e., corticomotoneuronal cells of the brain alter the trajectory of a limb in space by activating these reflex circuits involving agonist, antagonist, synergist, and neighbouring joint muscle groups. Feedback and feedforward mechanisms are employed by the cerebellum to assist plastic changes in the brain and spinal cord. Some stereotypical reflexes mediated by the spinal cord are state- or phase-dependent. For example, activation of Golgi tendon organs (GTOs) in the soleus and gastrocnemius muscles will trigger a different set of interneurons in the spinal cord, depending on whether the individual is in a state of locomotion or is non-ambulatory, and whether the individual is in the swing or stance phase of gait (Fig. 7.19).

This is analogous to the stumbling-correction reflex observed in cats. Sensory stimuli to the dorsum of the foot will activate a different set of interneurons, depending on whether the individual is in the stance or swing phase of gait. For example, during stance, the reflex

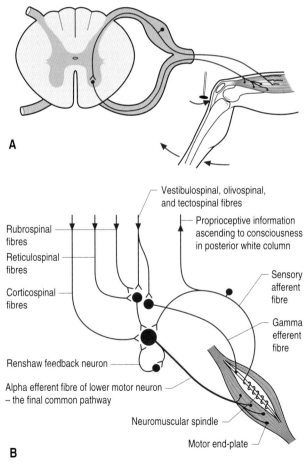

Fig. 7.19 (A) The simple muscle spindle (tendon) reflex. The reflex hammer strikes the tendon and causes a stretch of the muscle spindle fibres. This fires the afferent nerve pathway, which then synapses on the ventral horn cell, causing a depolarization of the ventral horn neuron, which in turn produces a contraction of the extrafugal muscles innervated by the ventral horn neurons. (B) The complex array of modulating inputs that the ventral horn neuron is exposed to at any given moment. Thus even the simple reflex arc that we are all familiar with is much more complex than first imagined.

would result in lower limb extension on that side, while during swing, the reflex would result in powerful flexion withdrawal response.

Flexor reflex afferent (FRA) responses result in a whole limb response of flexion and withdrawal. These FRA responses are stereotypical responses serving a protective function. An example includes the response to plantar stimulation of the foot, which results in the withdraw of the entire lower limb.

Clinical Symptoms and the Level of Decussation

When faced with motor or sensory signs and symptoms, it is important to consider the level of decussation in different pathways to assist in identifying the location of a lesion in the various planes of the neuraxis.

A unilateral spinal cord lesion may affect motor control, joint position sense, and discriminatory sensation ipsilaterally, while pain and temperature sensation may be affected contralaterally.

QUICK FACTS 8A   **Summary of Afferent Tracts**

Fig. 7.20 Summary of afferent tracts. The dorsal root neuron receptors that detect pain and temperature synapse on neurons in the substantia gelatinosa area of the grey matter. These neurons then cross the midline of the spinal cord to ascend in the contralateral spinothalamic tracts to the contralateral thalamus. In comparison, the dorsal root ganglion receptors that detect position and proprioception project ipsilaterally to the appropriate nucleus (gracilis/cuneatus) in the caudal medulla. The projections from the nuclear neurons then cross the midline and ascend in the contralateral medial lemniscal tracts to the contralateral thalamus. All of the neurons in the thalamus then project to the appropriate area of the somatosensory cortex. The representation of the somatotopic map of the body in the cortex is referred to as the sensory homunculus. Note the neurons in the trigeminal ganglia are the embryological homologues of the dorsal root ganglion neurons of the spinal cord.

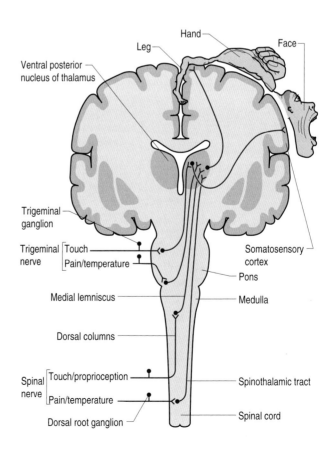

Fig. 7.21 Summary of efferent tracts. The pyramidal cells of the cortex form the output neurons of the motor cortex. The pyramidal axons that supply the muscles and effector organs of the face form the corticobulbar tracts and are referred to as the upper motor neurons of the cranial nerves. These projections are crossed for the most part but some ipsilateral projections are also present. The pyramidal axons that supply the muscles and effector organs of the rest of the body are referred to as the corticospinal tracts. The majority of the corticospinal projections or tracts cross the midline to synapse on effector neurons on the contralateral side to their origin, but as in the corticobulbar projections some ipsilateral projections are also present.

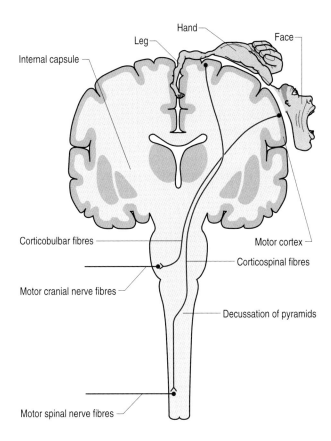

Laminar Organization in the Spinal Cord is Not Complete or as Accurate as Previously Thought

Laminar organization in the spinal cord is not complete or as accurate as previously thought. The traditional understanding of the laminar distribution of pathways in the white matter of the spinal cord was that the projections to and from the most distal areas of the body were more lateral in the spinal cord except in the dorsal columns where the reverse occurs. Some variability of these laminar patterns have been demonstrated; however, the general pattern in dorsal column, spinothalamic, and corticospinal tracts is important to understand from a clinical perspective.

The Spinal Nerves

There are 31 pairs of spinal nerves divided into cervical (8), thoracic (12), lumbar (5), sacral (5), and coccygeal (1) levels. The spinal nerves are composed of afferent ascending fibres from the dorsal root ganglion neurons and efferent descending fibres from the anterior and lateral horn neurons. These fibres are separated into sensory and motor fibres as the dorsal (sensory) and ventral (motor) roots of the spinal cord.

The spinal nerves represent the neural division of the embryological somite and contain motor, sensory, and autonomic components. The spinal nerves separate into dorsal and ventral rami as they exit the vertebral foramina (Fig. 7.22). The somatic component of the spinal nerve contains the motor nerves to skeletal muscle and the afferent information from a variety of receptors. The visceral component contains the afferent and efferent fibres of the autonomic nervous system.

The dorsal and ventral rami of the spinal nerves than continue to separate into smaller and smaller peripheral nerves, all of which contain both afferent and efferent fibres of the somatic and visceral components. The anatomy of the visceral or autonomic division is discussed in Chapter 8. The functional distribution of the muscular and sensory divisions, including dermatomes and motor actions of peripheral nerves, has been discussed in Chapter 4.

Peripheral Nerve Fibre Classification

The peripheral nerves are made up of nerve fibres of different diameters. Several schemes have attempted classifications of peripheral nerve fibres based on various parameters such as conduction velocity, function, fibre diameter, and other attributes. The two main classification systems in use are the Erlanger and Gasser system and the Lloyd system. Both schemes have two basic categories which divide the fibres into myelinated and unmyelinated groups. Over time and through convention a combination of the two classification systems has evolved: Erlanger and Gasser is used for efferent fibre classification and Lloyd for afferent fibre classification.

Erlanger and Gasser (1937) divided peripheral nerve fibres based on velocity of conduction. These are the three peaks seen on a compound nerve conduction velocity study and can be classified as follows.

A fibres, which are myelinated and have large diameters (22 μm), transport action potentials at the rate range of 120 to 60m/s. These are further divided into *efferent* and *afferent* type A fibres. Efferent type A fibres include:

Aα—to extrafusal muscle fibres;

Aβ—collaterals of Aα; and

Aγ—to intrafusal muscle fibres.

Afferent type A fibres include:

Aα—cutaneous, joint, muscle spindle, and large alimentary enteroreceptors;

Aβ—Merkel discs, pacinian corpuscles, Meissner corpuscles, Ruffini endings; and

Aγ—thermoreceptors and nociceptors in dental pulp, skin, and connective tissue.

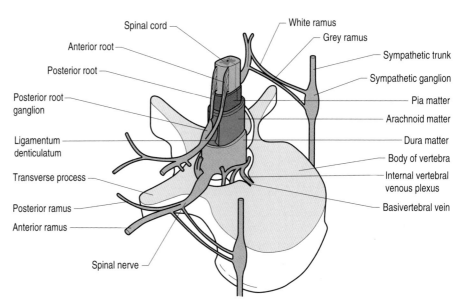

Fig. 7.22 A three-dimentional view of the spinal cord, spinal nerve roots, and paraspinal ganglia. Note the dural layers covering the spinal cord and spinal root pathways.

Peripheral Nerves   CELLS OF   **QUICK FACTS 9**

Fig. 7.23 Peripheral nerves. Peripheral nerves can be classified as cranial or spinal nerves. Each peripheral nerve consists of efferent and/or afferent fibres or both. They may be myelinated or non-myelinated, and have a series of connective tissue blankets called endoneurium, perineurium, and epineurium.

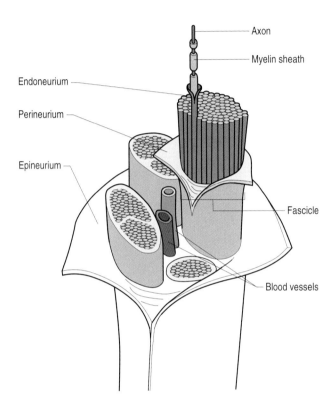

Axon

Myelin sheath

Endoneurium

Perineurium

Epineurium

Fascicle

Blood vessels

B fibres, which are myelinated and have diameters slightly smaller than that of the A fibres, transport action potentials at the rate of 30–4 m/s. *Efferent* type B fibres compose the fibres of preganglionic autonomic neurons.

C fibres, which are unmyelinated and of small diameter (1.5 μm), transport action potentials at the rate of 4–0.5 m/s. *Efferent* type C fibres are non-myelinated and compose the fibres of post-ganglionic autonomic neurons. *Afferent* C fibres are non-myelinated and convey information from thermoreceptors and nociceptors.

Lloyd's classification is based on fibre diameters ranging from 22 to 1.5 μm for myelinated fibres and 2–0.1 μm for non-myelinated fibres. Only afferent fibres were classified, and these were arranged into four groups. Myelinated fibres are divided into group I, II, and III, and non-myelinated fibres compose group IV (Table 7.1). Group or type I fibres, which have diameters ranging from 12 to 22 μm, are further divided into groups Ia and Ib. Group Ia fibres are larger, are heavily myelinated, and transmit information from muscle spindles and joint mechanoreceptors. Group Ib fibres are smaller, are moderately myelinated, and transfer information from Golgi tendon organs, and some joint mechanoreceptors.

Group or type II fibres have a diameter ranging from 6 to 12 μm, are moderately myelinated, and transmit information from secondary sensory fibres in muscle spindles. Group or type III fibres have a diameter ranging from 1 to 6 μm and are composed of unmyelinated nerve fibres ending in connective tissue sheaths which transmit information concerning pressure and pain.

Table 7.1 Lloyd's Classification of Nerve Fibres

Type	Receptor	Axon	Sensitive to...
Ia	Primary spindle endings	12–20	Muscle length and rate of change
Ib	Golgi tendon organs	12–20	Muscle tension
II	Secondary spindle endings	6–12	Muscle length
II	Non-spindle endings	6–12	Deep pressure
III	Free nerve endings	2–6	Pain, chemical, and thermal stimulation
IV	Free nerve endings	0.5–2 (non-myelinated)	Pain, chemical, and thermal stimulation

QUICK FACTS 10   **Conduction Speeds of Axons**

- Conduction speed depends largely on two factors:
  1. Axon diameter and
  2. Myelination.
- Large-diameter fibres conduct faster than small diameter fibres (A, B, C fibres).
- Myelinated fibres conduct faster than unmyelinated fibres.
- Small unmyelinated C fibres conduct at 0.25 m/s.
- Large myelinated fibres conduct at 100 m/s.

The largest diameter fibres have a number of clinically important, unique properties, which include the following:

1. They have the greatest nerve conduction velocity.
2. They are the most sensitive to hypoxia.
3. They are the most sensitive to compression.
4. They are the most sensitive to thermal changes.
5. They are the most sensitive to bacteraemia and viral toxaemia.
6. They have the lowest threshold to electrical stimuli.

The nociceptive C fibres are the most sensitive to chemicals such as anaesthetic agents.

Compression of Nerves Results in Retrograde Chromatolysis and Transneural Degeneration

Compression of a peripheral nerve affects the largest nerve fibres first: thus the Ia afferents and the alpha motor neurons. Compression, therefore, produces both sensory and motor losses because they both involve large axon types in proportion to the number of axons damaged. In a compression axonopathy, one cannot exist without the other, which is of diagnostic value. This concept can be extrapolated to all nerve fibres of a specific diameter under compression. For example, if a patient perceives pain, the type C nociceptive fibres are intact. This knowledge can be extrapolated to also mean that the type C autonomic fibres must also be intact.

Pressure on a peripheral nerve produces retrograde changes in the axons proximal to the site of compression and possibly in the neuronal cell bodies. There are four basic features of retrograde chromatolysis:

- Swelling of the cell due to failure of ionic pumps and loss of internal negativity, both allowing an influx of hydrated sodium;
- Eccentricity of the nucleus due to decreased tubulin, the supporting intracellular protein;

CELLS OF

Brown–Sequard Syndrome	**QUICK FACTS 11**

Damage to the lateral half of the spinal cord results in motor and sensory disturbances below the level of the lesion. Neural impairment involves:
- Ipsilateral motor paralysis;
- Ipsilateral loss of joint proprioception;
- Ipsilateral loss of vibration sense;
- Ipsilateral loss of two-point discrimination;
- Contralateral loss of pain sensation; and
- Contralateral loss of temperature sensation.

Brown–Sequard Syndrome: Causes	**QUICK FACTS 12**

- Syringomyelia
- Cord tumor
- Haematomyelia
- Trauma (knife/bullet)
- Radiation myelopathy

- Decreased rough endoplasmic reticulum and Nissl substance due to decrease of protein replication; and
- Decreased mitochondrial activity and population.

Repair of the axon and cell body can take place if there is sufficient protein substrate, sufficient mitochondrial capacity for producing adenosine triphosphate (ATP), sufficient fuel supply, and appropriate levels of stimulation received by the neuron. The axon will send out sprouts of protein which will be guided to the target end organ along the route of the damaged axon by the myelin sheath if it is intact. The time for repair is approximately 3–4 cm per month and is calculated from the site of injury to the point of synapse with the target organ, such as the muscle. Crush injuries to axons, which are much more common than transections through the axon, heal faster because the myelin sheath generally remains intact in crush injuries. If repair does not occur, macrophages migrate from the periphery and neutral proteases are activated, resulting in foamy necrosis of the nerve. There is an approximate 2-year window of repair and if the target organ has not been reached by the regenerating axon by that time, there will be neuronal death and permanent loss of end organ function.

Wallerian Degeneration Occurs in Six Stages
Wallerian degeneration refers to the segmental stages in the breakdown of a myelinated nerve fibre in the stump distal to a transection through the axon. A transection or transection-like injury to the axon can occur because of trauma, infarction, or acute poisoning. The six stages of Wallerian degeneration include the following:

1. Transection or transection-like event occurs to the axon, which results in a decreased axoplasmic flow and cessation of nutrient supply to the distal axon.
2. Dissolution of axon occurs within 2 days of the transection and breakdown of the axon into clumps within the myelin sheath starts to occur.
3. Secondary demyelination starts to occur and the myelin sheath starts to disintegrate at various points along its length referred to as 'Schmidt–Lantermann clefts' because of axon degeneration.
4. Resorption of the axon remains starts to occur via Schwann cell auto-phagocytosis of myelin/axon debris. The debris is phagocytosed and digested by lysosomal

---

QUICK FACTS 13   **Central Cord Syndrome (*Syringomyelia*)**

- It is a disease of the spinal cord.
- It has an unknown cause.
- It is associated with gliosis and cavitation of the spinal cord.
- Lower cervical roots are most commonly affected but lumbar and brainstem may also be involved.
- It is thought to occur because of inappropriate nest formation of glial cells in the central portion of the cord.
- Imperfect closure of the neural tube may also be linked.

---

activity into neutral lipid and transferred to macrophages for further degradation and removal. This process may take up to 3 months for completion.

5. Schwann cell proliferation starts to occur with the myelin debris acting as a mitogen. The rapidly developing Schwann cells form a column of cells called the 'bands of Bungner'.

6. Axonal regeneration will occur under the appropriate environmental conditions. If axonal regeneration fails, then endoneural fibrosis starts to occur, which results in atrophy of the Schwann cells and fibrosis of the endoneurium.

The Process of Axonal Regeneration Occurs in Three Stages
Axonal regeneration can occur as a reparative response of the proximal axonal stump and neural cell body under appropriate conditions. The potential to regenerate will depend on the central integrative state of the neuron involved. This process occurs in three stages:

QUICK FACTS 14   **Syringomyelia: Presentation**

- It presents clinically with muscular wasting and weakness.
- It also has a variety of sensory defects.
- Occurrence is frequently associated with:
  - Pigeon breast;
  - Scoliosis;
  - Cervical rib;
  - Hydrocephalus;
  - Gliomas;
  - Hemangiomas;
  - Fusion of cervical vertebra;
  - Wasting of the small muscles of the hands and painless burns on the fingers or forearms;
  - Horner's syndrome;
  - Loss of bladder function and ataxia;
  - Neuropathic (Charcot's) joints;
  - Morvan's syndrome (slowly healing painless infections of the hands and fingers); and
  - A rapid progression phase that slows to a chronic slowly progressing phase.
- Treatment, which usually proves ineffective, includes:
  - Surgery and
  - Radiation therapy.

1. The reactive stage involves the formation of a proximal axon stump. The formation of a proximal axon stump requires sealing of the axon stump, swelling of proximal stump, and the demyelination of one proximal internodal segment. Neuronal cell body undergoes central chromatolysis, which involves swelling of the cell due to failure of the sodium/potassium ionic pumps. This results in an increase in sodium concentration on the inside of the cell, which attracts water molecules by osmosis and swells the neuron. Eccentricity of nucleus occurs because of a decrease in the proteins necessary to manufacture microtubules and microfilaments, secondary to reduced rough endoplasmic reticulum volume, which maintains the shape and structure of the neuron including the central location of the nucleus. A reduction in both mitochondrial production levels and population also occurs.

2. The regenerative phase involves the regrowth of the distal axon. Axon regrowth usually occurs via terminal or collateral sprouting of the axon.

3. The remyelination phase starts to occur when the newly forming axon reaches 2 μm in diameter; then the axon starts to attract Schwann cells and the first myelin starts to form in the region of the bands of Bungner. The new axon sheath is thinner and has shorter internodal spaces than the original axon.

Fibrillations and Fasciculations on Electromyography (EMG)

Chronic partial denervation of a nerve results in increased branching of surviving axons. This increased branching results in an increase in motor unit size. Increased motor unit size produces giant units on electromyography (EMG).

- Fibrillations are spontaneous motor fibre contractions detectable via EMG because of muscle fibre irritability.
- Fasciculations are spontaneous quivering movements visible to the naked eye because of spontaneous motor unit firing.
- Muscle disease often results in the production of small polyphasic units on EMG.

Primary Demyelination Can Occur via Two Main Mechanisms

Primary demyelination involves the selective loss of the myelin sheath with sparing of the axon. It usually involves one or several internodes and results in blocks in conduction along the axon. This process can occur via two major mechanisms:

1. The direct destruction of myelin occurs in diseases such as Guillain–Barre polyneuropathy (GBP)—The hallmark of GBP is an autoimmune attack by sensitized macrophages on the myelin sheath with sparing of the Schwann cells.

2. The metabolic impairment of the Schwann cell—An example of this type of metabolic dysfunction can be seen with the exposure to diphtheria toxin. This toxin, which is manufactured by the bacterium *Corynebacterium diphtheriae*, acts to poison the respiratory mechanisms of the mitochondria, resulting in the inhibition of protein synthesis in Schwann cells, leading to segmental demyelination.

Classification of Nerve Injuries

There is no single classification system that can describe all the many variations of nerve injury. Most systems attempt to correlate the degree of injury with symptoms, pathology, and prognosis. In 1943, Seddon introduced a classification of nerve injuries based on three main types of nerve fibre injury and whether there is continuity of the nerve. The three types include *neuropraxia*, *axonotmesis*, and *neurotmesis*.

Neuropraxia is the mildest form of nerve injury, brought about by compression or relatively mild, blunt trauma. It is most likely a biochemical lesion caused by concussion or shock-like injuries to the nerve fibres. In this case there is an interruption in conduction of the impulse down the nerve fibre, and recovery takes place without Wallerian degeneration. There is a temporary loss of function which is reversible within hours to months of the injury (the average is 6–8 weeks) and there is frequently greater involvement of motor rather than sensory function with autonomic function being retained. This is the type of nerve injury seen in many practices. A common cause is compartment compression brought about by pyramidal paresis. Common sites of this type of compression block include the radial nerve, axillary nerve, median nerve, and the posterior interosseous nerve.

Axonotmesis occurs in somewhat more severe injuries than those that cause neuropraxia. There is usually an element of retrograde proximal degeneration of the axon, and for regeneration to occur this loss must first be overcome. The regeneration fibres must cross the injury site and regeneration through the proximal or retrograde area of degeneration may require several weeks. Regeneration occurs at a rate of 3–4 cm per month under ideal conditions. Loss in both motor and sensory nerves is more complete with axonotmesis than with neuropraxia, and recovery occurs only through regeneration of the axons, a process requiring time. EMG performed 2 to 3 weeks following the injury usually demonstrates fibrillations and denervation potentials in the musculature distal to the injury site.

Neurotmesis is the most severe axonal lesion with potential of recovering. It occurs with severe contusion, stretch, lacerations, etc. Not only the axon but the encapsulating connective tissues also lose their continuity. The last or greatest extreme degree of neurotmesis is transection, but most neurotmetic injuries do not produce gross loss of continuity of the nerve but rather the internal disruption of the architecture of the nerve sufficient to involve perineurium and endoneurium as well as axons and their covering. Denervation changes recorded by EMG are similar to those seen with axonotmetic injury. There is a complete loss of motor, sensory, and autonomic function. If the nerve has been completely divided, axonal regeneration causes a neuroma to form in the proximal stump.

For classifying neurotmesis, it may be better to use the Sunderland system. In Sunderland's classification, peripheral nerve injuries are arranged in ascending order of severity. In first-degree injury conduction along the axon is *physiologically interrupted* at the site of injury, but the axon is not actually disrupted (neuropraxia). In second-degree injury axonal disruption is present but the integrity of the endoneural tube is maintained (axonotmesis). Further degrees of injuries (third, fourth, fifth) are based on the increasing degrees of anatomic disruption of the fibres with or without rupture of the ensheathing membrane, until the final fifth-degree injury where total anatomical rupture of the whole nerve occurs (neurotmesis).

Diagnosis of Nerve Lesions

A complete diagnosis of a traumatic nerve lesion should include identification of the following.

- The nerve or nerves injured;
- The anatomical *level* of injury to the nerve;
- The pathological *type* of injury: neurotmesis, axonotmesis, or neuropraxia;
- Associated bone, vascular, and tendon injuries;
- Secondary effects like deformities and contractures; and
- Any evidence of recovery of the nerve palsy.

Clinical Examination of Nerve Injuries

The clinical examination of nerve injuries includes the recording of all clinical findings under the following headings:

1. Motor signs—Note any muscles paralysed distal to the lesion and the wasting of muscles. The muscle actions should be graded using the following scale:

   0—Nil, no power at all;

   1—Muscle flicker only present, no power to move the joint;

   2—Power to move a joint but only when gravity is eliminated;

   3—Power to move a joint against gravity;

   4—Power to move a joint against gravity and resistance; and

   5—Normal power.

2. Sensory signs—Sensory signs should be noted under both subjective and objective criteria. *Subjective criteria* can be obtained by asking the patient to describe the distribution of pain, tingling, or burning sensations and noting the responses. *Objective criteria* can be obtained by utilizing clinical tests to evoke a response from the patient such as blunting or loss of sensation to pinprick, cotton wool touch, and temperature.

3. Sudomotor signs—Sudomotor signs include involuntary responses to stimuli such as blushing. Anhidrosis can be detected by the area of dry skin it causes due to absence of sweating.

4. Vasomotor signs—Vasomotor signs such as cold or warm hands and feet can be used to gauge autonomic tone.

5. Trophic changes—Trophic changes can be detected by examining the skin for smoothness and shiny areas, ulceration, and subcutaneous tissue atrophy.

6. Reflexes—Loss of tendon reflexes can indicate afferent or efferent nerve damage or motor unit damage.

7. Recovery signs—Look and test for signs of recovery. The presence of Tinel's sign may indicate both damage and recovery in a nerve pathway.

Throughout the examination of the nerve injury, it is important to understand the central effects of such an injury.

Treatment of compressive lesions is threefold and involves assisting fuel and oxygen delivery, resetting the gain on the muscle spindles of the muscles with increased tone, and maximizing the function of the viable neurons within the injured nerve to promote regeneration and decrease iatrogenic loss of neurons during the repair process.

The Perception of Pain

Pain is a multidimensional phenomenon dependent on the complex interaction of several areas of the neuraxis. The link between pain and injury seems so obvious that it is widely believed that pain is always the result physical damage, and that the intensity of pain felt is proportional to the severity of the injury. For the most part, this relationship between pain and injury holds true in that a mild injury produces a mild pain, and a large injury produces great pain. However, there are many situations were this relationship fails to hold up. For example, some people are born without the ability to feel pain even when they are seriously injured. This condition is referred to as *congenital analgesia*. There are also people who experience severe pains not associated with any known tissue damage or that persist for years after injuries have apparently healed (Melzack & Wall 1996).

Clearly the link between injury and pain is highly variable. It must always be remembered that injury may occur without pain and pain may occur without injury. Let us now look at some examples of the variety of different pain syndromes that may be seen in practice.

Injury Without Pain

Congenital Analgesia

People who are born without the ability to feel pain often sustain extensive burns, bruises, and lacerations during childhood. They frequently bite deeply into their tongues during chewing and learn only with great difficulty to avoid inflicting severe wounds on themselves. Usually these people show severe pathological changes in the weight-bearing joints, especially of the hips, knees, and spine, which are attributed to the lack of protection to joints usually given by the sensation of pain. The condition of a joint that degenerates because of failure to feel pain is called the 'Charcot' or *neurotrophic* joint. It has long been known that if the nerves that normally innervate a joint are missing or defective, a condition in which the joint surfaces become damaged and the ligaments and other tissues become stretched and unstable develops. In many cases of congenital analgesia the cause remains a mystery (Melzack & Wall 1996). Histological and physical examination of the nerves and nerve activities surrounding this loss of pain show no abnormal nerve activity or abnormal concentrations of cerebrospinal endorphins.

Episodic Analgesia

Cases of congenital analgesia are rare. Much more common is the condition most have experienced at one time or another, that of sustaining an injury, but not feeling pain until many minutes or hours afterwards. Injuries may range from minor cuts and bruises to severe broken bones and even the loss of a limb. Soldiers in the heat of battle frequently described situations in which an injury has not produced pain. In studies performed on these injured soldiers, it was found that they were not in a state of shock nor were they totally unable to feel any pain, for they complained as vigorously as a normal man at an inept nurse performing vein punctures. Their lack of ability to feel pain was attributed to their sense of relief or euphoria at having escaped alive from the field of battle (Melzack & Wall 1996).

There are six important characteristics of episodic pain

1. The condition has no relation to the severity or location of injury. It may occur with small skin cuts on an arm or leg or with the arm or leg blown off by explosives.

2. It has no simple relationship to the circumstances. It may occur in the heat of battle, or when a carpenter cuts off the tip of his finger, trying to make an accurate cut.

3. The victim can be fully aware of the nature of the injury and of its consequences and still feel no pain.

4. The analgesia is instantaneous. The victim does not first feel pain and then bring it under control. These people are not confused, distracted, or in shock. They understand the extent of their injury and may even touch the injured area, and still do not feel pain.

5. The analgesia has a limited time course, usually by the next day all these people are in pain.

6. The analgesia is localized to the injury. People may complain about other more minor injuries at other locations on the body.

Pain Without Injury

In contrast to people who fail to feel pain at the time of injury are people that develop pain without apparent injury. Examples of conditions commonly seen in practice include tension headaches, migraines, fibromyalgia, trigeminal neuralgia, and back pain.

The mechanism of pain without cause is thought to occur through *central pain* mechanisms. In central pain, an arm or a leg that apparently has nothing wrong with it can hurt so much or feel so strange that patients struggle to describe the pain or the feelings that they perceive (Boivie 2005). Central pain syndrome is a neurological condition caused by damage to or dysfunction of the central nervous system (CNS), which includes the brain, thalamus, brainstem, and spinal cord. The thalamus, in particular, has been implicated as a causative lesion site in as high as 70% of cases presenting with central pain (Bowsher et al 1998). The characteristics of central pain include steady burning, cold, pins and needles, and lacerating or aching pain although no one characteristic is pathognomonic (Bowsher 1996). Central pain can be associated with breakthrough pain and decreased discriminative sensation. Onset can be delayed, particularly after stroke. There are considerable differences in the prevalence of central pain among the various disorders associated with it. The highest incidence of central pain occurs in multiple sclerosis (MS), stroke, syringomyelia, tumour, epilepsy, brain or spinal cord trauma, and Parkinson's disease (Boivie 1999; Siddall et al 2003; Osterberg et al 2005).

Treatment of central pain syndrome is difficult and often frustrating for both the patient and the practitioner. Anti-depressants and anti-convulsants may provide some relief. Pain medications are generally only partially effective. The functional neurological approach has been as effective as any therapies at decreasing the symptoms of central pain. The approach includes assessing the central integrated state of all levels of the neuraxis and determine how pain modulation may be achieved most effectively. The following questions are helpful as a guide to approaching the treatment necessary for each individual.

1. At what level of the neuraxis has the damage occurred?—This requires a full neurological exam as outlined in Chapter 4.

2. Is the damage reversible?—Evaluating the response of effectors to stimulation aimed at the relevant areas of the neuraxis can give an indication as to whether the lesion can be reversed.

3. At what level of the neuraxis has central sensitization or reorganization occurred?—A careful analysis of the results of the neurological exam will establish the level of the lesion in the neuraxis.

4. What options are available to influence these processes?—Several approaches are available for treatment alternatives (see Chapter 17).

Pain Disproportionate to the Severity of Injury

The kidney may, under certain conditions, concentrate some components in the urine so that these compounds precipitate out of the urine and form small kidney stones or renal calculi. Small pieces of the stones break off and pass into the ureter that leads from the kidney to the bladder. In size, they are not more than twice the size of the normal diameter of the normal ureter. Pressure builds up behind the plug formed by the stone, tending to drive it into the ureter and as a result, the muscle in the wall of the ureter goes into localized strong contraction. This band of contraction moves down the ureter to produce peristaltic waves to drive the stone down. During this process called 'passing a stone' agonizing spasms of pain sweep over the patient in such a way that even the toughest and most stoical of characters usually collapse. The patient is pale with a racing pulse knees drawn up, with a rigid abdomen and motionless. Even crying out because of the pain is restrained because all movement exaggerates the pain. As the stone passes into the bladder there is immediate and complete relief of the pain resulting in an exhausted patient. The reason for describing this event here is that in physiological terms, and mechanical terms, this is a rather trivial event. Furthermore, it occurs in a structure which is poorly innervated when compared to other areas of the body. This process of passing kidney stones is described by the patient as painful beyond any expectation that pain can reach such intensity (Melzack & Wall 1996).

Several terms are used to describe pain disproportionate to the injury or not appropriate to the stimulus causing the pain.

Hyperalgesia is the term used to describe an excessive response to noxious stimulation. Hyperalgesia can be classified as either primary or secondary in nature. Primary hyperalgesia results from the release of various chemicals at the site of injury, leading to sensitization of nociceptive afferents. Secondary hyperalgesia involves collateral branches of the nociceptive afferents at the level of the spinal cord, which results in the regions surrounding the site of injury becoming more sensitive to pain.

Allodynia is the term used to describe pain produced by normally innocuous stimulation. For example stroking the skin would not normally be painful; however, stroking the skin after a sunburn may produce pain. With allodynia there is no pain if there is no stimulus, unlike other types of pain that can occur spontaneously without the presence of a stimulus.

Pain after Healing of an Injury

Motorcycle accidents are typically associated with injuries of the head and shoulder. On hitting a solid structure such as the road or a light standard, the rider is catapulted forwards and hits the road or other obstacle at high-speed. Crash helmets have effectively decreased head injuries, but the next vulnerable point that hits the road is often the shoulder, which may be wrenched down the back. The arm is supplied by a network of nerves, the brachial plexus, which leaves the spinal cord at the level of the lower neck and upper chest and funnels into the arms. In the most severe of these injuries the spinal roots are avulsed, that is, ripped out of the spinal cord, and no repair is possible. When this type of injury occurs, the arm is commonly paralysed from the shoulder down to the hand. The muscles of the arm become thin and limp with no sensation in the arm. Occasionally people with this injury have reported feeling a phantom limb, in which they can sense very clearly as an entire arm, but which had no relationship to the real arm. These phantom arms seem to be placed in various positions, which do not coincide to the position of the real arm at their side. The phantom arm commonly feels as though it is on fire.

Occasionally people who have experienced amputations of limbs may feel the presence of that limb even though the limb has been amputated. This is known as phantom pain (Melzack & Wall 1996). This shows that in certain cases pain may persist long after all apparent physical healing has occurred.

The term *phantom limb* was introduced by Silas Weir Mitchell. It is used to describe malrepresentation of actual limb position or existence following amputation or nerve blocks and is recognized by the patient as an 'illusion' rather than being the patient's delusion (Ramachandran & Hirstein 1998). Phantoms occur in 90–98% of all amputees almost immediately, but less commonly in children.

The intensity of the phantom presence appears to depend on both the degree of cortical representation present and the subjective vividness of that part in one's body image prior to amputation. The perceived postures of phantom limbs are probably related to the patient's experience prior to amputation, or may be perceived as maintaining a spastic, causalgic, or dystonic posture. The phantom sensations tend to fade after anywhere between days and decades. Some people experience a bizarre sensation referred to as telescoping in which they perceive a gradual shrinking of the limb so that it remains as only the hand on a stump. It is thought that this may occur due to increased representation of the hand in the brain's somatotopic maps.

When one part of the body is used more than an adjacent part, the somatotopic representation of that part will begin to expand and the receptive fields of the adjacent lesser utilized region of the cortex will become smaller. When an area of the body is amputated, the area of the brain that normally responds to sensory activation of the amputated body part will then begin to respond to sensory activation of adjacent body parts. This process probably occurs because of thalamocortical arborization or unmasking of previously seldom used, occult synapses in the cortex.

The reduction in activity experienced by cortical neurons as a result of sensory deprivation reduces the amounts of the inhibitory neurotransmitter γ-aminobutyric acid (GABA) released from interneurons, which in turn may allow previously weak synapses to become disinhibited. These normally suppressed inputs probably originate from long-range horizontal collaterals of pyramidal neurons located in cortex adjacent to the area of cortex that has lost its afferent stimulus due to the removal of the limb (Ramachandran & Hirstein 1998). Conversely, high levels of GABA brought about by persistent intense sensory input can cause weak synapses to become even more strongly inhibited, resulting in a surround inhibition of cortical areas not of immediate concern. In other words the extensive use of the fingers of the left hand, as would be the case in learning to play the guitar, will 'focus' the cortical area representing the fingers of the left hand and inhibit adjacent areas of cortex representing the elbow and shoulder.

Tinnitus, which is the subjective sensation of noise in the ears, has also been referred to as a phantom auditory sensation that may occur due to reorganization of the auditory cortex following some degree of deafferentation from the cochlear of the inner ear. Cochlear lesions resulting in loss of a specific range of frequencies can lead to reorganization of the auditory cortex due to replacement of the corresponding cortical areas with neighbouring areas of sound representation (Sexton 2006).

Musical hallucinations have also occurred in patients who have previously experienced tinnitus and progressive hearing loss. The complex nature of these hallucinations supports the theory of central auditory involvement due to deafferentation, despite the fact that hallucinations represent inappropriate overactivity of auditory neurons.

The Anatomy of Pain

Several pathways that originate from neurons in the spinal cord and project to higher centres in the neuraxis have nociceptive components (Willis & Coggeshall 2004; Willis & Westlund 2004). These pathways include the following:

QUICK FACTS 15	Anterior Spinal Artery Syndrome

- Occlusion of this artery results in a characteristic clinical picture:
  - Sudden paraplegia;
  - Disturbance in bladder and bowel function;
  - Impaired pain and temperature sense; and
  - Spared proprioception and vibration sense.
- The syndrome occurs due to softening of the spinal cord (myelomalacia) following vascular occlusion.
- The anterior spinal artery supplies the anterior two-thirds of the spinal cord.
- It is formed from two small branches of the vertebral arteries.
- The posterior arteries supply the posterior third of the spinal cord.

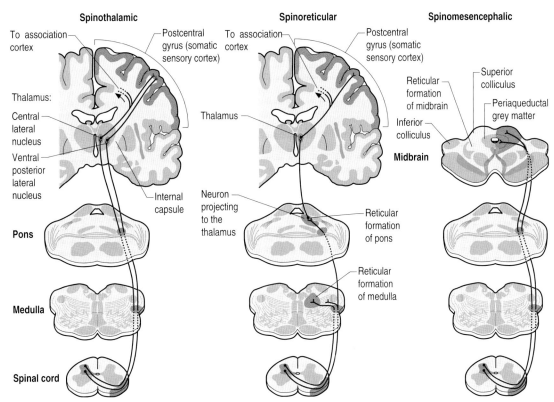

Fig. 7.24 Three of the major ascending pathways that transmit nociceptive information from the spinal cord to higher centres. The spinothalamic tract is the most prominent ascending nociceptive pathway in the spinal cord.

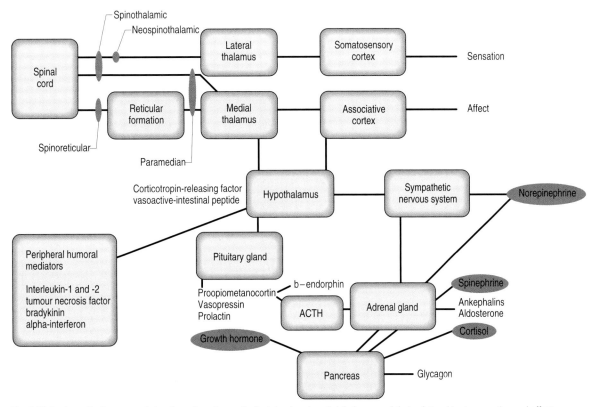

Fig. 7.25 A schematic diagram outlining the pain pathways to the lateral and medial thalamus and their relationships to sensation and affect. The diagram also includes the functional projections from the medial thalamus to the endocrine system and sympathetic nervous system.

1. Spinothalamic tract (STT) receives axons from neurons in laminae I and V–VII of the contralateral cord and project to the thalamus ipsilateral to the tract (Fig. 7.24). This tract has traditionally been recognized as the most important tract for the transmission of nociceptive information. The STT is thought to contribute to motivational and affective aspects of pain as well (Fig. 7.25). The axons of neurons in lamina I terminate on a number of nuclei in the thalamus including the ventroposterior lateral (VPL) nucleus, the ventral posterior inferior (VPI) nucleus, and the central lateral nucleus in the medial thalamus (Zhang et al 2000).

2. Spinoreticular tract receives axons from neurons in laminae VII and VIII. The tracts ascend bilaterally in the anterolateral system (Figs 7.26 and 7.27).

3. Spinomesencephalic tracts receive axons from neurons in laminae I and V and ascend in the anterolateral system bilaterally to synapse in the mesencephalic reticular formation and periaqueductal grey areas (Figs 7.26 and 7.27).

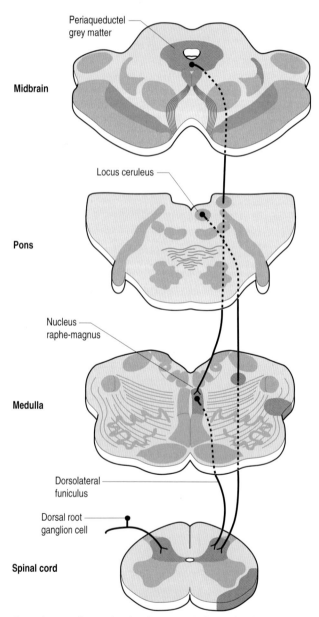

Fig. 7.26 A descending pathway regulates nociceptive relay neurons in the spinal cord. The pathway arises in the midbrain periaqueductal grey region and projects to the nucleus raphe magnus and other serotonergic nuclei (not shown), then via the dorsolateral funiculus to the dorsal horn of the spinal cord. Additional spinal projections arise from the noradrenergic cell groups in the pons and medulla and from the nucleus paragigantocellularis, which also receives input from the periaqueductal grey region. In the spinal cord these descending pathways inhibit nociceptive projection neurons through direction connections as well as through interneurons in the superficial layers of the dorsal horn.

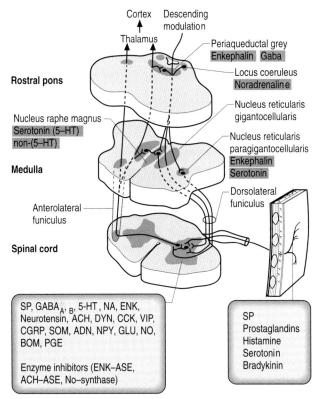

Fig. 7.27 The descending modulation of nociception, from the pons, medulla, and spinal cord.

4. Spinohypothalamic tracts receive axons from neurons in laminae I, V, and VIII, and project to supraspinal autonomic centres responsible for complex neuroendocrine and cardiovascular responses.

5. Postsynaptic dorsal column (PSDC) receives the majority of its axons from neurons in laminae III and IV but does receives additional axons from lamina X as well (Al-Chaer et al 1996; Willis & Coggeshall 2004). The projections from the PSDC first synapse on neurons in the dorsal column nuclei. Axons from the dorsal column nuclei cells project to the contralateral thalamus via the medial lemniscal tracts and to the brainstem (Wang et al 1999).

6. Spinocervical tracts receive axons from neurons in laminae III and IV and project to synapse on neurons of the lateral cervical nucleus.

7. Spinoparabrachial tract is a component of the spinomesencephalic tract that projects to the parabrachial nuclei and amygdala. This contributes to the affective component of pain.

Descending control of spinal projection neurons are mediated through pathways that descend from supraspinal areas into the spinal cord. Inhibition of STT in the spinal cord occurs through projections from the para aqueductal grey (PAG), nucleus raphe magnus, medullary reticular formation, anterior pretectal nucleus, ventrobasal thalamus, and postcentral gyrus. Excitation of the STT neurons can occur through stimulus from the motor cortex and isolated areas of the medullary reticular formation (Figs 7.26 and 7.27).

Pain...: Good or Evil?

From our above discussions, it seems that pain can serve three purposes:

1. Pain can occur before a serious injury as when one steps on a hot or otherwise potentially damaging object. This has a real survival value. It produces immediate withdrawal or some other action that prevents further injury.

2. Pain can also prevent further injury and act as the basis for learning to avoid injurious objects or situations, which may occur at a later time.

3. Pain due to damaged joints, abdominal infections or diseases, or serious injuries may also set limits on activity and enforce rest, which are often essential for the body's natural recuperative and disease-fighting mechanisms to work.

However, one also perceives pains that serve no useful survival value, such as the phantom pain described earlier. It is also commonly observed that very severe disease processes may develop to a very extensive state before pain is experienced by the individual (Melzack & Wall 1996). Why in this case did our sensation of pain fail us?

The Psychology of Pain

Pain is not simply a function of the amount of bodily damage done; rather, the amount and quality of pain one feels are also determined by:

1. Previous experiences and how well they are remembered;

2. One's ability to understand the cause of pain;

3. One's ability to grasp its consequences; and

4. Even the culture in which one is brought up plays an essential role in how one feels and responds to pain.

The above facts lead to the conclusion that the perception of pain cannot be defined simply in terms of a particular kind of stimuli; rather, the perception of pain is a highly personal experience depending on cultural learning, the meaning of the situation, and other factors unique to each individual in any given situation. There are a variety of stressors known to affect the perception of pain (Melzack & Wall 1996). These include ethnic/cultural values, age, environment, support systems, anxiety, and stress.

A number of recent studies have implicated the *cingulate gyrus* as the functional link between pain and emotional interactions (Rainville et al 1997; Sawamoto 2000). It is now known that the cingulate gyrus participates in pain and emotion processing. It has four regions, with associated subregions, and each makes a qualitatively unique contribution to brain functions. These regions and subregions are the subgenual (sACC) and pregenual (pACC) anterior cingulate cortex, the anterior midcingulate (aMCC) and posterior midcingulate cortex (pMCC), the dorsal posterior (dPCC) and ventral posterior cingulate cortex (vPCC), and the retrosplenial cortex (RSC) (Vogt et al 2006).

Pain processing is usually conceived in terms of two cognitive domains with sensory-discriminative and affective-motivational components. The ACC and MCC are thought to mediate the latter of these components. The nociceptive properties of cingulate neurons include large somatic receptive fields and a predominance of nociceptive activations, with some that even respond to an innocuous tap. These responses are predicted by the properties of midline and intralaminar thalamic neurons that project to the cingulate cortex, including the parafascicular, paraventricular, and reuniens nuclei that derive their nociceptive information from the spinal cord, the subnucleus reticularis dorsalis, and the parabrachial nuclei.

Rather than having a simple role in pain affect, the cingulate gyrus seems to have three roles in pain processing:

1. The pACC is involved in unpleasant experiences and directly drives autonomic outputs.

2. The aMCC is involved in fear, prediction of negative consequences, and avoidance behaviours through the rostral cingulate motor area.

3. The pMCC and dPCC are not involved in emotion but are driven by short-latency somatosensory signals that mediate orientation of the body in space through the caudal cingulate motor area.

In addition to these functions, nociceptive stimuli reduce activity in the vPCC and, therefore, activity in a subregion that normally evaluates the self-relevance of incoming visual sensations.

So, there is a complex interaction between pain and emotion. Moreover, hypoanalgesia and opioid and acupuncture placebos indicate mechanisms whereby the cingulate subregions can be engaged for therapeutic intervention.

Pain Thresholds

It is often believed that variations in pain experienced for person-to-person is due to different pain thresholds. There are four different thresholds related to pain, and it is important to distinguish between them.

1. Sensation threshold—this is the lowest stimulus value at which a sensation, such as tingling or heat, is first reported by the subject;

2. Pain perception threshold—this is the lowest stimulus value at which the person reports that the stimulation feels painful;

3. Pain tolerance—this is the lowest stimulus level at which the subject withdraws or asks to have the stimulation stopped; and

4. Encouraged pain tolerance—this is the same as the above, but the person is encouraged to tolerate higher levels of stimulation.

Combined Degeneration of the Spinal Cord	**QUICK FACTS 16**

- Corticospinal and posterior columns are affected.
- It is common in vitamin B_{12} deficiencies (e.g. pernicious anaemia).
- Degeneration of the spinal cord may occur before the clinical manifestations of pernicious anaemia.
- Clinical manifestations include:
  - Tingling;
  - Numbness; and
  - Pins and needles, occurring first in the toes and feet and later in the fingers.
- Psychological symptoms may also occur:
  - Hallucinations;
  - Disorientation;
  - Memory deficits; and
  - Personality changes.

There is now evidence that suggests that the majority of people, regardless of their cultural background, have a uniform sensation threshold. The sensory conduction apparatus appears to be essentially similar in all people so that a given critical level of input always elicits a sensation. The most striking effect of cultural background, however, is on pain tolerance levels. For example, women of Italian descent tolerate less shock than women of American or Jewish descent.

The importance of the meaning associated with the pain-producing situation is made particularly clear in experiments carried out by Pavlov on dogs. Dogs normally react violently when they are exposed to electric shocks to one of their paws, Pavlov found, however, that when he consistently presented food to a dog after each shock the dog developed an entirely new response. Immediately after each shock the dog would salivate, wag its tail, and turn eagerly towards the food dish. The electric shock now fails to evoke any responses indicative of pain and has become a signal meaning that food was on the way. This type of condition behaviour was observed as long as the same paw was shocked. If the shocks were applied to another paw the dog reacted violently. This study shows very convincingly that stimulation of the skin is localized, identified, and evaluated before it produces perceptual experience and overt behaviour (Melzack & Wall 1996). The meaning of the stimulus acquired during earlier conditioning modulates the sensory input before it activates brain processes that underlie perception and response.

If a person's attention is focused on a painful experience the pain perceived is usually intensified. In fact, the mere anticipation of pain is usually sufficient to raise the level of anxiety and thereby the intensity of the perceived pain. In contrast, it is well known that distraction of attention away from the pain can diminish or abolish it. This may explain why athletes sometimes sustained severe injuries during the excitement of the sport without being aware that they have been hurt.

The power of suggestion on pain is clearly demonstrated by studies using placebos. Clinical investigators have found that severe pain such as postsurgical pain can often be relieved by giving patients a placebo (usually some non-analgesic substance such as sugar or salt in place of morphine or other analgesic drugs). About 35% of the patients report marked relief of pain after being given a placebo (see below).

When psychological factors appear to play a predominant role in a person's pain, the pain may be labelled as *psychogenic pain*. The person is presumed to be in pain because they need or want it.

Pain Can Be Caused by Nociceptive or Neuropathic Mechanisms

The pain produced by nociceptive mechanisms involves direct activation of nociceptors. This is the commonly understood mechanism of pain production, where receptors sensitive to damage-causing activities, classified as nociceptive receptors or nociceptors, are stimulated and transmit excitatory information to the substantia gelatinosa neurons of the dorsal horn for integration and processing.

Neuropathically produced pain involves direct injury to nerves in the peripheral nervous system (PNS) or the CNS which has a burning or electric quality. Some examples of syndromes or conditions where neuropathic pain is thought to be involved include complex region pain syndrome (CRPS) (see below), post-herpetic neuralgia, phantom limb pain, and anaesthesia dolorosa, which is a condition where pain is perceived in the absence of sensation following treatment for chronic pain. Some neuropathic pains are thought to be sustained, at least in part, by sympathetic efferent activity via the expression of alpha-adrenergic receptors on injured C-fibres (see below).

Inflammatory pain is related to tissue damage. Damage to neurons can result in the release of neurotransmitters, and neuropeptides that can result in *neurogenic inflammation*. The proinflammatory substance prostaglandin E2 (PGE2) is released from damaged neurons and other cells. PGE2 is a metabolite of arachidonic acid via the cyclo-oxygenase pathway. The cyclo-oxygenase enzyme can be blocked by the use of nonsteroidal anti-inflammatory drugs (NSAIDs) and aspirin and is thought to be the mechanism by which these medications exert their effect. Bradykinin, which is also an extremely active proinflammatory and pain-activating substance, is also released when tissue is damaged. Bradykinin activates Aδ and C fibres directly and causes synthesis and release of prostaglandins from nearby cells.

Other proinflammatory substances released following injury include substance P and calcitonin-gene-related-peptide (CGRP), which both act on venules to spread inflammation and release histamine from mast cells.

Descriptions of pain

Transient Pain

Pains of brief duration are usually recognized as having little consequence and rarely produce more than fleeting attention. These momentary transient pains are often felt as two types of pains. For example, if you drop a heavy book on your foot you experience an immediate pressure-type sensation, followed by the secondary pain that will arrive shortly and when it does it wells up in your consciousness and obliterates all thoughts for the moment.

Acute Pain

The characteristics of acute pain are tissue damage, pain, and anxiety. Acute pain is usually related to an identifiable injury or disease focus and self-limited, resolving over hours to days or in a period associated with a reasonable period for healing. It is generally composed of the transitional period between coping with the cause of the injury and preparing for recovery. It is usually of short duration of days to weeks. Acute pain usually responds well to treatment. An injury should be considered to be in the acute phase during the natural history of normal healing for that injury. For example, the natural history of healing for a broken bone could be expected to range from 4 to 6 weeks. Pain experienced during the initial 4–6 weeks should be thought of as acute. However, if pain persists for longer than 6 weeks, the chronic classification should be applied.

Chronic Pain

This type of pain persists even after all possible physiological healing has occurred. It is no longer a symptom of injury but a pain syndrome. It may reflect separate mechanisms from the original insult and not reflect actual tissue damage or focal disease. The patient will often use vague descriptions of pain with difficulty in describing timing and localization of the pain.

Patients are beset with a sense of hopelessness or helplessness and often the pain is described in terms that have emotional associations. Marked alteration in behaviour with depression and/or anxiety often result, which may reflect a more cognitive aspect of pain. This condition is usually present for months to years in duration, with the patient experiencing marked reduction in daily activities, excessive amounts of medications, fragmentation of medical services, history of multiple non-productive tests, treatments, and surgeries.

Placebo Effect

A *placebo* is a substance or procedure thought to have no intrinsic therapeutic value which is given to an individual to satisfy a physiological or psychological need for treatment. The effects of placebos often produce the same or better results than treatments thought to have an intrinsic value. It was once thought that the effects of placebo were predominantly psychosomatic but current research has revealed that the placebo is indeed a real effect. For example, placebo analgesia can be blocked by naloxone, an opioid antagonist, suggesting that endogenous analgesia systems are likely to be activated during placebo analgesia.

Spinal Muscular Atrophy   **QUICK FACTS 17**

- Motor neuron disease
- Characterized by skeletal muscle wasting due to progressive degeneration of anterior horn cells
- Sensation and cerebellar function are conserved.
- Two basic forms:
  1. Infantile form (floppy baby syndrome)—also known as Werdnig–Hoffman syndrome
     - Parachute test to evaluate baby's muscle tone and extensor integrity
  2. Childhood form—also known as Wohlfart–Kugelberg–Welander disease.
     - Progressive muscular atrophy that begins in early childhood
     - Symptoms include proximal muscle atrophy, weakness, and fasciculations
     - Cause unknown

The gold standard in best practice therapeutics is that the treatment should significantly outperform the placebo effect in order to be considered a viable option for therapy. In the treatment of pain, production of analgesia or loss of pain sensation is the desired effect (Zhuo 2005).

As mentioned above endogenous analgesia systems are a likely component of the placebo effect. The anterior cingulate gyrus (ACC) has been found to be involved in this placebo analgesia. It has been theorized that ACC activation is responsible for facilitating descending inhibitory systems. However, electrical stimulation or glutamate synaptic activation in the ACC has actually been observed to increase nociceptive reflexes at the level of the spinal cord, and enhanced synaptic transmission and long-term plasticity have been found in ACC neurons after tissue injury, which suggests that the ACC may actually enhance any existing nociceptive effects. This would act in the opposite of the placebo effect and actually increase pain! Several theories have been advanced to incorporate these findings into a model that still allows the involvement of the ACC as a component in the generation of the placebo effect (Zhuo 2005).

The first theory involves the inhibition of pain-producing neurons in the ACC. Many neurons in the ACC respond to acute pain and the amount of this activation is related to pain unpleasantness. Activation of inhibitory neuron in the ACC can affect the excitability of these neurons by releasing GABA onto their postsynaptic receptors. Consequently, the excitability of ACC neurons is reduced, and neurons respond less to noxious stimuli.

The second theory involves the activation of local opioid-containing neurons in the ACC. Similar to the first theory, neurons containing opioid peptides may be activated. Opioid may act presynaptically and/or postsynaptically to inhibit excitatory synaptic transmission and reduce neurons responses to subsequent peripheral noxious stimuli. This mechanism could explain the fact that some placebo effects are sensitive to blockade by naloxone.

A third possibility involves the inhibition of descending facilitatory modulation from the ACC. The release of the inhibitory neurotransmitter GABA and/or opioids will reduce the excitability of ACC neurons that send descending innervations directly or indirectly to rostral ventral medulla (RVM) neurons. Consequently, descending facilitatory influences will be reduced.

The final theory involves a mixed activation of excitatory and inhibitory transmission by placebo treatment with the net result within the ACC being reduced excitatory transmission.

Complex Regional Pain Syndromes

The description of CRPS dates back to at least 1864 when Mitchell first described this condition. Mitchell coined the term 'causalgia', meaning burning pain. The most striking feature of this condition is pain that is disproportional to an injury. The onset of CRPS typically follows minor injuries such as sprains, fractures, or surgery. Other names for this condition include:

- Reflex sympathetic dystrophy syndrome (RSD/RSDS);
- Sudeck's atrophy;
- Shoulder–hand syndrome;
- Algodystrophy;
- Peripheral trophoneurosis;
- Sympathetically maintained pain;
- Sympathetically independent pain;
- Post-traumatic pain syndrome;
- Sympathalgia; and
- Sympathetic overdrive syndrome.

Due to confusion arising from the many names for this set of symptoms, the International Association for the Study of Pain (IASP) developed nomenclature to more accurately describe chronic pain. IASP coined the term chronic regional pain syndrome and broke CRPS into two categories;

CRPS I—Consists of pain, sensory abnormalities, abnormal sweating and blood flow, abnormal motor system function and trophic changes (thickening of the skin and nails, coarse thin hair growth), and atrophy of the superficial and deep tissues (skin, muscle, bone). The most common form is RSD and may not present with an identifiable nerve injury.

CRPS II—Same as CRPS I but presents with an identifiable nerve injury. Symptoms include burning pain made worse by light touch, temperature changes, or motion of the limb. These findings are most common in the foot or hand following partial injury to the nerve. The affected area appears cool, reddish, and clammy. The superficial and deep tissue structures may also begin trophic changes.

The key symptom of CRPS is continuous, intense pain out of proportion to the severity of the injury, which gets worse rather than better over time. CRPS most often affects one of the arms, legs, hands, or feet. Often the pain spreads to include the entire arm or leg. Typical features include dramatic changes in the colour and temperature of the skin over the affected limb or body part, accompanied by intense burning pain, skin sensitivity, sweating, and swelling.

The cause is unknown but CRPS affects from 2.3 to 3 times more women than men and is a major cause of disability in that only one in five patients is able fully to resume prior activities. Equally frightening is the increasing diagnosis of CRPS in children and adolescents; although there have been no large-scale studies on the incident of CRPS in children, some generalizations can be made about the children who get this condition. Published case studies indicate that the incident of CRPS increases dramatically between 9 and 11 years old, and it is found predominantly in young girls.

A recent web-based epidemiological survey of 1,610 people with CRPS, sponsored by the Reflex Sympathetic Dystrophy Association of America (RSDSA) and conducted by Johns Hopkins University, showed that common events leading to the syndrome were surgery (29.9%), fracture (15%), sprain (11%), and crush injuries (10%). There have also been some reports of increased occurrence of CRPS following the administration of general aesthetic.

Nearly all drugs currently used during the course of general anaesthesia may lead to hypersensitivity reactions of various types. There may be an acute type I allergic reaction or a more or less severe pseudoallergic reaction, in rare cases with lethal outcome.

In some cases the sympathetic nervous system has been implicated as an important component in sustaining the pain. These abnormal changes in the sympathetic nervous system seem to be responsible in some patients for constant pain signals to the brain, which alters the cortical areas of their brain responsible for pain and sensory reception of those areas of the body. Abnormal function of the sympathetic nervous system can also lead to movement disorders. Recent evidence, however, does not support that the pain of CRPS is solely sympathetically mediated; therefore, a thorough investigation examining the central integrated state of all levels of the neuraxis should be undertaken to determine the true nature of the patient's persistent or severe pain syndrome. An updated theory concerning the mechanism behind CRPS is that it is caused by supersensitivity of sympathetic nerve neurotransmitters and their metabolites (Rowbotham et al 2006). Patients with CRPS have been found to have decreased concentrations of noradrenalin in the venous effluent of the affected limb. This suggests that it is not due to increased output of the sympathetic nervous system. CRPS patients have increased concentrations of bradykinin and other local non-specific inflammatory mediators. Sympathetic inhibition may lead to up-regulation of beta-adrenergic receptors on the peripheral nociceptive fibres, making the afferents more sensitive to normal or lower levels of the neurotransmitter. It is more common to observe an initial increase in skin temperature followed by a chronically decreased skin temperature and trophic changes later in the course of the condition. The generation and maintenance of *central sensitization* are dependent on the actions of transmitter/receptor systems in the peripheral cord. Activation of receptor systems and second messenger systems leads to changes in receptor sensitivity, which increases the excitability of neurons (Schaible et al 2002). This is a form of physiological wind-up.

This process can be summarized into six steps:

1. Sensitization of C-nociceptors after initial pain-evoked sympathetic reflex vasoconstriction, which results in the activation of glutamatinergic N-methyl-D-aspartate (NMDA) receptors that cause increased Ca^{++} ion flux into the neurons which activated second messengers and increase sensitivity of the neuron to stimulus (Neugebauer et al 1993);

2. Nociceptors up-regulate expression of alpha-1 adrenoreceptors, which increases the action of catecholamines on the neuron;

3. Activation by tonic release of norepinephrine by sympathetic efferents, which bind to the increased receptor population and magnify the response;

4. Receptive field changes of central projecting pain neurons, resulting in increased pools of neuron activation and inappropriate spread of the initial stimulus;

5. Activity-dependent neuronal plasticity, allowing the system to function over long periods (Schaible & Grubb 1993); and

6. Central sensitization, resulting in wind up of pain neurons.

Pain is not the only reason why patients have difficulty moving. Patients state that their muscles feel stiff and that they have difficulty initiating movement.

Paediatric patients present unique challenges. For example, children have not had sufficient time to develop the psychosocial skills necessary to cope with the pain and suffering due to CRPS. The fear and anxiety that this syndrome produces in a child leads to a further lowering in the child's pain threshold, making activities of normal life even more painful. The presence of these seemingly unexplainable symptoms has led to a great deal of confusion and frustration among children and their families. Another theory is that CRPS is caused by a triggering of the immune response, which leads to the characteristic inflammatory symptoms of redness, warmth, and swelling in the affected area (Romanelli & Esposito 2004).

General Features of CRPS

- Discomfort: spontaneous pain or hyperalgesia/hyperaesthesia;
- Distribution: Not limited to single nerve territory;
- Disproportionate to inciting event;
- Other associated features on affected limb, especially distal;

QUICK FACTS 18   **Amyotrophic Lateral Sclerosis (ALS)**

- Both upper and lower motor neuron involvement;
- Aetiology unknown;
- Characterized by progressive degeneration of the corticospinal tracts and anterior horn cells;
- Onset: 40–60 years (offspring born before knowledge of disease in many cases);
- Progressive and fatal: 2–6 yrs;
- Symptoms include:
  - No sensory findings (no pain, numbness);
  - Fasciculations;
  - Muscle cramps;
  - Segmental, asymmetrical weakness;
  - Upper and lower motor neuron signs;
  - Tongue fasciculations;
  - Bladder and bowel function spared; and
  - Deep tendon reflexes usually spared in early phase.

EMG conduction velocities remain near normal even in the presence of severe atrophy. This separates this disorder from peripheral motor neuropathies in which the conduction velocity is reduced.

QUICK FACTS 19   **ALS: Classic Presentation**

- Painless weakness;
- Atrophy of the hands;
- Fasciculations in the entire upper extremities;
- Spasticity and reflex hyperactivity of the legs; and
- Extensor plantar sign (Babinski present).

- Oedema;
- Skin blood flow (temperature) or sudomotor abnormalities;
- Motor symptoms;
- Trophic changes;
- Types:
    - CRPS I: No definable nerve lesion
    - CRPS II: Nerve lesion present.

Motor Disorders

- Sense of weakness with complex motor tasks (79%): 'Give-way';
- Difficulty initiating movements;
- Limited range of motion: wrist; ankle;
- Involuntary movements;
- More common with nerve lesions;
- Tremor (48%);
- Irregular myoclonic jerks, dystonia, or muscle spasm (30%); and
- Tendon reflexes: increased, on affected side 46%.

Treatment

Treatments for CRPS type I supported by evidence of efficacy and little likelihood for harm are topical dextramethasone (DMSO) cream, IV bisphosphonates, and limited courses of oral corticosteroids. Despite some contradictory evidence, physical therapy, joint manipulation, and calcitonin (intranasal or intramuscular) are likely to benefit patients with CRPS type I.

Patients with CRPS and intractable pain showed a shrinkage of cortical maps on primary (SI) and secondary somatosensory cortex (SII) contralateral to the affected limb. This was paralleled by an impairment of the two-point discrimination thresholds. Behavioural and psychomotor stimulation over 1–6 months consisting of graded sensorimotor retuning led to a persistent decrease in pain intensity, which was accompanied by a restoration of the impaired tactile discrimination and regaining of cortical map size in contralateral SI and SII. This suggests that the reversal of tactile impairment and cortical reorganization in CRPS can be accomplished by increasing the appropriate sensory stimulation to cortical areas. Nutritional supplementation with a variety of supplements including vitamin C and calcitonin has also been shown to be effective.

References

Al-Chaer ED, Lawand NB, Westlund KN et al 1996 Pelvic visceral input into the nucleus gracilis is largely mediated by the post-synaptic dorsal column pathway. Journal of Neurophysiology 76:2675–2690.

Barson AJ 1970 The vertebral level of termination of the spinal cord during normal and abnormal development. Journal of Anatomy 106:489–497.

Boivie J 1999 Central pain. In: Wall PD, Melzack R (eds) Textbook of pain, 4th edn. Churchill Livingstone, Edinburgh, p 879–914.

Boivie J 2005 Central pain. In: Mersky H, Loeser JD, Dubner R (eds) The paths of pain 1975–2005. IASP Press, Seattle, WA.

Bowsher D 1996 Central pain: clinical physiological characteristics. Journal of Neurology, Neurosurgery, and Psychiatry 61:62–69.

Bowsher D, Leijon G, Thomas K-A 1998 Central post-stroke pain: correlation of MRI with clinical pain characteristics and sensory abnormalities. Neurology 51:1352–1358.

Chusid JG 1982 The brain. In: Correlative neuroanatomy and functional neurology, 19th edn. Lange Medical, Los Altos, CA, p 19–86

Erlanger J, Gasser HS 1937 Electrical signs of nervous activity. University of Pennsylvania Press, Philadelphia.

Fulton JF, Sheenan D 1935 The uncrossed lateral pyramidal tract in higher primates. Journal of Anatomy 69:181–187.

Jit I, Charnalia J 1959 The vertebral level of the termination of the spinal cord. Journal of Anatomical Society India 8:93–101.

Melzack R, Wall PD 1996 The challenge of pain. Penguin, New York.

Neugebauer V, Lucke T, Schaible HG 1993 N-Methyl-D-aspartate (NMDA) and non-NMDA receptor antagonists block the hyperexcitability of dorsal horn neurons during development of acute arthritis in rat's knee joint. Journal of Neurophysiology 70:1365–1377.

Nyberg-Hansen R 1965 Sites and mode of termination of reticulospinal fibers in the cat. An experimental study with silver impregnation methods. Journal of Comparative Neurology 124:71–100.

Nyberg-Hansen R 1969 Cortico-spinal fibres from the medial aspect of the cerebral hemisphere in the cat. An experimental study with the Nauta method. Experimental Brain Research 7:120–132.

Osterberg A, Boivie J, Thuomas K-A 2005 Central pain in multiple sclerosis-prevalences, clinical characteristics and mechanisms. European Journal of Pain 9:931–942.

Rainville P, Duncan GH, Price DD et al 1997 Pain affect encoded in human anterior cingulate but not somatosensory cortex. Science 277:968–971.

Ramachandran VS, Hirstein W 1998 The perception of phantom limbs. The D. O. Hebb lecture. Brain 121:1603–1630.

Rexed B 1964 Some aspects of the cytoarchitectonics and synaptology of the spinal cord. Progress in Brain Research 11:58–90.

Romanelli P, Esposito V 2004 The functional anatomy of neuropathic pain. Neurosurgery Clinics of North America 15:257–268.

Rowbotham MC, Kidd BL, Porreca F 2006 Role of central sensitization in chronic pain: osteoarthritis and rheumatoid arthritis compared to neuropathic pain. In: Flor H, Kalso E, Dostrvsky J (eds) Proceedings 11th World Congress on Pain. IASP Press, Seattle, WA.

Sawamoto N, Honda M, Okada T et al 2000 Expectation of pain enhances responses to nonpainful somatosensory stimulation in the anterior singulate cortex and parietal operculum/

posterior insula: an event-related functional magnetic resonance imaging study. Journal of Neuroscience 20:7438–7445.

Schaible HG, Grubb BD 1993 Afferent and spinal mechanisms of joint pain. Pain 55:5–54.

Schaible HG, Ebersberger A, Von Banchet GS 2002 Mechanisms of pain in arthritis. Annals of the New York Academy of Science 966:343–354.

Sexton SG 2006 Forehead temperature asymmetry: A potential correlate of hemisphericity. (Personal communication).

Siddall PJ, McClelland JM, Rutkowski SB et al 2003 A longitudinal study of the prevalence and characteristics of pain in the first 5 years following spinal cord injury. Pain 103:249–257.

Szentagothai J 1948 Anatomical considerations of monosynaptic reflex arcs. Journal of Neurophysiology 11:445–454.

Vogt BA, Porro CA, Faymonville ME 2006 Pain processing and modulation in the cingulated gyrus. In: Flor H, Kalso E, Dostrvsky J (eds) Proceedings 11th World Congress on Pain. IASP Press, Seattle, WA.

Wang CC, Willis WD, Westlund KN 1999 Ascending projections from the central, vixceral processing region of the spinal cord: and PHA-L study in rats. Journal of Comparative Neurology 415:341–362.

Willis WD, Coggeshall RE 2004 Sensory mechanisms of the spinal cord. Kluwer Academic/Plenum, New York.

Willis WD, Westlund KN 2004 Pain system. In: Paxinos G, Mai JK (eds) The human nervous system. Elsevier, Amsterdam, p 1125–1170

Zhang X, Wenk HN, Honda CN et al 2000 Locations of spinothalamic tract axons in cervical and thoracic spinal cord white matter in monkeys. Journal of Neurophysiology 83:2869–2880.

Zhuo M 2005 Central inhibition and placebo analgesia. Molecular Pain 1:21.

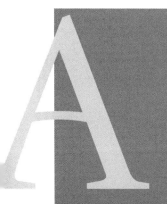

Clinical Case Answers

Case 7.1

7.1.1 The *spinothalamic* pathway, from a clinical standpoint, carries pain and temperature sensation from the entire body, excluding trigeminal distributions, to the thalamus. Primary afferent fibres have cell bodies located in the dorsal root ganglion (DRG) and their central processes synapse in the dorsal horn laminae I, II, and V predominately. Secondary afferents, which form the spinothalamic tract proper, decussate (cross the spinal cord) about 2–3 levels higher in the spinal cord and ascend in the anterolateral funiculus to the ventral posterior lateral (VPL) nucleus of the thalamus. Sensory modulation can occur in the brain, thalamus, or spinal cord, especially in lamina II, and is also influenced by visceral afferents in lamina V where convergence of afferent information can result in referred pain phenomena.

7.1.2
1. Unrecognized fracture;
2. Soft tissue calcification;
3. Complex region pain syndrome;
4. Psychogenic; and
5. Coincidental pathology such as a bone or soft tissue tumour.

7.1.3 The presentation CRPS includes the following signs and symptoms which usually occur following an injury of some sort to a peripheral limb:

General Features
- Discomfort: spontaneous pain or hyperalgesia/hyperaesthesia;
- Distribution: Not limited to single nerve territory;
- Disproportionate to inciting event;
- Other associated features on affected limb, especially distal;
- Oedema;
- Skin blood flow (temperature) or sudomotor abnormalities;
- Motor symptoms;
- Trophic changes;
- Types:
  ○ CRPS I: No definable nerve lesion
  ○ CRPS II: Nerve lesion present.

Motor Disorders
- Sense of weakness with complex motor tasks (79%): 'Give-way';
- Difficulty initiating movements;
- Limited range of motion: wrist; ankle;
- Involuntary movements;
- More common with nerve lesions;
- Tremor (48%);
- Irregular myoclonic jerks, dystonia, or muscle spasm (30%); and
- Tendon reflexes: increased, on affected side 46%.

In this case the young lady has all of the features of CRPS except the involuntary movements spind tremors.

Case 7.2

7.2.1

Muscle spindle receptors in the muscles and the joint receptors in the joints relay information to the spinal cord concerning movement and proprioception. The *ventral spinocerebellar* pathway conveys information about the ongoing status of interneuronal pools in the spinal cord to the cerebellum. It therefore provides continuous monitoring of ascending and descending information concerning locomotion and posture. The neurons of this tract originate in laminae V–VII between L2 and S3. Their projection axons decussate to the other side so that they ascend in the contralateral anterolateral funiculus. These fibres then decussate again via the superior cerebellar peduncle to synapse on neurons in the anterior part of the ipsilateral cerebellum (Fig. 7.12).

The *dorsal spinocerebellar* tract neurons originate medially to the IML column of the spinal cord between C8 and L2/3.

The primary afferent cell bodies are located in the DRG and their central processes synapse with the above-mentioned neurons near the entry level or after ascending for a short distance in the dorsal columns. Secondary afferents ascend in the ipsilateral dorsolateral funiculus, lateral to the corticospinal tracts, and enter the ipsilateral cerebellum via the inferior cerebellar peduncle. Via this pathway, the cerebellum is provided with ongoing information about joint and muscle activity in the trunk and limbs. The cuneocerebellar pathway carries the same type of information from the upper limb and cervical spine via the cuneate fasciculus of the dorsal columns.

7.2.2

1. Cervical disc protrusion;
2. Soft tissue swelling around the injury resulting in spinal compression;
3. Bone displacement due to the fracture, resulting in cord compression;
4. Brachial plexus injury not diagnosed; and
5. Intracranial haemorrhage.

Chapter 8

Autonomic Nervous System

Clinical Cases for Thought

Case 8.1   A 14-year-old girl presents with her mother who is concerned that her child has unequal pupils. She first became aware of this following the child's school photos.

Questions
8.1.1   You explain to the mother that this finding is called anisocoria. She then asks you 'What causes it?' Outline your answer.

Case 8.2   A 56-year-old woman is referred by her cardiologist because she is experiencing cardiac dysrhythmia for which he can find no cause.

Questions
8.2.1   Outline a possible mechanism for the dysrhythmia this woman is experiencing involving the autonomic innervation of the heart.

Introduction

There are three components of the autonomic nervous system.

1. Sympathetic system;
2. Parasympathetic system; and
3. Enteric system.

The sympathetic nervous system can function more generally with respect to its less precise influence on physiology as it mediates whole-body reactions involved in the 'fight and flight' responses. Both the sympathetic and parasympathetic systems are tonically active to help maintain a stable internal environment in the face of changing external conditions which is best described as homeostasis.

Both the sympathetic and parasympathetic systems comprise preganglionic and postganglionic neurons. The cell bodies of preganglionic neurons in the sympathetic system are located in the intermediolateral cell column (IML) of the spinal cord between T1 and L2. The axons of these neurons exit the spinal cord via the ventral root with the motor neurons of the ventral horn. A branch known as the white rami communicans (myelinated) carries these fibres to the sympathetic chain ganglia where many of the preganglionic cells synapse with postganglionic cells. At cervical and lumbar levels, postganglionic sympathetic neurons form grey rami communicans (unmyelinated and slower conducting) that are distributed to vascular smooth muscle, pilo erector muscle, and sweat glands via the spinal nerves and their branches. At cervical levels, some of the postganglionic neurons also project to the eye, blood vessels, and glands of the head and face via the carotid and vertebral arterial plexi. The cell bodies of parasympathetic preganglionic neurons are located in discrete nuclei at various levels of the brainstem and at the IML column of levels S2–4 in the spinal cord (vertebral level L1–2). In contrast to the sympathetic system, the preganglionic parasympathetic neurons are generally longer than the postganglionic neurons as they synapse in ganglia further from their origin and closer to the effector than the postganglionic neurons innervate.

Organization of the Autonomic Nervous system

The autonomic nervous system comprises the major autonomous or non-volitional efferent outflow to all organs and tissues of the body with the exception of skeletal muscle. Anatomically, the autonomic outflow from the spinal cord to the end organ occurs through a chain of two neurons consisting of a pre- and postganglionic component. The preganglionic component neurons live in the grey matter of the spinal cord. The postganglionic component neurons vary in location with some living in the paraspinal or sympathetic ganglia, and others in ganglia distant from the cord known as stellate ganglia. Although historically only the efferent connections were considered, all of the projections of the autonomic nervous system are reciprocal in nature and involve both afferent and efferent components. The autonomic system can be divided into three functionally and histologically distinct components: the parasympathetic, sympathetic, and enteric systems. All three systems are modulated by projections from the hypothalamus. Hypothalamic projections that originate mainly from the paraventricular and dorsal medial nuclei influence the parasympathetic and sympathetic divisions as well as the enteric division of the autonomic nervous system. These descending fibres initially travel in the medial forebrain bundle and then divide to travel in both the periaqueductal grey areas and the dorsal lateral areas of the brainstem and spinal cord. They finally terminate on the neurons of the parasympathetic preganglionic nuclei of the brainstem, the neurons in the intermediate grey areas of the sacral spinal cord, and the neurons in the intermediolateral cell column of the thoracolumbar spinal cord. Descending autonomic modulatory pathways also arise from the nucleus solitarius, noradrenergic nuclei of the locus ceruleus, raphe nuclei, and the pontomedullary reticular formation (PMRF).

The parasympathetic system communicates via both efferent and afferent projections within several cranial nerves including the oculomotor (CN III) nerve, the trigeminal (CNV) nerve, the facial (CNVII) nerve, the glossopharyngeal nerve, and the vagus (CN X) and accessory (CN XI) nerves (Fig. 8.1). The vagus nerve and sacral nerve roots compose the major output route of parasympathetic enteric system control (Furness & Costa 1980). Axons of the preganglionic nerves of the parasympathetic system tend to be long, myelinated, type II fibres and the postganglionic axons tend to be some what shorter, unmyelinated, C fibres (see Chapter 7). The cell bodies of parasympathetic preganglionic neurons are located in discrete nuclei at various levels of the brainstem as described above and in the intermediolateral cell column of levels S2–4 in the spinal cord or vertebral level L1–2. In contrast to the sympathetic system, the preganglionic parasympathetic neurons are generally longer than the postganglionic neurons as they synapse in ganglia that are further from their origin and closer to the effector than the postganglionic neurons innervate.

The neurotransmitter released both pre- and postsynaptically is acetylcholine. Cholinergic transmission can occur through G-protein coupled mechanisms via muscarinic receptors or through inotropic nicotinic receptors. The activity of ACh is terminated by the enzyme acetylcholinesterase, which is located in the synaptic clefts of cholinergic neurons. To date, seventeen different subtypes of nicotinic receptors and five different subtypes of muscarinic receptors have been identified (Nadler et al 1999; Picciotto et al 2000).

Cholinergic, nicotinic receptors are present on the postsynaptic neurons in the autonomic ganglia of both sympathetic and parasympathetic systems. Cholinergic, muscarinic receptors are present on the end organs of postsynaptic parasympathetic neurons (Fig. 8.2).

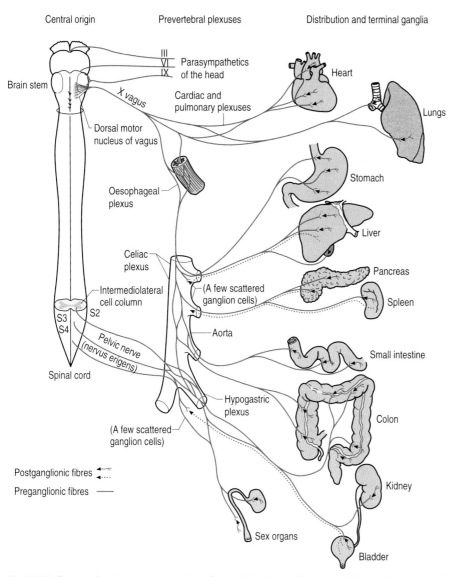

Central origin   Prevertebral plexuses   Distribution and terminal ganglia

Fig. 8.1 This figure outlines the parasympathetic outflow to the body including the cranial nerves III, VII, and IX, the vagus nerve (CNX) and the pelvic division of spinal nerves.

The neurological output from the parasympathetic system is the integrated end product of a complex interactive network of neurons spread throughout the mesencephalon, pons, and medulla. The outputs of the cranial nerve nuclei including the Edinger–Westphal nucleus, the nucleus tractus solitarius, the dorsal motor nucleus, and nucleus ambiguus are modulated via the mesencephalic reticular formation (MRF) and PMRF. This complex interactive network receives modulatory input from wide areas of the neuraxis including all areas of cortex, limbic system, hypothalamus, cerebellum, thalamus, vestibular nuclei, basal ganglia, and spinal cord (Walberg 1960; Angaut & Brodal 1967; Brodal 1969; Brown 1974; Webster 1978). The relationship of the parasympathetic outflow to the immune system has received very little study to date and as a consequence very little is known about the influence of the parasympathetic or the enteric system on immune function.

Supraspinal Modulation of Autonomic Output

Monosynaptic connections between two structures suggest an important functional relationship between the two structures in question. Polysynaptic connections may be

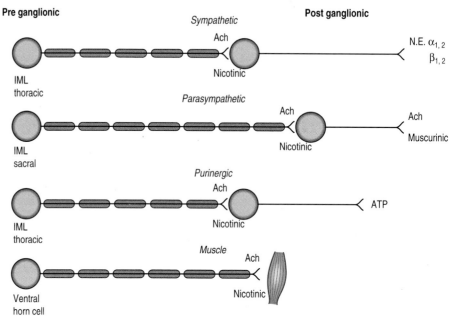

Fig. 8.2 This figure outlines the pre-ganglionic and post-ganglionic neurotransmitters and receptors of the sympathetic and parasympathetic divisions of the autonomic nervous system. It also includes the transmitter (ACH⁻) of the ventral horn cell and the (nicotinic) receptors in muscle. Note that all preganglionic axons are myelinated and all post ganglionic axons are unmyelinated.

important as well but are not as well understood as monosynaptic connections. Monosynaptic connections have been demonstrated to exist between a variety of nuclei in the medulla, pons, diencephalon, and the preganglionic neurons of the IML (Smith & DeVito 1984; Natelson 1985). Nuclei with monosynaptic connections with the neurons of the IML include:

- Areas of the ventral lateral reticular formation including neuron pools in the ventral pons and ventral lateral medulla;
- Neuron pools in the locus ceruleus of the dorsal rostral pons;
- Serotonergic neurons of the raphe nucleus;
- Epinephrine-producing neurons of the caudal ventrolateral medulla;
- Neuron pools of the parabrachial complex;
- Neuron pools of the central grey area and the zona incerta; and
- Neuron pools in the paraventricular and dorsal medial nuclei of the hypothalamus.

The hypothalamus is the only structure with direct monosynaptic connects to the nuclei of the brainstem and to the neurons of the IML. This suggests that the influence of the hypothalamus on autonomic function is substantial.

The projections from the cerebral cortex and their role in modulation of autonomic function are not well understood. However, existence of direct projections from the cortex to subcortical structures regulating autonomic function has been established (Cechetto & Saper 1990). Neurophysiological studies demonstrating autonomic changes with stimulation and inhibition of the areas of cortex also suggest a regulatory role. The following outlines the established areas of cortex and their projection areas:

1. Medial prefrontal cortex has direct projections to the amygdala, hypothalamus, brainstem, and spinal cord areas involved in autonomic control.

2. The cingulate gyrus has direct projections to the amygdala, hypothalamus, brainstem, and spinal cord areas involved in autonomic control.

3. The insular and temporal pole areas of cortex also demonstrate direct projections to the amygdala, hypothalamus, brainstem, and spinal cord areas involved in autonomic control.

4. Primary sensory and motor cortex are thought not to control autonomic activity directly but to coordinate autonomic outflow with higher mental functions, emotional overlay, and holistic homeostatic necessities of the system.

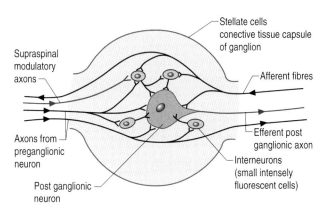

Fig. 8.3 This figure illustrates the synaptic connections of afferent and efferent axons fibres on the ganglion cells. Note that both afferent and efferent information modulates the activity of the ganglion cell, both directly and indirectly through interneurons.

Most Areas Modulating the Autonomic Systems are Bilateral Structures

It is worth noting at this point that with the exception of a few midline structures in the brainstem, the locus ceruleus, and the raphe nuclei, all other structures that modulate the autonomic output are bilateral structures. This presents the possibility that asymmetric activation or inhibition lateralized to one side or the other may translate to the activity of the end organs and produce asymmetries of function from one side of the body to the other (Lane & Jennings 1995). Accurately assessing the asymmetric functional output of the autonomic nervous system is a valuable clinical tool in evaluating asymmetrical activity levels of cortical or supraspinal structures that project to the output neurons of the autonomic system.

The Autonomic Ganglion

The autonomic ganglion is the site at which the presynaptic neurons synapse on the postsynaptic neurons. The sympathetic ganglia are situated paraspinally in the sympathetic trunk or prespinally in the celiac and superior mesenteric ganglia. The parasympathetic ganglia are situated in close proximity to the target structures that they innervate. The autonomic ganglia consist of a collection of multipolar interneurons surrounded by a capsule of stellate cells and connective tissue.

Incoming and outgoing nerve bundles are attached to the ganglion (Fig. 8.3). The incoming bundles contain afferent fibres from the periphery returning to the spinal cord, preganglionic axons that synapse on the postganglionic neurons in the ganglion, preganglionic axons that pass through the ganglion giving off collateral axons to the interneurons as they do so, and descending axons from cholinergic neurons in the spinal cord that modulate the activity of the interneurons in the ganglion. The interneurons in the ganglion are referred to as small intensely fluorescent cells and they are thought to be dopaminergic in nature. The outgoing bundle contains postganglionic axons, and afferent fibres from the periphery entering the ganglion (Snell 2001). The presence of such a complex structure in the ganglion has lead to the suspicion that the ganglion are not just relay points but integration stations along the pathway of the autonomic projections.

Parasympathetic Efferent Projections

The *oculomotor parasympathetic fibres* commence in the midbrain. These fibres are the axon projections of neurons located in the Edinger–Westphal (EWN) or accessory oculomotor nuclei. The parasympathetic projections travel with the ipsilateral oculomotor nerve and exit with the nerve branch to the inferior oblique muscle and enter the ciliary ganglion where they synapse with the postganglionic neurons. The axons of the postganglionic neurons then exit the ganglion via the short ciliary nerves and supply the ciliary muscle and the sphincter pupillae. Activation of the postganglionic neurons causes contraction of both the ciliary muscle, resulting in relaxation of the lens, and the sphincter pupillae muscle, resulting in constriction of the pupil. These actions can be stimulated separately or simultaneously as in the accommodation reflex (Fig. 8.4).

Functionally, the Edinger–Westphal nucleus receives the majority of its input from the contralateral field of vision. This involves the stimulus of the ipsilateral temporal and contralateral nasal hemiretinas, which results in the constriction of the ipsilateral pupil. For example, a shining light from the right field of vision will stimulate the left nasal hemiretina and the right temporal hemiretina which project through the left optic tract to the left EWN. The left EWN stimulation results in constriction of the ipsilateral (left) pupil. Some fibres from the left optic tract also synapse on the right EWN, effectively resulting in constriction of both pupils. This constitutes the consensual pupil reflex. Comparison between the time to activation (TTA) and time to fatigue (TTF) in each pupil following stimulation from the contralateral field of vision can be used to estimate the central integrative state of the respective EWN. This in addition to further evaluation of the oculomotor and trochlear function can then be used to estimate the central integrative state (CIS) of the respective mesencephalon. In situations where the CIS of the EWN is healthy one would expect rapid TTA and normal TTF response times, relatively, equal in both pupils. In situations where the CIS of one EWN is undergoing transneural degeneration of relatively short duration, one would expect an extremely rapid TTA followed by a relatively short TTF in the ipsilateral eye when compared to the contralateral eye. In situations where the CIS of one EWN is such that transneural degeneration, long-standing in nature, is present then one would expect the pupil of the ipsilateral EWN to show an increased TTA and a decreased TTF in comparison with the contralateral eye. On prolonged stimulus a pupil in this condition will often fluctuate the pupil size between normal and partial constriction. This is referred to as hippus.

The parasympathetic efferent projections of the *facial nerve* involve motor axons to the submandibular gland and the lacrimal gland. The motor fibres project in two different pathways and to two different ganglia. The motor projections to the *submandibular gland*

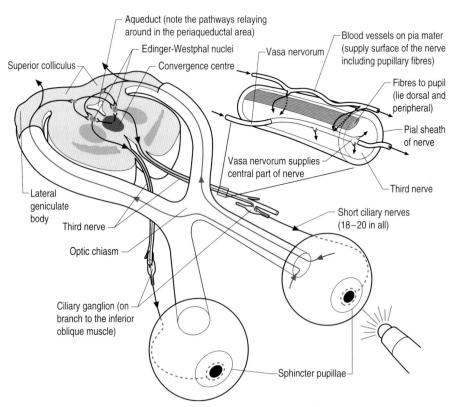

Fig. 8.4 This figure outlines the anatomical relationships of the optic and oculomotor nerves, as well as the mesencephalic nuclei of the third nerve. Note the inset that shows the detailed anatomy of the oculomotor nerve.

arise from neurons in the superior salivatory nucleus in the medulla. The axons of these neurons emerge from the brainstem in the nervous intermedius and join the facial nerve until the stylomastoid foramen where they separate as the chorda tympani, which traverse the tympanic cavity until they reach and join with the lingual nerve. They travel with the lingual nerve until they reach and synapse on the postganglionic neurons of the submandibular ganglion. The axons from these neurons project to the submandibular glands via the lingual nerve supplying the secretomotor fibres to the gland. Activation of the postganglionic neurons results in dilatation of the arterioles of the gland and increased production of saliva (Fig. 8.5).

The motor projections to the *lacrimal gland* travel in the greater petrosal nerve through the pterygoid canal and synapsing on the neurons of the pterygopalatine ganglion. The axons of the neurons in the pterygopalatine ganglion project their axons with the zygomatic nerve to the lacrimal gland and form direct branches from the ganglion to the nose and palate.

The efferent projections of the glossopharyngeal nerve contain axons that are secretory motor to the parotid gland. The projections start in the neurons of the inferior salivatory nucleus of the medulla and travel in the glossopharyngeal nerve through the tympanic plexus where they separate and travel with the lesser petrosal nerve to synapse on the neurons in the otic ganglion. The axons of these neurons then travel in the auriculotemporal nerve to the parotid gland. Activation of the neurons of the otic ganglion produces vasodilation of the arterioles and increased saliva production in the gland.

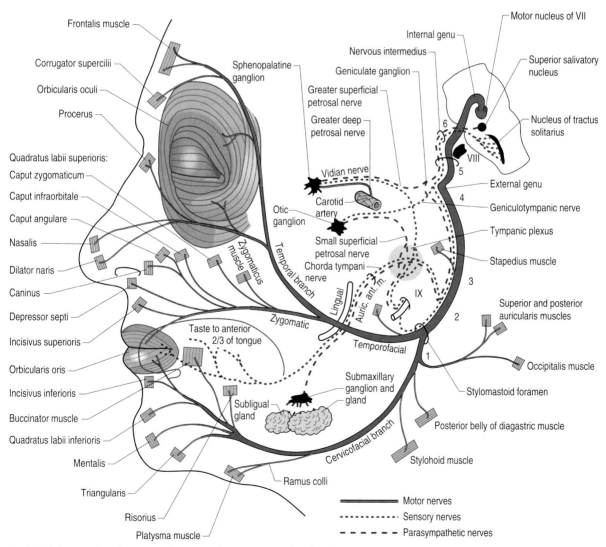

Fig. 8.5 This figure outlines the motor and parasympathetic projections of the facial nerve (CN VII).

The motor projections of the *vagus nerve* arise from the neurons of the dorsal motor nucleus and the nucleus ambiguous of the medulla. The *cardiac branches* are inhibitory, and in the heart they act to slow the rate of the heartbeat. The *pulmonary branch* is excitatory and in the lungs they act as a broncho constrictor as they cause the contraction of the non-striate muscles of the bronchi. The *gastric branch* is excitatory to the glands and muscles of the stomach but inhibitory to the pyloric sphincter. The *intestinal branches*, which arise from the postsynaptic neurons of the mesenteric plexus or Auerbach's plexus and the plexus of the submucosa or Meissner's plexus, are excitatory to the glands and muscles of the intestine, caecum, vermiform appendix, ascending colon, right colic flexure, and most of the transverse colon but inhibitory to the ileocaecal sphincter (Fig. 8.6).

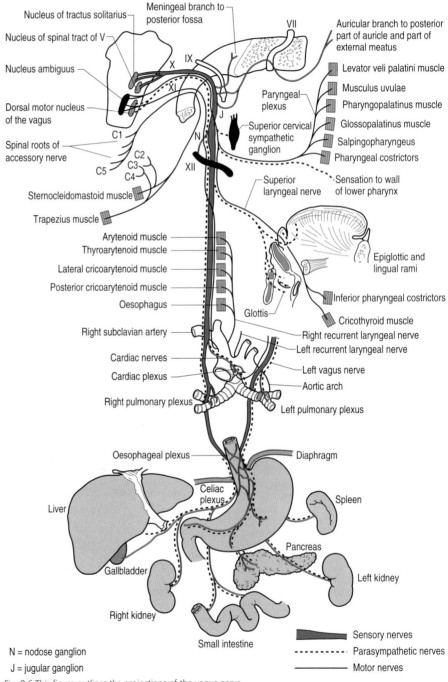

N = nodose ganglion

J = jugular ganglion

Fig. 8.6 This figure outlines the projections of the vagus nerve.

The *pelvic splanchnic* nerves are composed of the anterior rami of the second, third, and fourth sacral spinal nerves. These nerves diverge, giving off several collateral branches to supply the pelvic viscera. Most of the projections merge with fibres of the sympathetic pelvic plexus and pass to ganglia located adjacent to their target structures, where they synapse with their postganglionic components.

Functionally, the CIS of the medulla can be estimated by examining the activities of the cranial nerves, which mediate the effector functions of end organs that can be measured. For example, a patient that presents with excessive watering of the eyes, increased salivation and nasal mucus production, difficulty in taking deep breaths, decreased heart rate, stomach pain, intestinal cramping, and frequent loose bowel movements may indicate an overactive medullary region. An underactivated medullary region may present with dry eyes, dry mouth, dry nasal cavities, increased heart rate, and constipation. This highlights the importance of conducting a thorough neurological examination of both the motor and visceral functions of the cranial nerves and relating the findings in a functional manner back to the neuraxial structures involved.

The *sympathetic system* enjoys a wide-ranging distribution to virtually every tissue of the body (Fig. 8.7). The presynaptic neurons live in a region of the grey matter of the spinal

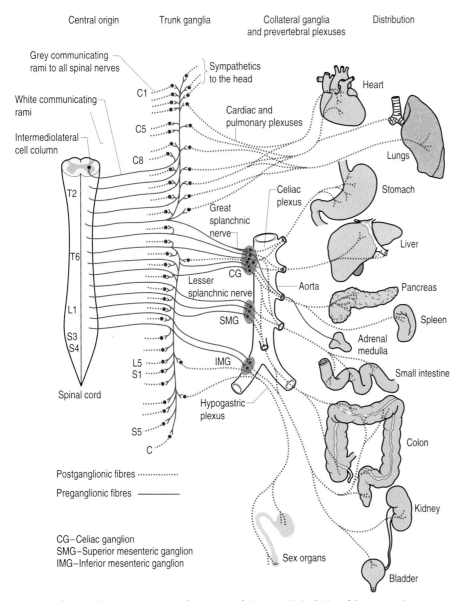

Fig. 8.7 This figure outlines the wide range of projections of the sympathetic division of the autonomic nervous system.

cord called the intermediomedial and intermediolateral cell columns located in lamina VII. Axons of these neurons exit the spinal cord via the ventral rami where they further divide to form the white rami communicantes. The fibres then follow one of several pathways (Fig. 8.8):

1. They synapse in the paravertebral or prevertebral ganglia segmentally.

2. They synapse in segmental regions of the paravertebral or prevertebral ganglion other than those at which they exited.

3. They do not synapse in the prevertebral or paravertebral ganglia and continue as presynaptic myelinated fibres into the periphery (Williams & Warwick 1984).

The output of the preganglionic neurons of the sympathetic system is the summation of a complex interactive process involving segmental afferent input from dorsal root ganglion and suprasegmental input from the hypothalamus, limbic system, and all areas of cortex via the MRF and PMRF (Donovan 1970; Webster 1978; Williams & Warwick 1984). Most postganglionic fibres of the sympathetic nervous system release norepinephrine as their neurotransmitter. The adrenergic receptors bind the catecholamines norepinephrine (noradrenalin) and epinephrine (adrenalin).

These receptors can be divided into two distinct classes, the alpha adrenergic and beta adrenergic receptors (Fig. 8.2). The chromaffin cells of the adrenal medulla which are embryological homologues of the paravertebral ganglion cells are also innervated by preganglionic sympathetic fibres which fail to synapse in the paravertebral ganglia as described above. When stimulated these cells release a neurotransmitter/neurohormone that is a mixture of epinephrine and norepinephrine with a 4:1 predominance of epinephrine (Elenkov et al 2000).

Both epinephrine and norepinephrine are manufactured via the tyrosine-dihydroxyphenylalanine (DOPA)-dopamine pathway and are called catecholamines. When the body is in a neutral environment, catecholamines contribute to the maintenance of homeostasis by regulating a variety of functions such as cellular fuel

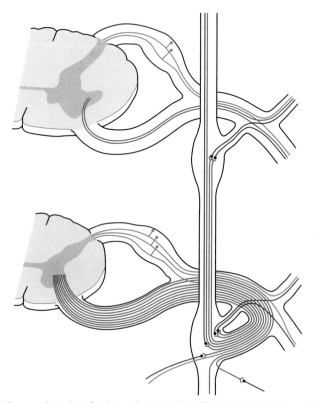

Fig. 8.8 This figure illustrates the variety of pathways that sympathetic fibres may take in the paraspinal ganglion. Pre-synaptic fibres may pass directly through the ganglion and not synapse until they reach other ganglion usually deep in the tissues of the gut. Other pre-synaptic fibres may synapse with their post-synaptic cells at the same level as they exit the spinal cord. Other pre-synaptic fibres may travel up or down in the ganglionic chains to synapse many levels distant to the level they exited the spinal cord. The superior cervical ganglia are examples of this type of projection.

metabolism, heart rate, blood vessel tone, blood pressure and flow dynamics, thermogenesis, and as explained below, certain aspects of immune function. When a disturbance in the homeostatic state is detected, both the sympathetic nervous system and the hypothalamus–pituitary–adrenal axial system become activated in the attempt to restore homeostasis via the resulting increase in both systemic (adrenal) and peripheral (postganglionic activation) levels of catecholamines and glucocorticoids. In the1930s Hans Selye described this series of events or reactions as the general adaptation syndrome or generalized stress response (Selye 1936). Centrally, two principal mechanisms are involved in this general stress response, these are the production and release of corticotrophin releasing hormone produced in the paraventricular nucleus of the hypothalamus and increased norepinephrine release from the locus ceruleus norepinephrine releasing system in the brain stem. Functionally, these two systems cause mutual activation of each other through reciprocal innervation pathways (Chrousos & Gold 1992). Activation of the locus ceruleus results in an increase release of catecholamines, of which the majority is norepinephrine, to wide areas of cerebral cortex, subthalamic, and hypothalamic areas. The activation of these areas results in an increased release of catecholamines from the postganglionic sympathetic fibres as well as from the adrenal medulla.

Functional Effects of Sympathetic Stimulation

Postganglionic sympathetic fibres that course to the periphery with peripheral motor nerves usually only supply the blood vessels of the muscle of the peripheral nerve. Activation of these fibres produces vasodilation. Sympathetic fibres that course to the periphery in peripheral sensory nerves usually supply the vasoconstrictor muscles of blood vessels, the secretomotor fibres of sweat glands, and the motor fibres of the piloerector muscles of hair follicles in areas supplied by the nerve. Stimulation of these fibres results in vasoconstriction of the blood vessels, usually an increase in sweat gland, and piloerector activity.

Sympathetic projections that innervate structures in the cranial region arise from preganglionic neurons in the spinal IML at the level of T1. Axons from these neurons exit the spinal column and pass uninterrupted through the cervicothoracic ganglion to reach the superior cervical ganglion where they terminate on the postganglionic neurons in the ganglion. Axons from these neurons then project via the internal carotid nerve, which courses with the carotid artery through the carotid canal into the cranium, where it enlarges to form the carotid plexus. Fibres emerging from the carotid plexus accompany all of the cranial nerves to innervate the blood vessels in the distribution of the cranial nerves. Visceromotor and vasomotor fibres course with the oculomotor nerve to the ciliary ganglion where they pass through uninterrupted to form the long ciliary nerves which course to the eyeball. The vasomotor fibres control the extent of vasoconstriction of the arterioles supplying the eyeball. The visceromotor fibres terminate on the dilatator pupillae muscle of the iris where activation results in pupillary dilation (Fig. 8.9). Some fibres course to the levator palpebrae superioris muscles of the upper eyelid also known as Muller's smooth muscle. Activation of these fibres results in the contraction of these muscles which retract the eyelid. The sympathetic supply to this muscle only composes a partial segment of the innervation, which is also contributed to by motor fibres in the oculomotor nerve. Other fibres emerge from the ciliary ganglia to innervate the ciliary muscles. Activation of these fibres results in contraction of the ciliary muscles, which causes the lens to relax for better focus of near objects.

Vestibuloautonomic Reflexes

Vestibulosympathetic reflexes are varied in nature due to the extensive interaction between the vestibular system, midline components of the cerebellum, and autonomic control centres. Major regions that mediate autonomic function and receive inputs from the vestibular system include the nucleus tractus solitarius (NTS), parabrachial nuclei

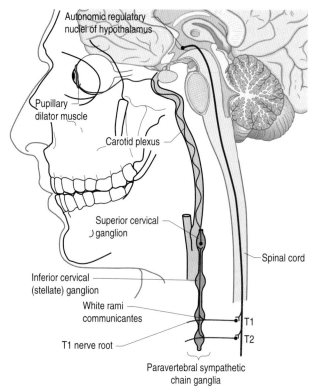

Fig. 8.9 This figure illustrates the sympathetic projection system from the hypothalamus to the pupil of the eye. Projections from the hypothalamus to the pre-ganglionic cells located in the IML cell columns of the spinal cord between the levels of T1 and L2 modulate the activation of the these pre-ganglionic cells, which then project axons to the post-ganglionic cells in the superior cervical ganglion. Post-synaptic cell axons then follow the carotid arteries into the head and branch to follow the oculomotor nerve to the eye.

(pons and midbrain), hypothalamic nuclei, rostral and caudal ventrolateral medulla (RVLM and CVLM), dorsal motor nucleus (DMN) of the vagus, nucleus ambiguus, and locus coeruleus. Other parasympathetic nuclei such as the superior salivatory nucleus (SSN) of the pons and the Edinger–Westphal nucleus of the midbrain also receive direction projections leading to salivation and tearing, and pupil constriction, respectively.

The effect of vestibular activation on the sympathetic system is mediated largely through the CVLM and RVLM. The RVLM is a region of the medullary reticular formation that contains tonic vasomotor neurons—i.e. neurons that exert tonic excitation of the IML. The CVLM can be activated by the vestibular system and higher nervous system centres directly, or indirectly via the NTS. It contains neurons that inhibit the RVLM.

Therefore, there are two phases to vestibulosympathetic reflexes—excitatory and inhibitory phases. In some instances, vestibulosympathetic reflexes will consist of an early excitatory phase and a late inhibitory phase. This type of reflex helps to protect the individual from the effects of orthostatic stress, which occurs when one stands up quickly. Therefore, orthostatic hypotension is not only dependent on baroreceptor activity, but also on vestibulosympathetic reflexes.

These reflexes are very complex and it appears that certain neurons within the vestibular system may have a greater effect on the excitatory phase and others have a greater effect on the inhibitory phase. Whatever the case, it should be clear that increased output from the vestibular nucleus or vestibular receptors can increase both sympathetic and parasympathetic activity at the same time. For example, this may result in a rise in blood pressure and sweating due to activation of the RVLM and hypothalamus and increased tearing and bowel activity due to activation of the SSN and the DMN of the vagus. A loss of vestibular activity may lead to orthostatic hypotension due to poor maintenance of vasomotor tone when changing posture. Significant overactivity of the vestibular system could also create the symptoms of light-headedness due to excessive vasomotor tone throughout the carotid tree.

Horner's Syndrome

Disruption of the sympathetic chain at any point from the hypothalamic or supraspinal projections to the oculomotor nerve can result in a spectrum of symptoms referred to as Horner's syndrome. The classic findings in this syndrome include ptosis, miosis, and anhidrosis but a number of other abnormalities may also be present. Ptosis or drooping of the upper eyelid is caused by the interruption of the sympathetic nerve supply to the muscles of the upper eyelid. Miosis or decreased pupil size is a result of the decreased action of the dilator muscles of the iris due to decreased sympathetic input. This results in the constrictor muscles acting in a relatively unopposed fashion, resulting in pupil constriction. A Horner's pupil will still constrict when light is shined on the pupil although careful observation is sometimes required to detect the reduced amount of constriction that occurs. Another test that can be used in these cases utilizes the ciliospinal reflex, which results in pupil dilation in response to pain. A pinch applied to the neck region will result in bilateral pupil dilation under normal conditions. However, in the case of unilateral disruption of the sympathetic innervation as in Horner's syndrome, the pupil on the effected side will show decreased or absent dilation response. Occasionally the appearance of enophthalmos or retraction of the eyeball into the eye socket occurs because of the relaxation of the eyelid muscles. Anhidrosis or reduced sweating capability sometimes also occurs on the ipsilateral face and neck in Horner's syndrome. The affected skin will usually appear shiny and will feel smooth to the touch compared with the non-involved areas. Anhidrosis is usually not associated with postganglionic lesions or lesions above the superior cervical ganglion because sympathetic projections to the face and neck emerge from the sympathetic chain prior to the superior cervical ganglion. However, if the disruption occurs in the hypothalamic projections to the IML, anhidrosis may actually be present on the entire upper quarter on the ipsilateral side. The causes of Horner's syndrome can be multiple and varied and include (Fig. 8.10):

- Infarcts or haemorrhage of the lateral brainstem;
- Trauma to the spinal cord;
- Apical lung tumour, also referred to as Pancoast tumour or syndrome;
- Trauma or tumour of the neck region;
- Injuries or pathology of the carotid plexus including carotid dissection;
- Interruption of the cavernous sinus including thrombus, aneurysm, or neoplasm;
- Fracture or infection of the orbit; and
- Physiological asymmetry of sympathetic function.

The Distribution of the Sympathetic System is Widespread

The distribution of the sympathetic projections is widespread and in fact includes all tissues of the body. Distribution from the major ganglia is discussed below.

The *superior cervical ganglion* arises from the axons of preganglionic neurons located in the spinal cord levels T1–2 and is physically located at the second and third cervical vertebral levels. Postganglionic axons project to the structures of the head and neck including:

- Vasomotor fibres to the brain and eyeball;
- Motor fibres to the pupil and smooth muscles of the upper eyelid;
- Motor fibres to the ciliary muscles of the lens;
- Vasomotor fibres to the meninges of the posterior cranial fossa;
- Vasomotor fibres to the carotid bodies;
- Vasomotor and visceromotor fibres to the sweat glands of the face; and
- Vasomotor fibres to the blood vessels of the face.

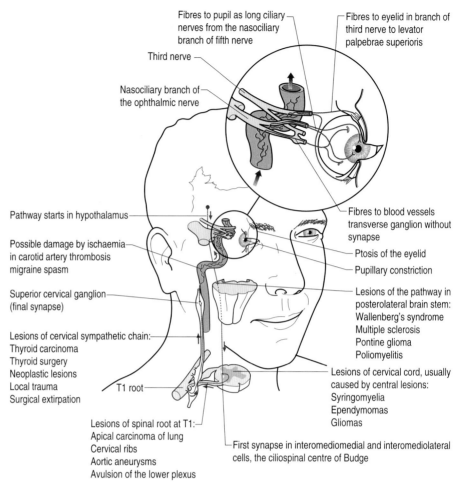

Fibres to pupil as long ciliary nerves from the nasociliary branch of fifth nerve

Fibres to eyelid in branch of third nerve to levator palpebrae superioris

Third nerve

Nasociliary branch of the ophthalmic nerve

Pathway starts in hypothalamus

Possible damage by ischaemia in carotid artery thrombosis migraine spasm

Superior cervical ganglion (final synapse)

Lesions of cervical sympathetic chain:
Thyroid carcinoma
Thyroid surgery
Neoplastic lesions
Local trauma
Surgical extirpation

T1 root

Lesions of spinal root at T1:
Apical carcinoma of lung
Cervical ribs
Aortic aneurysms
Avulsion of the lower plexus

Fibres to blood vessels transverse ganglion without synapse

Ptosis of the eyelid

Pupillary constriction

Lesions of the pathway in posterolateral brain stem:
Wallenberg's syndrome
Multiple sclerosis
Pontine glioma
Poliomyelitis

Lesions of cervical cord, usually caused by central lesions:
Syringomyelia
Ependymomas
Gliomas

First synapse in interomediomedial and interomediolateral cells, the ciliospinal centre of Budge

Fig. 8.10 This figure outlines the anatomy and location of a variety of causes of Horner's syndrome. The inset shows the detailed anatomy of the fibres innervating the pupil.

The *middle cervical ganglion* arises from the axons of the preganglionic neurons in the IML of spinal cord levels T2–4 and is physically located at the sixth cervical vertebral level. Postganglionic axons project to structures of the neck including:

- Both vasomotor and visceromotor fibres to the thyroid gland;
- Both vasomotor and visceromotor fibres to the parathyroid glands;
- Motor and vasomotor fibres to the trachea;
- Motor and vasomotor fibres to the oesophagus; and
- Vasomotor fibres that accompany the C4 and C5 cervical spinal nerves.

The cervicothoracic or stellate ganglion arises from the axons of preganglionic neurons in the IML at the spinal cord levels T5–6 and is physically located at the vertebral levels C7–T1. Postganglionic axons project to structures of the neck and upper chest including:

- Vasomotor fibres to the vertebral arteries;
- Vasomotor fibres to the C4, C5, C6, C7 spinal nerves; and
- Vasomotor fibres to the common carotid arteries.

Sympathetic distribution in the thoracic area is consistent with the projections of the paraspinal ganglia at each vertebral segmental level. However, the formation of the splanchnic nerves deserves mention. The splanchnic nerves are formed by preganglionic myelinated fibres that pass through the paraspinal ganglia without synapsing, although some evidence suggests that collateral branching of these fibres which do synapse in the ganglia may occur (Fig. 8.3).

The *greater splanchnic nerve* is formed from preganglionic fibres of IML neurons located at the spinal cord levels T5–9. These axons project to the celiac and aorticorenal ganglia and the suprarenal glands where they synapse with their respective postganglionic counter parts. The *lesser splanchnic nerve* arises from the preganglionic neurons in the IML at the spinal cord levels T9–10. These axons project to the aorticorenal ganglion. The sympathetic projections of the lumbar area are formed from axons of the IML neurons at the levels T8–12 and project to the intermesenteric and superior hypogastric plexuses. The postganglionic fibres from this level, arising from the paraspinal ganglia, form the projections that course with the obturator and femoral nerves to the thigh.

The pelvic sympathetic projections are formed from the axons of the preganglionic neurons of the IML at the spinal cord levels T10–L2. These axons project to a series of four ganglia that lie adjacent to the sacrum. Postganglionic fibres of these ganglia course with the tibial, pudendal, inferior, and superior gluteal nerves to their respective distributions.

The autonomic innervation of several clinically important areas will be considered in detail.

Innervation of the Heart

Preganglionic parasympathetic neurons that modulate the heart rate reside in the medulla and synapse with postganglionic neurons adjacent to the heart. Parasympathetic fibres project from the nucleus tractus solitarius, dorsal vagal nucleus, and the nucleus ambiguous and course to the periphery in the glossopharyngeal (CN IX) and vagus (CN X) cranial nerves. Direct connections exist between the sensorimotor cortex and the NTS, DMV, and RVLM. These direct cortical projections to the NTS/DMV provide the anatomical basis for cortical influences on both the baroreceptor reflex and cardiac parasympathetic control (Zamrini et al 1990). These connections also display an ipsilateral predominance.

The neurons of the NTS, DMN, and nucleus ambiguous also send projection fibres to the preganglionic sympathetic neurons in the IML and to other brainstem nuclei that modulate sympathetic outflow (Lane & Jennings 1995). The right and left vagal projections demonstrate an asymmetric distribution with the right vagal projections innervating some aspects of the anterior right and left ventricles and the left vagal projections innervating the posterior lateral aspects of the ventricles. However, the predominant innervation of the vagal projections terminates on the atrial aspects of the heart and include the sinus (SA) node, which usually determines the rate of the heartbeat. The influence of the vagal projections on the ventricles appears to be limited to counteracting the sympathetic innervation (Rardon & Bailey 1983).

Sympathetic innervation of the heart can be separated into left and right sympathetic limbs based on physiological studies. The right postganglionic sympathetic projections arising from the paravertebral sympathetic ganglia including the stellate ganglia course to the heart and innervate the atria and the anterior surfaces of the right and left ventricles. The left sympathetic projections have a more posterior lateral distribution and innervate the atrioventricular (AV) node and the left ventricle (Levy et al 1966; Randall & Ardell 1990). Stimulation of the sympathetic projections results in different physiological effects on the heart. Stimulation of the right stellate ganglia produces mainly chronotropic effects such as increases in heart rate, and stimulation of the left stellate ganglia mainly results in inotropic effects such as altered contractility, changes in rhythm, and increase in systemic blood pressure (Levy et al 1966; Rogers et al 1978) (Fig. 8.11). Increased stimulation to either or both ganglia results in a decreased fibrillation threshold (Schwartz 1984; Swartz et al 1994). With respect to cortical control of cardiovascular function, the research suggests that asymmetries in brain function can influence the heart through ipsilateral pathways. It is quite clear that stimulation or inhibition at various levels on the right side of the neuraxis results in greater changes in heart rate, while increased sympathetic tone on the left side of the neuraxis results in a lowered ventricular fibrillation threshold. This occurs because parasympathetic mechanisms are dominant in the atria, while sympathetic mechanisms are dominant in the ventricles (Lane et al 1992).

Innervation of the Lungs

The postganglionic sympathetic fibres projecting to the lungs arise from the paravertebral ganglia at the vertebral levels T2–5 and project to the bronchi and blood vessels of the lung. Excitation of the sympathetic fibres causes dilation of both the bronchi and the blood vessels.

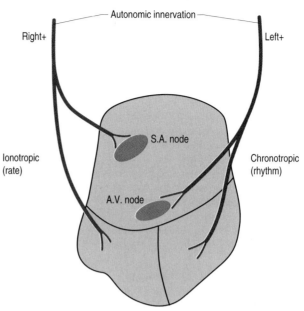

Fig. 8.11 This figure outlines the autonomic innervation to the heart. The different projection patterns of the left and right nerve supplies may explain the different clinical findings of right and left autonomic dystonia.

Parasympathetic supply arises from the DMN of the vagus nerve and courses to the lung in the vagus nerve, where the fibres synapse in the numerous pulmonary plexuses located throughout the lung tissues. Postganglionic fibres then project to the bronchi, secretory glands, and blood vessels of the lung. Excitation of the parasympathetic fibres results in constriction of the bronchi and blood vessels and increased production of secretions from the glands.

Innervation of the Kidneys

Postganglionic fibres arise from the renal plexus and course to synapse on the vasomotor structures of the renal arteries. Excitation of these fibres results in constriction of the renal arteries. Parasympathetic projections arise from the vagus nerve and course to the vasomotor structures of the renal artery. Excitation of these fibres results in dilation of the renal arteries.

Medulla of the Adrenal Glands (Suprarenal Glands)

The sympathetic fibres that arrive at the medulla of the adrenals are presynaptic in nature, usually coursing through the greater splanchnic nerve. The fibres synapse on the secretory cells of the medulla, which are embryological homologues of the postganglionic neurons in the paraspinal ganglia and act as the postganglionic component for the preganglionic projections. The neurotransmitter released is acetylcholine as it is in all other preganglionic autonomic synapses. Excitation of these fibres results in an increased production and secretion of the catecholamines norepinephrine and epinephrine from the adrenal medulla.

Innervation of the Urinary Bladder

The innervation of the bladder is complex. Afferent sympathetic fibres emerge from the muscle tissue of the bladder, the detrusor muscle, and course through the hypogastric nerve to the upper lumbar sympathetic ganglia. They then course with the posterior nerve roots to the IML neurons at the levels T9–L2 in the spinal cord. These fibres probably transmit proprioceptive and nociceptive information from the bladder. Efferent sympathetic fibres project from the IML neurons at the levels T11–12 and course with the white rami to the hypogastric plexus where they synapse and join the hypogastric nerve to reach the detrusor muscle and internal sphincter of the bladder. Excitation of these fibres results in contraction of the internal sphincter muscle and inhibition of the detrusor muscle. Parasympathetic innervation involves both afferent and efferent projections. The afferent projections arise from the bodies of the detrusor and internal sphincter muscles and course with the pudendal nerve to the S2–4 posterior nerve roots, terminating in the anterolateral grey areas of the spinal cord at these levels. These fibres probably carry proprioceptive, nociceptive, touch, temperature, and muscle stretch information from the bladder tissues. The efferent parasympathetic fibres pass from the S2–4 segments of the spinal cord to the hypogastric plexus where they synapse and project to the detrusor and internal sphincter muscles. Excitation of these fibres results in excitation of the detrusor and inhibition of the internal sphincter muscles.

The external sphincter is innervated by the pudendal nerve, which arises from the anterior horns of the S2–4 spinal roots. These fibres are under voluntary control and excitation results in contraction of the external sphincter muscle. Afferent fibres carried by the pudendal nerve relay proprioceptive and nociceptive information from the external sphincter muscle and posterior urethra.

Cortical control over micturition also exists. Areas in the paracentral lobule of the cortex evoke excitation of bladder contractions; this may play a role in the voluntary control over micturition (Chusid 1982) (Fig. 8.12).

The sympathetic nerves to the detrusor muscle have little or no action on the smooth muscle of the bladder wall and are mainly distributed to the blood vessels. In the male, sympathetic activation results in contraction of the sphincter and bladder neck during ejaculation in order to prevent seminal fluid from entering the bladder. Urination is brought about by activation of the parasympathetic system that results in contraction of the detrusor muscle and relaxation of the internal sphincter along with voluntary relaxation of the external sphincter through cortical stimulus.

Erection of the Penis and Clitoris

The parasympathetic system controls the engorgement of the penile and clitoral tissues. Engorgement of these tissues results in erection of the penis and expansion of the clitoris.

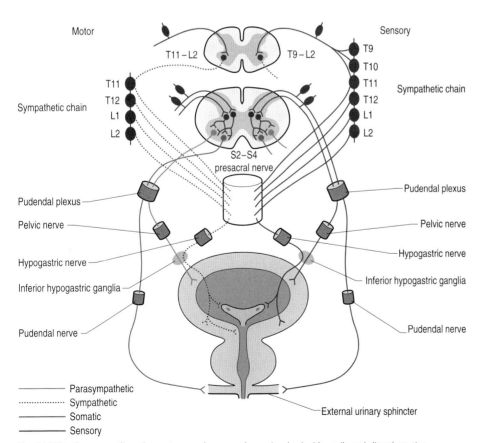

Fig. 8.12 This diagram outlines the anatomy and nerve pathways involved with penile and clitoral erection.

The preganglionic parasympathetic fibres arise from the lateral grey area of the sacral spinal cord levels S1–4 and synapse in the hypogastric plexus. The postganglionic projections course with the pudendal arteries to innervate the tissue of the penis and clitoris. Excitation of the postganglionic fibres results in massive increases in blood flow to the tissues and results in erection.

Ejaculation is accomplished through the action of the sympathetic nervous components that arise in the grey matter of the spinal cord at the spinal cord levels L1–2. The preganglionic fibres synapse in the lumbar ganglia. The axons of the postganglionic neurons then course to the vas deferens, the seminal vesicles, and the prostate gland through the hypogastric plexuses. Excitation of the postganglionic projections results in waves of contraction of the smooth muscles of these structures and the ejaculation of sperm (Snell 2001).

Innervation of the Uterus

The innervation of the uterus is mainly through the preganglionic neurons that arise from the T12–L1 levels of the spinal cord. The preganglionic fibres course through the paraspinal ganglion to the inferior hypogastric plexus where they synapse. The axons of the postganglionic neurons then project to the smooth muscle of the uterus were excitation results in vasoconstriction and muscular contraction. Parasympathetic preganglionic fibres arise from neurons in the spinal cord levels S2–4 and synapse in the hypogastric plexuses before projecting to the smooth muscle of the uterus. Excitation of these fibres results in relaxation of the uterine muscles and dilation of the blood vessels. The uterus is also under a high degree of hormonal control as well as neuronal control (Snell 2001).

Referred Visceral Pain

Since most of the viscera is only innervated by autonomic projections, afferent autonomic nerve pathways must relay nociceptive, temperature, and proprioceptive information back to the central nervous system. Usually visceral pain is poorly localized and difficult to qualitatively describe. Frequently information transferred by afferent autonomic fibres is perceived in other areas of the body also innervated by the same segmental levels. This phenomenon is called referred pain. Certain areas of the body have been consistently identified with referred pain from specific organs. These are referred to as a referred pain patterns (Fig. 8.13).

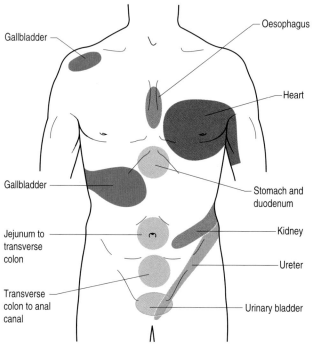

Fig. 8.13 This figure outlines the referred pain patterns from a variety of organs.

Sympathetic Control of Blood Flow

Flow rate is directly proportional to the pressure gradient and inversely proportional to the resistance. For example, if resistance increases because of narrowing of the blood vessel, the flow rate will decrease if the pressure gradient remains constant. Resistance would increase if the vessel reduced its diameter, because a greater proportion of the blood would then come into contact with the surface area of the vessel, therefore creating greater friction. The resistance increases with the length and diameter of the vessel(s). As the length of the vessel increases or the diameter decreases, a given amount of blood will come into contact with the vessel wall more often and thus increase the resistance to flow. Pressure is greater nearer the heart because resistance is less due to the large diameter of the vessels and the relatively short distance the blood has flown at that point. The pressure gradient depends on the pressure at the beginning and the end of the system, not on the absolute pressure within the vessel. When resistance increases, so too must the pressure gradient to maintain the same flow rate. The heart would therefore have to work harder.

To summarize:

1. Viscosity of the blood;
2. Vessel length; and
3. Vessel radius

all influence resistance of the vessel.

- A slight change in diameter of the vessel can bring about a large change in flow rate because of the resistance being inversely proportional to the fourth power of the radius.
- The arterial system acts as a pressure reservoir to maintain flow rate when the heart is relaxing—i.e., the large vessels extend and then compress because of the presence of large amounts of elastin in the walls of the vessel. A greater amount of blood enters the same than leaves it during systole—about a third of the amount leaves.
- Capillary flow stays the same during the cardiac cycle.
- Mean arterial pressure is the main driving force of flow rate. It is equal to diastole + $\frac{1}{3}$ diastole.
- Mean arterial pressure = cardiac output × total peripheral resistance.
- Arterioles are the main resistance vessels—capillaries do not offer as much resistance.
- There is a significant drop in mean pressure in the arterioles because of a high degree of arteriolar resistance (from ~93 to 37mmHg). This helps to create the pressure differential and the driving force for blood flow.

With an increased arteriolar vasoconstriction, this will increase mean arterial pressure upstream, thereby increasing the driving force of blood flow to other regions. Other local factors will also then influence the actual level of fuel delivery to any one region.

Sympathetic innervation causes constriction in most vessels, but heart and skeletal muscle are capable of strongly overriding the vasoconstrictor effect through powerful local metabolic mechanisms. For example, an increase in exercise-induced sympathetic innervation to the heart leads to a greater cardiac output and increased overall sympathetic vasoconstrictor tone. Vessels in the heart and active skeletal muscle will dilate in response to greater metabolic activity and benefit from an overall increase in upstream driving force. Skeletal and heart muscle also have beta2 receptors for epinephrine (adrenalin) that is released from the adrenal medulla in response to increased sympathetic innervation—beta2 receptor activation reinforces the metabolically induced vasodilation in these areas.

Vasoconstriction is prominent in the digestive tract during exercise to accommodate the increased driving force to metabolically active organs (heart and muscle).

Sympathetic innervation to smooth muscle of the arterial tree helps to maintain a constant driving force (or head of pressure) of blood flow to the brain and heart.

In short, cerebral blood flow is largely dependent on local metabolic factors as there is no sympathetic innervation to most of the arterioles in the brain. In response to greater metabolic demand there is a change in blood flow velocity through the internal carotid vessels and major branching vessels (ACA, MCA, PCA etc.) such that velocity increases. As cardiac output is not changing, there is a compensatory decrease in velocity of blood in other vessels supplying metabolically inactive regions of the brain or those areas that are inhibited. Research has shown an increase in blood flow velocity in the internal carotid vessels accompanying ablation (destruction) of ipsilateral sympathetic ganglia and also in cases whereby brain metabolism was expected to increase on that same side (e.g. right or left brain cognitive activities). A compensatory decrease in velocity is often observed contralaterally.

Other research shows an increase in blood flow through vessels to the eye (ophthalmic artery is a branch of the internal carotid artery) on the same side as sympathetic denervation. The forehead vessels receive their sympathetic innervation via the same plexus, and forehead skin temperature asymmetry correlates with research showing internal carotid blood flow asymmetry in migraine sufferers (some conflicts, however)—internal carotid or MCA dilation and forehead skin temperature increase during the headache phase of the migraine.

Forehead skin temperature would therefore be expected to decrease in response to sympathetically mediated vasoconstriction or a decrease in blood flow through supply arteries—this would be associated with relative vasoconstriction of all associated vessels in that vascular tree. This may have a large influence on some aspects of visual function related to both retinal and cortical mechanisms.

In summary, and based on much broader literature searches, the best bet at this point seems to be that hemisphericity will more likely (and in more cases) be associated with decreased forehead skin temperature on the same side. Do not forget also that if hemisphericity is associated with a loss of inhibition of ipsilateral IML, then one would expect to see greater vasoconstriction of forehead vessels anyway. The integrity of the PMRF and vestibular systems is vital in all this. Sometimes, forehead skin temperature will be seen to be decreased on the same side as vestibular escape because of excitatory vestibulosympathetic reflexes—however, the side of vestibular escape will often be the same side as decreased hemisphericity due to decreased contralateral vestibulocerebellar function (Sexton 2006).

Clinical Examination of Autonomic Function

What components of the neurological, physical, or orthopaedic examinations allow one to gain information about autonomic function? Complete examination techniques are covered in Chapter 4. However, due to the importance of the autonomic examination in determining the functional state of the neuraxis the autonomic examination is reviewed again here.

Pupil Size and Pupil Light Reflexes

These are dependent on sympathetic and parasympathetic tone. Vestibular, cerebellar, and cortical influences on both sympathetic and parasympathetic tone should be considered. Some of these influences are discussed earlier in the manual.

Width of Palpebral Fissure (Ptosis)

This is dependent on both sympathetic and oculomotor innervation. Therefore, one needs to differentiate between a Horner's syndrome, oculomotor nerve lesion, or physiological changes in the CIS of the MRF.

Blood Pressure

Blood pressure should always be measured on both arms. Blood pressure is dependent in part on the peripheral resistance, which can be different on either side of the head and body due to asymmetrical control of vasomotor tone. Increased vasomotor tone can occur because of decreased integrity or CIS of the ipsilateral PMRF, or because of excitatory vestibulosympathetic reflexes.

Skin Condition

Increased peripheral resistance may result in decreased integrity of skin particularly at the extremities.

Ophthalmoscopy—Vein to Artery (V:A) Ratio and Vessel Integrity

Ophthalmoscopy is useful for assessing the vascularity of the optic disc and retina. This should accompany measurement of the blind spot size as changes in the morphology of the optic disc and peripapillary region of the retina could explain the shape or size of the blind spot. Changes that occur before and after an adjustment or other activity are functional in nature.

The V:A ratio refers to the difference in size of the veins and arteries that branch from the central retinal artery. A large difference may be due to increased sympathetic output, which causes greater peripheral resistance and constriction of arteries. The condition of blood vessels can also be helpful as an indicator of cerebrovascular integrity (Figs 8.14 and 8.15).

Nystagmus can also be detected very easily.

Heart Auscultation

Arrhythmias and changes in heart sounds can occur due to altered CIS of the PMRF. A detailed discussion is beyond the scope of this book.

Bowel Auscultation

This can be particularly useful during some treatment procedures to monitor the effect of stimulation on vagal function (e.g., caloric irrigation—further instruction required, adjustments and visual stimulation or exercises, etc).

Skin and Tympanic Temperature and Blood Flow

This is particularly useful as a pre- and post-adjustment check. Profound changes in skin temperature asymmetry can occur following an adjustment. These changes are side dependent. An adjustment on the side of decreased forehead skin temperature will commonly result in greater symmetry or reversed asymmetry. Conflicting results are likely to be dependent on a number of factors, which are currently being investigated further. Remember that forehead skin temperature depends on fuel requirements of the brain, and vestibular and cortical influences on autonomic function among other things (Sexton 2006).

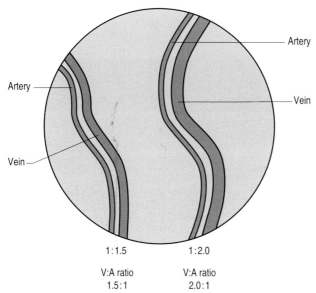

1:1.5   1:2.0

V:A ratio   V:A ratio
1.5:1   2.0:1

Fig. 8.14 This figure illustrates the concept of the vein to artery ratio (V:A ratio) in the arteries of the retina. A normal ratio is 1.5:1 which indicates that the vein is slightly larger than the artery. If the V:A ratio increases it may mean the vein has expanded or the artery has contracted. A common cause of an increased V:A ratio is sympathetic over activation.

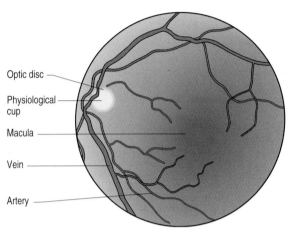

Fig. 8.15 This figure demonstrates the normal anatomy of the retina.

Dermatographia—The 'Flare' or Red Response

The red response is often observed in patients who suffer from chronic inflammatory conditions or heightened sensitivity to pain. See complex regional pain syndrome in Chapter 7.

Lung Expansion, Respiratory Rate, and Ratio

An inspiration: expiration ratio of 1:2 is considered to represent approximately normal sympathovagal balance—i.e., expiration should take twice as long as inspiration. This is difficult to achieve for some patients at first and requires some training.

Shallow and rapid breathing can result in respiratory alkalosis, which leads to hypersensitivity in the nervous system. CO_2 is blown off at a higher rate, resulting in decreased [H^+] ions in the blood. Lower [Ca^{++}] follows, causing [Na^+] to rise in extracellular fluid. This can be seen clinically by the presence of percussion myotonia, which is seen in various metabolic and hormonal disorders, or due to changes in segmental or supraspinally mediated innervation. Percussion myotonia can be tested by striking the thenar eminence of the thumb and watching for involuntary flexion of the thumb or spasmatic contraction of the thenar muscles for a prolonged period of greater than a second or two.

References

Angaut P, Brodal A 1967 The projection of the vestibulo-cerebellum onto the vestibular nuclei of the cat. *Archives de Italiennes de Biologie* 105:441–479.

Brodal A 1969 Neurological anatomy. Oxford University Press, London.

Brown LT 1974 Corticorubral projections in the rat. Journal of Comparative Neurology 154:149–168.

Cechetto D, Saper C 1990 Role of the cerebral cortex in autonomic function. In: Loewy A, Spyer K (eds) Central regulation of autonomic functions. Oxford University Press, New York, p 208–223.

Chrousos GP, Gold PW 1992 The concepts of stress and stress system disorders: Overview of physical and behavioral homeostasis. Journal of the American Medical Association 267:1244–1252.

Chusid JG 1982 The brain. In: Correlative neuroanatomy and functional neurology, 19th edn. Lange Medical, Los Altos, CA, p 19–86.

Donovan BT 1970 Mammillian neuroendocrinology. McGraw-Hill, New York.

Elenkov IJ, Wilder RL, Chrousos GP et al 2000 The sympathetic nerve—An integrative interface between two supersystems: The brain and the immune system. Pharmacological Review 52:595–675.

Furness JB, Costa M 1980 Types of nerves in the enteric nervous system. Neuroscience 5:1–20.

Lane RD, Jennings JR 1995 Hemispheric asymmetry, autonomic asymmetry, and the problem of sudden cardiac death. In: Davidson RJ, Hugdahl K (eds) Brain asymmetry. MIT Press, Cambridge, MA.

Lane RD, Wallace JD, Petrosky P et al 1992 Supraventricular tachycardia in patients with right hemisphere strokes. Stroke 23:362–366.

Levy MN, Ng ML, Zieske H 1966 Functional distribution of the peripheral cardiac sympathetic pathways. Circulation Research 14:650–661.

Nadler LS, Rosoff ML, Hamilton SE et al 1999 Molecular analysis of the regulation of muscarinic receptor expression and function. Life Science 64:375–379.

Natelson BH 1985 Neurocardiology—an interdisciplinary area for the 80s. Archives of Neurology 42:178–184.

Picciotto M, Caldarone BJ, King SL et al 2000 Nicotinic receptors in the brain: links between molecular biology and behaviour. Neuropsychopharmacology 22:451–465.

Randall WC, Ardell JL 1990 Nervous control of the heart: anatomy and pathophysiology. In: Zipes DP, Jalife J (eds) Cardiac electrophysiology. WB Saunders, Philadelphia.

Rardon D, Bailey J 1983 Parasympathetic effects on electrophysiologic properties of cardiac ventricular tissue. Journal of the American College of Cardiology 2:1200–1209.

Rogers MC, Battit G, McPeek B 1978 Lateralization of sympathetic control of the human sinus node: ECG changes of stellate ganglion block. Anesthesiology 48:139–141.

Schwartz P 1984 Sympathetic imbalance and cardiac arrhythmias. In: Randall W (ed) Nervous control of cardiovascular function. Oxford University Press, New York.

Selye H 1936 Thymus and the adrenals in the response of the organism to injuries and intoxications. British Journal of Experimental Pathology 17:234–238.

Sexton SG 2006 Forehead temperature asymmetry: A potential correlate of hemisphericity (personal communication).

Smith OA, DeVito JL 1984 Central neural integration for the control of autonomic responses associated with emotion. Annual Review of Neuroscience 7:43–65.

Snell RS 2001 The autonomic nervous system. In: Clinical neuroanatomy for medical students. Lippincott Williams and Wilkins, Philadelphia.

Swartz CM, Abrams R, Lane RD et al 1994 Heart rate differences between right and left hand unilateral electro-convulsive therapy. Journal of Neurology, Neurosurgery, and Psychiatry 57:97–99.

Walberg F 1960 Further studies on the descending connections to the inferior olive. Reticulo-olivary fibers: an experimental study in the cat. Journal of Comparative Neurology 114:79–87.

Webster KE 1978 The brainstem reticular formation. In: Hemmings G, Hemmings WA (eds) The biological basis of schizophrenia. MTP Press, Lancaster.

Williams PL, Warwick R 1984 Gray's anatomy. Churchill Livingston, Edinburgh.

Zamrini EY, Meador KJ, Loring DW et al 1990 Unilateral cerebral inactivation produces differential left/right heart rate responses. Neurology 40:1408–1411.

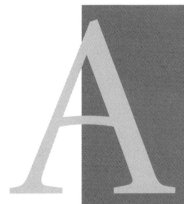

Clinical Case Answers

Case 8.1

8.1.1 Anisocoria can be caused by asymmetric activation of the pupil muscles. This in turn can result from dilation of one pupil or constriction in one pupil. Horner's syndrome is caused by a dysfunction in the sympathetic input to the eye, resulting in a constricted pupil on the ipsilateral side as the dysfunction. Increased sympathetic input can result from wind-up of the IML cells of the spinal cord or decreased parasympathetic input. This young lady may also have a congenital anisocoria, which has been present since birth and represents no physiological dysfunction. Asking the mother to produce photos of the child from infancy may solve the mystery.

Case 8.2

8.2.1 Preganglionic parasympathetic neurons that modulate the heart rate reside in the medulla and synapse with postganglionic neurons adjacent to the heart. The neurons of the NTS, DMN, and nucleus ambiguous also send projection fibres to the preganglionic sympathetic neurons in the IML and to other brainstem nuclei that modulate sympathetic outflow (Lane and Jennings 1995). The right and left vagal projections demonstrate an asymmetric distribution with the right vagal projections innervating some aspects of the anterior right and left ventricles and the left vagal projections innervating the posterior lateral aspects of the ventricles. However, the predominant innervation of the vagal projections terminate on the atrial aspects of the heart and include the sinus (SA) node, which usually determines the rate of the heartbeat. The influence of the vagal projections on the ventricles appears to be limited to counteracting the sympathetic innervation.

Sympathetic innervation of the heart can be separated into left and right sympathetic limbs based on physiological studies. The right postganglionic sympathetic projections arising from the paravertebral sympathetic ganglia including the stellate ganglia course to the heart and innervate the atria and the anterior surfaces of the right and left ventricles. The left sympathetic projections have a more posterior lateral distribution and innervate the atrioventricular (AV) node and the left ventricle. Stimulation of the sympathetic projections results in different physiological effects on the heart. Stimulation of the right stellate ganglia produces mainly chronotropic effects such as increases in heart rate, and stimulation of the left stellate ganglia mainly results in inotropic effects such as altered contractility, changes in rhythm, and increase in systemic blood pressure. Increased stimulation to either or both ganglia results in a decreased fibrillation threshold. With respect to cortical control of cardiovascular function, the research suggests that asymmetries in brain function can influence the heart through ipsilateral pathways. It is quite clear that stimulation or inhibition at various levels on the right side of the neuraxis results in greater changes in heart rate, while increased sympathetic tone on the left side of the neuraxis results in a lowered ventricular fibrillation threshold. This occurs because parasympathetic mechanisms are dominant in the atria, while sympathetic mechanisms are dominant in the ventricles.

The Cortex

Clinical Cases for Thought

Case 9.1   A patient presents after jogging headfirst into a stop sign. They complain of a severe headache, 'vagueness' of thought, and nausea. After performing a full neurological examination, the only significant finding appears to be absence of the corneal reflex on the left.

Questions

9.1.1   What are some important aspects of the history that might lead one to take further action with this patient? What could that further action be?

9.1.2   List at least five differential diagnostic considerations one would have for this patient.

Case 9.2   A 49-year-old female patient presents with complaints of bilateral paresis and sensory loss in the legs with loss of micturition control. During the history session you notice that she also exhibits a flat affect, decreased motivation, and delayed initiation of movement.

Question

9.2.1   Develop a list of at least five differential diagnoses.

Introduction

The cortex is encased in a boney protective covering and cushioned by several membranous structures referred to as the meninges. The meninges are composed of three layers; the dura mater, the arachnoid mater, and the pia mater. These membranes are involved in a variety of functions such as production and resorption of cerebral spinal fluid, cushioning the brain, and transmitting a variety of blood vessels to the brain. The cortex itself is a complex conglomeration of neurons, axons, dendrites, blood vessels, and glial cells. Although traditionally we have spoken of functional localization of a variety of areas of cortex, in reality the functional systems of the neuraxis work in conjunction with each other to produce the best possible outcome for the circumstances at hand. For example, the thought processes that we will attribute to the frontal cortex need to interact with the basal ganglion in order to flow and unfold in a meaningful way. In this chapter a variety of disease processes that can affect the meninges and the cortex proper and cortical dysfunctions such as Alzeimer's disease and epilepsy and the result of these dysfunctions will be discussed. The functional projections and networks of the cortex, as well as ways of clinically measuring the activation levels of these systems, will also be examined.

Embryological Development

Neuronal fate in the mammalian cortex is influenced by the timing of cell differentiation, which is dependent on both genetic and environmental factors (see Chapter 2). The cerebral cortex neurons are generated in the ventricular zone by the epithelial layer of progenitor cells that line the lateral ventricles. They migrate to the cortical plate, which eventually develops into the grey matter of the cortex. The final position assumed by these neurons depends on their 'birthmoment' or time of last division. The migration occurs along radially organized glial cells called radial glia, which guide the migrating neurons to the cortex. The layering of the neurons in the cerebral cortex is established with an inside-first, outside-last manner so that the newest neurons must pass over and around the more mature neurons probably gaining information from the previously established neurons as they pass.

The Meninges

The meninges are layered structures that contain cerebrospinal fluid and give protection to the brain and spinal cord. The meninges are composed of three layers; the dura mater, the arachnoid mater, and the pia mater (Figs 9.1 and 9.2).

The *dura mater* is the tough fibrous outer component of the meninges and is composed of two layers. The periosteal layer is intimately attached to the inner surface of the skull bones. The second layer is the meningeal layer of the dura. The periosteal and meningeal layers of the dura are tightly connected in most areas except where the meningeal layer projects deep into the cranial cavity and forms tough fibrous sheets, the falx cerebri and the tentorium cerebelli, that divide the cranial space into well-defined sections. The falx cerebri divides the cerebral hemispheres along the median plane of the skull. The tentorium cerebelli forms a sheet-like structure that separates the cerebellum from the rest of the brain. This is an important landmark as anatomical structures are referred to as infratentorial if they are below or inferior to the tentorium and supratentorial if they are superior or above the tentorium. Several important structures must pass through the tentorium in order to enter the brainstem and spinal cord. These structures pass through

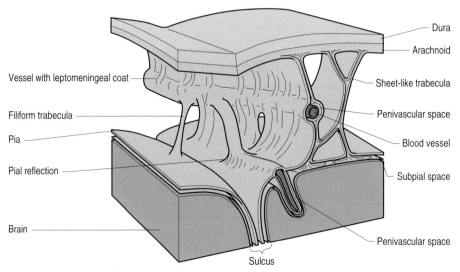

Fig. 9.1 The relationships of the three layers forming the meninges.

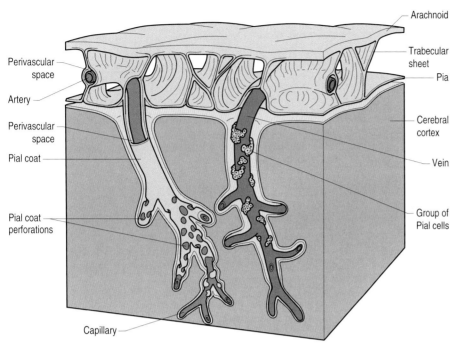

Fig. 9.2 The relationship between the arachnoid and pia.

an opening in the tentorium referred to as the tentorial notch. This is an important clinical point because structures put under increased pressure because of space-occupying lesions or cerebral spinal fluid blockage can be squeezed into the notch, resulting in damage and dysfunction of the tissues passing through the notch and of the tissues forced into the notch. The falx cerebri is another structure that can be potentially damaging to neural tissue that gets forcibly pushed into or under it by increased intracranial pressure.

The *arachnoid layer* is composed of thin spider web-like attachments to the dura superiorly and the pia inferiorly. The *pia mater* adheres very closely to the surface parenchyma of the brain. This layer follows the surface of the brain into all of the surface gyri and sulci. Vessel must past through the pia to get to the parenchyma of the brain. As an artery enters the cortex, a layer of pia mater accompanies the vessel into the brain. With decreasing size of the vessel, the pial coating becomes perforated and finally disappears at capillary level. The perivascular space between the artery and the pia mater inside the brain is continuous with the perivascular space around the meningeal vessel. Veins do not have a similar coating of pia mater.

The way in which the meninges connect to each other and the structures that they attach to gives rise to three clinically important spaces or potential spaces, the epidural space, the subarachnoid space, and the subdural space. The *epidural space* is a potential space that can form between the dura and the bone of the skull. The meningeal arteries run in the space between the tightly adherent dura and the skull. The middle meningeal artery passes the temporal bone, which is the thinnest bone of the skull and thus the most easily fractured. Trauma to the temporal bone can cause tears in the meningeal arteries and result in blood escaping into the potential epidural space. As the blood builds up it forces the periosteal layer of dura away from the bone and bulges into the arachnoid and pia layers, eventually exerting pressure on the brain. This process is referred to as an epidural haematoma (Fig. 9.3).

Epidural haematomas are usually rapidly growing and expanding as the arterial pressure spreads the periosteal dura from the bone of the skull. The dural separation continues until it reaches a cranial suture where the dura is much more tightly joined to the skull. This results in an expansile lesion that takes the shape of a biconcave lens. Clinically the patient may experience a lucid interval following trauma to the skull where they may not have any symptoms. Within a few hours the expanding haematoma starts to compress the brain and results in increased intracranial pressure and death if not treated.

The *subdural space* is clinically important because of the many bridging veins leaving the brain parenchyma and exiting through the dura to the venous sinuses. *Subdural haematoma* (SDH) results when the bridging veins flowing from the cortex parenchyma to

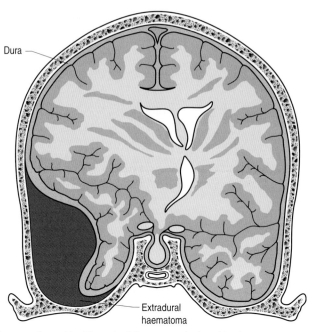

Fig. 9.3 The development of an epidural (extradural) haematoma in the epidural space.

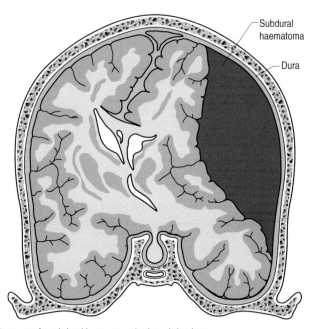

Fig. 9.4 The development of a subdural haematoma in the subdural space.

the sagittal sinus experience a trauma severe enough to tear them. This results in a slow-growing, low-pressure haematoma in the potential space between the dura and the arachnoid layers which often occurs in the parietal area of the cortex. There is no classic pattern of presenting symptoms but they are often trauma induced. The trauma need not be extreme and in fact, trivial trauma is suspected in over 50% of cases.

The symptoms of SDH often mimic other cerebrovascular events or space-occupying lesions. Alcohol consumption reduces clotting mechanisms and often results in head trauma from falls. Anticoagulants can also increase the risk of SDH from minor trauma in the elderly (Fig. 9.4). *Chronic subdural haematomas* can take weeks to months in the elderly before they start to experience symptoms. This is mainly due to the low-pressure, slow leak from the veins and the fact that brain tissue shrinks somewhat as we age and allows a greater space for the blood to occupy before interference with function occurs. *Acute subdural haematomas* require a considerable amount of traumatic force to occur and as such are usually associated with other serious brain injuries like traumatic subarachnoid haemorrhage and brain contusions.

The *subarachnoid space*, which is the space between the pia and arachnoid layers, is divided by trabeculae and contains the cerebrospinal fluid and the major blood vessels of the brain. A major clinical consideration of this area is the possibility of a *subarachnoid haemorrhage*. These most commonly occur when a pre-existing aneurysm located on the arteries traversing the subarachnoid space fails and blood leaks out into the space. The aneurysm can develop a slow leak or simply burst. Less than 15% of patients have symptoms prior to rupture, but following rupture the symptoms include the simultaneous onset of severe headache with nausea and vomiting. The headache is often described as the worse headache of their life. Photophobia and neck stiffness may also accompany the other symptoms. Because of the similarity of presentation with meningitis and migraine these must be considered as differential diagnoses until ruled out.

Any process that causes an increase in *intracranial pressure*, such as intracranial tumours, haemorrhages, oedema, and altered cerebrospinal fluid pressures, can result in compression of brain tissue. The portion of brain that becomes compressed and the way in which it responds to the compression is dependent on the *mass effect*. The mass effect can result in numerous ramifications in different individuals; however, three clinically relevant situations involving compression of brain tissues through anatomically ridged structures, a process called herniation, will be outlined below.

1. Transtentorial herniation involves the compression and protrusion of the medial temporal lobe, usually the uncus or periuncal areas, inferiorly through the tentorial notch (Fig. 9.5). Because of the pressure exerted on the mesencephalic area and the peduncles of the cerebrum, oculomotor dysfunction and hemiplegia can result. The oculomotor damage usually results in a dilated pupil ipsilateral to the side of the lesion due to the unopposed action of the sympathetic nerves. The hemiplegia usually occurs on the side opposite the lesion. Damage to the mesencephalic reticular system can also lead to loss of consciousness and coma.

2. Central herniation is the downward displacement of the brainstem. The action of the downward displacement may traction the abducens nerve (CN VI) and cause lateral rectus palsy (Fig. 9.5).

3. Tonsillar herniation occurs when increased intracranial pressure forces the tonsillar region of the cerebellum down through the foramen magnum of the skull. Because of the high pressure experienced in the medullary region this condition usually results in respiratory arrest, blood pressure instability, and death (Fig. 9.5).

4. Subfalcine herniation results when the cingulate gyrus is pushed under the falx cerebri and into the other half of the brain. No specific clinical signs may be present with this condition (Fig. 9.5).

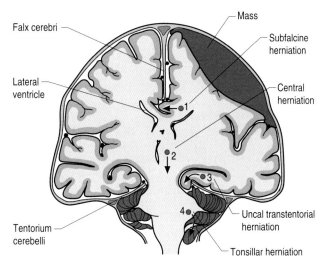

Fig. 9.5 The effect of unequal distribution of intracranial pressure that may result in the shifting of position of brain structures known as the mass effect.

Cerebral Spinal Fluid (CSF)

Cerebral spinal fluid is normally a clear, colourless, and odourless fluid that diffuses over the brain and spinal cord. CSF probably functions to cushion the brain and spinal cord from external jarring or shocking forces that may be transmitted through the tissues to reach these structures. CSF may also function in some capacity as a metabolic transport medium, transporting nutrients to the neuraxial cells and metabolic waste products away from the neuraxial components. CSF may also function as a pressure distributor in cases where changes in intracranial volume have occurred such as in postoperative lesions where the removed tissue area fills with CFS. The CSF is formed by the dialysis of blood across the tissues of the choroid plexuses found in the ventricle of the brain and brainstem. The circulation of CSF occurs in two systems, the internal system which includes the two lateral ventricles, the interventricular foramens, the third ventricle, the cerebral aqueduct, and the fourth ventricle, and the external system, which includes all of the external spaces surrounding the brain and spinal cord including the various cisterns. Communication between the internal and external systems occurs via two lateral apertures in the fourth ventricle referred to as the foramens of Luschka, and a medial aperture also in the fourth ventricle referred to as the foramen of Magendie. The total volume of CSF in all systems measures about 150 cm^3. The CSF is formed at the rate of about 20 cm^3/hr or about 480 cm^3/day. This means that all of the CSF in your body is replaced about 3.2 times per day. This is accomplished via absorption of the CFS by the arachnoid granulations located along the superior longitudinal sinus which allow the CSF to enter the venous drainage system and return to the general circulation (Fig. 9.6).

QUICK FACTS 1	Summary of CSF Examination

Finding	Suspected Condition
Neutrophils and decreased glucose	Acute bacterial meningitis
Neutrophils and normal glucose	Brain abscess
Lymphocytes and decreased glucose	Virus, tuberculosis, or cryptococcal
Lymphocytes and normal glucose	Virus, brain tumour, syphilis

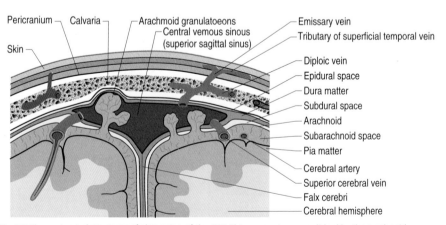

Fig. 9.6 The anatomical structures of absorption of the CSF. This process is accomplished by the arachnoid granulations located along the superior longitudinal sinus which allow the CSF to enter the venous drainage system and return to the general circulation.

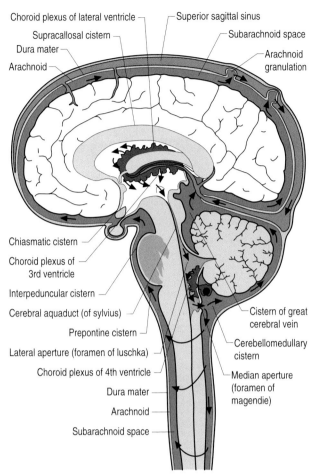

Fig. 9.7 The flow of CSF through the CSF system. Note the presence of choroid plexus in all of the ventricles.

The CSF circulates from the lateral ventricles, through the third ventricle, to the fourth ventricle where it then enters the external system and bathes the spinal cord and the external surface of the brain (Fig. 9.7).

Clinical Examination of Cerebral Spinal Fluid

Examination of the CSF can be a valuable tool in the diagnosis of several conditions such as infection that can affect the neuraxis. A common procedure utilized to obtain CSF is the lumbar puncture. This procedure provides direct access to the subarachnoid space of lumbar cistern which contains the CSF (Fig. 9.8). This procedure can be used to obtain samples of CSF, measure the pressure of the CSF, remove excess CSF if necessary, and act as a conduit for the administration of medication or radiographic contrast material. The CSF is examined for a variety of different elements:

1. CSF pressure—Normal value is 100–200 mmH$_2$O (7.7–15.4 mmHg). Elevated CSF pressure may be caused by blockage of the ventricular drainage system, overproduction, or space-occupying lesions. The two most common causes are meningitis and subarachnoid haemorrhage. Brian tumours and abscesses will cause an increase after a delay of days to weeks.

2. CSF appearance—Normal CSF is clear and colourless. CSF is generally white or cloudy if significant white blood cells (WBC) are present (over 400/mm^3). CSF may appear red or pink if red blood cells (RBC) are present; however, if RBC have been in the CSF for more than 4 hours the fluid may appear yellow (xanthochromia). This is due to the breakdown of haemoglobin.

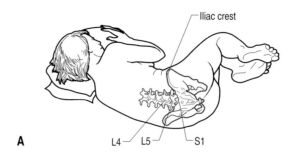

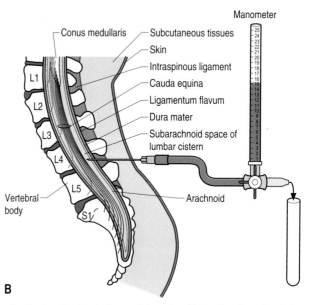

Fig. 9.8 (A) Position of patient and landmarks for needle insertion. (B) Location of needle relative to structures of the lumbar cistern. Switch between measurement of CSF pressure or collection of CSF samples can be selected with a three-way stopcock, as shown.

3. CSF glucose—Normal is 45 mg/100 ml or higher. The most significant clinical finding is a decrease in glucose concentration. This occurs in virtually every case of bacterial meningitis. Other causes of decreased glucose include:

   • Bacterial invasion;

   • Fungal invasion;

   • Tuberculosis; and

   • Subarachnoid haemorrhage (due to release of glycolytic enzymes).

   Since a relationship exists between blood glucose and CSF glucose levels, a blood glucose concentration measure should be performed at the same time as the CSF sample is taken.

4. CSF protein—Normal value is considered to be 15–45 mg/100 ml in adults. In newborns it may range as high as 150 mg/100 ml. The most significant clinical finding is an elevation of protein concentration. Causes of increased protein concentration include:

   • Cerebral trauma;

   • Brain or spinal cord tumour;

   • Brain abscess;

   • Systemic lupus;

   • Multiple sclerosis;

   • Uraemia; and

   • Bacterial invasion.

5. CSF cell count—Normally the CSF contains no more than $5\,cells/mm^3$. Under normal conditions virtually all of the cells present should be lymphocytes. Usually the highest leukocyte counts are found in acute bacterial infections such as meningitis. Usually the cell type most contributing to the leukocytosis in bacterial infections is the polymorphonuclear cell or neutrophil.

Clinical Syndromes Involving the Meninges

Meningiomas

Meningiomas account for approximately 20% of all intracranial tumours. They arise from the dura, especially where the dura adheres densely to bone. A variety of different types of meningiomas include:

- Acoustic and hypoglossal neuromas (neurofibroma);
- Parasagittal meningiomas;
- Surface meningiomas;
- Sphenoid ridge;
- Olfactory groove;
- Tuberculum sella; and
- Tentorial meningioma.

Cerebral Abscesses

A brain abscess is a focal suppurative process within the brain parenchyma. Abscesses may have a wide variety of causes including *Staphlococcus aureus* and *Streptococcus*. The majority of abscesses are mixed infections involving both Gram +ve and Gram –ve bacteria. These infections occur most commonly in association with three clinical settings:

1. Resulting from a contiguous site of focal infection, i.e. dental infection, sinusitis, otitis;
2. Resulting from a distant site, usually haematogenous spread from a lung infection; and
3. Following head injury or surgery.

The classic triad of headache, fever, and focal nerve deficit is present in about 50% of cases. Other symptoms include seizures, papilloedema, nausea and vomiting, and nuchal rigidity (Vogel 1994).

Meningitis

Meningitis is an inflammatory response to pathogen infection of the dura, arachnoid, and pia maters and the CSF. Leptomeningitis involves the pia–arachnoid layers and pachymeningitis involves the dura layer. Since the subarachnoid space and thus the CSF is continuous throughout the brain, spinal cord, and optic nerves the entire neuraxis is usually affected.

Are They Petechiae or Not?	QUICK FACTS 2

The glass test involves pressing a glass against the skin to see if the red spots fade. Petechiae will not fade when pressed.

Access to the intracranial compartment is by way of the bloodstream, whereas access to the CSF is through the choroid plexus or directly through the blood vessels of the pia mater. Although the pia appears to be delicate and fragile it actually forms a remarkably efficient barrier against the spread of infection, and it generally prevents involvement of the underlying brain tissue.

Once a pathogen gains entrance to the CSF the immune system's counterattack is severely hampered, until a substantial population of the pathogen stimulates neutrophilic pleocytosis in the case of bacteria invasion or lymphocytic pleocytosis in the case of a virus invasion (Scheld 1994; Pryor 1995). Bacteria gain entrance to the CSF by one of three proposed mechanisms:

1. Chemicals released from the bacteria cause relaxation of the intercellular tight junction between the cells forming the blood–brain barrier.
2. Bacteria enter through the fenestrations of the choroid plexus.
3. Bacteria enter inside of macrophages or other cells normally circulating through the CNS.

The primary results of bacterial invasion are:

1. CSF neutrophilic pleocytosis;
2. Increased permeability of the choroid plexus leading to increased CSF pressure, which results in an increased intracranial pressure;
3. Decreased cerebral blood flow;
4. Cortical hypoxia;
5. CSF acidosis; and
6. Neutrophilic invasion of the subarachnoid space.

Normal concentration of WBC in the CSF is 0–5 cells/mm^3, and almost all are normally lymphocytes.

Meningitis may be caused by a variety of organisms, including *Cryptococcus neoformans*, which is a yeast found in the soil with a worldwide distribution. The incidence is about 5/1,000,000 and it is most often found in people with a compromised immune system. Risk factors of immune compromise include lymphoma, diabetes, and AIDS. Symptoms of cryptococcal meningitis include:

- Headache;
- Fever;
- Nausea and vomiting;
- Stiff neck (Kernig's and Brudzinski's signs may be positive—Fig. 9.9);
- Photophobia;
- Mental status changes; and
- Hallucinations.

Diagnosis
- Lumbar puncture must be performed.
- CSF stains may show yeast.
- CSF culture grows the yeast.

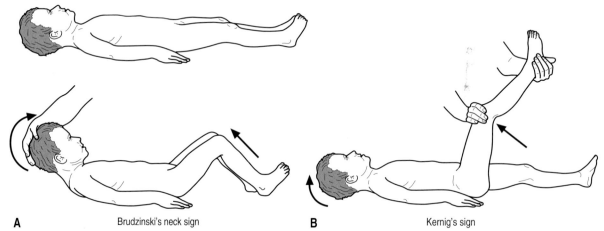

A Brudzinski's neck sign   **B** Kernig's sign

Fig. 9.9 (A) The performance of Brudzinski's neck sign. With the patient lying relaxed the neck is quickly flexed and when dural irritation is present the patient's knee will bend to reduce the stretch of the meninges. (B) Kernig's sign. With the patient lying quietly and relaxed the leg is slowly raised, flexed at the knee, then the leg is suddenly straightened. In cases of meningeal irritation the patient will suddenly bring their neck into a flexed position.

- CSF may be positive for cryptococcal antigen.
- Blood test shows positive serum cryptococcal antigen

Treatment
- Antifungal agents are used to treat this infection.
- Intravenous amphotericin B is the most common.
- In cases where the above is ineffective, intrathecal (injection into the spinal canal) of the medication is necessary.
- High oral doses of fluconazole are sometimes effective.

Treponema Pallidum **(Syphilis)**
This condition can develop as a complication of untreated or poorly treated syphilis. It is characterized by changes in mental status and nerve function which involves a form of meningovascular neurosyphilis, which is a progressive life-threatening complication of syphilis infection. This condition resembles meningitis caused by other organisms but involves serious damage to the vascular structures of the brain, which result in stroke in a large percentage of patients. The symptoms include:

- Headache;
- Nausea and vomiting;
- Stiff neck (Kernig's and Brudzinski's signs may be positive—Fig. 9.9);
- Neck pain;
- Stiffness of shoulders and arms;
- Fever;
- Photophobia;
- Sensitivity to noise;
- Mental status changes including confusion, disorientation, decreased attention, irritability, sleepiness, and lethargy;
- Vision changes; and
- Seizures.

Diagnosis
Focal neurological deficits, which are localized loss of nerve function, are common findings. Neurological exam may also show reduced cranial nerve function, especially nerves controlling eye movements (abducens CN IV, trochlear CN VI, oculomotor CN III). Examination should also include electroencephalogram (EEG) if seizures are present, head CT or MRI, CSF examination, serum venereal disease research laboratory (VDRL), or serum rapid plasma reagin (RPR) which are screening tests for syphilis. If the screening tests are positive, then a fluorescent treponemal antibody absorption (FTA-ABS) test is necessary to confirm.

Treatment
Treatment goals are to cure the infection, reduce progression of the disorder, and reduce nerve damage as any existing nerve damage is permanent. Penicillin, tetracycline, and erythromycin are the drugs of choice. Dramatic improvement of symptoms may occur after treatment. However, a progressive disability may result.

Haemophilus influenzae
Bacteria *Haemophilus influenzae* type B is the most common agent involved. This condition is the leading cause of meningitis in children from 1 month to 5 years of age, with the peak incidence from 6 to 9 months. The organism usually spreads from somewhere in the respiratory tract to the blood stream and then onto the meninges.
   Risk factors for the development of this condition include recent history of otitis media, sinusitis, or pharyngitis. This also includes the history of a family member infected with *H. influenzae* in the past. Symptoms and examination finds may include:

- Irritability, poor feeding in infants;
- Fever;
- Below normal temperature in young infants;
- Severe headache (loud screeching scream);

Age	Agent
Less than 1 month	Group B strep.
1 month to 5 years	H. Influenzae
5–29 years	N. meningitidis
Over 29 years	S. pneumoniae

- Nausea and vomiting;
- Stiff neck or crying when neck flexed (Kernig's and Brudzinski's may be positive—Fig. 9.9);
- Unusual body posture;
- Pain in the back when neck is flexed or chin brought to chest;
- Photophobia;
- Bulging of the fontanelles (soft spots in the skull) of infants;
- Opisthotonos (lying with the back arched, head back, and chin up);
- Seizures;
- Stupor, coma; and
- Elevated WBC numbers in blood and CSF.

Antibiotic treatment must be started as soon as meningitis is expected. Steroid medication may also be given to reduce damage to the auditory nerves, which occurs in about 20% cases. The mortality of the condition is quite high with 3–5% of patients not surviving. Of those who do survive, some will develop brain damage, hydrocephalus, learning disorders, and behavioural problems. It is recommended that all family members start chemoprophylaxis as soon as possible.

Meningococcus

This condition is caused by the bacteria *Neisseria meningitis*, also known as the meningococcus. This is the most common cause of meningitis in people 5–29 years of age. The development of this condition usually occurs following an upper respiratory infection or sore throat. The onset of disease may be rapid and progress to critical or life-threatening in hours. The symptoms include a distinctive rash with pinpoint red spots referred to as petechiae (Fig. 9.10), as well as the following:

- High fever;
- Severe headache;
- Nausea and vomiting;
- Stiff neck (Kernig's and Brudzinski's may be positive);
- Photophobia; and
- Mental status changes.

A specific physical exam will reveal low blood pressure, tachycardia, stiff neck, and rash, while blood tests will show elevated WBC. Blood culture grows meningococci. Spinal tap shows increased WBC, low glucose, and high protein. Complications can include brain damage, shock, increased CSF pressure, myocarditis, hydrocephalus, deafness, muscular paralysis, and mental retardation.

Streptococcus pneumoniae (Pneumococcus)

This condition is caused by infection by the bacteria *Streptococcus pneumoniae* or pneumococcus. It is the most common cause in adults over 29 years of age. The onset of symptoms is usually rapid (within hours to days). Risk factors for contracting this condition include recurrent meningitis, leakage of CSF, head injury, diabetes, alcohol abuse, recurrent pneumonia, infection of heart valves, recurrent ear infections, and recent

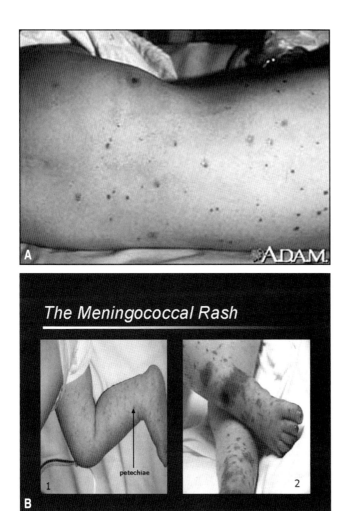

Fig. 9.10 (A) The symptoms of meningitis include a distinctive rash with pinpoint red spots referred to as petechiae. (B) A further example of the distinctive rash with pinpoint red spots referred to as petechiae often seen in meningitis.

upper respiratory infection. The signs and symptoms are similar to those of other types of meningitis and include:

- Tachycardia;
- Increased temperature;
- Stiff neck (Kernig's and Brudzinski's may be positive);
- Severe headache;
- Nausea and vomiting;
- Photophobia; and
- Mental status changes.

Diagnosis
Spinal tap (lumbar puncture) will often reveal Gram +ve bacteria (pneumococcus), elevated protein, and low glucose levels. CT scan or MRI is usually normal unless high intracranial pressures have developed. Serum and CSF cultures may grow pneumococcus.

Treatment
Antibiotic therapy should be started as soon as possible. Ceftriaxone is the most commonly used drug. If the bacteria show resistance, than vancomycin or rifampin may be used. Corticosteroid therapy is often also utilized especially in children. Even with early treatment, 20% of people who contract the disease will die and 50% will suffer from serious long-term complications.

Staphylococcus (aureus, epidermidis)

This condition is usually caused by the bacteria *Staphylococcus aureus* or *Staphylococcus epidermidis*. It may develop as a complication from surgery or from haematogenous spread from another site. Risk factors include brain surgery, CSF shunts, infections of the heart valves, and previous brain infections such as an abscess or encephalitis. The symptoms include:

- Fever;
- Severe headache;
- Nausea and vomiting;
- Stiff neck;
- Photophobia; and
- Rash (septicaemia).

CSF and serum cultures may show staph, and infections of this type often result in death.

Mycobacterium tuberculosis

This condition is caused by *Mycobacterium tuberculosis*. This condition usually spreads from another site in the body. Symptom onset is usually gradual. This is a very rare disorder that usually only occurs in people with a compromised immune system; however, it is fatal if untreated.

Aseptic Meningitis

This type of meningitis shows all the signs and symptoms of bacterial meningitis but no bacteria can be isolated as the cause. Many pathogens other than bacteria have been implicated as the cause of aseptic meningitis. These include viruses, fungi, tuberculosis, and medication-induced. The enterovirus family, which includes the Coxsackie virus and the echovirus, account for about 50% of cases of aseptic meningitis. Other enteroviruses such as the mumps virus also contribute a significant portion of the aseptic cases.

Herpes virus, both type 1 and 2, can cause aseptic meningitis in infants and young children, or in people with compromised immune system function.

Rabies virus and the AIDS virus (HIV) have been found as causes of meningitis also. Interestingly a few medications have also been linked to the development of aseptic meningitis including antibiotics and some over-the-counter anti-inflammatory medications. All of the signs and symptoms of bacterial meningitis may be present.

There is an elevated WBC count in the CSF, and serum and CSF cultures do not grow bacteria. No specific treatment is available, and people usually have a full recovery 5–14 days after the onset of symptoms.

Gram –ve Organisms

Causative agents include *Pseudomonas aeruginosa*, *Escherichia coli*, *Enterobacter aerogenes*, *Proteus morganii*, and *Klebsiella pneumoniae*. All the signs and symptoms previously listed for Gram +ve bacterial meningitis may be present. IV antibiotics is the treatment of choice, and 40–80% of patients do not survive this type of meningitis.

Migraine

Some evidence suggests that pain-sensitive dura and middle meningeal artery wall may contribute to the pain of migraine headaches. (See headache section later in this chapter.)

Encephalitis

Encephalitis is an inflammatory response involving both the meninges and the brain parenchyma. Several organisms can cause encephalitis including bacteria, fungi, and viruses. By far viruses are the most common cause. Most common causes of viral encephalitis are enterovirus, herpes simplex type 1 virus, mumps virus, and arbovirus. In addition to the symptoms indicative of meningitis the patient with encephalitis may also present with:

- Mental state abnormalities including delirium, confusion, and disorientation;
- Focal or diffuse neurological signs (evidence of upper motor neuron involvement); and
- Aphasia, ataxia, hemiparesis, and cranial nerve deficits.

The treatment of encephalitis is mostly supportive. Acyclovir, which is an antiviral agent, is sometimes effective in cases of herpes encephalitis. The prognosis varies with the age of the patient: under 30 years, the survival rate is 67–100%, and over 30 years, it is 64%.

Vascular Accidents

Intracerebral Haemorrhage

Intracerebral haemorrhage occurs when the vessels in the brain parenchyma fail and blood leaks into the brain tissues. The haemorrhage often involves lenticulostriate arteries in the region of the external capsule underlying the cortex. The haemorrhage may be traumatic or non-traumatic but it often produces a sudden fulminating headache with rapid deepening loss of consciousness. Tentorial herniation is also common due to asymmetrical pressures from one hemisphere to the other.

Subarachnoid Haemorrhage

A subarachnoid haemorrhage most commonly occurs when a pre-existing aneurysm located on the arteries traversing the subarachnoid space fails and blood leaks out into the space. The aneurysm can develop a slow leak or simply burst. Less than 15% of patients have symptoms prior to rupture, but following rupture the symptoms include the simultaneous onset of severe headache with nausea and vomiting. The headache is often described as the worst headache of their life. Photophobia and neck stiffness may also accompany the other symptoms.

Arteriovenous Malformation (AVM)

These are congenital malformations of the arteriovenous junctions that result in large tangled areas that are often structurally delicate and can be ruptured with relatively minor trauma. The haemorrhage occurs in sinusoidal vessels that are under low pressure. These types of

Blood Supply of the Cortex

QUICK FACTS 4

Fig. 9.11 (A) The lateral surface of the left cerebral hemisphere, showing the areas supplied by the cerebral arteries. (B) The medial surface of the left cerebral hemisphere, showing the areas supplied by the cerebral arteries. Here the area supplied by the anterior cerebral artery is coloured blue, that by the middle cerebral artery pink, and that by the posterior cerebral artery is yellow.

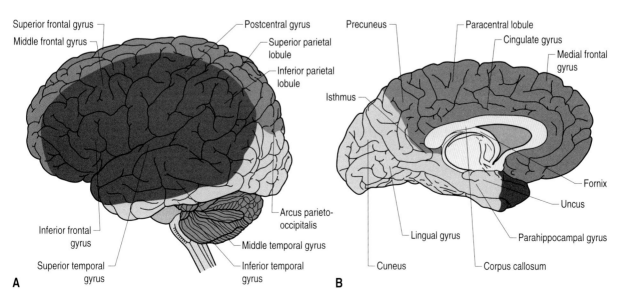

haemorrhage often result in focal neurological signs and headache, epilepsy, and occasionally hydrocephalus. The arachnoid villi can become blocked by blood from repeated subarachnoid haemorrhages and therefore impair CSF resorption, which leads to hydrocephalus.

QUICK FACTS 5	Aneurysm Sites

- Anterior communicating artery (28%)
- Posterior communicating artery (25%)
- Middle cerebral artery (12%)
- Ophthalmic, anterior, and posterior cerebral (13%)
- Other sites (22%)

Hydrocephalus

Hydrocephalus is caused by excess CSF in the intracranial cavity. This condition can develop from an excess in production of CSF, an obstruction to the flow of CSF, or decreased resorption of CSF.

Communicating hydrocephalus is caused by blockage of the arachnoid granulations by blood products because of subarachnoid bleeding, meningitis, or other factors that decrease the ability of the granulations to function adequately. *Noncommunication hydrocephalus* involves a blockage of the flow of CSF in the ventricular system. Blockages usually occur in the small foramina or the cerebral aqueduct.

Normal pressure hydrocephalus is sometimes seen in older individuals and involves chronically enlarged ventricles and cortical atrophy. The following triad of symptoms is also commonly seen:

- Memory disturbance and confusion;
- Progressive gait disability; and
- Difficulty with urinary control.

Differential diagnostic considerations should include:

- Various dementias;
- Parkinson's disease;
- Subdural, extradural, subarachnoid haematomas;
- Multi-infarct dementia;
- Hypoglycaemia;
- Toxicity;
- Infection;
- Renal and hepatic failure; and
- Hypercalcaemia.

The Cortex

The cortex in humans is composed of several well-identified functional areas, interspersed in the cortical matter referred to as association cortex. Although we will speak of functional localization of a variety of areas of cortex, in reality the functional systems of the neuraxis work in conjunction with each other to produce the best possible outcome for the circumstances at hand. For example, the thought processes attributed to the frontal cortex need to interact with the basal ganglion in order to flow and unfold in a meaningful way. The hippocampus and amygdala are essential functional areas for the fusion of emotions and behavioural response which are attributed to cortical functions. Movement, controlled by the motor cortex in the frontal lobe, is meaningless and random without the feedback supplied by the spinal cord and cerebellum. The cortex can be divided into the lobar areas outlined in the following.

Layers of Cerebral Cortex   QUICK FACTS 6

- It is convenient for learning purposes to divide the cerebral cortex into layers that may be distinguished by cell types, cell functions, cell density, and cell arrangements.
- These layers include six levels of cortex (layers I–VI) also named from superficial to deep:
  - Molecular layer (plexiform layer)
  - External granular layer
  - External pyramidal layer
  - Internal granular layer
  - Ganglionic layer (internal pyramidal layer)
  - Multiform layer (layer of polymorphic cells)

The Frontal Lobes

The frontal lobe is concerned with sophisticated operations such as higher order sensory processing, planning, implementation, language processing, abstract thought, and regulation of movement, cognition, emotion, and behaviour. The most anterior part of the frontal lobe is involved in complex cognitive processes like reasoning and judgment. Collectively, these processes may be called *biological intelligence*. A component of biological intelligence is *executive function*. Executive function regulates and directs cognitive processes. Decision making, problem solving, learning, reasoning, and strategic thinking are all components of executive function. The prefrontal cortex also serves as the attentional control system, which regulates information flow into two separate rehearsal systems and facilitates retrieval of stored memories:

1. Articulatory loop—language (words and numbers etc); and
2. Visuospatial sketchpad—vision and action.

Anatomically, the frontal lobe is bounded posteriorly by the fissure of Rolando or central sulcus, and inferiorly by the fissure of Sylvius or the lateral fissure. The frontal lobe can be divided into two main areas the precentral area and the prefrontal area. The precentral area contains areas 4 and 6 of the cortex and is composed of the precentral gyrus and the posterior portions of the superior, middle, and inferior frontal gyri. The prefrontal area is composed by the remainder of the frontal lobes and is traversed by two sulci that divide the prefrontal area into three gyri, the superior, middle, and inferior frontal gyri. The cortex varies between 1.5 and 4.5 mm in thickness and is always thicker on the exposed surface of the gyri than in the deep sulci areas.

Types of Cells in the Cortex   QUICK FACTS 7

- Martinotti cells
- Neurogliaform
- Basket cells
- Horizontal cells
- Fusiform cells
- Stellate cells
- Pyramidal cells

QUICK FACTS 8 | **Pyramidal Cells**

- Pyramid cells are named for the shape of their bodies, which resemble a pyramid.
- Most pyramidal cells are 10–50 μm in width.
- However, giant pyramidal cells (Betz cells), which may expand to 120 μm in width, are found in the precentral gyrus of the frontal lobe (motor cortex).
- The apices of the pyramidal cells are orientated towards the pial surface of the cortex.
- Extending from the apex of each pyramidal cell is a large apical dendrite that rises towards the pia, giving off multiple collateral branches as it climbs.
- Other dendrites pass laterally into the surrounding neuropil.
- From the base arises a single axon that either synapses in deeper cortical layers or exits via the white fibre tracts as a projection, association, or commissural fibre.

QUICK FACTS 9 | **Stellate Cells**

- These cells are sometimes referred to as granule cells because of their small size.
- They are polygonal (star) in shape and measure about 8 μm in width.
- These cells have multiple branching dendrites and relatively short axons that terminate on nearby cells.

QUICK FACTS 10 | **Fusiform Cells**

- These cells have their long axis orientated vertical to the cortical surface.
- They are usually concentrated only in the deepest cortical layers.
- Dendrites arise from each pole of the cell body.
- The inferior dendrite synapses within the same layer of cortex as the cell body. The superior dendrite rises up through several layers of cortex to the superficial layers.
- Axons arise from the inferior body and descend in white fibre tracts as association, commissural, or projection fibres.

QUICK FACTS 11 | **Horizontal Cells**

- These cells are small, fusiform, and orientated horizontally to the cortical surface.
- They are usually found in the most superficial layers of cortex.
- Dendrites emerge from each end of the cell body and axons run horizontally (parallel) to the cortical surface and synapse on pyramidal cells.

Cells of Martinotti   **QUICK FACTS 12**

- These are small, multipolar cells present in all levels of cortex.
- The cell has short dendrites; the axon is orientated to the cortical surface, and gives off a few colateral axons as it rises to superficial layers of cortex.

The structure of the cortex is laminar in nature, with six distinct layers present throughout most of the cortex. The thickness, number of cells, and predominant cell types in each layer vary over different areas of cortex. Listed from most superior to most inferior, these layers are the molecular layer, the external granular layer, the internal pyramidal layer, the internal granular layer, the ganglionic layer, and the fusiform or multiform layer (Fig. 9.12). The *molecular layer* or layer 1 is the most superior layer of the cortex. It contains the cell bodies of neuroglial cells, and axons and dendrites of neurons from deeper layers of cortex. The *external granular layer* or layer 2 is very dense and contains small granular cells and small pyramidal cells that project to neurons in other levels of cortex. The *external* or *medial pyramidal layer*, layer 3, contains pyramidal cells arranged in row formation. A variety of neurons projecting axons to other layers of cortex which form the association projections arise from this layer. The *internal granular layer*, layer 4, is thin, but its cell structure is the same as that of the external granular layer. The *ganglionic layer* or *internal pyramidal layer*, level 5, contains small granular cells, large pyramidal cells, and the cell bodies of some association fibres. The association fibres that originate here form two large tracts, *the Bands of Baillarger and Kaes Bechterew*. The neurons of this layer project to subcortical structures other than the thalamus including the basal ganglia, the midbrain,

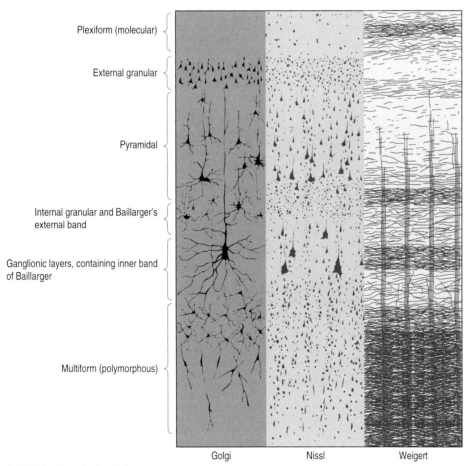

Plexiform (molecular)

External granular

Pyramidal

Internal granular and Baillarger's external band

Ganglionic layers, containing inner band of Baillarger

Multiform (polymorphous)

Golgi   Nissl   Weigert

Fig. 9.12 A schematic of cortical structure.

and the spinal cord. The *fusiform layer* is also known as the *multiform layer*, layer 6; neurons in this layer primarily project to the thalamus. All layers are present in all parts of the cortex. However, they do not have the same relative density in all areas. Depending upon the function of a particular area, some of these layers will be thicker than others in that location. The most common classification scheme used to differentiate areas of cortex based on structural and functional differences is that composed by Korbinian Brodmann in 1909. Based on microscopic evaluations of the cortex he divided the cortex into 52 different cytoarchitecturally different areas, known as Brodmann areas (Fig. 9.13). The cytoarchitectural divisions described by Brodmann have been shown to match quite closely to the functional output areas of the cortex. Some of these are outlined in Table 9.1.

The Motor Cortex

The motor cortex is located anterior to the central sulcus of Rolando and continues medially into the paracentral lobule. The primary area of motor cortex is Brodmann's area 4 and is in the precentral gyrus. The motor cortex is somatotopically organized so that areas in the cortex correspond to areas of the body. These connections are depicted by the motor homunculus of man. The amount of tissue in the precentral gyrus dedicated to the innervation of a particular part of the body is proportional to the amount of motor control needed by that area, not just its physical size on the body. For example, much more of the motor strip is dedicated to the control of the fingers than to the legs even though the legs are much larger in physical mass of the body. Monosynaptic connections

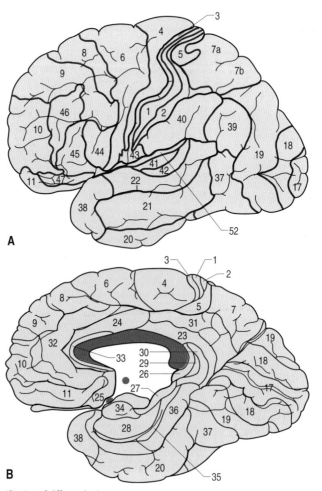

Fig. 9.13 The classification of different brain areas.

Table 9.1 Brodmann's Areas of the Cortex

Brodmann's Area	Functional Area	Location	Function
1–3	Primary somatosensory cortex	Postcentral gyrus	Touch
4	Primary motor cortex	Precentral gyrus	Voluntary movement control
5	Tertiary somatosensory cortex; posterior parietal association area	Superior parietal lobule	Limb and eye movement planning
6	Supplementary motor cortex; supplementary eye field; premotor cortex; frontal eye fields	Precentral gyrus and rostral adjacent cortex	Visuomotor; perception
7	Posterior parietal association area	Superior parietal lobule	Visuomotor; perception
8	Frontal eye fields	Superior, middle frontal, gyri, medial frontal lobe	Saccadic eye movements
9–12	Prefrontal association cortex; frontal eye fields	Superior, middle frontal, gyri, medial frontal lobe	Thought, cognition, movement planning
17[a]	Primary visual cortex	Banks of calcarine fissure	Vision
18	Secondary visual cortex	Medial and lateral occipital gyri	Vision; depth
19	Tertiary visual cortex, middle temporal visual area	Medial and lateral occipital gyri	Vision, colour, motion, depth
20	Visual inferotemporal area	Inferior temporal gyrus	Form vision
21	Visual inferotemporal area	Middle temporal gyrus	Form vision
22	Higher order auditory cortex	Superior temporal gyrus	Hearing, speech
23–27	Limbic association cortex	Cingulate gyrus, subcallosal area, retrosplenial area and parahippocampal gyrus	Emotions
28	Primary olfactory cortex; limbic association cortex	Parahippocampal gyrus	Smell, emotions
29–33	Limbic association cortex	Cingulate gyrus and retrosplenial area	Emotions
34–36	Primary olfactory cortex; limbic association cortex	Parahippocampal gyrus	Smell, emotions
37	Parietal-temporal-occipital association cortex; middle temporal visual area	Middle and inferior temporal gyri at junction of temporal and occipital lobes	Perception, vision, reading, speech
38	Primary olfactory cortex; limbic association cortex	Temporal pole	Smell, emotion
39	Parietal-temporal-occipital association cortex	Inferior parietal lobule (angular gyrus)	Perception, vision, reading, speech
40	Parietal-temporal-occipital association cortex	Inferior parietal lobule (supramarginal gyrus)	Perception, vision, reading, speech
41	Primary auditory cortex	Heschl's gyri and superior temporal gyrus	Hearing

(Continued)

Table 9.1 Brodmann's Areas of the Cortex—Cont'd

Brodmann's Area	Functional Area	Location	Function
42	Secondary auditory cortex	Heschl's gyri and superior temporal gyrus	Hearing
43	Gustatory cortex (?)	Insular cortex, frontoparietal operculum	Taste
44	Broca's area; lateral premotor cortex	Inferior frontal gyrus (frontal operculum)	Speech, movement planning
45	Prefrontal association cortex	Inferior frontal gyrus (frontal operculum)	Thought, cognition, planning, behaviour
46	Prefrontal association cortex (dorsolateral prefrontal cortex)	Middle frontal gyrus	Thought, cognition, planning behaviour, aspects of eye movement control
47	Prefrontal association cortex	Inferior frontal gyrus (frontal operculum)	Thought, cognition, planning, behaviour

Source: Martin (1996).
[a]Areas 13–16 are part of the insular cortex.

QUICK FACTS 13   **Classification of Cortical Neurons**

1. Interneurons
   - Neurons that have axons that do not leave the cortex.
   - E.g., Stellate (granule) cells
   - Horizontal cells
   - Cells of Martinotti
   - Small pyramidal cells of layers 2 and 3
2. Association Neurons
   - Send axons through white fibre tracts to other regions of cortex, usually to adjacent gyri, e.g. small pyramidal cells of layers 3 and 5.
3. Efferent Neurons
   - Axons leave the cortex to innervate structures in diencephalon, brainstem, cerebellum, or spinal cord.
   - These cells usually send their axons via the white fibre tracts; i.e. corpus callosum, corona radiata, or internal capsule. Some cells send co-lateral axons through all three fibre tracts.
   - E.g., Giant pyramidal cells (Betz cells) of layer 5

with ventral horn neurons are important for individuated finger movements. Indirect connections with interneurons are important for controlling larger groups of muscles in behaviours such as reaching and walking. Motor activity is modulated by a continuous stream of tactile, visual, and proprioceptive information, which arrives via the thalamus, needed to make voluntary movement both accurate and properly sequenced. Motor association areas are also modulated by the cerebellum and basal ganglia, which then project to the primary motor areas.

Functional Projections of the Motor Cortex

The motor cortex projects ipsilaterally to the reticular formation of the mesencephalon and the neostriatum of the basal ganglion where activation of glutaminergic neurons produces excitation. Reciprocal projections between the mesencephalon and the cortex ensure that the cortex will receive stimulation whenever the mesencephalon is excited. The cortex also projects to the ipsilateral pontomedullary reticular formation (PMRF) and the contralateral cerebellum via the pontine nuclear groups and the pontine reticular formation. Excitation of the PMRF results in a number of functional activities including an increase in activation of the ipsilateral gamma motor neurons that result in an increase in sensitivity of ipsilateral muscle spindle fibres. This results in an increased feedback to the contralateral cortex via the cerebellum and thalamus. This functional circuit can be utilized to stimulate areas of contralateral cortex clinically (Fig. 9.14). The mesencephalon and basal ganglia are sometimes referred to as areas of singularity. This means that there are fewer sources of integration than in other areas like the PMRF, and changes in frequency of firing (FOF) may have a more profound impact on the function of these areas of the nervous system. Decreased cortical activity can lead to a lack of modulation of primitive behaviour that originates in the mesencephalic motor centres and mesolimbic circuits, which is referred to as a release phenomenon. Writer's cramp, spasmodic torticollis, and facial tics are all conditions that may be caused by defects in basal ganglionic circuits and unchecked responses originating in the mesencephalon or cerebral cortex. Another example is the impulsive behaviour of children who have been diagnosed with ADHD and the inability of their brain to inhibit irrelevant signals through corticostriatothalamic circuits. These children are functioning at a more subcortical level (Melillo & Leisman 2004).

Broca's area is found on the inferior third frontal gyrus in the hemisphere dominant for language. This area is involved in the coordination or programming of motor movements for the production of speech sounds. While it is essential for the execution of the motor movements involved in speech it does not directly cause movement to occur. The firing of neurons here does not generate impulses for motor movement; that is the function of neurons in the motor strip. The neurons in Broca's area generate motor programming patterns when they fire. This area is also involved in syntax, which involves the ordering of words in speech. Injuries to Broca's area may cause apraxia or Broca's aphasia (Fig. 9.15).

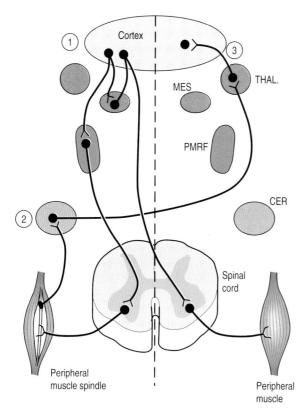

Fig. 9.14 A schematic of some of the functional motor cortical circuits.

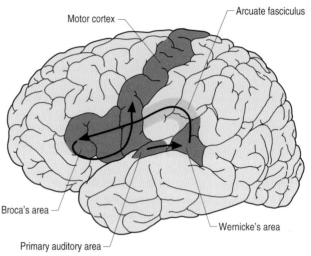

Fig. 9.15 The anatomical location of Broca's and Wernicke's areas in the cortex.

The *angular gyrus* lies near the superior edge of the temporal lobe, immediately posterior to the supramarginal gyrus. It is involved in the recognition of visual symbols. This area may be one of the most important cortical areas of speech and language and may act as the master integration centre for all other association cortices. The angular gyrus is also a very human portion of the brain as it is not found in non-human species. Fibres of many different types travel through the angular gyrus, including axons associated with hearing, vision, and the meaning of these stimuli to the individual at any given moment. The arcuate fasciculus, the groups of fibres connecting Broca's area to Wernicke's area in the temporal lobe, also projects and receives projections from this area. The following disorders may result from damage to the angular gyrus in the hemisphere dominant for speech and language: anomia, which is difficulty with word-finding or naming; alexia with agraphia, which is difficulty with reading and writing; left–right disorientation, the inability to distinguish right from left; finger agnosia, which is the lack of sensory perceptual ability to identify by touch; and acalculia which refers to difficulties with arithmetic (Fig. 9.16).

The Cortex Receives Axons from Four Major Transmitter-Dependent Projection Systems

The cortex, thalamus, and brainstem receive neuromodulating projection axons from a variety of projections systems located in the brainstem. These projection systems are involved in a diverse array of activities including modulation of:

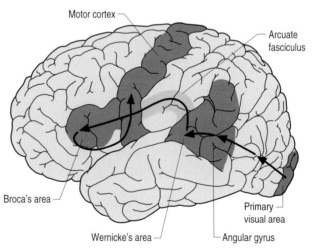

Fig. 9.16 The projections from the primary visual cortex to the angular gyrus and Broca's area.

Clinical Tests Indicating Decreased Dopamine Function	**QUICK FACTS 14**

- Decreased blink rate and loss of modulation of blink reflexes during glabellar tap reflex.
- Increased withdrawal reflexes.
- Altered modulation of pupillary tone with cognitive activity.
- Poor fixation and loss of visual stability.
- Anti-saccadic and OKN testing can reveal abnormalities in frontal and basal ganglionic circuits that reflect these behaviours.
- Turning behaviour (tendency to turn in a particular direction) is dependent on asymmetries in dopaminergic transmission. It is thought that individuals (and dogs!) have a tendency to turn away from the side of greater dopaminergic transmission.
- Slow-wave cortical responses (P300s) can also more objectively reveal abnormalities in EEG responses to sensory stimuli in a range of cognitive and mood disorders.

- Levels of consciousness;
- Sleep–wake cycles;
- Emotional states;
- Motor behaviour; and
- Cortical response activity.

The projection systems are classified according to the neurotransmitters that they release. These projection systems include the cholinergic projection system, the dopaminergic projection system, the noradrenergic projection system, the serotonergic projection system, and the histaminergic projection system.

The *cholinergic projection system* consists of three different neuron pools that project to different functional areas. Two of the groups project axons directly to cortical areas and the third group projects to the cortex indirectly through the thalamus. The first group of neurons is located in the basal forebrain in a nuclear group referred to as the nucleus basalis of Meynert. This nuclear group contains neurons that project cholinergic axons directly to widespread areas of cortex. The second group of neurons project almost exclusively to the hippocampal formation and arise from neurons in the medial septal nuclei and the nucleus of the diagonal band of Broca. The cholinergic activity of these two groups of neurons is usually facilitory in nature. The third group of cholinergic projection axons arises from neurons located in two areas of the pontomesencephalic region of the brainstem. The first group of neurons is located in the lateral portion of the reticular formation and periaqueductal grey areas in a nuclear group of neurons referred to as the pedunculopontine tegmental nuclei. The second group of neurons is located at the junction between the midbrain and pons referred to as the laterodorsal tegmental nuclei. Projection axons from both of these nuclear groups terminate in various nuclei, including the intralaminar nuclei of the thalamus. The postsynaptic thalamic neurons then project to widespread areas of cortex (Fig. 9.17).

The *dopaminergic projection system* consists of three different neuron pools, the mesostriatal, the mesolimbic, and the mesocortical groups that project to different functional areas (Fig. 9.18). The mesostriatal group of neurons is located in the substantia nigra pars compacta of the midbrain and projects mainly to the caudate and putamen. Lesions to this pathway result in movement disorders such as Parkinson's disease. Some evidence for the asymmetric distribution of dopamine in this projection system has been documented. The close association of dopamine and motor control has led to the speculation that dopamine should be more concentrated in the hemispheres dominating motor control. This is the left hemisphere for the majority of humans. Several studies

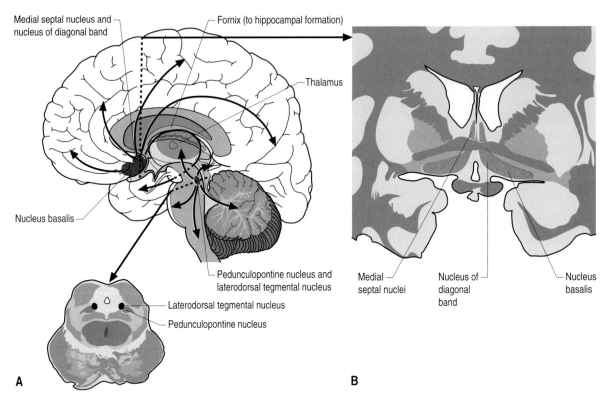

Fig. 9.17 (A) A lateral view of the cholinergic projection system. (B) An anteroposterior view of the same systems described in (A).

have demonstrated that this is in fact the case (Rossor et al 1980; Glick et al 1982; Wagner et al 1983). Other studies have demonstrated that factors related to dopamine metabolism and dopamine-specific activation of adenylate cyclase have also been asymmetrical with higher activity levels in the contralateral hemisphere to hand preference (Glick et al 1983; Yamamoto & Freed 1984).

The mesolimbic projection pathway arises from neurons in the ventral tegmentum of the midbrain and projects to the medial temporal cortex, the amygdala, the cingulate gyrus, and the nucleus accumbens, all areas associated with the limbic system. Lesions or dysfunction of these projections is thought to contribute to the positive symptoms of schizophrenia such as hallucinations.

The mesocortical projection pathway arises from neurons in the ventral tegmental and substantia nigral areas of the midbrain and terminates in widespread areas of prefrontal cortex. The projections seem to favour motor cortex and association cortical areas over sensory and primary motor areas (Fallon & Loughlin 1987). Dopaminergic neurons do not discharge in response to movement, but instead in relation to conditions involving probability and imminence of behavioural reinforcement and reward. Firing of reward neurons shifts from time of reward to presentation of the cue, or from unconditional to conditioned stimulus. This suggests that dopaminergic modulation is involved with higher integrative cortical functions and the regulation of cortical output activities (Clark et al 1987). Damage or dysfunction in these projections may contribute to the cognitive aspects of Parkinson's disease and the negative symptoms of schizophrenia. Clinical measures of dopamine activity can be very important in monitoring patients with disorders of dopamine function such as in movement disorders and schizophrenia.

Blink rate has been shown to be an accurate biophysical correlate of dopamine function (Gallois et al 1985). A faster blink rate is observed in individuals who have higher dopaminergic output. A faster blink rate is also observed during visual and vestibular stimulation in individuals who have signs of vestibulocerebellar dysfunction. Decreased blink rate as demonstrated by the glabellar tap reflex and loss of modulation of blink reflexes can be an accurate sign of dopamine deficiency or dysfunction.

The *noradrenergic projection system* consists of neurons in two different locations in the rostral pons and the lateral tegmental area of the pons and medulla. The neurons in the rostral pons area are referred to as the locus ceruleus and together with the neurons in the lateral tegmental area of the pons and medulla project to all areas of the entire

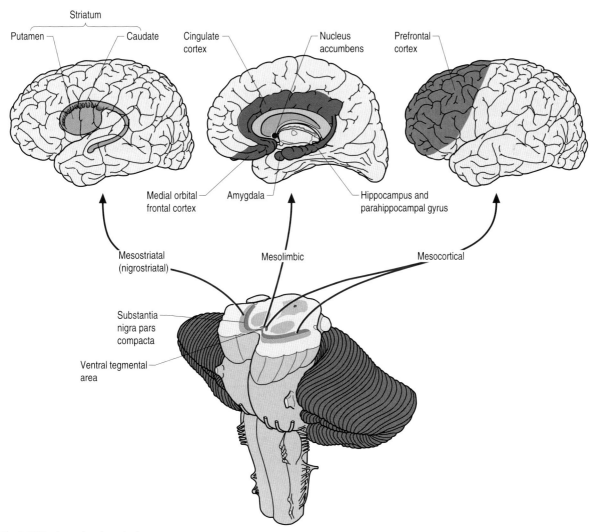

Fig. 9.18 The dopaminergic projection system.

forebrain including the limbic areas as well as to the cerebellum, brainstem, and spinal cord (Fig. 9.19). The noradrenergic projection system seems to be involved in the cerebral regulation of arousal, attention-related functions, and adaptive responses of the individual to environmental stresses (Clark et al 1987; Morilak et al 1986). The noradrenergic system is also involved in the modulation of affective behaviour. Norepinephrine concentrations are decreased in some types of depression (see Chapter 16). This system is also involved in neuroimmuno regulation (see Chapter 15).

The *serotinergic projection system* consists of a group of nuclei in the midbrain pons and medulla referred to as the raphe nuclei and additional groups of neurons in the area postrema and caudal locus ceruleus. These nuclei can be divided into rostral and caudal groups. The rostral raphe nuclei project ipsilaterally via the median forebrain bundle to the entire forebrain where serotonin can act as either excitatory or inhibitory in nature, depending on the situation (Fallon & Loughlin, 1987). The caudal raphe nuclei project to the cerebellum, medulla, and spinal cord (Fig. 9.20). Serotonin projection pathways are thought to play a role in a variety of psychological activities. Dysfunction of serotonin modulation can lead to depression, anxiety, obsessive-compulsive behaviour, aggressive behaviour, and eating disorders (Arora & Meltzer 1989; Spoont 1992). Serotonin activity has also been shown to be asymmetrical in nature with a predominance towards the right hemisphere (Arato et al 1987, 1991; Demeter et al 1989).

The *histaminergic projection system* has only recently been identified. It consists of scattered neurons in the area of the midbrain reticular formation as well as a more defined

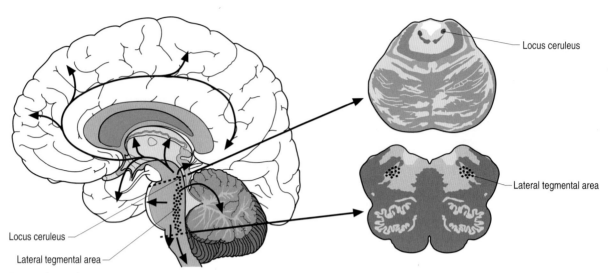

Fig. 9.19 The noradrenergic projection system.

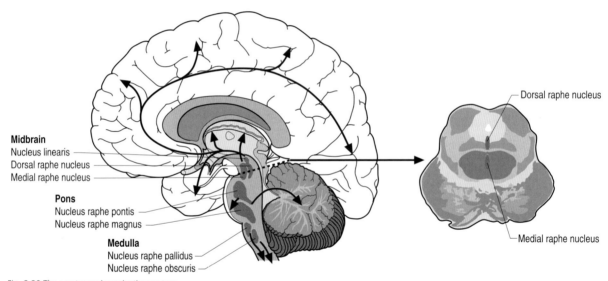

Fig. 9.20 The serotonergic projection system.

group of neurons in the tuberomammillary nucleus of the hypothalamus. These neurons project to the forebrain and are probably involved in the modulation of the alert state of the brain (Fig. 9.21).

The nature of the above neurotransmitter projection systems seems to suggest that the transmitter activities follow the psychological asymmetrical distribution of cortical or hemispheric function. Neurotransmitters closely associated with up-regulation or down-regulation of autonomic or psychological arousal such as norepinephrine and serotonin are more concentrated in the right hemisphere, emphasizing the well-known role of the right hemisphere in arousal. In contrast, neurotransmitters more closely associated with control of movement such as dopamine are more concentrated in the dominant movement hemisphere, which is on the left in the majority of people (Wittling 1998).

The Parietal Lobes

The post-central gyrus which represents the primary sensory areas composes Broadmann's areas 3(a, b), 1, 2. The primary somatosensory area is 3b. Because of convergent and divergent connections in relay nuclei of the thalamus, the receptive area of neurons in area 3b represents inputs from about 300–400 mechanoreceptive afferents. In some cortical

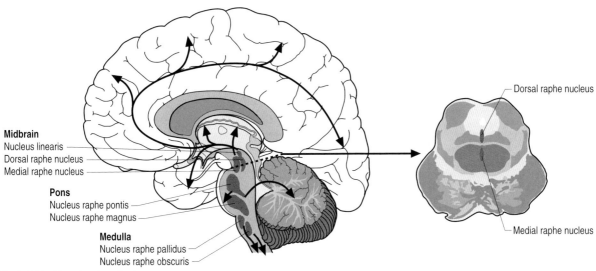

Midbrain
Nucleus linearis
Dorsal raphe nucleus
Medial raphe nucleus

Pons
Nucleus raphe pontis
Nucleus raphe magnus

Medulla
Nucleus raphe pallidus
Nucleus raphe obscuris

Dorsal raphe nucleus

Medial raphe nucleus

Fig. 9.21 The histaminergic projection system.

Areas Involved in Processing Somatic Receptive Input in the Somatosensory Cortex

QUICK FACTS 15

1. Basic processing of tactile information occurs in area 3.
2. More complex higher order processing occurs in area 1.
3. Tactile and limb position information combine to mediate the tactile recognition of objects in area 2.

---

areas the number of receptors is actually even larger. Cortical receptive fields can be modified by experience or sensory nerve injury. They respond best to excitation in the middle of its receptive field.

The somatosensory association areas, which are located more posterior than the primary sensory areas in the posterior parietal cortex, compose Brodmann's areas 5 and 7, which receive information particularly from the lateral nuclear group of the thalamus and the pulvinar. They are involved in sensory initiation and guidance of movement. Area 5 is also involved in tactile discrimination and proprioceptive integration, from both hands. Many neurons in area 5 receive input from adjacent joints and muscle groups of entire limbs and, therefore, information about posture of the entire limb, which is important for sensory guidance of movement such as would be required when reaching for an object. Area 7 is involved with tactile and visual integration, which includes stereognosis and eye–hand coordination.

Neurons in the primary somatosensory cortex also somatotopically represent areas of the body. This is referred to as the somatosensory homunculus of man. In the homunculus, there are approximately 100 times the cortical tissue per square centimetre of skin on the fingers than in the abdomen skin representation. The primary somatosensory area has four complete maps of the body surface due to four topographically organized sets of inputs from the skin that project to Brodmann's areas 3a, 3b, 1, and 2.

The parietal lobes provide a representation of external and intrapersonal space by integrating somatic, visual, and auditory evoked potentials from neighbouring lobes. The parietal areas are also an essential source of presynaptic inputs for frontal and limbic association areas and subcortical structures. Therefore, damage can lead to changes in cognition, mood, and behaviour just as a cerebellar or frontal lobe lesion can. The parietal lobes can be divided into superior and inferior functional areas. The superior parietal area is involved in visually guided action in the context of intact perception and awareness and the inferior parietal area is involved with visual perception and awareness. The angular gyrus and supramarginal gyrus of the inferior lobe may also be involved in the development of neglect syndromes. The somatosensory association area projects information to higher order somatosensory association areas include parahippocampal, temporal association, cingulate cortices, and the premotor cortex where it is integrated for use in motor control, eye–hand coordination, memory-related tactile experience, and touch.

QUICK FACTS 16	Somatic Sensibility

1. Discriminative touch
2. Proprioception
3. Nociception
4. Temperature sense

QUICK FACTS 17	Epicritic Sensations

1. Fine touch/localization (topognosis)
2. Vibration (determine freq. and amp.)
3. Spatial detail/two-point discrimination
4. Recognition of shapes (stereognosis)
5. Receptors are encapsulated and well myelinated.

QUICK FACTS 18	Protopathic Sensations

1. Pain and temperature.
2. Itch and tickle.
3. Receptors are non-encapsulated and unmyelinated.

Somatic sensibility comprises a description of the nature of different types of afferent information. There are four major classes of somatic information: discriminative touch, proprioception, nociception, and temperature sense. There are two classes of somatic sensation, epicritic and protopathic, that are detected by encapsulated and unencapsulated receptors respectively (see Chapter 5).

Clinical Neglect Syndromes
Neglect syndromes include a variety of different manifestations in which certain afferent input fails to integrate appropriately and does not emerge into consciousness or the meaning of the input fails to be recognized.

Hemineglect is the unwillingness to acknowledge one side of the body or one side of the universe in which one finds oneself. It may occur in the form of sensory or motor neglect. Hemineglect is usually associated with lesions of the right parietal lobe and thus the sensory and motor manifestations occur on the left side of the body. Left-sided parietal lesions are usually much less severe and can go unnoticed by a careless or incomplete examination. Hemi-sensory neglect involves the patient neglecting sensory input such as sound, vision, touch, position sense, or pain on one side of the body. This condition can best be demonstrated by simultaneously stimulating receptors on both sides of the body.

Clinical Tests for Hemineglect   QUICK FACTS 19

- Visual fields
- Two-point discrimination and joint position sense
- Optokinetic pursuit
- Smooth visual tracking
- Finger to nose in each visual field
- Best hand test
- Stereognosia/atopognosia/agraphognosia
- Sensory extinction/inattention
- Visual searching tasks

In a hemineglect syndrome the patient will not acknowledge the sensation of the neglected side; in some cases even when it is pointed out to them that both sides are being stimulated they will deny any sensation. This condition occurs significantly more commonly in right brain lesions than in left brain lesions. Therefore, left hemiplegia or left hemianopia is much more commonly found. Anosognosia is an example of a type of hemineglect syndrome. Anosognosia may express a total lack of knowledge of a disease or disability on one side of their body. The prerequisite for anosognosia is a lesion involving the angular gyrus and junction with supramarginal gyrus.

The Temporal Lobes

The *temporal lobes* are involved in the central processing of vision (ventral stream), hearing, smell, taste, and vestibular input and are also heavily involved in memory, behaviour, and emotion. The temporal lobe is inferior to the lateral fissure and anterior to the occipital lobe. It is separated from the occipital lobe by an imaginary line rather than by any

What Does It Mean?   QUICK FACTS 20

- *Anomia* is a difficulty with word-finding or naming. Someone suffering from anomia can list the functions of an object and explain its meaning, but cannot recall its name.
- *Alexia with agraphia* refers to difficulties with reading and writing.
- *Left–right disorientation* is an inability to distinguish right from left.
- *Finger agnosia* or *tactile agnosia* is the lack of sensory perceptual ability to identify by touch.
- *Acalculia* refers to difficulties with arithmetic.

Clinical Testing of Temporal Function   QUICK FACTS 21

- Smell
- Visual fields
- Anomia
- Associative agnosia
- Hearing
- Digit span (forwards/backwards)

natural boundary. The temporal lobe can be divided into three gyri, the superior, middle, and inferior, and by two sulci, the superior and inferior. It is also involved in semantics, or word meaning, as Wernicke's area is located there. *Wernicke's area* is located on the posterior portion of the superior temporal gyrus (Fig. 9.15). In the hemisphere dominant for language, this area plays a critical role in the ability to understand and produce meaningful speech. A lesion here will result in Wernicke's aphasia. *Heschl's gyrus*, area 41, which is also known as the anterior transverse temporal gyrus, is the *primary acoustic area*. There are two *secondary acoustic* or *acoustic association areas* which make important contributions to the comprehension of speech. They are not completely responsible for this ability, however, as many areas, including Wernicke's area, are involved in this process.

Kluver-Bucy Syndrome

Damage to the front of the temporal lobe and the amygdala just below it can result in the strange condition called Kluver-Bucy Syndrome. Classically, the person will try to put anything to hand into their mouths and typically attempt to have sexual intercourse with it. A classic example is of the unfortunate chap arrested whilst attempting to have sex with the pavement. Effectively, it is the 'what' pathway that is damaged with regards to foodstuff and sexual partner. Monkeys with surgically modified temporal lobes have great difficulty in knowing what prey is, what a mate is, what food is, and in general what the significance of any object might be.

Other symptoms may include visual agnosia (inability to visually recognize objects), loss of normal fear and anger responses, memory loss, distractibility, seizures, and dementia. The disorder may be associated with herpes encephalitis and trauma, which can result in brain damage.

Temporal lobe lesions also produce tameness or hypo-emotionality, visual agnosia, and changes in dietary and sexual behaviour.

The Occipital Lobes

The *occipital lobe*, which is the most posterior lobe, has no natural boundaries. It is involved in vision. The *primary visual area* is divided by the calcarine sulcus and receives input from the optic tract via the thalamus (Fig. 9.16). The superior visual field is represented below the calcarine sulcus. The inferior visual field is represented above the calcarine sulcus. The visual-processing units in the visual cortex are composed of horizontal columns of neurons called hypercolumns with a variety of interneuron projections from surrounding horizontal neurons. Hypercolumns are the processing modules of all information about one part of the visual world. Columnar units are linked by horizontal connections within the same layer, particularly cells that respond to similar orientations of stimuli but belong to different receptive fields. The horizontal neuronal projections from horizontal interneurons are thought to mediate the 'physiological fill-in effect' and the 'contextual effect' whereby we evaluate objects in the context in which we see them.

QUICK FACTS 22	Temporal Lobe Activation in Rehabilitation

- Naming/viewing pictures of animals and tools—bilateral ventral temporal activation
- Animals—Left medial temporal lobes
- Tools—Left premotor area (also activated by hand movements)

The *secondary visual areas* integrate visual information, giving meaning to what is seen by relating the current stimulus to past experiences and knowledge. A lot of memory is stored here. These areas are superior to the primary visual cortex. Damage to the primary visual area causes blind spots in the visual field, or total blindness, depending on the extent of the injury. Damage to the secondary visual areas could cause *visual agnosia*. People with this condition can see visual stimuli, but cannot associate them with any meaning or identify their function. This represents a problem with meaning, as compared to anomia, which involves a problem with naming, or word-recall.

Cortical Asymmetry

Cortical asymmetry is characterized by asymmetry in sensory, motor, and autonomic signs in addition to imbalances in the expression of hemispheric specializations. This includes aspects of personality, mood, and cognition.

Cerebral Asymmetry (Hemisphericity)

The study of brain asymmetry or hemisphericity has a long history in the behavioural and biomedical sciences but is probably one of the most controversial concepts in functional neurology today. The fact that the human brain is asymmetric is fairly well established in the literature (Geschwind & Levitsky 1968; LeMay & Culebras 1972; Galaburda et al 1978; Falk et al 1991; Steinmetz et al 1991). The exact relationship between this asymmetric design and the functional control exerted by each remains controversial.

The concept of hemispheric asymmetry or lateralization involves the assumption that the two hemispheres of the brain control different aspects of a diverse array of functions and that the hemispheres can function at two different activation levels. The level at which each hemisphere functions is dependent on the central integrative state (CIS) of each hemisphere, which is determined to a large extent by the afferent stimulation it receives from the periphery as well as nutrient and oxygen supply. The afferent stimulation is gated through the brainstem and thalamus, both of which are asymmetric structures themselves, and indirectly modulated by their respective ipsilateral cortices.

Traditionally the concepts of hemisphericity were applied to the processing of language and visuospatial stimuli. Today, the concept of hemisphericity has developed into a more elaborate theory that involves cortical asymmetric modulation of such diverse constructs as approach versus withdrawal behaviour, maintenance versus interruption of ongoing activity, tonic versus phasic aspects of behaviour, positive versus negative emotional valence, asymmetric control of the autonomic nervous system, and asymmetric modulation of sensory perception, cognitive, attentional, learning, and emotional processes (Davidson & Hugdahl, 1995).

The cortical hemispheres are not the only right- and left-sided structures. The thalamus, amygdala, hippocampus, caudate, basal ganglia, substantia nigra, red nucleus, the cerebellum, brainstem nuclei, and peripheral nervous system all exist as bilateral structures with the potential for asymmetric function.

Hemisphericity does not relate strictly to the handedness of the patient and there is poor correlation between handedness and eyedness—another measure of hemisphere-specific dominance. Classic symptoms of decreased left hemisphericity include depression and dyslexia, while decreased right hemisphericity can present with attention deficits and behavioural disorders. A variety of brain functions have been attributed to the right or left hemisphere; see Table 9.2. Autonomic asymmetries are an important indicator of cortical asymmetry as this reflects fuel delivery to the brain and the integrity of excitatory and inhibitory influences on sympathetic and parasympathetic function. Large projections from each hemisphere project to the ipsilateral PMRF with smaller projections to the mesencephalic RF. Therefore, other signs of altered PMRF or mesencephalic CIS may indicate hemisphericity. During tests of cerebellar function, slowness of movement in a limb (rather than breakdown of reciprocal actions) will often represent a decrease in cortical function—rather than a cerebellar cause. Of course, the two problems may coexist because of diaschisis occurring in hemisphericity. Therefore, cortical hemisphericity is often dependent on the presence of a series of findings related to subcortical output, fuel delivery, cognition, mood, and behaviour.

Examination
In addition, and most importantly from a functional neurological perspective, asymmetry or dysfunction in three of the most influential components of the nervous system should be considered. These areas include:

1. Vestibulocerebellar system;
2. Autonomic nervous system; and
3. Cerebral neuronal activity.

Table 9.2 Brain Functions per Hemisphere

Left Hemisphere	Right Hemisphere
Analytical—Assesses detail	Global—Assesses the big picture
Processes information in sequential or linear order	Processes information randomly or in variable order
Verbal processing	Visuospatial processing
Comprehension of words	Comprehension of tone, gestures, and body language
Motor and cognitive control of speech	Tone of voice and gestures
Plans an ordered response and reacts logically	Responds impulsively or emotionally
Mediates thought patterns based on fact and knowledge	Mediates thought patterns based on instinct and feelings Mediates creativity
Fine motor control and sensory processing	Gross motor control and spatial orientation
Prefers familiar environment	Responds to novel environments
Prefers processing high temporal and spatial frequency information (e.g., higher speed and detail)	Prefers processing low temporal and spatial frequency information (e.g., lower speed and detail)

Asymmetrical Autonomic Functional Considerations

Cardiovascular Function

With respect to cortical control of cardiovascular function, several studies have demonstrated that asymmetries in brain function influence the heart through ipsilateral pathways. These studies have shown that stimulation or inhibition at various levels on the right side of the neuraxis results in greater changes in heart rate, while increased sympathetic tone on the left side results in a lowered ventricular fibrillation threshold (Lane et al 1992). These finding have been explained by the fact that parasympathetic mechanisms appear to be dominant in the atria, while sympathetic mechanisms are dominant in the ventricles. Direct connections were traced between the sensorimotor cortex and the nucleus of tractus solitarius (NTS), dorsal motor nucleus of the vagus (DMV), and the rostral ventrolateral medulla (RVLM). These direct cortical projections to the NTS/DMV provide the anatomical basis for cortical influences on the baroreceptor reflex and cardiac parasympathetic control. These connections were also noted to have an ipsilateral predominance.

The preferential innervation of the sinoatrial node by the right vagus and the AV node by the left vagus might predict that parasympathetic effects of left hemisphere lesions would be expressed less strongly at the sinoatrial node than those of right hemisphere lesions (Barron et al 1994). These alterations in heart rate may be due in part to an imbalance in relative descending influences of the right and left brain on autonomic outflow (Zamrini et al 1990).

Measuring Cortical Hemisphericity

Best-Hand Test (Bilateral Line-Bisection Test)

It is known that patients with right hemisphere infarcts tend to bisect a horizontal line significantly to the right of the midline, while left hemisphere infarcts results in a less severe error to the left of the midline. Pseudoneglect occurs in 'normal' subjects with errors to the left of the midline.

The determined midpoint of a horizontal line depends on the hemisphere that is dominantly activated. Which brain side estimate is delivered depends upon which hand is chosen as the messenger. The hand giving the most accurate estimate is driven by the most behaviourally predominant side of the brain. Thus, properly utilized, two-hand line-bisection can be another biophysical window on hemisphericity (Morton 2003a).

Conducting the Line-Bisection Test

Type 20 staggered horizontal lines 1 cm apart on two vertical 215 × 280 mm pages. Line lengths differ by 10 mm from 70 to 160 mm (top to middle of page), and then in reverse

Clinical Examination for Parietal Dysfunction Should Include the Following Procedures

QUICK FACTS 23

- Visual fields
- Two-point discrimination and joint position sense
- Optokinetic pursuit
- Smooth visual tracking
- Finger to nose in each visual field
- Best-hand test
- Stereognosia/atopognosia/agraphagnosia
- Sensory extinction/inattention
- Visual searching tasks

order to the bottom of the page. Start by marking the midpoint of each line with your right hand and then with your left hand on the second page. Measure the distance (to 0.5 mm precision) from the true midpoint (include – (left) or + (right)) and tally each page independently. Divide totals by 20.

The two-hand line-bisection task is an attractive hemisphericity-type test because of the great variety of highly stable performances between normal subjects on this task. Apparently, these stable individual differences between right and left hand midline judgment become visible because the distal end of each appendage is controlled by a different cerebral hemisphere, each of which independently makes its midline judgment known. It is interesting to note that subjects tend to not be aware of their off-centre marks until placing the pen in the other hand.

Motor Strength and Tone
Muscle tone will often be diminished on the side of decreased brain function in all muscles. Loss of inhibition to the flexor muscle above solar plexus and extensor muscles below the solar plexus results in a mild flexion of the ipsilateral arm and extension of the ipsilateral leg, a posture referred to as parietal paresis.

Limb Control
Loss of coordination that appears cerebellar in nature may be due to loss of cortical function on the contralateral side.

Other Release Phenomena
The exaggeration of flexor reflex afferent reactions is a motor release phenomenon that may be caused by decreased function of the contralateral cortex. The expression of inappropriate emotions or the occurrence of vivid nightmares may be caused by limbic release phenomenon which occurs as a result of ipsilateral decreased cortical function.

Spontaneous Lateral Eye Movements
A certain level of cortical activity is necessary to prevent random or meaningless lateral saccadic activity of the eyes. When this movement dysfunction is present it can indicate a decreased cortical function (see Chapter 13).

Remembered Saccades
Remembered saccades are controlled by the contralateral frontal cortical areas. Decreased functionality in these areas results in inaccurate saccades (see Chapter 13).

Forehead Skin Temperature
Forehead temperature, if taken in the supraorbital regions, is supplied by branches of the internal carotid system, the same system that supplies the cortical areas of the brain. Asymmetry in skin temperature on the forehead may be associated with asymmetry in brain activity. The exact relationship is still controversial but an increased temperature seems to suggest the side of greatest activation.

Tympanic Temperature

Many studies have tried to link tympanic temperature to brain activation. The exact relationship is still controversial; however, it appears that as cortical activation levels increase the tympanic temperature decreases (Cherbuin & Brinkman 2004). This is due to the counter current cooling mechanisms that exist in this system so that as carotid flow and thus activation increases, the temperature decreases.

Asymmetric Autonomic Responses

The cortex stimulates the activation of a variety of areas of the PMRF that result in the inhibition of intermediolateral (IML) neurons that are the presynaptic neurons of sympathetic function. The projections from the cortex to the PMRF are ipsilateral for the most part and thus asymmetrical inhibition patterns that can be detected clinically can develop. For example the artery to venous ratio (A:V ratio) of retinal vessels may be different form eye to eye, indicating asymmetrical sympathetic activation. Changes in heart rate versus heart rhythm may indicate asymmetrical activation of the sympathetic or parasympathetic systems.

Blind Spot Sizes

Blind spot measurements can be an indication of asymmetrical cortical or thalamic activation.

Cerebellum Testing

The large projections systems between the cortex and cerebellum make each susceptible to decreased activation occurring in the other. This process is referred to as diaschisis. Clinical findings of decreased cerebellar function may be secondary to decreased contralateral cortical function and vice versa. Tests such as Rhomberg's and Facuda's march test can be useful in evaluating the asymmetrical differences.

Speech Patterns

Speech is a complex process that involves a variety of cortical areas that must function in a cohesive manner for successful speech production. Alterations in these patterns in conjunction with other findings can suggest decreased hemispheric function.

Cognitive and Behavioural Testing

Various human functions have been attributed to certain hemispheric areas. Dysfunction in these areas can often be clinically observed and act as a guide to activations states of each hemisphere. (See Table 9.3 and questionnaire in Appendix 9.1.)

Table 9.3 Typical Brain Behaviours		
Left Hemisphere Behaviour		**Right Hemisphere Behaviour**
Names	Recognizes	Faces
Verbal	Instructions	Visual or Kinesthetic
Inhibited	Emotions	Strong
Words	Meaning	Body Language
Logical	Thoughts/ideas	Humorous
Sequentially	Process information Problem solving	Subjectively, patterns
Serious	Appeals	Playful
Details and facts	Reading/listening	Main idea, big picture
Systematic plans	Learning	Exploration
Well-structured	Assignments	Open-ended
Outline	Remembers	Summarize

Diffuse Neuronal and Axonal Injuries Involving the Cortex

Severe TBI may result in widespread damage to axons, termed diffuse axonal injury (DAI) (Olsson et al 2004). DAI is one of the most common and important pathologic features of traumatic brain injury and can be caused from almost any type of head trauma ranging from direct blunt force trauma to the head, to the impact of coup/contra-coup injuries resulting from whiplash type trauma. The result of these injuries to the head may develop into closed head injuries ranging from mild to severe.

DAI caused by mild closed head injury (CHI) is likely to affect the neural networks concerned with the planning and execution of a variety of cortical functions, one of which includes the sequences of memory-guided saccades. This dysfunction of saccadic activity is very sensitive and can be used to identify the presence of diffuse axonal and neuronal injury following head trauma. CHI subjects show more directional errors, larger position errors, and hypermetria of primary saccades and final eye position. No deficits are usually seen in temporal accuracy including timing and rhythm of the saccades (Heitger et al 2002). Using saccadic testing combined with the history of head injury and any of the following symptoms which have been shown to often present with traumatic brain injury can give a fairly accurate estimation of the degree of axonal injury suffered by the patient:

- Psychomotor slowing;
- Central auditory pathway dysfunction involving tinnitus, hearing deficits, and hyperacusis;
- Deficits in facial emotion perception;
- Abnormal saccadic sequence control of remembered saccades; and
- Attention deficits.

Brain trauma is accompanied by regional alterations of brain metabolism, reduction in metabolic rates, and possible energy crisis. Positron emission tomography (PET) for metabolism of glucose and oxygen reveals that traumatic brain injury leads to a state of persistent metabolic crisis as defined by an elevated lactate/pyruvate ratio that is not related to ischaemia (Vespa et al 2005). These increases in lactate are typically more pronounced in patients with a poor outcome (Clausen et al 2005).

Brain tissue acidosis is known to mediate neuronal death (Marion et al 2002).

Severe human traumatic brain injury (TBI) profoundly disturbs cerebral acid–base homeostasis. The observed pH changes persist for the first 24 hours after the trauma. Brain tissue acidosis is associated with increased tissue PCO_2 and lactate concentration. These pathobiochemical changes are more severe in patients who remain in a persistent vegetative state or die. In brain tissue adjacent to cerebral contusions or underlying subdural haematomas, even brief periods of hyperventilation, which decreases pH and increases CO_2 and lactate concentrations, can significantly increase extracellular concentrations of mediators of secondary brain injury. These hyperventilation-induced changes are much more common during the first 24–36 hours after injury than at 3–4 days (Marion et al 2002).

Over one million whiplash injuries occur in the USA every year. Neuropsychological disturbances are often reported in whiplash patients but are largely ignored because of their borderline nature. Patients often complain of headache, vertigo, auditory disturbances, tinnitus, disturbances in concentration and memory, difficulties in swallowing, impaired vision, and temporomandibular dysfunction (Spitzer et al 1995). This syndrome has become known as 'whiplash brain'.

Patients who had received a whiplash injury to the neck consistently showed evidence of hypoperfusion and hypometabolism in parieto-occipital regions of the brain (Otte et al 1997). This was hypothesized to be due to DAI from acceleration forces or increases in spinotrigeminal nociceptive inputs from the cervical spine. Spinotrigeminal and vestibular afferents are capable of altering cerebral homodynamics and frequency of firing of monoaminergic neurons in the brainstem reticular formation.

The susceptibility of axons to mechanical injury appears to be due to both their viscoelastic properties and their high organization in white matter tracts. Although axons are supple under normal conditions, they become brittle when exposed to rapid deformations associated with brain trauma. Accordingly, rapid stretch of axons can damage the axonal cytoskeleton, resulting in a loss of elasticity and impairment of axoplasmic transport. Subsequent swelling of the axon occurs in discrete bulb formations or in elongated varicosities that accumulate transported proteins (Smith et al 2003).

Ultimately, swollen axons may become disconnected and contribute to additional neuropathologic changes in brain tissue. DAI may largely account for the clinical manifestations of brain trauma. However, DAI is extremely difficult to detect noninvasively and is poorly defined as clinical syndrome. Future advancements in the diagnosis and treatment of DAI will be dependent on our collective understanding of injury biomechanics, temporal axonal pathophysiology, and its role in patient outcome (Henderson et al 2005).

A growing body of evidence indicates that spondylotic narrowing of the spinal canal and abnormal or excessive motion of the cervical spine results in increased strain and shear forces that cause localized axonal injury within the spinal cord. During normal motion, significant axial strains occur in the cervical spinal cord. At the cervicothoracic junction, where flexion is greatest, the spinal cord stretches 24% of its length. This causes local spinal cord strain. In the presence of pathological displacement, strain can exceed the material properties of the spinal cord and cause transient or permanent neurological injury. Stretch-associated injury is now widely accepted as the principal etiological factor of myelopathy in experimental models of neural injury, tethered cord syndrome, and DAI (Henderson et al 2005).

Axonal injury reproducibly occurs at sites of maximal tensile loading in a well-defined sequence of intracellular events: myelin stretch injury, altered axolemmal permeability, calcium entry, cytoskeletal collapse, compaction of neurofilaments and microtubules, disruption of anterograde axonal transport, accumulation of organelles, axon retraction bulb formation, and secondary axotomy. Stretch and shear forces generated within the spinal cord seem to be important factors in the pathogenesis of cervical spondylotic myelopathy.

Alzheimer's disease (AD) is characterized by synaptic and axonal degeneration together with senile plaques (SP). SP are mainly composed of aggregated beta-amyloid, which are peptides derived from the amyloid precursor protein (APP). Apart from TBI in itself being considered a risk factor for AD, severe head injury seems to initiate a cascade of molecular events also associated with AD (Olsson et al 2004).

Seizures and Epilepsy

Epilepsy is a disorder in which an individual has the predisposing tendency to suffer unprovoked recurrent seizures. A seizure is an episode of desynchronized bursts of brain activity that result in abnormal activity or experiences in the individual. The seizures in some forms of epilepsy may arise in the entire brain and result in generalized seizures. Other forms both start and are limited to a particular region or focus in the brain. These type of seizures are referred to as partial or focal seizures. Seizures can start as a focal seizure in any area of the brain and spread to other areas to become secondary generalized seizures. Partial seizures can be further classified as simple or complex.

Simple partial seizures can occur in any area of the brain and the symptoms generated will depend on the area of the brain involved. The one common characteristic of a simple partial seizure is that consciousness is spared. The individual can recall the events before, during, and after the seizure and may be aware of the seizure activity itself. For example, a simple partial seizure involving the right motor cortex may produce a slight twitching of the left hand. This twitching is referred to as a positive symptom because it increases activity. However, a simple partial seizure in the left frontal lobe in the area of Broca may result in impaired speech. This is referred to as a negative symptom because activity is impaired. The time that the seizure is actually taking place is referred to as the ictal period and the time period immediately following the seizure is the postictal period (Wyllie 1993).

Complex partial seizures result in a disruption in consciousness, most probably because of interference with the reticular activation system in the brainstem or because of widespread areas of cortical involvement. Complex partial seizures may occur in any area of the brain but most commonly occur in the temporal lobe. Although there are multiple causes for temporal lobe epilepsy the most common form is referred to as mesial temporal lobe epilepsy syndrome (MTLE) or limbic epilepsy (Engel 1993). It is common for people with MTLE to experience an aura prior to the complete onset of seizure activity.

The aura may manifest as an order or mental sensation such as déjà vu or as repetitive motor tasks such as lip smacking or petting motions of the hands. These types of repetitive tasks are referred to as automatisms. With MTLE the ipsilateral basal ganglia are commonly also involved and can result in contralateral dystonias or immobility. Postictal recovery may take from minutes to hours and may include confusion, amnesia, agitation, tiredness, aggression, or depression.

Generalized seizures are usually tonic–clonic type seizures, which begin with the tonic stage, which involves generalized contraction of most muscle groups and loss of consciousness. Clonic phase involves rhythmic jerking motions that occur bilaterally. They usually start quite aggressively and then diminish as time passes. In this stage biting and or swallowing the tongue is a real concern. Postictal recovery may take minutes to hours and includes exhaustion, amnesia, headache, and confusion.

Generalized seizures have no preceding aura or focal seizure and involve both hemispheres from the onset. The mechanism is related rhythmic activity by neuronal aggregates in the upper brainstem or thalamus that project diffusely to the cortex. In partial and secondarily generalized seizures, the abnormal electrical activity originates from a seizure focus that results in enhanced excitability due to altered cellular properties or synaptic connections due to scar, blood clot, tumour, etc. Epilepsy very rarely occurs due to tumour, especially in the case of children.

Alzheimer's Disease

Alzheimer's disease is a progressive degenerative brain disease. It is the most common cause of dementia in the elderly. The prevalence of Alzheimer's disease increases rapidly over the age of 65 when the prevalence is about 1% to the age of 85 were the prevalence about 40% (Blumenfeld 2002). The clinical symptoms of Alzheimer's include:

- Impairment of memory;
- Impairment of language;
- Apraxia;
- Progressive cognitive impairment;
- Psychosis;
- Depression; and
- Personality changes.

Alzheimer's Disease	QUICK FACTS 24

- Alzheimer's disease is the most common progressive degenerative brain disease in the elderly.
- Alzheimer's disease is characterized by synaptic and axonal degeneration together with senile plaques (SP). SP are mainly composed of aggregated beta-amyloid (Aβ), which are peptides derived from the amyloid precursor protein (APP).
- Apart from TBI in itself being considered a risk factor for AD, severe head injury seems to initiate a cascade of molecular events also associated with Alzheimer's disease.

The initial symptoms of memory loss common in Alzheimer's disease are usually very mild, not unlike the memory loss common in the normal aging process.

Initially only the recent memory is affected and long-term memory is spared. Individuals can actually perform quite well even as the disease has advanced considerably by maintaining a consistent and non-variable routine, or as quite often occurs a family member will cover up the progressively more frequent lapses of memory and cognition.

Inevitably, the symptoms progress to the point where the individual starts to experience difficulty with the tasks of daily living even in their routine and with family support (McKhann et al 1984).

In order for the diagnosis of Alzheimer's disease to be established, the individual must have dementia, a progressive loss of memory, and at least one other cognitive impairment that impairs their normal daily functions. Often the diagnosis is only made when all other forms of dementia have been ruled out which can be quite difficult clinically. The average life expectancy from the initial diagnosis is approximately 10 years although a great deal of variation is common.

The neuropathology of the disease is the formation of neuritic plaques and neurofibrillary tangles. The neuritic plaques are composed of an insoluble protein called beta-amyloid and apolipoprotein E, which is enveloped in a cluster of abnormal axons and dendrites called dystrophic neurites. The neurofibrillary tangles are composed of intracellular accumulations of hyperphosphorylated microtubule associated proteins or paired helical proteins referred to as tau proteins (Blumenfeld 2002). Severe head injury seems to initiate a cascade of molecular events also associated with the development of neurofibrillary tangles and neuritic plaques and thus Alzheimer's disease.

Headache Syndromes

Headaches are a common neurological symptom that may indicate a serious pathological condition. The majority of headaches, however, do not signal a major pathology but are benign in nature. The brain parenchyma itself is not able to detect painful stimulus. The pain of headache must therefore come from the other structures inside the head such as the blood vessels, meninges, and scalp or be referred from some other structures closely aligned, in a neurological sense, with the above structures. The trigeminal nerve supplies the nociceptive reception of the anterior face and most of the supratentorial internal structures of the skull such as the dura and blood vessels, except for the infratentorial posterior cranial fossa for which the vagus and glossopharyngeal nerves supply the nociceptive input. Headaches are usually classified into two groups, those being primary and secondary in nature. Primary headaches are not associated with other pathology and are, with the exception of the pain and disability they cause, usually benign. Secondary headaches are by definition associated with other usually serious pathology that should not be missed on examination.

Primary Headaches

Primary headache syndromes are diagnosed by defining the clinical features of the patient's headaches and applying those to established definitions. If care is taken during the history and examination to identify any warning signs that may also be present, then the chances of missing a secondary headache is substantially reduced. Common warning signs that must be investigated thoroughly if found include:

- Development of a first-time headache in someone who does not usually get headaches;
- Sudden onset or thunderclap headache;
- Initial onset of headaches after age 50 years;
- Association of headache with other systemic signs or symptoms such as fever, myalgias, or weight loss;
- Changes in headache pattern such as frequency, severity, timing, or type of pain; and
- Associated neurological signs or symptoms such as changes in personality, or cognitive dysfunctions.

Some common primary headaches are outlined below.

Cluster Headache
This type of headache is relatively uncommon and occurs in men with a greater frequency than women. Men between the ages of 30 and 40 years are usually affected to a greater degree than other age ranges. There is a genetic predisposition with the occurrence of this

headache. The pain is described as severe unilateral orbital, suborbital, or temporal and lasting from 15 to 180 minutes without treatment. Associated symptoms include conjunctival injections, lacrimations, congestion, rhinorrhea, ptosis, miosis, and eyelid oedema.

Migraine Headache

The classical features of a migraine type headache include a frequent association with the menstrual cycle in women, characteristic triggers that set off the migraine process, family history of migraine, reversible attacks of cognitive impairment related to the headaches, and associated dizziness, vertigo, nausea, and vomiting. The typical migraine type headache will progress through a series of phases that have been referred to as the prodrome, aura, headache, and postdrome phases.

The *prodrome phase* usually includes changes such as elation of mood, irritability, depression, sense of hunger or thirst, drowsy feelings, mental or physical slowing, and occasionally abdominal bloating. The *aura phase* usually precedes the actual headache and terminates before the start of the headache and involves visual features such as scotomas, fortification spectra, and scintillations. It may also include physical alterations including hemiparesis and numbness. The *headache phase* usually involves a moderate to severe unilateral temporal throbbing pain that is aggravated by activity. Associated symptoms may include nausea, vomiting, photophobia, phonophobia, and osmophobia.

Tension Headache

Tension headaches are the most common and least distinct type of headache. They may occur episodically or chronically and are usually described as dull, achy, bilateral in nature, with the sensation of squeezing or pressing of the head. Activity does not usually aggravate tension type headaches and phonophobia, photophobia, nausea, and vomiting are not usually associated. Tension headaches can be classified by their frequency and chronicity of occurrence.

New Daily Persistent Headache

This headache occurs greater than 15 days per month. The onset has been less than 1 month in duration. The headaches occur for greater than 4 hours each and the patient has had no prior history of migraine headache in the past. The initial onset of the headache usually involves a constant headache in a constant location for more than 3 days duration.

Hemicrania Continua

This type of headache is present for greater than 1 month but less than 6 months. They are usually constant in location, which is unilateral in nature. The pain is continuous and there appear to be no precipitating factors involved in initiating the headache.

Chronic Tension Type Headache

This headache occurs greater than 15 days per month. The headaches are over 4 hours in duration and have been occurring for the past 6 months. These patients usually have a history of episodic tension type headaches with a gradual increase in severity and frequency over the past 3 months.

Chronic Transformed Migraine Headache

This headache has the same criteria as the chronic tension type headache but some of the symptoms of migraine headache also occur.

Causes of Secondary Headaches

A variety of pathological conditions or traumatic events can be associated with headaches. Some of the more common of these include:

- Tumours;
- Meningitis;
- Giant cell arteritis;
- Fasting;
- Head trauma;
- Intracranial haemorrhage;
- Cerebral infarct;
- Carotid or vertebral artery dissection;

- Venous sinus thrombus;
- Postictal headache;
- Hydrocephalus;
- Low CSF pressure;
- Toxic poisoning;
- Metabolic imbalances;
- Epidural abscess;
- Vasculitis;
- Trigeminal neuralgia; and
- Tooth ache.

Appendix 9.1 Right or Left Brain-Oriented? The Asymmetry Questionnaire

Name: _____

For each of these 15 pairs of statements, mark an × at the *start* of the *one* statement that is *most* like you.

Statement A	Statement B
1. I often talk about my and others' feelings of emotion.	1. I tend to avoid talking about emotional feelings.
2. I am good at finishing projects.	2. I am a strong starter of projects.
3. I organize parts into the whole (synthetic, creative).	3. I break the whole into parts (reproductive–reductionistic).
4. I am quick-acting in emergency.	4. I methodically solve problems by process of elimination.
5. I think and listen interactively–vocally, and talk a lot.	5. I think and listen quietly, keep my talk to a minimum.
6. I don't read other people's minds very well.	6. I am very good at knowing what others are thinking.
7. I see the big picture (project data beyond, can predict).	7. I am analytical (stay within the limits of the data).
8. I tend to be independent, hidden, private, and indirect.	8. I tend to be interdependent, open, public, and direct.
9. I usually design original outfits of clothing.	9. I dress for success and wear high status clothing.
10. I need to be alone and quiet when upset.	10. I need closeness and to talk things out when upset.
11. I praise others, and also work for praise from others.	11. I do not praise others, nor need the praise of others.
12. I'm more interested in objects and things.	12. I tend to be more interested in people and feelings.
13. I seek frank feedback from others.	13. I avoid seeking evaluation by others.
14. I often feel my partner (or closest friend/s) talks too much.	14. I feel my partner (or closest friend(s)) doesn't talk or listen to me enough.
15. I'm strict when given some authority—people (or my children) obey me and work for my approval.	15. I am not strict when given authority.

Source: Morton BE 2003b Asymmetry questionnaire outcomes correlate with several hemisphericity measures. Brain and Cognition 51:372–374.

References

Arato M, Frecska E, Tekes K et al 1991 Serotonergic inter-hemispheric asymmetry: gender difference in the orbital cortex. Acta Psychiatrica Scandinavica 84:110–111.

Arato M, Tekes K, Palkovits M et al 1987 Serotonergic split-brain and suicide. Psychiatry Research 21:355–356.

Arora RC, Meltzer HY 1989 Serotonergic measures in the brains of suicide victims: 5-HT$_2$ binding sites in the frontal cortex of suicide victims and control subjects. American Journal of Psychiatry 146:730–736.

Barron SA, Rogovski Z, Hemli J 1994 Autonomic consequences of cerebral hemisphere infarction. Stroke 25:113–116.

Blumenfeld H 2002 Higher order cerebral function. In: Neuro-anatomy through clinical cases. Sinauer Associates, Sunderland, MA.

Cherbuin N, Brinkman C 2004 Cognition is cool: can hemispheric activation be assessed by tympanic membrane thermometry? Brain Cognition 54(3):228–231.

Clark CR, Geffen GM, Geffen LB 1987 Catecholamines and attention. I: animal and clinical studies. Neuroscience and Biobehavioural Reviews 11:341–352.

Clausen T, Khaldi A, Zauner A et al 2005 Cerebral acid-base homeostasis after severe traumatic brain injury. Journal of Neurosurgery 103(4):597–607.

Davidson RJ, Hugdahl K 1995 Brain asymmetry. MIT Press, Cambridge, MA/London.

Demeter E, Tekes KL, Majorossy K et al 1989 The asymmetry of ^{3}H-imipramine binding may predict psychiatric illness. Life Sciences 44:1403–1410.

Engel J (ed) 1993 Surgical treatment of the epilepsies. Raven, New York.

Falk D, Hildebolt C, Cheverud J et al 1991 Human cortical asymmetries determined with 3D-MR technology. Journal of Neuroscience Methods 39(2):185–191.

Fallon JH, Loughlin SE 1987 Monoamine innervation of cerebral cortex and a theory of the role of monoamines in cerebral cortex and basal ganglia. In: Peters A, Jones EG (eds) Cerebralo cortex. Plenum Press, New York, vol 6 p 41–127

Galaburda AM, LeMay M, Geschwind N 1978 Right-left asymmetries in the brain. Science 199:852–856.

Gallois P, Hautecoeur P, Ovelacq E et al 1985 The gaze and functional hemispheric activation in normal subjects. Revue Neurologique 141(11):735–739.

Geschwind N, Levitsky W 1968 Human brain: Left-right asymmetries in temporal speech regions. Science 161:186–187.

Glick SD, Meibach RC, Cox RD et al 1983 Multiple and interrelated functional asymmetries in rat brain. Life Sciences 32:2215–2221.

Glick SD, Ross DA, Hough LB 1982 Lateral asymmetry of neurotransmitters in human brain. Brain Research 234:53–63.

Heitger MH, Anderson TJ, Jones RD 2002 Saccade sequences as markers for cerebral dysfunction following mild closed head injury. Progress in Brain Research 140:433–448.

Henderson FC, Geddes JF, Vaccaro AR et al 2005 Stretch-associated injury in cervical spondylotic myelopathy: new concept and review. Neurosurgery 56(5):1101–1113; discussion 1101–1113.

Lane RD, Wallace JD, Petrosky PP et al 1992 Supraventricular tachycardia in patients with right hemisphere strokes. Stroke 23:362–366.

LeMay M, Culebras A 1972 Human Brain morphological differences in the hemispheres demonstrable by carotid arteriography. New England Journal of Medicine 287:168–170.

McKhann G, Drachman DA, Folstein M et al 1984 Clinical diagnosis of Alzheimer's disease; report of the NINCDS-ADRDS Work Group under the auspices of the Department of Health and Human Services Task Force on Alzheimer's Disease. Neurology 34:939–944.

Marion DW, Puccio A, Wisniewski SR et al 2002 Effect of hyperventilation on extracellular concentrations of glutamate, lactate, pyruvate, and local cerebral blood flow in patients with severe traumatic brain injury. Critical Care Medicine 30(12):2619–2625.

Martin JH 1996 Neuroanatomy text and atlas. McGraw-Hill, New York.

Melillo R, Leisman G 2004 Neurobehavioral disorders of childhood. Kluwer Academic/Plenum, New York.

Morilak DA, Fornal C, Jacobs BL 1986 Single unit activity of noradrenergic neurons in locus coeruleus and serotonergic neurons in the nucleus raphe dorsalis of freely moving cats in relation to the cardiac cycle. Brain Research 399(2):262–270.

Morton BE 2003a Two-hand line-bisection task outcomes correlate with several measures of hemisphericity. Brain and Cognition 51:305–316.

Morton BE 2003b Asymmetry questionnaire outcomes correlate with several hemisphericity measures. Brain and Cognition 51:372–374.

Olsson A, Csajbok L, Ost M, Hoglund K et al 2004 Marked increase of beta-amyloid (1–42) and amyloid precursor protein in ventricular cerebrospinal fluid after severe traumatic brain injury. Journal of Neurology 251:(7):870–876.

Otte A, Ettlin TM, Nitzsche EU et al 1997 PET and SPECT in whiplash syndrome: a new approach to a forgotten brain?. Journal of Neurology, Neuosurgery and Psychiatry 63:386–372.

Pryor D 1995 Common CNS infections. New Ethicals 32(11)

Rossor M, Garrett N, Iversen L 1980 No evidence for lateral asymmetry of neurotransmitters in post-mortem human brain. Journal of Neurochemistry 35:743–745.

Scheld WM 1994 Acute bacterial meningitis in Harrison's principles of internal medicine, 13th edn.

Smith DH, Meaney DF, Shull WH 2003 Diffuse axonal injury in head trauma. Journal of Head Trauma Rehabilitation 18(4):307–316.

Spitzer WO, Skovron ML, Salmi LR 1995 Scientific monograph of the Quebec task force on whiplash associated disorders: redefining 'whiplash' and its management. Spine 20(Suppl 8): 1s–73s.

Spoont MR 1992 Modulatory role of serotonin in neural information processing: Implications for human psychopathology. Psychological Bulletin 112:330–350.

Steinmetz H, Volkmann J, Jancke L et al 1991 Anatomical left-right asymmetry of language-related temporal cortex is different in left-handers and right handers. Annals of Neurology 29(3):315–319.

Vespa P, Bergsneider M, Hattori N et al 2005 Metabolic crisis without brain ischemia is common after traumatic brain injury: a combined microdialysis and positron emission tomography study. Journal of Cerebral Blood Flow Metabolism 25(6):763–774.

Vogel FS 1994 The central nervous system. In: Rubin E, Farber J (eds) Pathology, 2nd edn.

Wagner HN, Burns DH, Dannals RF et al 1983 Imaging dopamine receptors in the human brain by positron tomography. Science 2211:1264–1266.

Wittling W 1998 Brain asymmetry in the control of autonomic-physiologic activity. In: Davidson R, and Hugdahl K (eds) Brain asymmetry. MIT Press: Cambridge, MA.

Wyllie E 1993 The treatment of epilepsy; principles and practice. Lea & Febiger, Philadelphia.

Yamamoto BK, Freed CR 1984 Asymmetric dopamine and serotonin metabolism in nigrostriatal and limbic structures of the trained circling rat. Brain Research 297:115–119.

Zamrini EY, Meador KJ, Loring DW et al 1990 Unilateral cerebral inactivation produces differential left/right heart rate responses. Neurology 40:1408–1411.

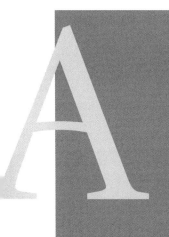

Clinical Case Answers

Case 9.1

9.1.1 With any head injury the possibility of an internal haemorrhage of some sort has occurred. The headache, the absent corneal reflex, and nausea are all consistent with an intracranial haemorrhage. In order to further evaluate this young man a CT scan of his head should be performed immediately.

9.1.2
1. Concussion
2. Subdural haematoma
3. Epidural haematoma
4. Skull fracture
5. Cerebral contusion

Case 9.2

9.2.1
1. Cauda equina syndrome
2. Frontal lobe epilepsy
3. Frontal lobe tumour
4. Parkinson's disease
5. Ablative frontal lobe stroke

Chapter 10

The Thalamus and Hypothalamus

Clinical Cases for Thought

Case 10.1   A 23-year-old young lady presents with a chief complaint of excessive weight gain. She reports that she has gained 15 kg in the past 12 weeks. Pregnancy tests were negative. She has also experienced visual disturbances over the past week.

Questions

10.1.1   Outline three differential diagnostic concerns you have concerning her presentation.

10.1.2   Which nuclei of the hypothalamus are thought to play a role in hunger control?

Case 10.2   A 45-year-old woman presents with the chief complaint of visual disturbances. When she closes one eye she has blank areas in her visual field.

Questions

10.2.1   What are the causes of an enlarged physiological blind spot?

10.2.2   Explain the mechanism by which in normal circumstances we are not aware of our physiological blind spots.

Introduction

1. The thalamus and hypothalamus have traditionally been thought of as a simple relay system and the master control over the pituitary gland respectively. But as our understanding of the functions of these areas of the neuraxis grows so too does the variety of functions these areas contribute to human function. The thalamus is now thought to play a vital role in the innate stimulatory patterns of wide areas of cortex that allow consciousness. We can record this activity with an electro-encephalogram. The hypothalamus seems to be the control centre for certain aspects of the sympathetic nervous system and is also involved in certain types of learning and memory.

    In this chapter we will explore the anatomy and neurological functional circuits of these interesting and clinically relevant areas of the neuraxis.

Anatomy of the Thalamus

The diencephalon encloses the third ventricle and includes the thalamus with its lateral and medial geniculate bodies, the subthalamus, the epithalamus, and the hypothalamus. Each cerebral hemisphere contains a thalamus, which is a large egg-shaped mass of grey matter, in the dorsal portion of the diencephalon (Fig. 10.1). The thalamus is an important link between sensory receptors and cerebral cortex for all modalities except olfaction.

The rostral end of the thalamus, also known as the anterior tubercle, is narrower than the posterior portion of the thalamus which contains a medial enlargement referred to as the pulvinar and a lateral enlargement referred to as the lateral geniculate body. The medial surface of the thalamus forms the lateral wall of the third ventricle and forms a connection to the medial surface of the opposite thalamus through a short communicating projection of grey matter called the massa intermedia or the central thalamic adhesion (Chusid 1982). The thalamus receives extensive projections from all of the main subcortical areas of the nervous system including spinal cord, hypothalamus, cerebellum, and the basal ganglia and forms reciprocal projections with the majority of the cerebral cortex. The connections to and from the cortex, also known as the thalamic radiations, are carried in four fibre tracts referred to as peduncles or stalks. These projections form a considerable portion of the internal capsule (Fig. 10.2). The anterior thalamic peduncle carries projection fibres from the anterior and medial thalamic nuclei to all areas of the frontal cortex. The superior peduncle carries projection fibres to and from the ventral and lateral thalamic nuclei to the pre- and postcentral gyri and premotor and presensory areas of the cortex. The posterior peduncle caries projection fibres to and from the posterior and lateral thalamic areas including the lateral geniculate body and the

| QUICK FACTS 1 | The Hypothalamus Acts on Four Major Systems |

1. Autonomic nervous system
2. Endocrine system
3. Limbic/emotional component
4. Homeostatic controls

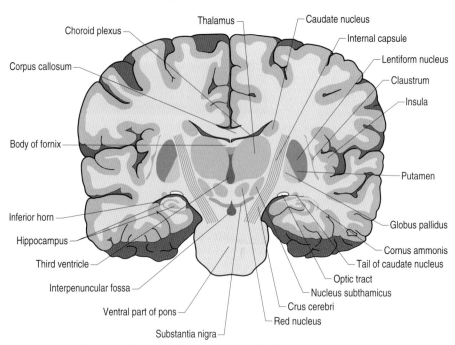

Fig.10.1 A cross-sectional view of the anatomical relationships of the diencephalon.

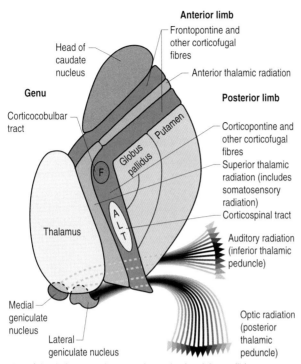

Fig. 10.2 The relationship of the thalamus to the internal capsule, the globus pallidus, putamen, and the caudate nucleus, and the location in the internal capsule of a variety of efferent and afferent pathways.

pulvinar to the posterior and occipital cortical areas. The inferior thalamic peduncle connects the posterior thalamic areas including the medial geniculate body to the temporal areas of cortex (Williams & Warwick 1984). The external medullary laminae are layers of myelinated fibres on the lateral surface of the thalamus immediately adjacent to the internal capsule (Fig. 10.3). The internal medullary lamina is a vertical sheet of white matter deep in the substance of the thalamus that bifurcates in the anterior portion of the thalamus to divide the substance of the thalamus into lateral, medial, and anterior segments (Fig. 10.3). The thalamus has seven groups of nuclei organized with respect to the internal medullary lamina. These include

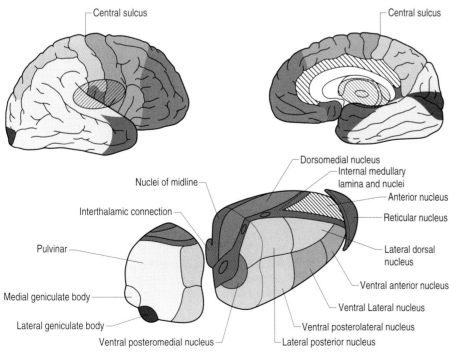

Fig. 10.3 The thalamic nuclei and their main projections to the cortex.

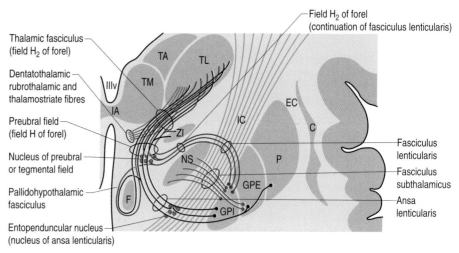

Fig.10.4 The formation of the thalamic fasciculus from the ansa lenticularis and the fasciculus lenticularis. Note that the anterior nuclear group receives input from the ipsilateral mammillary nuclei of the hypothalamus via the mammillothalamic tract and from the presubiculum of the hippocampal formation.

the anterior nuclear group located rostrally, the nuclei of the midline, the medial nuclei, the ventral nuclei, lateral nuclear mass which expands posteriorly to include the pulvinar, the intralaminar nuclear group, and the reticular nuclei (Fig. 10.3). Several nuclei of the thalamus are considered to be areas of singularity dependent on neural activation from the cortex to survive. These nuclei show marked transneural degeneration if the areas of cortex that project to them are damaged, understimulated, or subject to excessive inhibition (Williams & Warwick 1984). This process is an example of diaschisis, where reduced output from one area of the neuraxis results in degeneration of the downstream neuron pools.

The *anterior nuclear group* receives input from the ipsilateral mammillary nuclei of the hypothalamus via the mammillothalamic tract and from the presubiculum of the hippocampal formation (Fig. 10.4). Neurons in the anterior thalamic group project to regions of the cingulate and frontal cortices, mainly areas 23, 24, and 32. The anterior group of nuclei is a principal limbic component in linking the hippocampus and the hypothalamus and is involved with the modulation of memory and emotion.

Recent advances in our understanding of this area of the neuraxis have lead to the conclusion that an intact and normally functioning hippocampal-fornical-mammillo-thalamic-limbo-cortical pathway is essential for the establishment of recent memory. The *medial nuclei* are composed of a number of small nuclei including the parafascicular, submedius, paracentralis, and paralateralis. However, the medial nuclei are dominated by the nucleus medius dorsalis. The medial nuclei form reciprocal projections from the hypothalamus, the frontal cortex, the amygdaloid complex, the corpus striatum, and the brainstem reticular formation. These nuclei also form reciprocal projections with all other thalamic nuclei. Dysfunction of the medial nuclei in man results in complex changes in motivational drive, in problem-solving ability, and in emotional stability.

The *ventral nuclear group* is composed of three nuclei, the ventral anterior (VA), the ventral posterior (VP), and the ventral intermedius (VI). The ventral posterior nucleus is further divided into the functionally important ventral posterior lateral (VPL) and ventral posterior medial (VPM) nuclei. The vast majority of the fibres reaching the ventral group are from the afferent fibres of the sensory system of man. The VPL receives projections from the contralateral cuneate and gracile nuclei via the medial lemniscal pathway and both contralateral and ipsilateral spinothalamic projections via the anterolateral system. The VPM receives projections from the trigeminal and gustatory lemnisci. These nuclei project reciprocally via the posterior limb of the internal capsule to the somatosensory areas including areas 1, 2, and 3 of cortex (Fig. 10.2). The VI nuclei receive extensive projections from the dentate and interpositus nuclei of the cerebellum and from the basal ganglia. The VI projects to other thalamic nuclei and to the motor areas of cortex namely areas 4 and 6. The VA nucleus receives extensive projections from the globus pallidus via the thalamic fasciculus and from the dentate nucleus of the cerebellum. The VA nucleus is therefore very important in the integration or modulation of projections from the basal ganglia and the cerebellum on the cortical areas of motor function.

The midline nuclei are composed of the paraventricular, parataenial, and reuniens nuclei. The afferent and efferent projections of these nuclei are very difficult to elucidate but they, along with the intralaminar nuclei, most probably mediate cortical arousal.

The *lateral nuclear group* is composed of the lateral dorsal (LD) nucleus, the lateral posterior (LP) nucleus, and the pulvinar, which on its own occupies approximately 25% of the whole caudal thalamic area. The pulvinar is relatively late in phylogeny and only occurs in higher primates and man. The pulvinar is thought to receive projections from the lateral and medial geniculate bodies as well as direct projections from retinal cells of the optic tracts. The pulvinar reciprocally projects to the temporal, occipital, and parietal cortices. The LD nucleus reciprocally projects to the inferior parietal and posterior cingulate cortices. The LP nucleus reciprocally projects to the parietal and postcentral gyri areas of cortex.

The *reticular nuclei* form an outer shell around the lateral aspects of the thalamus. All afferent and efferent projection fibres, to and from the thalamus, pass through this reticular nuclear area. The neurons of this nucleus are predominantly GABA-ergic in nature, while other thalamic nuclei are mainly excitatory and glutaminergic. The reticular nuclei appear not to have direct projections to the cortex but only to other nuclei of the thalamus (Destexhe & Sejnowski 2003).

The *intralaminar nuclei* include several small clusters of neurons contained within the substance of the internal medullary laminae. These nuclei include paracentralis, centralis lateralis and centralis limitans, and the much larger central medial nucleus. The function of these nuclei is still not clear.

The nuclei of the midline are small islands of neurons usually in the area of the interthalamic adhesion. These nuclei receive a predominance of their projections from the reticular formation of the brainstem and project to the corpus striatum and cerebellum. The functional significance of these nuclei remains a mystery.

The *lateral geniculate nucleus* (LGN) appears as a swelling on the rostral surface of the pulvinar and receives afferent input from the axons of the retinal ganglion cells of the temporal half of the ipsilateral eye and the nasal half of the contralateral eye. The LGN neurons then project axons to the ipsilateral primary visual cortex via the optic radiations. The nucleus consists of six layers of nerve cells and is the terminus of about 90% of the fibres of the optic tract. The remaining 10% of fibres terminate in the pretectal areas of the mesencephalon, the superior colliculus of the tectum of the mesencephalon, and some fibres synapse directly on neurons in the hypothalamus (Snell 2001). Only 10–20% of the projections arriving in the LGN are derived directly from the retina. The remaining projections arise from the brainstem reticular formation, the pulvinar, and reciprocal projections from the striate cortex. These projections between the LGN and the striate cortex are important for a number of reasons but may play a major role in the process of physiological completion or 'fill in' that occurs during visual processing in the cortex.

The *medial geniculate nucleus* (MGN) or body is the tonotopically organized auditory input to the superior temporal gyrus. It appears as a swelling on the posterior surface of the pulvinar. Afferent fibres arriving in the medial geniculate body from the inferior colliculus form the inferior brachium. The inferior colliculus receives projections from the lateral lemniscus. The MGN receives auditory information from both ears but predominantly from the contralateral ear. The efferent projection fibres of the MGN form the auditory radiations that terminate in the auditory cortex of the superior temporal gyrus (Snell 2001).

The Physiological 'Blind Spot'

The visual image inverts and reverses as it passes through the lens of the eye and forms an image on the retina. Image from the upper visual field is projected onto the lower retina and that from the lower visual field onto the upper retina. The left visual field is projected to the right hemiretina of each eye in such a fashion that the right nasal hemiretina of the left eye and the temporal hemiretina of the right eye receive the image. The central image or focal point of the visual field falls on the fovea of the retina, which is the portion of the retina with the highest density of retinal cells and as such produces the highest visual acuity. The fovea receives the corresponding image of the central 1°–2° of the total visual field but represents about 50% of the axons in the optic nerve and projects to about 50% of the neurons in the visual cortex. The macula comprises the space surrounding the fovea and also has a relatively high visual acuity. The optic disc is located about 15° medially or towards the nose on each retina and is the convergence point for the axons of retinal cells as they leave the retina and form the optic nerve. This area although functionally important has no photoreceptors. This creates a blind spot in each eye about 15° temporally from a central fixation point. When both eyes are functioning, open, and focused on a central fixation point, the blind spots do not overlap so all of the visual field is represented in the cortex and one is not aware of the blind spot in one's visual experience. The area of the visual striate cortex, which is the primary visual area of the occipital lobe, representing the blind spot and the monocular crescent which are both in the temporal field, does not contain alternating independent ocular dominance columns. This means that these areas only receive information from one eye. If that eye is closed, the area representing the blind spot of the eye remaining open will not be activated because of the lack of receptor activation at the retina.

It is expected that when one eye is closed the visual field should now have an area not represented by visual input and the absence of vision over the area of the blind spot should be apparent. However, this does not occur. The cortical neurons responsible for the area of the blind spot must receive stimulus from other neurons that create the illusion that the blind spot is not there. This is indeed the case and is accomplished by a series of horizontal projecting neurons located in the visual striate cortex that allow for neighbouring hypercolumns to activate one another. The horizontal connections between these hypercolumns allow for perceptual completion or 'fill in' to occur (Gilbert & Wiesel 1989; McGuire et al 1991).

The blind spot is therefore not strictly monocular, but it is dependent on the frequency of firing (FOF) of horizontal connections from neighbouring neurons. These may be activated via receptors and pathways from either eye.

Perceptual completion refers to the process whereby the brain fills in the region of the visual field that corresponds to a lack of visual receptors. This explains why one generally is not aware of the blind spot in everyday experience. The size and shape of the blind spots can be mapped utilizing simple procedures as outlined in Chapter 4.

The size and shape of the blind spots are dependent to some extent on the central integrative state (CIS) of the horizontal neurons of the cortex that supply the stimulus for the act of completion to occur. The integrative state of the horizontal neurons is determined to some extent by the activity levels of the neurons in the striate cortex in general. Several factors can contribute to the CIS of striate cortical neurons; however, a major source of stimulus results from thalamocortical activation via the reciprocal thalamocortical optic radiation pathways. It is clear from the above that the majority of the projection fibres reaching the LGN are not from retinal cells. This strongly suggests that the LGN acts as a multimodal sensory integration convergence point that in turn activates neurons in the striate cortex appropriately. The level of activation of the LGN is temporally and spatially dependent on the activity levels of all the multimodal projections that it receives.

In 1997, Professor Frederick Carrick discovered that asymmetrically altering the afferent input to the thalamus resulted in an asymmetrical effect on the size of the blind spot in each eye. The blind spot was found to decrease on the side of increased afferent stimulus. This was attributed to an increase in brain function on the contralateral side because of changes in thalamocortical activation that occurred because of multimodal sensory integration in the thalamus.

The stimulus utilized by Professor Carrick in his study was a manipulation of the upper cervical spine, which is known to increase the FOF of multimodal neurons in areas of the thalamus and brainstem that project to the visual striate cortex. These reciprocal connections lower the threshold for activation of neurons in the visual cortex. By decreasing the threshold for firing of neurons in the visual cortex, the manipulation resulted in a smaller blind spot because the area surrounding the permanent geometric blind spot zone is more likely to reach threshold and respond to the receptor activation that occurs immediately adjacent to the optic disc on the contralateral side. The size and shape of the blind spot will also be associated with the degree of activation of neurons associated with receptors adjacent to the optic disc. The receptors surrounding the optic disc underlie the neurons that form the optic nerve exiting by way of the optic disc. The amplitude of receptor potentials adjacent to the optic disc may therefore also be decreased because of interference of light transmission through the overlying fibres even though they should have lost their myelin coating during development; otherwise, interference would be even greater. This interference results in decreased receptor amplitude, which in turn results in decreased FOF of the corresponding primary afferent nerve. This may result in a blind spot that is physiologically larger than the true anatomical size of the blind spot.

This lead to the understanding that the size and shape of the blind spots could be used as a measure of the CIS of areas of the thalamus and cortex due to the fact that the amplitude of somatosensory receptor potentials received by the thalamus will influence the FOF of cerebello-thalamocortical loops that have been shown to maintain a CIS of cortex.

Therefore, muscle stretch and joint mechanoreceptor potentials will alter the FOF of primary afferents that may have an effect on visual neurons associated with the cortical receptive field of the blind spot when visual afferents are in a steady state of firing. Professor Carrick proposed that 'A change in the frequency of firing of one receptor-based neural system should effect the central integration of neurons that share synaptic relationships between other environmental modalities, resulting in an increase or decrease of cortical neuronal expression that is generally associated with a single modality' (Carrick 1997).

Care should be taken not to base too much clinical significance on the blind spot sizes until any pathological or other underlying cause that may have resulted in the changes in blind spot size are ruled out. The blind spot has been found to increase in size because of the following conditions:

- Multiple evanescent white dot syndrome;
- Acute macular neuroretinopathy;
- Acute idiopathic blind spot enlargement (AIBSE) syndrome;
- Multifocal choroiditis;
- Pseudo presumed ocular histoplasmosis;
- Peripapillary retinal dysfunction; and
- Systemic vascular disease.

An ophthalmoscopical examination is therefore an important component of the functional neurological examination. There are several other valuable ophthalmoscopic findings discussed in Chapter 4 that can assist with estimating the CIS of various neuronal pools.

Functions of the Thalamus

The thalamus receives input from every afferent sensory modality with the exception of olfaction. Olfactory perception occurs in the primary and secondary olfactory areas of the cortex, thus bypassing the thalamus.

Thalamic Dysfunction May Result in Profound Effects Including Sensory Loss, Thalamic Pain, and Involuntary Movements

Lesions of the VPL or VPM usually result in *sensory loss* in all modalities of sensation of the contralateral side of the body including light touch, tactile localization and discrimination, and proprioception.

Spontaneous, contralateral, pain that is often excessive in nature to the stimulus may follow thalamic lesions such as infarction. This type of pain is referred to as *thalamic pain* and is usually not responsive to even powerful doses of analgesic drugs.

Movement disorders involving choreoathetoid movements may result following thalamic lesions. The movement disorder is probably due to a loss of integration of information from the corpus striatum and may also be due to loss of proprioceptive integration due to a lesion involving the VPL or VPM nuclei.

Processing of Thalamic Input

Sensory input from all modalities except olfaction do not reach the cerebral cortex directly but first synapse on thalamocortical relay neurons in specific regions of the thalamus. These relay neurons in turn project to their respective areas of sensory cortex via reciprocal pathways that result in a topographically organized thalamocortical loop projection system (Jones 1985). The thalamocortical relay neurons also form reciprocal connections with thalamic reticular neurons which are inhibitory. These reticular neurons also receive projections from all other afferent or efferent projections coming into or leaving the thalamus. This network thus receives bidirectional excitatory stimulus from the thalamocortical and corticothalamic loops and inhibitory input from the reticular collaterals. In addition to relaying sensory input the thalamic relay neurons also have intrinsic properties that allow them to generate endogenous threshold activity and exhibit complex firing patterns (Sherman 2001). They relay information to the cortex in the usual integrate and fire pattern unless they have recently undergone a period of inhibition. Following a period of inhibition stimulus, in certain circumstances they can produce bursts of low-threshold spike action potentials referred to as post-inhibitory rebound bursts. This activity seems to be generated endogenously and may be responsible for production of a portion of the activation of the thalamocortical loop pathways thought to be detected in encephalographic recordings of cortical activity captured by electroencephalograms (EEG) (Destexhe & Seinowski 2003). In addition to displaying integrate and fire and burst and tonic modes of behaviour, the relay neurons can also generate sustained oscillation activity in the delta frequency range of 0.5–4 Hz. (Curro Dossi et al 1992). The thalamic reticular neurons also produce oscillatory activity but in the range 8–12 Hz (Contreras 1996). The control of the thalamic neuronal oscillations appears to be under the modulation of the cortex (Blumenfeld & McCormick 2000). In fact it appears that cortical feedback is necessary to maintain the thalamic oscillations. One theory suggests that the thalamic oscillations are utilized by a variety of structures in the brain to promote neuroplastic change through the constant repetition of synaptic stimulation that would result from the periods of oscillations in a neural circuit. One such example would be in the formation of long-term memory. The hippocampus recalls events that have happened throughout the day and presents them to the cortex. The cortex could then stimulate the thalamus to form oscillatory excitation patterns that would result in synaptic plasticity that may constitute long-term memory (Destexhe & Sejnowski 2001).

It is clear from the above discussions that the thalamic integration of multimodal projections and the complex firing patterns seen in thalamic neurons position the thalamus as a key integrator and functional element in the neuraxis and not a simple relay centre as once thought.

Anatomy of the Hypothalamus

The hypothalamus lies below or ventral to the thalamus and forms the floor and lateral inferior walls of the third ventricle.

The hypothalamus is composed of a number of structures including the mammillary bodies, the tuber cinereum, the infundibulum which arises from the tuber cinereum and continues inferiorly as the pituitary stalk, the optic chiasm, and a number of nuclear groups of neurons (Chusid 1982). The nuclear groups of the hypothalamus are divided by the fornix and the mammillothalamic tract into medial and lateral zones. The *medial zone* contains eight distinct groups of nuclei including the preoptic nucleus, the anterior nucleus, a section of the suprachiasmatic nucleus, the paraventricular nucleus, the dorsal medial nucleus, the ventromedial nucleus, the infundibular or arcuate nucleus, and the posterior nucleus (Fig. 10.5).

The *lateral zone* contains six distinct groups of nuclei including a section of the preoptic nucleus, a section of the suprachiasmatic nucleus, the supraoptic nucleus, the lateral nucleus, the tuberomammillary nucleus, and the lateral tuberal nuclei.

The hypothalamus receives information from the rest of the body in a variety of ways that include information from the nervous system, information from the blood stream, and information from the cerebrospinal fluid (Fig. 10.5).

Afferent Inputs to the Hypothalamus

Afferent projections to the hypothalamus can take two basic forms. Direct projections, which form fairly distinct anatomical pathways, and multisynaptic collateralized projections, which are known to exist but difficult to identify as distinct pathways. The hypothalamus receives collateralized and direct afferent projections from wide-ranging areas of the neuraxis including:

- The tegmentum and periaqueductal grey area of the mesencephalon;
- The subthalamic nuclei;

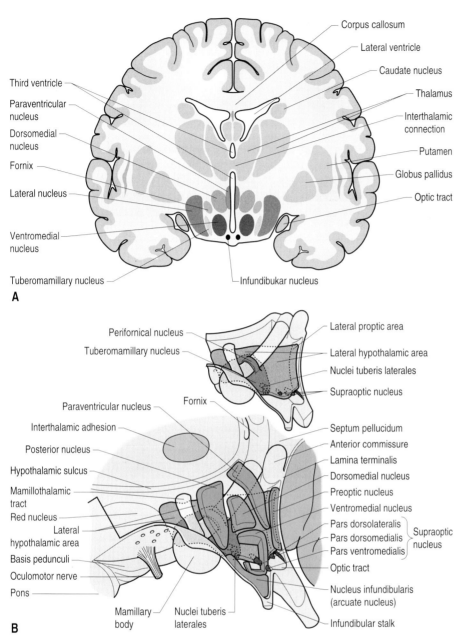

Fig.10.5 The (A) medial and (B) lateral nuclear groups of the hypothalamus.

- The globus pallidus;
- Various thalamic nuclei;
- The hippocampal formation;
- Areas of the anterior olfactory cortex;
- The amygdaloid nuclear complex;
- The septal nuclei;
- Prefrontal areas of cortex;
- The hypophysis cerebri;
- Direct retinal projections;
- The cerebellum;
- The pontomedullary reticular formation;
- Collaterals from the lemniscal somatic afferents; and
- Certain regions of the limbic cortex including the orbital frontal cortex, insular cortex, anterior cingulate cortex, and areas of the temporal cortex.

The Hypothalamus Receives a Number of Prominent Projections from Limbic System Structures

The hypothalamic nuclei receive projections from a variety of areas of the neuraxis known to contribute to functional aspects of the limbic system.

The *fornix* is a fibre bundle that projects from the hippocampal formation to the mammillary bodies. The fornix receives collateral contributions from the cingulate gyrus and many of the septal nuclei as it curves ventrally towards the anterior commissural area. The fornix divides into two columns or crura at the anterior commissural area (Fig. 10.6). The hippocampal commissure is a collection of transverse fibres connecting the two crura throughout most of the length of the fornix. Before the anterior commissure intersects with the crural fibres the fornix gives rise to precommissural projections to the preoptic regions of the hypothalamus. The postcommissural fornix gives rise to projections to the dorsal, lateral, and periventricular regions of the hypothalamus before terminating in the mammillary bodies of the hypothalamus.

The *amygdaloid complex* projects to the preoptic regions and to a variety of other hypothalamic nuclei via the amygdalohypothalamic fibres that arise from two different pathways, the stria terminalis and the ventral amygdalofugal tract (Fig. 10.7).

The *medial forebrain bundle* constitutes the main longitudinal pathway of the hypothalamus and contains both afferent and efferent fibres. Fibres from the septal nuclei, the olfactory cortex, and orbitofrontal cortex descend in this tract to the hypothalamic nuclei. Fibres from the pontomedullary reticular formation, the ventral tegmental cholinergic and noradrenergic projection systems, and mesolimbic dopamine projection system ascend in the medial forebrain bundle (Fig. 10.7).

Efferent Projections of the Hypothalamus

The three major efferent projection systems of the hypothalamus include:

1. Reciprocal limbic projections;
2. Polysynaptic projections to autonomic and motor centres in the brainstem and spinal cord; and
3. Neuroendocrine communication with the neurohypophysis and adenohypophysis of the pituitary gland.

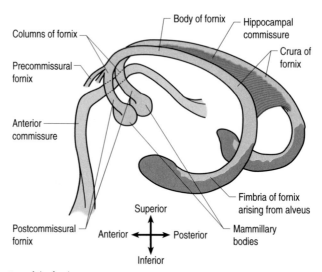

Fig.10.6 The structure of the fornix.

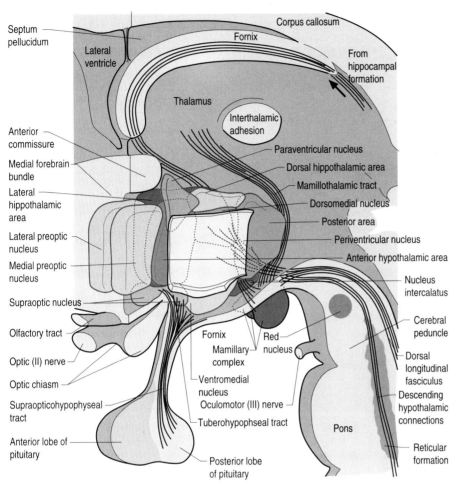

Septum pellucidum
Corpus callosum
Fornix
Lateral ventricle
From hippocampal formation
Thalamus
Interthalamic adhesion
Anterior commissure
Paraventricular nucleus
Medial forebrain bundle
Dorsal hippothalamic area
Lateral hippothalamic area
Mamillothalamic tract
Dorsomedial nucleus
Lateral preoptic nucleus
Posterior area
Periventricular nucleus
Medial preoptic nucleus
Anterior hypothalamic area
Supraoptic nucleus
Nucleus intercalatus
Olfactory tract
Fornix
Red nucleus
Cerebral peduncle
Mamillary complex
Optic (II) nerve
Ventromedial nucleus
Dorsal longitudinal fasciculus
Optic chiasm
Oculomotor (III) nerve
Supraopticohypophyseal tract
Tuberohypophseal tract
Descending hypothalamic connections
Pons
Anterior lobe of pituitary
Posterior lobe of pituitary
Reticular formation

Fig.10.7 The structure of the amygdaloid complex and the medial forebrain bundle.

Functions of the Hypothalamus

The hypothalamus functions to modulate a diverse array of bodily functions including autonomic, limbic, homeostatic, and endocrine activities.

Hypothalamic projections that originate mainly from the paraventricular and dorsal medial nuclei influence both parasympathetic and sympathetic divisions of the autonomic nervous system. These descending fibres initially travel in the medial forebrain bundle and then divide to travel in both the periaqueductal grey areas and the dorsal lateral areas of the brainstem and spinal cord. They finally terminate on the neurons of the parasympathetic preganglionic nuclei of the brainstem, the neurons in the intermediate grey areas of the sacral spinal cord, and the neurons in the intermediolateral cell column of the thoracolumbar spinal cord. Descending autonomic modulatory pathways also arise from the nucleus solitarius, noradrenergic nuclei of the locus ceruleus, raphe nuclei, and the pontomedullary reticular formation.

The hypothalamus may play an important function in the emotional modulation of autonomic pathways and immune system function through influences of the limbic system projections it receives (Beck 2005).

A variety of homeostatic functions are also modulated by the hypothalamus. The suprachiasmatic nucleus regulates circadian rhythms; the lateral hypothalamus regulates appetite and body weight set points; the ventromedial nucleus inhibits appetite, where dysfunctions in this nucleus can result in obesity; the anterior regions of the hypothalamus regulate thirst, and both anterior and posterior hypothalamic regions

QUICK FACTS 2   **The Hypothalamus Serves the Following Homeostatic Functions**

1. Blood pressure and electrolyte maintenance
   a. Drinking and salt appetite
   b. Blood osmolality
   c. Vasomotor tone
2. Body temperature regulation
3. Energy metabolism regulation
   a. Feeding
   b. Digestion
   c. Metabolic rate
4. Reproductive functions
   a. Mating and sexual desire
   b. Pregnancy
   c. Lactation
5. Emergency responses to stress
   a. Adrenal stress hormones
   b. Physical and immunological responses

are involved in thermoregulation. Sexual desire and other complex emotional states are also modulated by hypothalamic nuclei. Neuroendocrine control mechanisms operate mainly through the pituitary. Parvocellular neurons project to the median eminence to control the anterior pituitary gland. The hypothalamus does this indirectly via release of neurotransmitters and peptides into the highly fenestrated portal venous system and promotes the release of 'releasing hormones' and 'release-inhibiting hormones'. Magnocellular neurons continue down the stalk to the posterior pituitary gland, directly into its general circulation. The hypothalamus promotes the release of oxytocin and vasopressin (Figs 10.8 and 10.9). The intimate relationship between the hypothalamus, the pituitary gland, and the adrenal gland, which is modulated by hormones released by the pituitary gland, is referred to as the hypothalamus–pituitary–adrenal axis. This system is responsible for numerous homeostatic responses of the neuraxis and has been implicated in the negative aspects of the stress response. When a disturbance in the homeostatic state is detected, both the sympathetic nervous system and the hypothalamus–pituitary–adrenal axial system become activated in the attempt to restore homeostasis via the resulting increase in both systemic (adrenal) and peripheral (postganglionic activation) levels of catecholamines and glucocorticoids. In the1930s Hans Selye described this series of events or reactions as the general adaptation syndrome or generalized stress response (Selye 1936). Centrally, two principal mechanisms are involved in this general stress response; these are the production and release of corticotrophin-releasing hormone produced in the paraventricular nucleus of the hypothalamus and increased norepinephrine release from the locus ceruleus norepinephrine-releasing system in the brainstem. Functionally, these two systems cause mutual activation of each other through reciprocal innervation pathways (Chrousos & Gold 1992). Activation of the locus ceruleus results in an increase release of catecholamines, of which the majority is norepinephrine, to wide areas of cerebral cortex and subthalamic and hypothalamic areas. The activation of these areas results in an increased release of catecholamines from the postganglionic sympathetic fibres as well as from the adrenal medulla.

This results in a number of catecholamine-mediated responses such as increased heart rate, increased blood pressure, and increased glucose release into the blood (see Chapter 8 for a more complete list of responses).

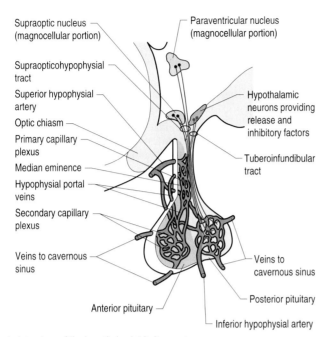

Supraoptic nucleus
(magnocellular portion)

Paraventricular nucleus
(magnocellular portion)

Supraopticohypophysial
tract

Superior hypophysial
artery

Hypothalamic
neurons providing
release and
inhibitory factors

Optic chiasm

Primary capillary
plexus

Median eminence

Tuberoinfundibular
tract

Hypophysial portal
veins

Secondary capillary
plexus

Veins to cavernous
sinus

Veins to
cavernous sinus

Anterior pituitary

Posterior pituitary

Inferior hypophysial artery

Fig.10.8 Anatomical structure of the hypothalamic/pituitary system.

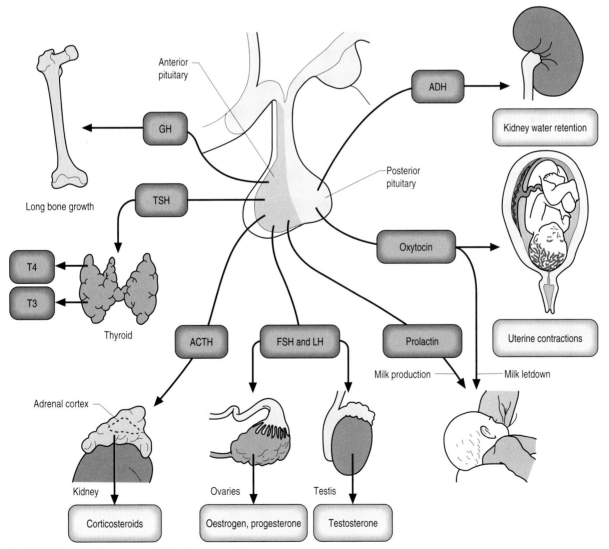

Anterior
pituitary

ADH

Kidney water retention

GH

Long bone growth

TSH

Posterior
pituitary

Oxytocin

T4

T3

Thyroid

ACTH

FSH and LH

Prolactin

Uterine contractions

Milk production

Milk letdown

Adrenal cortex

Kidney

Ovaries

Testis

Corticosteroids

Oestrogen, progesterone

Testosterone

Fig.10.9 A diagrammatic summary of pituitary hormone actions.

References

Beck RW 2005 Psychoneuroimmunology. In: Beirman R (ed) Pathology made simple, Macquarie University.

Blumenfeld H, McCormick DA 2000 Corticothalamic inputs control the pattern of activity generated in thalamocortical networks. Journal of Neuroscience 20:5153–5162.

Carrick FR 1997 Changes in brain function after manipulation of the cervical spine. Journal of Manipulative and Physiological Therapeutics 20:(8):529–545.

Chrousos GP, Gold PW 1992 The concepts of stress and stress system disorders: Overview of physical and behavioral homeostasis. Journal of American Medical Association 267: 1244–1252.

Chusid JG 1982 The brain. In: Correlative neuroanatomy and functional neurology,19th edn. Lange Medical, Los Altos, CA, p 19–86.

Contreras D 1996 Oscillatory properties of cortical and thalamic neurons and generation of synchronized rhythmicity in the corticothalamic networks. PhD thesis, Laval University, Quebec, Canada.

Curro Dossi R, Nunez A, Steriade M 1992 Electrophysiology of a slow (0.5–4 Hz) intrinsic oscillation of cat thalamocortical neurons in vivo. Journal of Physiology 447:215–234.

Destexhe A, Seinowski TJ 2001 Thalamocortical assemblies. Oxford University Press, Oxford.

Destexhe A, Seinowski TJ 2003 Interactions between membrane conductances underlying thalamocortical slow wave oscillations. Physical Reviews 83:1401–1453.

Gilbert CD, Wiesel TN 1989 Columnar specificity of intrinsic horizontal and corticocortical connections in the cat visual cortex. Journal of Neuroscience 9:2432–2442.

Jones EG 1985 The thalamus. Plenum, New York.

McGuire BA, Gilbert CD, Rivlin PK 1991 Targets of horizontal connections in macaque primary visual cortex. Journal of Comparative Neurology 305:370–392.

Selye H 1936 Thymus and the adrenals in the response of the organism to injuries and intoxications. British Journal of Experimental Pathology 17:234–238.

Sherman SM 2001 A wake up call from the thalamus. Nature Neuroscience 4:344–346.

Snell RS 2001 The thalamus and its connections. In: Clinical neuroanatomy for medical students. Lippincott Williams and Wilkins, Philadelphia,

Williams P, Warwick R 1984 The diencephalon or 'Interbrain'. In: Gray's anatomy. Churchill-Livingston, Edinburgh, p 953–990.

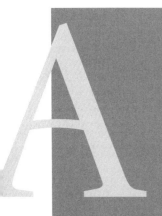

Clinical Case Answers

Case 10.1

10.1.1
1. Pituitary tumour;
2. Hypothalamic tumour; and
3. Psychosomatic.

10.1.2 The lateral nuclei of the hypothalamus regulates appetite and body weight set points.

Case 10.2

10.2.1 The blind spot has been found to increase in size because of the following conditions:
- Multiple evanescent white dot syndrome;
- Acute macular neuroretinopathy;
- Acute idiopathic blind spot enlargement (AIBSE) syndrome.
- Multifocal choroiditis;
- Pseudo-presumed ocular histoplasmosis;
- Peripapillary retinal dysfunction;
- Systemic vascular disease; and
- Decreased cortical activity contralaterally to the enlarged blind spot.

10.2.2 It is expected that when one eye is closed the visual field should now have an area not represented by visual input and the absence of vision over the area of the blind spot should be apparent. However, this does not occur. The cortical neurons responsible for the area of the blind spot must receive stimulus from other neurons that create the illusion that the blind spot is not there. This is indeed the case and is accomplished by a series of horizontal projecting neurons located in the visual striate cortex that allow for neighbouring hypercolumns to activate one another. The horizontal connections between these hypercolumns allow for perceptual completion or 'fill in' to occur.

The blind spot is therefore not strictly monocular, but it is dependent on the frequency of firing (FOF) of horizontal connections from neighbouring neurons. These may be activated via receptors and pathways from either eye.

Perceptual completion refers to the process whereby the brain fills in the region of the visual field that corresponds to a lack of visual receptors. This explains why one generally is not aware of the blind spot in everyday experience.

Chapter

11

The Basal Ganglia

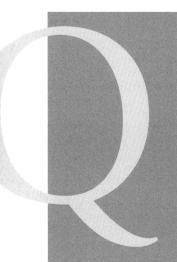

Clinical Cases for Thought

Case 11.1   A 61-year-old woman presents with a chief complaint of mild change in personality and wild involuntary jerks and flinging movements of her left arm. She has noticed the personality changes for a few months now but the arm motions started 2 weeks prior to presentation but have been getting progressively worse.

Questions

11.1.1   What are dyskinesias? Give several examples.

11.1.2   Explain the theoretical dysfunction in the basal ganglionic pathways that could explain this situation.

Case 11.2   A 56-year-old dentist presents with a chief complaint of a slight tremor in his right hand. He has noticed the tremor getting progressively worse over the past few months and is concerned that he will injure one of his patients should the tremor get worse. On examination you note rigidity of motion at the elbow and the wrist. You also note that his thumb and first finger are moving in a 'pill rolling' motion at rest but stop when he moves his hand. On further questioning he admits that both his father and brother have recently been diagnosed with idiopathic Parkinson's disease.

Questions

11.2.1   What are the cardinal classic symptoms of idiopathic Parkinson's disease? Which of these does this man exhibit?

11.2.2   Describe the neuronal circuits of the basal ganglia thought to be responsible for hypokinetic dyskinesias.

11.2.3   What treatment options are available for this patient?

Case 11.3   A 13-year-old girl was brought to your office by her mother with a chief complaint of extremely fidgeting and restlessness to the point that it is interrupting her schoolwork and her sleeping patterns. She describes difficulty in concentrating over the past few weeks and is extremely moody. On further questioning you discover that she was treated for a group A streptococcal infection while on a school holiday in Europe about 5 months ago.

Introduction

The activation pathways of the cortico-neostriatal-thalamo-cortical system are thought to operate as through parallel segregated circuits that maintain their segregation throughout the neostriatal-thalamo-cortical projections. Several loops including a motor loop, a limbic loop, and a frontal cortical loop function to modulate motor, limbic, and frontal cortical activities, respectively.

The thalamus, in normal circumstances, exerts an excitatory influence on the target neurons of the cortex to which it projects. The basal ganglia with its high rates of spontaneous inhibitory discharge maintain the thalamic target nuclei in a state of tonic inhibition. The inhibitory output nuclei of the basal ganglia are themselves modulated by two parallel pathways, one inhibitory and one excitatory that are themselves modulated by input from excitatory cortical neurons.

Under normal conditions the inhibition and excitation of the thalamus from the basal ganglia occurs at the appropriate time and in the appropriate amounts to support the activities of the cortex. However, in certain circumstances dysfunction of the basal ganglionic circuits can result in a number of conditions that affect movement and thought processes: Idiopathic Parkinson's disease (PD), Huntington's disease (HD), Sydenham's chorea (SC), Tourette's syndrome (TS), ballismus, dystonias, obsessive compulsive disorders (OCD), attention deficit hyperactivity disorders (ADHD), schizophrenia, depression, substance abuse disorders, and temporal lobe epilepsy (Marsden 1984; Swerdlow & Koob 1987; Javoy-Agid et al 1984; Reiner et al 1988; Modell et al 1990; Swerdlow 1996; Castellanos 1997; Van Paesschen et al 1997; Leckman et al 1998).

In this chapter we will consider the neurocircuitry of the cortico-thalamo-thalamic-cortico system and the disorders of movement that can arise from dysfunctions of this system. Other non-motor dysfunctions are discussed in Chapter 16.

Anatomy of the Basal Ganglia

The basal ganglia consist of a group of five principal subcortical nuclei. These include the caudate nucleus, the putamen, globus pallidus, subthalamic nucleus, and substantia nigra. From a functional point of view, the nucleus accumbens and the ventral pallidum may also be included as part of the basal ganglia as they are also involved in a variety of basal ganglionic activities mostly involving limbic functions.

The caudate nucleus and the putamen are embryological homologues that have maintained similar morphological structure and function as they matured. For this reason these two nuclei, and the nuclei formed by the merger of these structures, the ventral striatum, are grouped into a single functional structure called the neostriatum (Kandel et al 2000) (Fig. 11.1).

The neostriatum receives projection axons from virtually all areas of cortex and acts as the gatekeeper for all input to the basal ganglia. The caudate nucleus is a large C-shaped

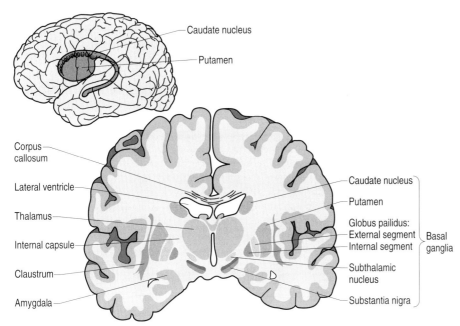

Fig. 11.1 The anatomical relationship of the basal ganglia and related structures from an anterior to posterior perspective.

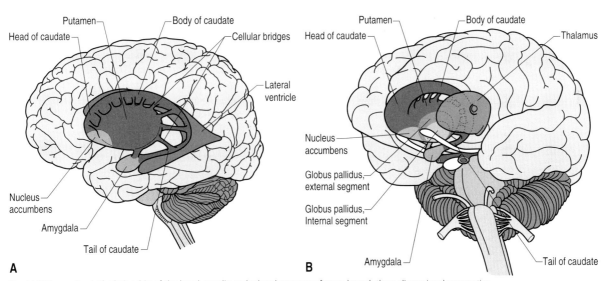

Fig. 11.2 The anatomical relationship of the basal ganglia and related structures from a lateral, three-dimensional perspective.

structure composed of a head, body, and tail that maintains a constant relationship with the lateral ventricle of the brain. Except for an area located anterior and ventrally where these two nuclei merge as the ventral striatum, the caudate nucleus and the putamen are separated by the fibre tracts of axons of the internal capsule. Most of the area composing the ventral striatum, which receives projections from areas of the limbic system, is taken up by the nucleus accumbens (Blumenfeld 2002) (Fig. 11.2).

Although the cauda nucleus and putamen are separated by the internal capsule they remain in communication with each other via small projections of axons called cellular bridges. These bridging structures give the region a striped appearance when anatomically sectioned, and thus lead to the name 'striatum'.

The putamen is a large nucleus that forms the lateral most aspect of the basal gangliar nuclei. Together with the globus pallidus, which lies just medial to the putamen, these two nuclei form the lentiform nucleus.

The globus pallidus is formed from two distinct nuclei, the globus pallidus pars internus (GPi) and the globus pallidus pars externus (GPe). The external nuclear region lies lateral to the internal nuclear region. The globus pallidus pars internus lies immediately lateral to the internal capsule, which separates it from the thalamus, the subthalamic nuclei, and the substantia nigra of the midbrain.

The subthalamic nucleus, or body of Luys, is a cylindrical mass of grey substance dorsolateral to the upper end of the substantia nigra and extending posteriorly as far as the lateral aspect of the red nucleus. It receives projection fibres from the globus pallidus pars externus and forms part of the indirect pallidal pathway.

The substantia nigra is a broad layer of pigmented grey substance separating the ventral portion of the mesencephalon from the tectum and extending from the upper surface of the pons to the hypothalamus. The substantia nigra can be separated into two areas which have different cell types. The most ventral area is referred to as the substantia nigra pars reticulata (SNr) and the more dorsal portion the substantia nigra pars compacta (SNc). The SNc contains a large population of dopaminergic neurons that contain a darkly pigmented grey substance, neuromelanin, which accumulates with age in dopaminergic neurons. The neuromelanin is thought to be composed of oxidized polymers of dopamine that accumulate in lysosomal storage granules in the neurons (Kandel et al 2000).

The ventral tegmental area of the mesencephalon also contains a population of dopaminergic neurons that are homologues of the neurons in the SNc.

The Neostriatum is the Input Nucleus of the Basal Ganglia

The neostriatum, which is composed of the caudate nucleus and the putamen, is the major input nucleus of the basal ganglia. The neostriatum has been estimated to contain some 110 million neurons per hemisphere (Alexander & DeLong 1992) compared to the 12 million neurons receiving cortical projections in each half of the basis pontis (Tomasch 1969). The striatum receives excitatory glutaminergic topographic projections from all areas of cortex and the intralaminar (centromedian and parafascicular) nuclei of the thalamus (Kunzle 1975, 1977; Selemon & Goldman-Rakic 1985). Dopaminergic input projections are also received from the SNc via the nigrostriatal pathway. The influence of this pathway on the neostriatal neurons involves complex interactions with various classes of dopamine receptors that result in excitation in some neurons and inhibition in others. Serotonergic axons from the raphe nuclei also project to the neostriatum.

The neostriatum contains a variety of different neurons including medium-spiny projection neurons, large cholinergic neurons, and small interneurons.

Medium-spiny projection neurons, which comprise about 90–95% of the neurons in the neostriatum, release gamma-aminobutyric acid (GABA). These GABA-ergic inhibitory neurons receive the majority of the cortical input to the neostriatum and are the sole output neurons of the neostriatum. Thus all output from the neostriatum to the globus pallidus and substantia nigra is inhibitory in nature.

These neurons can be further divided into two more basic groups. One group projects to the globus pallidus pars externus and in addition to GABA also releases the neuropeptides enkephalin and neurotensin. The second group projects to the globus pallidus pars internus or the substantia nigra pars reticulata and in addition to releasing GABA also releases the neuropeptides substance P and dynorphin (Kandel et al 2000).

The large cholinergic interneurons release ACh and have extensive collateral branching systems with the medium-spiny projection neurons and are thought to excite the inhibitory output neurons.

The small cell group of interneurons releases a variety of inhibitory neuroactive substances such as somatostatin, neuropeptide Y, and nitric oxide synthase (Fig. 11.3).

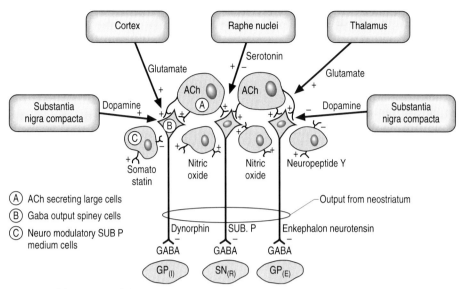

Fig. 11.3 Cellular structure of the neostriatum.

(A) ACh secreting large cells
(B) Gaba output spiney cells
(C) Neuro modulatory SUB P medium cells

Direct and Indirect Pathways from the Neostriatum to the GPi and SNr Can Modulate Inhibition of the Thalamus and Pontomedullary Reticular Formation

There are two predominant pathways from the neostriatum to the output nuclei of the basal ganglia, the globus pallidus pars internus and the substantia nigra pars reticulata. Understanding the inhibition and excitation circuits involved in these two pathways will help one understand the spectrum of functional disorders ranging from hyperkinetic to hypokinetic, involving movement and thought processes caused by basal ganglia disorders.

In the direct pathway, the output neurons of the neostriatum project axons that synapse on the neurons of the GPi and/or on the neurons in the SNr. These projections, arising from the neostriatum, release GABA, substance P, and dynorphin, which act in an inhibitory fashion on the target neurons in the GPi and the SNr.

In the indirect pathway, axons from the neurons of the neostriatum project to neurons in the GPe where they release the neurotransmitter GABA, enkephalin, and neurotensin, which act in an inhibitory nature on the neurons of the GPe. The neurons of the GPe in turn project to the neurons located in the subthalamic nucleus of Luys (STN), where they release the neurotransmitter GABA and act to inhibit the output neurons of the subthalamic nuclei. The neurons of the subthalamic nuclei project to the neurons of the GPi via the subthalamic fasciculus where they release glutamate and are excitatory in nature. The subthalamic output neurons are the only excitatory neurons in the basal ganglionic circuits. These STN neurons project to neurons in the GPi.

The output neurons in the GPi and SNr are inhibitory in nature and release the neurotransmitter GABA (Fig. 11.4).

The neurons in GPi project axons via the anterior thalamic fasciculus to the ventral lateral and ventral anterior nuclei of the thalamus. These projections are mainly associated with motor control functions of the body below the head and neck. GPi neurons also project to the intralaminar nuclei (centromedian and parafascicular) and the mediodorsal nuclei of the thalamus. These projections are largely associated with limbic activities (Fig. 11.5). Output projections of the GPi reach the thalamic fasciculus via two different pathways. The first pathway called the ansa lenticularis loops ventrally and passes beneath the internal capsule before swinging dorsally to join the thalamic fasciculus and reach the thalamus.

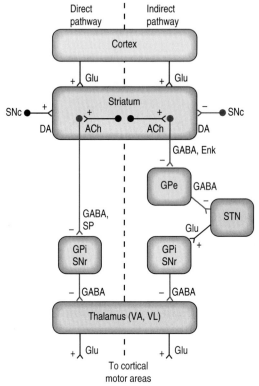

Fig. 11.4 Two predominant pathways from the neostriatum to the output nuclei of the basal ganglia, the globus pallidus pars internus (GPi) and the substantia nigra pars reticulata (SNr).

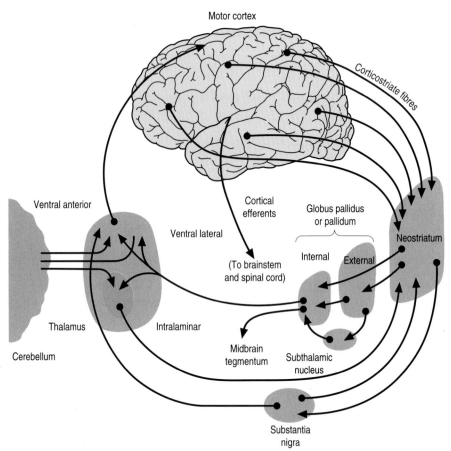

Fig. 11.5 The complex functional projection systems involved in the corticostriatal-basal ganglionic-thalamocortical loops in the neuraxis. Note that wide-ranging areas of cortex project to the neostriatum and that the thalamus also receives projections from the cerebellum.

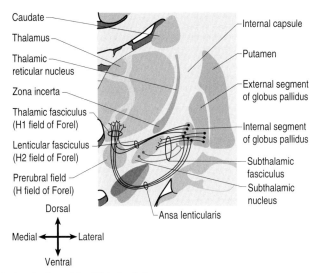

Fig. 11.6 The output projections of the GPi to the thalamus.

The second pathway called the lenticular fasciculus passes straight through the internal capsule to join the ansa lenticularis to form the thalamic fasciculus and enter the thalamus (Chusid 1982). The point at which the two pathways combine to form the thalamic fasciculus is sometimes referred to as the H fields of Forel. The H1 field of Forel refers to the thalamic fasciculus, the H2 field of Forel refers to the lenticular fasciculus, and the H or prerubral field of Forel refers to the area where the ansa lenticularis joins the thalamic fasciculus (Fig. 11.6). Finally the GPi neurons also project to the complex reticular neurons in the pons and medulla known as the pontomedullary reticular formation (PMRF). These projections are involved in the modulation of the reticulospinal tracts (Afifi 1994).

The neurons in the SNr also project to the ventral anterior and ventrolateral nuclei of the thalamus. These projections are associated with motor control of the head and neck. The SNr neurons also project to the superior colliculus where they modulate actions of the tectospinal pathways. Finally, the SNr neurons project to the PMRF, where they also modulate the output of the reticulospinal tract neurons (Fig. 11.5).

The neuron in the substantia nigra pars compacta release dopamine as their neuromodulators. These neurons project to the neostriatum where they have complex modulatory effects on the output neurons of the neostriatum. The net effect of the SNc release of dopamine in the neostriatum is an excitation of the output neurons of the direct pathway and an inhibition of the output neurons of the indirect pathway (Parent & Cicchetti 1998).

Functional Modulatory Outputs of the Direct and Indirect Pathways may result in Movement and Cognitive Dysfunctions

The activation pathways of the cortico-neostriatal-thalamo-cortical system are thought to operate through parallel segregated circuits that maintain their segregation throughout the neostriatal-thalamo-cortical projections. Several loops including a motor loop, a limbic loop, and a frontal cortical loop function to modulate motor, limbic, and frontal cortical activities respectively (Fig. 11.7).

Cortical activation of the direct basal ganglionic pathway results in a net excitation of the thalamus and subsequently excitation of the cortical areas that receive thalamic projections. Cortical activation of the indirect basal ganglionic pathway results in inhibition of the thalamus and subsequently inhibition of the cortical areas receiving thalamic projections (Fig. 11.4). The large ACh-releasing neurons in the neostriatum tend to preferentially form excitatory synapses on the output neurons of the indirect pathway; thus, excitation of these neurons would result in an increased activation of the indirect pathway or an inhibition of movement and thought processes.

QUICK FACTS 1	Summary of Outputs from Basal Ganglionic Structures
Neostriatum (caudate, putamen)	All inhibitory
Globus pallidus pars internus	All inhibitory
Globus pallidus pars externus	All inhibitory
Subthalamic nucleus	All excitatory
Substantia nigra pars reticulata	All inhibitory
Substantia nigra pars compacta	Both excitatory and inhibitory

QUICK FACTS 2 — Components of the Direct and Indirect Pathways

Direct Pathway

Neostriatum–Globus pallidus interna–Thalamus–Cortex and other targets

Indirect Pathway

Neostriatum–Globus pallidus externa–Subthalamic nuclei–Globus pallidus interna–Thalamus–Cortex and other targets

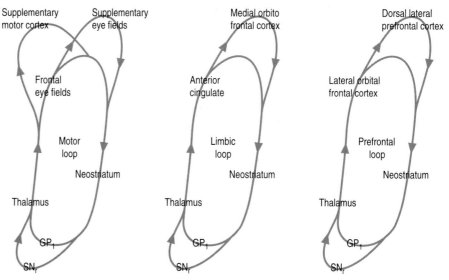

Fig. 11.7 Loops of the neostriatal-thalamo-cortical system.

Under normal conditions the inhibition and excitation of the thalamus from the basal ganglia occurs at the appropriate time and in the appropriate amounts to support the activities of the cortex. However, in certain circumstances dysfunction of the basal ganglionic circuits can result in a number of conditions that affect movement and thought processes. These include idiopathic Parkinson's disease (PD), Huntington's disease (HD), Sydenham's chorea (SC), Tourette's syndrome (TS), ballismus, dystonias, obsessive compulsive disorders (OCD), attention deficit hyperactivity disorders (ADHD), schizophrenia, depression, substance abuse disorders, and temporal lobe epilepsy (Marsden 1984; Javoy-Agid et al 1984; Swerdlow & Koob 1987; Reiner et al 1988; Modell et al 1990; Baxter et al 1992; Swerdlow 1996; Castellanos 1997; Van Paesschen et al 1997; Leckman et al 1998).

Idiopathic Parkinson's Disease

Idiopathic Parkinson's disease (PD) is associated with the degeneration of the dopaminergic neurons of the SNc, which as stated previously have an excitatory effect on the direct pathway and an inhibitory effect on the indirect pathway. A loss of dopaminergic stimulation in the neostriatum would result in a net inhibition of movement through both direct and indirect pathways (Fig. 11.8). The onset of PD is gradual in nature, but slowly and progressively continues until eventual severe disability. The cardinal signs and symptoms include tremor at rest, Bradykinesia (slowness of movement), muscular rigidity, akinesia (impairment in initiation and poverty of movement), and loss of postural reflexes (Wichmann & DeLong 2002). The clinical diagnosis of PD can only be tentative because the major symptoms described above are not specific for PD. Some degree of certainty of the diagnosis can be achieved if the patient responds favourably to levodopa, a precursor in the formation of dopamine synthesis.

The Effects of Excitation and Inhibition on the Direct and Indirect Basal Ganglionic Pathways		QUICK FACTS 3
Excitation of direct pathway	Excitation of thalamus	Movement, thought, limbic excitement
Excitation of indirect pathway	Inhibition of thalamus	Inhibition of movement, thought, limbic activity
Inhibition of direct pathway	Inhibition of thalamus	Inhibition of movement, thought, limbic activity
Inhibition of indirect pathway	Excitation of thalamus	Movement, thought, limbic excitement

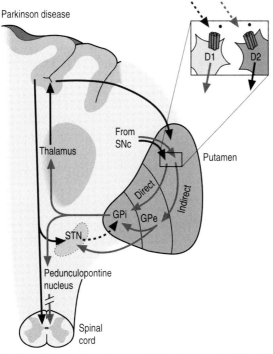

Fig. 11.8 Pathological function of the dopaminergic neurons in the development of idiopathic Parkinson's disease (PD).

PD must be distinguished from other disorders with extrapyramidal, cerebellar, or oculomotor features resembling PD, which are referred to as atypical Parkinson's or Parkinson-plus syndromes. These disorders include progressive supranuclear palsy, olivopontocerebellar atrophy, corticobasalar ganglionic degeneration, and Shy-Drager syndrome, all of which can frequently be identified by specific clinical features. In addition to the motor abnormalities, patients with PD frequently have cognitive and affective disturbances. Depression is common in PD and in many patients predates the extrapyramidal features. Dementia also commonly occurs in PD patients; prevalence data suggest that about 50% of PD cases have significant cognitive impairment. This too seems to be an integral part of the spectrum of clinical manifestations of PD.

QUICK FACTS 4	What Do They Mean?

- Dyskinesia—abnormal movements
- Bradykinesia—slowing of movements
- Hypokinesia—reduced amounts of movements
- Akinesia—absence of movement
- Rigidity—increased resistance to passive movement of a limb or joint
- Paratonia—active resistance against movement of limbs
- Dystonia—prolonged muscle spasms resulting in distorted positions or postures
- Athetosis—slow, twisting movements of the face, limbs, or trunk
- Chorea—dance-like movements that have a fluid, jerky, constant quality
- Ballismus—flinging, ballistic movements of the limbs
- Tremor—slow or fast rhythmic or semirhythmic oscillating movements

The pathological hallmark of PD is intracellular inclusions called *Lewy bodies*. These occur inside the dopamine-producing neurons in the substantia nigra pars compacta. These inclusions probably accumulate in neurons as breakdown products of dopamine and probably increase in concentration in neurons undergoing degeneration. During the past decade it has become clear that Lewy bodies are not limited to the substantia nigra in PD, but may occur in a widespread distribution in the cortex. Diffuse Lewy body disease is a pathological entity whose clinical correlates have not yet been defined. Patients commonly have cognitive decline and Parkinsonian features, and either one may dominate the picture (Korczyn 2000).

The number of dopamine (DA)-producing neurons progressively diminishes in PD over time. It is important to note that only DA neurons in the substantia nigra whose axons are destined to go to the putamen (less so to the caudate) in the nigrostriatal tract are affected. Chemical analysis shows progressive loss of DA in the striatum with the clinical symptoms first becoming apparent when DA content in the striatum is reduced by about 70%. This process may take as long as 20 years before symptoms become apparent (Hornykiewicz 1988; Scherman et al 1989).

Other neurotransmitter systems are also affected in PD. These include norepinephrine (NE) loss in the cell bodies of the locus coeruleus, serotonin (5-hydroxytryptamine (5-HT)) loss in the raphe nuclei, and cholinergic cell loss in the nucleus basalis of Meynert. These deficiencies probably contribute to the affective and cognitive changes in PD but may also be involved in motor dysfunction.

The etiology of PD is uncertain but is most probably multifactorial in nature with both genetic and environmental factors contributing to the development of the disease. One theory that has gained some popularity recently is that excessive concentrations of excitatory amino acids, particularly glutamate, may be involved in causing irreversible neuronal damage (Sonsalla et al 1989). This is particularly relevant for PD because of the massive cortical, glutaminergic innervation received by the corpus striatum.

The neurotoxicity is thought to be produced by over- or sustained activation of N-methyl-D-aspartate (NMDA) receptors on the neuron membranes. One environmental hypothesis suggests that a selective increase in lipid peroxidation in the substantia nigra neurons may occur in PD. This process may lead to excessive production of free radicals, which may in turn result in cellular damage and death (Ben Shachar et al 1991). A particularly relevant fact concerning this theory is that DA degradation may involve the sequestration of iron in free radical formation in the process of lipid peroxidation. Both the substantia nigra and globus pallidum are rich in iron, and the iron concentration increases with age, particularly in PD.

The gold standard treatment of PD is replacement of DA using levodopa. Levodopa is absorbed from the gastrointestinal tract and converted to DA in both the brain and the periphery by the enzyme 1-amino acid decarboxylase (1-AAD) (Clough 1991). The peripheral conversion of levodopa to DA can be inhibited by the actions of benserazide and carbidopa. Most patients today are treated by a combination of levodopa and benserazide or carbidopa. The aim of using this combination is to prevent the peripheral conversion of levodopa to DA, because DA may act in the periphery to produce undesirable side effects such as orthostatic hypotension and nausea (Cederbaum et al 1991).

Surgical interventions of PD include ablative and transplanting approaches. Targets for functional stereotactic neurosurgical lesions, which reduce tremor, are the ventrolateral thalamus and the posteroventral pallidum. There has been extensive interest in transplanting DA tissue removed from aborted foetal midbrains into the caudate or putamen in PD; however, the results remained confusing because of small cohort sizes and disease severity issues of the participants (Widner & Rehncrona 1993).

The prevalence of dementia in PD is far greater than that in the general population. PD dementia may be preceded by mild memory loss, transient confusional episodes, or hallucinosis. The progression of the cognitive decline is unrelated to that of the motor disability, and the only robust predictor for the development of dementia is the patient's age. Clinically, the dementia of PD differs from that of Alzheimer's disease (AD). PD patients rarely develop dysfunctions of the isocortical association areas, such as dysphasia or agnosia, and their dementia resembles a 'frontal' type of dementia.

Depression is also rather common in PD. Because depression is potentially treatable, every patient with PD *must* be assessed for possible depressive symptomatology (Cummings 1992). Several tests are available for diagnosing depression. These include neuropsychological evaluations, self-reports, and projection tests. However, while all these tests have important roles in research, none is superior to the clinical assessment by a competent clinician. The clinical evaluation of the affective state of PD patients may be difficult because the motionless face, the slowness of movement, and the bradyphrenia may create an erroneous impression of depression. The distinction from depressive motor retardation is obviously very important.

Huntington's Disease

In *Huntington's disease* (HD) the neurons in the neostriatum degenerate. The degeneration appears to be more pronounced in the output neostriatal neurons of the indirect pathway (Albin et al 1992). This results in the disinhibition of the GPe, which in turn results in an overinhibition of the subthalamic nucleus. The functional overinhibition of the subthalamic nucleus results in a situation that resembles an ablative lesion to the subthalamic nucleus and results in a hyperkinetic movement disorder (Fig. 11.9). In the latter stages of HD

Hallmark Signs and Symptoms of Parkinson's Disease	QUICK FACTS 5

1. Akinesia—Global impairment of movement initiation including gait
2. Bradykinesia—Global slowing of movement
3. Rigidity—'Cogwheel' rigidity superimposed over subclinical tremor
4. Tremor—4–5 Hz at rest; tremor is suppressed by voluntary movement initiation

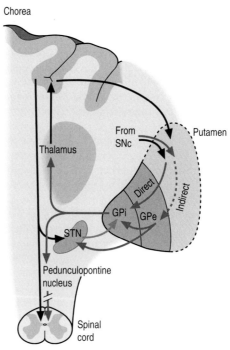

Fig. 11.9 The pathology observed in Huntington's disease (HD) in which the neurons in the neostriatum degenerate.

neostriatal degeneration spreads to include the output neurons of both the direct and indirect pathways, resulting in hypokinetic Parkinson-like activities (Young et al 1986).

Although a juvenile form of HD does occur and the onset of HD can range from as young as 2 years to as old as 80 years, disease onset typically occurs in adults in their mid-thirties to mid-forties. The disease affect men and women in equal frequencies, ranging from 5 to 10 per 100,000 (Kandel et al 2000). The disorder is characterized by insidious onset of both neurological and psychiatric symptoms. Initial symptoms include personality change and the gradual appearance of small involuntary movements; as the disease progresses, chorea becomes more obvious and incapacitating (Harper 1996). Over time, motor symptoms worsen such that walking, speaking, and eating becomes more difficult, and weight loss is common because of the extra energy required for movement and an increase in their basal metabolic rate. A large percentage of HD patients eventually succumb to aspiration pneumonia, resulting from the inability to coordinate pharyngeal muscles and vocal cords, which results in swallowing difficulties. It has a large genetic component.

The juvenile form of HD, which is also referred to as the Westphal variant form of HD, occurs in about 10% of reported cases. The initial presentation is more Parkinsonian in nature with bradykinesia, rigidity, and tremor rather than chorea as the prominent symptoms. Juvenile onset HD is usually the result from paternal transmission and in individuals who develop symptoms before age 10; more than 90% have an affected father (Folstein 1989). There is a unique tendency for juvenile HD to have a younger age of onset in successive generations, which is referred to as anticipation. Anticipation in juvenile HD is especially pronounced in cases of paternal transmission.

Within the striatum, HD differentially affects subpopulations of neurons, with projection neurons rather than interneurons preferentially being lost (DiFiglia 1990). Consistent with the finding of loss of projection neurons is the fact that GABA levels are markedly reduced in the caudate-putamen of HD patients. Of the two populations of striatal projection neurons, the neurons of the indirect pathway are affected first; thus, the indirect pathway is predominantly disrupted. With interruption of the indirect pathway, the current models of basal ganglionic circuitry predict an overall increase in movement, manifested as chorea and ballism. The functional result of degeneration of both the direct and indirect pathways is a rigid bradykinetic state, which occurs in the later stages of adult

HD. In the case of juvenile HD where the symptoms resemble Parkinson's disease early in the presentation, degeneration of both direct and indirect pathway striatal neurons occurs from the onset (Albin et al 1989).

The mode by which neurons die in HD is still unclear although the process of apoptosis or preprogrammed cell death may be the final common pathway through which neurons are terminated. Prior to the discovery of the HD gene, the leading hypotheses concerning the pathogenesis of HD implicated either excitotoxicity or metabolic dysfunction. The protein huntingtin, which is coded for by the huntingtin gene, has no clear relationship to excitatory amino acid neurotransmission, nor to mitochondrial energetics. The normal function of huntingtin is not completely known, although it has been implicated in membrane recycling (DiFiglia et al 1995). Thus, the influence of the huntingtin protein remains unclear as it relates to these hypotheses.

Excitotoxicity is the process in which neuronal cells die as a result of excessive excitatory amino acid neurotransmission. This process has been well documented with respect to overstimulation or excessive stimulation of glutaminergic NMDA receptors. This overstimulation can result excessive amounts of Ca^{++} ions entering neurons and triggering pre-programmed genetic termination pathways in the neuron. Glutamate has been postulated to trigger neuron death in a number of neurological disorders, including hypoxia-ischaemia, head trauma, epilepsy, schizophrenia, and neurodegenerative disorders such as Alzheimer's disease, Parkinson's disease, and amyotrophic lateral sclerosis (Fagg et al 1986; Choi & Rothman 1990; Kornbuber & Wiltfang 1998).

Mitochondrial dysfunction has also been implicated as a pathologic mechanism in HD, potentially rendering cells vulnerable to normal ambient levels of extracellular glutamate (Albin & Greenamyre 1992). Positron emission tomography and MRI spectroscopy studies have demonstrated abnormalities in glucose metabolism in HD patients (Mazziotta et al 1987). The impact or contribution of mitochondrial dysfunction in the development of HD remains under investigation; however, at least one study has demonstrated that administration of coenzyme Q_{10}, an essential cofactor of the mitochondrial electron transport chain, lowers elevated cortical lactate levels in HD patients back to levels seen in normal controls (Koroshetz et al 1997). This suggests that mitochondrial energetic processes are in some way contributing to the development of HD.

The discovery of the huntingtin gene was unusual in that the usual genetic mutations observed in human diseases include point mutations, deletions, duplications, or missense mutations. The mutation in the huntingtin gene (IT-15 gene), however, resides in an unstable region of the gene, where mutation can result in an expansion of a normally appearing trinucleotide repeat motif present in the alleles of HD patients. CAG is the codon for glutamine, and the trinucleotide repeat of this motif gives rise to a polyglutamine moiety within the *huntingtin* protein. Normal huntingtin alleles contain from 6 to 35 CAG repeats, giving rise to 6 to 35 glutamines in the mature protein. Patients with Huntington's disease invariably have alleles with greater than 35 repeats. While repeats greater than 40 invariably give rise to Huntington's disease, there is a 'grey area', between 35 and 39 repeats, where some uncertainty whether the disease will develop exists (Cha & Young 2000).

There are currently no effective therapies for preventing the onset or slowing the progression of HD. Current therapies are symptomatic, and include the use of neuroleptics to decrease chorea, and the use of psychotropic medications to address depression, obsessive compulsive symptoms, or psychosis. In addition, speech therapy and physical therapy are useful in addressing the swallowing and walking difficulties that many HD patients experience (Ranen et al 1993).

Ballismus

Ballismus or ballism includes a group of conditions characterized by flinging, large amplitude, rotary movements, usually involving the proximal limb muscles. The most common form of this condition occurs unilaterally and is referred to as hemiballism. The cause is classically a basal ganglionic lesion in the contralateral subthalamic nucleus, but contralateral lesions in the neostriatum can also result in ballismic dyskinesia (Provenzale & Schwarzschild 1994) (Fig. 11.10).

Hallmarks of Huntington's Disease

1. Autosomal dominant neurodegenerative condition
2. Progressive development of choreiform movements, dementia, psychiatric disturbances which ultimately result in death
3. Progressive degeneration of the neostriatum
4. Dysfunction of all three loops of basal ganglionic involvement

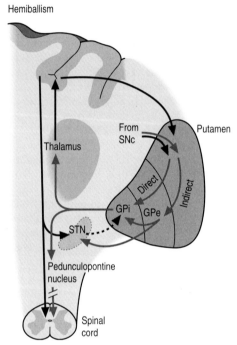

Fig. 11.10 The pathology seen in ballismus or ballism.

Sydenham's Chorea (SC)

This syndrome develops after an infection with group A streptococcal bacteria that has not been treated with the appropriate antibiotics. The most frequently involved population is adolescent females. The onset is usually 4–5 months following the infection and begins with an increased feeling of restlessness and increased periods of fidgeting. Occasionally, periods of emotional lability and obsessive-compulsive behaviours will also accompany the motor symptoms. The symptoms become gradually worse over weeks to months and then subside. The symptoms will recur in about 20% of those affected in later life. The cause is thought to involve a cross reaction of anti-streptococcal antibodies with receptors on striatal neurons.

Tourette's Syndrome (TS)

The diagnosis of TS is based solely on the patient history presented. The DSM-IV diagnostic criteria for TS is the frequent occurrence of multiple motor tics and one or more types of vocal tic present and occurring over a continuous interval for most of one year. Usually the onset of symptoms must have occurred early in life, before the age of 21 to be considered as TS (American Psychiatric Association 1994).

Tics are sudden, rapid, recurrent, nonrhythmic, stereotyped movements or vocalizations. Simple tics are brief circumscribed movements or sounds that resemble 'chunks' of movement or sounds rather than meaningful or recognizable actions.

These may include facial grimaces, mouth movements, head jerking, and shoulder, arm, and leg jerks. Complex tics are more sustained and elaborate movements or more recognizable words or sounds that can give the perception of being intentionally produced (Swerdlow & Leckman 2002). In a small percentage (10%) of those with TS vocal tics can involve vulgar or obscene expletives. This form of expression is referred to as coprolalia. Tics can be voluntarily suppressed but like obsessive-compulsive tendencies the suppression builds up anxiety and results in a more forceful expression when the tic eventually is expressed. Many children express tics as a normal activity as they pass through various phases of development. These normal or developmental tics have usually completely disappeared by 18 years of age (Shapiro et al 1978).

The usual presentation of TS typically begins between the ages of 3 and 8 years old, with periods of worsening and remission of the tics throughout childhood. The period of 8–12 years of age seems to be the period of greatest severity in most children with a steady decline to the age of 18 years where as many as 50% of the children will present as tic free (Leckman et al 1998). For those who maintain their tics into adulthood a more predicable pattern usually emerges with the frequency and intensity of the tics increasing during periods of increased stress or emotional excitement and generally over time.

The cause of TS has a high degree of concordance with a genetically generated dysfunction that has been postulated to involve the cortico-neostriatal-thalamo-cortical circuits in a variety of locations and in a variety of ways that seem to affect the function of the whole system rather than any one part of the system. Four areas of dysfunction have been suggested:

1. Intrinsic neostriatal neuron abnormalities such as increased packing density of the neurons in the neostriatum (Balthasar 1957);

2. A decrease in the activity of the output neurons of the direct pathway (Haber & Wolfer 1992);

3. Increased dopaminergic innervation of the neostriatum, with increased density of dopamine transporter sites (Singer et al 1992); and

4. Reduction in the glutaminergic output of the subthalamic nucleus (Anderson et al 1992).

Treatment of TS is aimed at developing flexible, integrated biosocial and biopsychological strategies to allow the build-up of anxiety to be dissipated in a controlled fashion, and control the excitement in emotional situations.

Dystonia

The characteristic features of dystonia are the distorted postures and movements caused by spasmodic muscular activity in people with this condition. If the spasmodic muscular activity is maintained for long periods it is referred to as dystonic posturing. If the spasmodic muscular activity results in slowly changing repetitive activity then it is referred to as dystonic movements (Rothwell et al 1983).

The hallmarks of dystonia include:

1. Excessive contraction of antagonistic muscles during voluntary movement;

2. Overflow of contraction to remote muscles not usually involved in the attempted movement; and

3. Development of spontaneous spasms on contraction of muscles.

The excessive involvement of antagonistic muscles and overflow of contraction suggest that the normal spinal inhibitory feedback mechanisms are dysfunctional in this condition. However, this does not appear to be the case. The classic spinal disynaptic pathway involving 1a reciprocal inhibition of antagonist muscles remains intact in dystonic patients (Nakashima et al 1989). However, the presynaptic or supraspinal inhibition of these reflexes is dysfunctional. The cause of the dysfunctional descending inhibition is thought to be due to altered function of the basal ganglionic circuits that relay back to the cortex via the thalamus.

Dystonias can be described in terms of the extent of spasmodic involvement. Focal dystonias include torticollis, which is spasm of the neck muscles; blepharospasm, which is spasm of the orbicularis oris muscle surrounding the eye; spasmodic dysphonia, which involves the muscles of the larynx and vocal cords; and writer's cramp, which involves the muscles of the hand. Generalized dystonias involve large areas of the body and can be unilateral or bilateral in nature.

The syndrome of primary idiopathic torsional dystonia (ITD) is a rare hereditary generalized dystonia that can affect most muscles of the body, although usually the muscles controlling eye movement and the sphincter muscles are spared. The cause of ITD is thought to involve the DYT1 gene on the chromosome 9q34. This gene codes for the enzyme dopamine beta-hydroxylase (DBH). The activity of the gene is thought to be related to the stimulus activity of neurons in the basal ganglia in such a way that when activation levels fall below a certain frequency the gene is activated. Such a situation might occur following an injury. It has been postulated that peripheral trauma may be a precipitating event to the development of ITD in gene carriers.

References

Afifi AK 1994 Basal ganglia: functional anatomy and physiology. Part 1. Journal of Child Neurology 9:(3):249–260.

Albin RL, Greenamyre JT 1992 Alternative excitotoxic hypotheses. Neurology 42:733–738.

Albin RL, Young AB, Penney JB 1989 The functional anatomy of basal ganglia disorders. Trends in Neuroscience 12:366–375.

Albin RL, Reiner A, Anderson KD et al 1992 Preferential loss of striato-external pallidal projection neurons in presymptomatic Huntington's disease. Annals of Neurology 31:425–430.

Alexander GE, DeLong MR 1992 Central mechanisms of initiation and control of movement. In: Asbury AK, McKhann GM, McDonald IW (eds) Diseases of the nervous system: clinical neurobiology. WB Saunders, Philadelphia, p 285–308.

American Psychiatric Association 1994 Diagnostic and statistical manual of mental disorders, 4th edn. American Psychiatric Association, Washington DC.

Anderson GM, Pollak ES, Chatterjee D et al 1992 Postmortem analysis of subcortical nomoamines and amino acids in Tourette syndrome. Advances in Neurology 58:123–133.

Balthasar K 1957 Uber das anatomische Substrat der geralisierten Tic-Krankheit (maladie des tics, Billes de la Tourette): Entwicklungshemmung des Corpus striatum. Archiv für Psychiatrie und Nervenkrankheiten vereinigt mit Zeitschrift für gesamte Neurologie und Psychiatrie 195:531–549.

Baxter LR, Schwartz JM, Bergman, et al 1992 Caudate glucose metabolic rate changes with both drug and behaviour therapy for obsessive-compulsive disorder. Archives of General Psychiatry 49:681–689.

Ben Shachar D, Riederer P, Youdim MBH 1991 Iron melanin interaction and lipid peroxidation: implication for Parkinson's disease. Journal of Neurochemistry 57:1609–1614.

Blumenfeld H 2002 Basal ganglia in neuroanatomy through clinical cases. Sinauer Associates, Sunderland, MA.

Castellanos FX 1997 Toward a pathophysiology of attention-deficit/hyperactivity disorder. Clinical Pediatrics 36:381–393.

Cederbaum JM, Gardy SE, McDowell FH 1991 'Early' initiation of levodopa treatment does not promote the development of motor response fluctuations, dyskinesias or dementia in Parkinson's disease. Neurology 41:622–629.

Cha JJ, Young AB 2000 Huntington's disease. In: Bloom FE, Kupfer DJ (eds.) Psychopharmacology: the fourth generation of progress. American College of Neuropsychopharmacology.

Choi DW, Rothman SM 1990 The role of glutamate neurotoxicity in hypoxic-ischemic neuronal death. Annual Review of Neuroscience 13:171–182.

Chusid JG 1982 The brain. In: Correlative neuroanatomy and functional neurology, 19th edn. Lange Medical, Los Altos, CA, p 19–86.

Clough CG 1991 Parkinson's disease: management. Lancet 337:1324–1327.

Cummings JL 1992 Depression and Parkinson's disease: review. American Journal of Psychiatry 149:443–454.

DiFiglia M 1990 Excitotoxic injury of the neostriatum: a model for Huntington's disease. Trends in Neuroscience 13:286–289.

DiFiglia M, Sapp E, Chase K et al 1995 Huntingtin is a cytoplasmic protein associated with vesicles in human and rat brain neurons. Neuron 14:1075–1081.

Fagg GE, Foster AC, Ganong AH 1986 Excitatory amino acid synaptic mechanisms and neurological function. Trends in Pharmacological Science 357–363.

Folstein S 1989 Huntington's disease: A disorder of families. Johns Hopkins University Press, Baltimore.

Haber SN, Wolfer D 1992 Basal ganglia peptidergic staining in Tourette syndrome: a follow-up study. Advances in Neurology 48:145–150.

Harper PS (ed) 1996 Huntington's disease. Major problems in neurology. WB Saunders, Philadelphia,

Hornykiewicz O 1988 Neurochemical pathology and the etiology of Parkinson's disease: basic facts and hypothetical possibilities. Mount Sinai Journal of Medicine 55:11–20.

Javoy-Agid F, Ruberg M, Taquet H et al 1984 Biochemical neuropathology of Parkinson's disease. Advances in Neurology 40:189–198.

Kandel ER, Schwartz JH, et al 2000 The basal ganglia. In: Kandel ER, Schwartz JH, Jessell TM (eds) Principles of neural science, 4th edn. McGraw-Hill, New York, p 853–867.

Korczyn AD 2000 Parkinson's disease. In: Bloom FE, Kupfer DJ (eds) Psychopharmacology: the fourth generation of progress. American College of Neuropsychopharmacology.

Kornbuber J, Wiltfang J 1998 The role of glutamate in dementia. Journal of Neural Transmission Supplementum 53:277–287.

Koroshetz WJ, Jenkins BG, Rosen BR et al 1997 Energy metabolism defects in Huntington's disease and effects of coenzyme Q_{10}. Annals of Neurology 41:160–165.

Kunzle H 1975 Bilateral projections from precentral motor cortex to the putamen and other parts of the basal ganglia. An autoradiographic study in Macaca fascicularis. Brain Research 88:195–209.

Kunzle H 1977 Projections from the primary somatosensory cortex to basal ganglia and thalamus in the monkey. Experimental Brain Research 30:481–492.

Leckman JF, Zhang H, Vitale A 1998 Course of tic severity in Tourette syndrome: the first two decades. Pediatrics 102:14–19.

Marsden CD 1984 Motor disorders in basal ganglia disease. Human Neurobiology 2:245–255.

Mazziotta JC, Phelps ME, Pahl JJ et al 1987 Reduced cerebral glucose metabolism in asymptomatic subjects at risk for Huntington's disease. New England Journal of Medicine 316:357–362.

Modell JG, Mountz JM, Beresford TP 1990 Basal ganglia/limbic striatal and thalamocortical involvement in craving and loss of control in alcoholism. Journal of Neuropsychiatry and Clinical Neurosciences 2:123–144.

Nakashima K, Rothwell JC, Day BL et al 1989 Reciprocal inhibition between forearm muscles in patients with writer's cramp and other occupational cramps, symptomatic hemidystonia and hemiparesis due to stoke. Brain 112:681–697.

Parent A, Cicchetti F 1998 The current model of basal ganglia organization under scrutiny. Movement Disorders 13:(2):199–202.

Provenzale JM, Schwarzschild MA 1994 Hemiballism. American Journal of Neuroradiology 15:(7):1377–1382.

Ranen NG, Peyser CE, Folstein SE 1993 A physician's guide to the management of Huntington's disease: pharmacologic and non-pharmacologic interventions. Huntington's Disease Society of America, New York.

Reiner A, Albin RL, Anderson KD, et al 1988 Differential loss of striatal projection neurons in Huntington disease. Proceedings of the National Academy of Science USA 85:5733–5737.

Rothwell JC, Obeso JA, Day BL, et al 1983 Pathophysiology of dystonias. In: Desmedt JE (ed) Motor control mechanisms in health and disease. Raven Press, New York, p 851–863.

Scherman D, Desnos C, Darchem F et al 1989 Striatal dopamine deficiency in Parkinson's disease: role of aging. Annals of Neurology 26:551–557.

Selemon LD, Goldman-Rakic PS 1985 Longitudinal topography and interdigitation of cortico-striatal projections in the rhesus monkey. Journal of Neuroscience 5:776–794.

Shapiro AK, Shapiro ES, Braun RD et al 1978 Gilles de la Tourette syndrome. Raven, New York.

Singer HS, Hahn IH, Moran TH 1992 Abnormal dopamine uptake sites in post-mortem striatum from patients with Tourette's syndrome. Annals of Neurology 58:123–133.

Sonsalla PK, Nicklas WJ, Heikkila RE 1989 Role for excitatory amino acids in methamphetamine-induced nigrostriatal dopaminergic toxicity. Science 243:398–400.

Swerdlow NR 1996 Cortico-striatal substances of cognitive, motor and sensory gating: speculations and implications for psychological function and dysfunction. In: Panksepp J (ed) Advances in biological psychiatry. JAI, Greenwich, CT, p 179–208.

Swerdlow NR, Koob GF 1987 Dopamine, schizophrenia, mania and depression: toward a unified hypothesis of cortico-striato-pallido-thalamic function. The Behavioral and Brain Sciences 10:197–245.

Swerdlow NR, Leckman JF 2002 Tourette syndrome and related tic disorders. In: Neuropsychopharmacology: the fifth generation of progress. American College of Neuropsychopharmacology.

Tomasch J 1969 The numerical capacity of the human corticopontocerebellar system. Brain Research 13:476–484.

Van Paesschen W, Revesv T, Duncan JS et al 1997 Quantitative neuropathology and quantitative magnetic resonance imaging of the hippocampus in temporal lobe epilepsy. Annals of Neurology 42:756–766.

Wichmann T, DeLong MR 2002 Neurocircuitry of Parkinson's disease. In: Neuropsychopharmacology: the fifth generation of progress. American College of Neuropsychopharmacology.

Widner H, Rehncrona S 1993 Transplantation and surgical treatment of Parkinsonian syndromes. Current Opinion in Neurology and Neurosurgery 6:344–349.

Young AB, Penney JB, Starosta-Rubenstein S et al 1986 Pet scan investigations of Huntington's disease: cerebral metabolic correlates of neurological features and functional decline. Annals of Neurology 20:296–303.

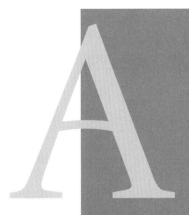

Clinical Case Answers

Case 11.1

11.1.1 Dyskinesias are disorders of movement, usually involving the basal ganglionic–cortical loops. Several types of dyskinesias have been identified including tics, athetosis, choreiform, ballismus.

11.1.2 This woman's symptoms are most likely the result of a dysfunction in the subthalamic nucleus. Understanding the inhibition and excitation circuits involved in direct and indirect pathways of the basal ganglia will help one to understand the spectrum of functional disorders ranging from hyperkinetic to hypokinetic, involving movement and thought processes caused by basal ganglia disorders.

In the direct pathway, the output neurons of the neostriatum project axons that synapse on the neurons of the globus pallidus pars internus (GPi) and/or on the neurons in the substantia nigra pars reticulata (SNr). These projections, arising from the neostriatum, release GABA, substance P, and dynorphin, which act in an inhibitory fashion on the target neurons in the GPi and the SNr.

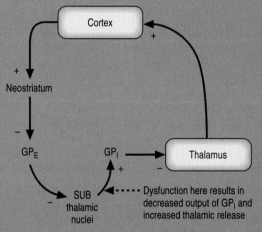

Fig. 11.1.2

In the indirect pathway, axons from the neurons of the neostriatum project to neurons in the globus pallidus pars externa (GPe) where they release the neurotransmitter GABA, enkephalin, and neurotensin, which act in an inhibitory nature on the neurons of the GPe. The neurons of the GPe in turn project to the neurons located in the subthalamic nucleus of Luys (STN), where they release the neurotransmitter GABA and act to inhibit the output neurons of the subthalamic nuclei. The neurons of the subthalamic nuclei project to the neurons of the GPi via the subthalamic fasciculus where they release glutamate and are excitatory in nature. The subthalamic output neurons are the only excitatory neurons in the basal ganglionic circuits. These STN neurons project to neurons in the GPi.

Dysfunction in this nucleus allow the thalamus to escape from the inhibition of the GPi and result in ballistic movements (see Fig 11.1.2).

Case 11.2

11.2.1   Idiopathic Parkinson's disease (PD) is associated with the degeneration of the dopaminergic neurons of the substantia nigra pars compacta (SNc), which as stated previously have an excitatory effect on the direct pathway and an inhibitory effect on the indirect pathway. A loss of dopaminergic stimulation in the neostriatum would result in a net inhibition of movement through both direct and indirect pathways. The onset of PD is gradual in nature, but slowly and progressively continues until eventual severe disability. The cardinal signs and symptoms include tremor at rest, Bradykinesia (slowness of movement), muscular rigidity, akinesia (impairment in initiation and poverty of movement), and loss of postural reflexes. This gentleman is exhibiting tremor at rest, and muscular rigidity.

11.2.2   Dysfunction in the direct pathway is thought to be responsible for hypokinesia. In the direct pathway, the output neurons of the neostriatum project axons that synapse on the neurons of the GPi and/or on the neurons in the SNr. These projections, arising from the neostriatum, release GABA, substance P, and dynorphin, which act in an inhibitory fashion on the target neurons in the GPi and the SNr (see Fig. 11.2.2).

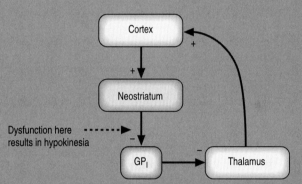

Fig. 11.2.2

11.2.3   The gold standard treatment of PD is replacement of DA using levodopa. Levodopa is absorbed from the gastrointestinal tract and converted to DA in both the brain and the periphery by the enzyme 1-amino acid decarboxylase (1-AAD). The peripheral conversion of levodopa to DA can be inhibited by the actions of benserazide and carbidopa. Most patients today are treated by a combination of levodopa and benserazide or carbidopa. The aim of using this combination is to prevent the peripheral conversion of levodopa to DA, because DA may act in the periphery to produce undesirable side effects such as orthostatic hypotension and nausea. Surgical interventions of PD include ablative and transplanting approaches. Targets for functional stereotactic neurosurgical lesions, which reduce tremor, are the ventrolateral thalamus and the posteroventral pallidum. There has been extensive interest in transplanting DA tissue removed from aborted foetal midbrains into the caudate or putamen in PD; however, the results remained confusing because of small cohort sizes and disease severity issues of the participants. Treatment aimed at increasing the cortical stimulus to the neostriatum may also be of benefit.

Case 11.3

11.3.1   Ballismus or ballism includes a group of conditions characterized by flinging, large amplitude, rotary movements, usually involving the proximal limb muscles. The most common form of this condition occurs unilaterally and is referred to as hemiballism. The cause is classically a basal ganglionic lesion in the contralateral subthalamic nucleus, but contralateral lesions in the neostriatum can also result in ballismic dyskinesia.

Chorea consists of repetitive, brief jerky large-scale dance-like, uncontrolled movements that start in one part of the body and move abruptly and unpredictably to other parts of the body.

Athetosis is a continuous stream of slow, sinuous, writhing movements, generally of the hands and feet.

11.3.2   Disorders of the indirect loop are thought to produce hyperkinetic movement disorders (see Fig. 11.1.2).

11.3.3   Huntington's disease is characterized by insidious onset of both neurological and psychiatric symptoms. Initial symptoms include personality change and the gradual appearance of small involuntary movements; as the disease progresses, chorea becomes more obvious and incapacitating (Harper 1996). Over time, motor symptoms worsen such that walking, speaking, and eating becomes more difficult, and weight loss is common because of the extra energy required for movement and an increase in their basal metabolic rate. A large percentage of HD patients eventually succumb to aspiration pneumonia, resulting from the inability to coordinate pharyngeal muscles and vocal cords which results in swallowing difficulties. It has a large genetic component.

Sydenham's chorea develops after an infection with group A streptococcal bacteria that has not been treated with the appropriate antibiotics. The most frequently involved population is adolescent females. The onset is usually 4–5 months following the infection and begins with an increased feeling of restlessness and increased periods of fidgeting. Occasionally, periods of emotional lability and obsessive-compulsive behaviours will also accompany the motor symptoms. The symptoms become gradually worse over weeks to months and then subside. The symptoms will recur in about 20% of those affected in later life. The cause is thought to involve a cross reaction of anti-streptococcal antibodies with receptors on striatal neurons.

Chapter 12

The Limbic System

Clinical Cases for Thought

Case 12.1   A 71-year-old man presents with a chief complaint of low back pain and knee pain. During the course of the examination you note that he has great difficulty remembering your questions and following directions. He repeatedly appears to forget your instructions. You decide to investigate his loss of short-term memory further and on questioning his wife you realize that he is displaying the symptoms of Alzheimer's disease.

Question

12.1.1   What neurophysiological circuits are involved in the establishment of short- and long-term memory?

Case 12.2   A 45-year-old man presents with a chief complaint of headache. The headache has progressively worsened over the past 2 months to the point that now he cannot function in his daily life. His wife, who has accompanied him, is very concerned about the headaches but is also concerned about a change in his personality that she has observed over the past 2 months. He has become increasingly aggressive and hypersexual, with sudden, violent outbursts. He immediately apologizes following the incident and cannot explain his actions.

Question

12.2.1   You suspect that this unfortunate man may have a brain tumour affecting certain components of his limbic system. What are the components of the limbic system and which areas are most likely to be involved in this man's situation?

Introduction

The limbic system was traditionally thought of as the integration system for olfaction and hence the old term rhinencephalon. It is now clear that the limbic structures are involved in a variety of functions that define us as human. The limbic system is involved in the complex integration of multimodal information concerning olfactory, visceral, and somatic input that emerges in the form of emotional and behavioural responses. This involves such behaviours as seeking and capturing prey, courtship, mating, raising children, the socialization of aggression, and the maintenance of human relationships. The limbic system also plays a role in the development of emotional drives and the establishment of memory.

Anatomical Components of the Limbic System

The exact components of the limbic system remain open to debate. For our purposes in this text the following structures will be considered as components of the limbic system (Figs 12.1 and 12.2):

- The olfactory nerves, bulb, and tract;
- The anterior olfactory nucleus;
- The olfactory striae and the olfactory gyri;
- The olfactory trigone;
- The anterior perforated substance;
- The olfactory tubercle;
- The piriform lobe;
- The amygdaloid complex of nuclei;
- Septum pellucidum and septum verum;
- The hippocampal formation;
- The fornix;
- The stria terminalis;
- The stria habenularis;
- The cingulated and parahippocampal gyri;
- The hypothalamus; and
- The medial and anterior thalamus.

The Olfactory Bulb, Tract, and Cortex

The olfactory bulb and tract develop from ectodermal extensions of the anteromedial part of the primitive cerebral hemisphere. The bulb is radial in structure with six defined layers, which include from the surface to the central core (Fig. 12.3):

1. The olfactory nerve fibre layer;
2. The area of synaptic glomeruli;
3. The molecular and external granule layers;
4. The mitral cell layer;
5. The internal granule layer; and
6. The fibres of the olfactory tract.

The olfactory nerves (CN I) emerge as the axons of the olfactory cells of the nasal mucosa. These axons are then collected into complex intercrossing bundles, which gather into about 20 nerve axon bundles that traverse the cribriform plate of the ethmoid bone to synapse in the glomeruli of the olfactory bulb (Fig. 12.4). The olfactory epithelium is bathed in lipid substance produced by Bowman's glands that dissolves particles in the air and makes them accessible to the receptors of the olfactory nerves.

The *glomeruli* of the olfactory bulb are composed of a complex of axons, dendrites, and neurons including the dendrites of external granule, mitral and tuft cells, and axons from the contralateral olfactory bulb and corticofugal fibres supplying descending modulation. The axons of the mitral and tuft cells course centrally through the olfactory tract to the anterior olfactory nucleus where some axons synapse and others project collaterals but continue with the postganglionic axons to form the olfactory stria. The axons continue posteriorly and divide into the medial and lateral olfactory stria at the junction of the anterior perforated substance circumventing the olfactory tubercle. The lateral olfactory stria project to the anterior perforated substance, the piriform lobe of the cerebrum, the lateral olfactory gyrus,

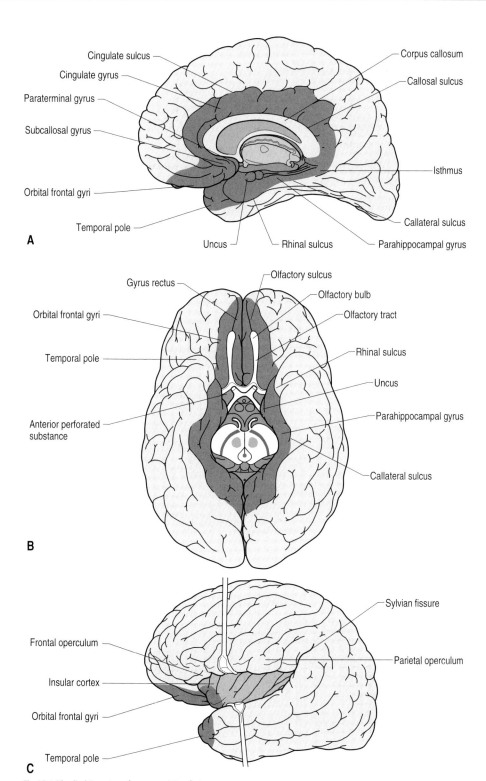

A

Cingulate sulcus
Cingulate gyrus
Paraterminal gyrus
Subcallosal gyrus
Orbital frontal gyri
Temporal pole
Uncus
Rhinal sulcus
Corpus callosum
Callosal sulcus
Isthmus
Callateral sulcus
Parahippocampal gyrus

B

Gyrus rectus
Orbital frontal gyri
Temporal pole
Anterior perforated substance
Olfactory sulcus
Olfactory bulb
Olfactory tract
Rhinal sulcus
Uncus
Parahippocampal gyrus
Callateral sulcus

C

Frontal operculum
Insular cortex
Orbital frontal gyri
Temporal pole
Sylvian fissure
Parietal operculum

Fig.12.1 The limbic system from a variety of views.

and the corticomedial group of amygdaloid nuclei. This group of structures is referred to as the *primary olfactory cortex* (Fig. 12.5). The medial olfactory stria give collaterals to the anterior perforated substance. Some fibres cross the midline via the anterior commissure and synapse in the contralateral anterior olfactory nucleus. These fibres are the only sensory fibres known to reach the cortex without synapsing in one of the thalamic nuclei. The entorhinal area of the parahippocampal gyrus, which forms the caudal area of the piriform lobe, is considered the *secondary olfactory cortex*. The secondary olfactory cortex mediates emotional and autonomic reflexes associated with smell, along with the hypothalamus. The primary and secondary olfactory cortical areas are responsible for the human perception of smell.

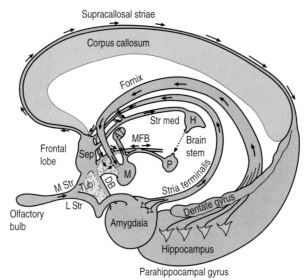

Fig.12.2 Three-dimensional representation of the limbic system.

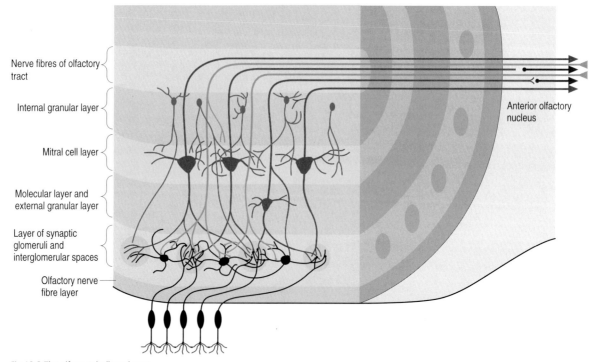

Fig.12.3 The olfactory bulb and tract.

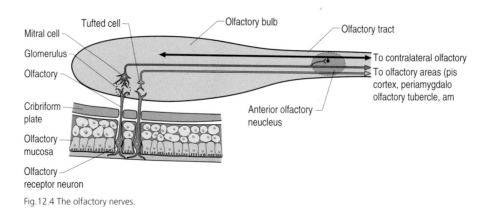

Fig.12.4 The olfactory nerves.

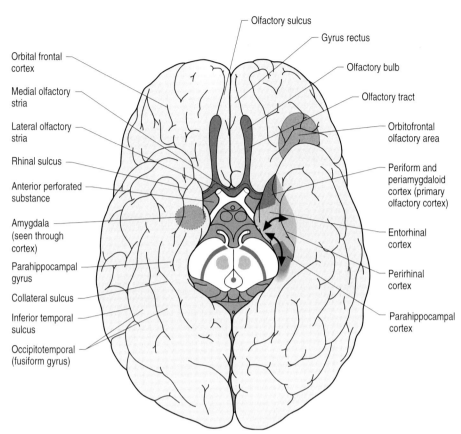

Olfactory sulcus

Gyrus rectus

Orbital frontal cortex

Medial olfactory stria

Lateral olfactory stria

Rhinal sulcus

Anterior perforated substance

Amygdala (seen through cortex)

Parahippocampal gyrus

Collateral sulcus

Inferior temporal sulcus

Occipitotemporal (fusiform gyrus)

Olfactory bulb

Olfactory tract

Orbitofrontal olfactory area

Periform and periamygdaloid cortex (primary olfactory cortex)

Entorhinal cortex

Perirhinal cortex

Parahippocampal cortex

Fig.12.5 Anatomical structures and locations of the primary and secondary olfactory cortices.

The Amygdala

The amygdala, so named because it resembles an almond in shape, is also referred to as the amygdaloid body or the amygdaloid nuclear complex. The amygdala is composed of groups of neurons and their associated nerve fibres in the dorsal medial part of the temporal lobe. The amygdaloid complex is composed of two main groups of nuclei, the corticomedial or basomedial circuit and the basolateral circuit. The corticomedial circuit is composed of the central, medial, and cortical amygdaloid nuclei, the nucleus of the lateral olfactory stria, and the anterior amygdaloid area. The corticomedial division contains irregular groups of pyramidal and granule neurons that resemble a rudimentary cortical structure. The basolateral circuit includes the lateral, basal, and accessory basal amygdaloid nuclei and through its transitional zone is continuous with the parahippocampal gyrus. The amygdala receives projections from the anterior olfactory nucleus, the olfactory bulb, the lateral olfactory stria, various hypothalamic nuclei, various thalamic nuclei, the reticular formation of the brainstem, and a number of areas of cortex. Some neurons of the amygdala project via the stria terminalis to the septal areas and preoptic areas of the hypothalamus, while others project their axons via the amygdalofugal fibres to many hypothalamic nuclei, the medial dorsal nucleus of the thalamus, and the mesencephalic reticular formation (Williams & Warwick 1982).

The Hippocampal Formation

The hippocampal formation is composed of a curved column of phylogenically ancient brain called the archipallium (Fig. 12.6). The hippocampal formation includes the hippocampus proper, the subiculum, and the dentate gyrus. Following the structure of the archipallium from a central point in the dentate gyrus in a radial clockwise fashion, the archipallium can be dived into three zones: the dentate gyrus, the cornu ammonis, and the subiculum (Fig. 12.7). The dentate gyrus and cornu ammonis display the three-layered

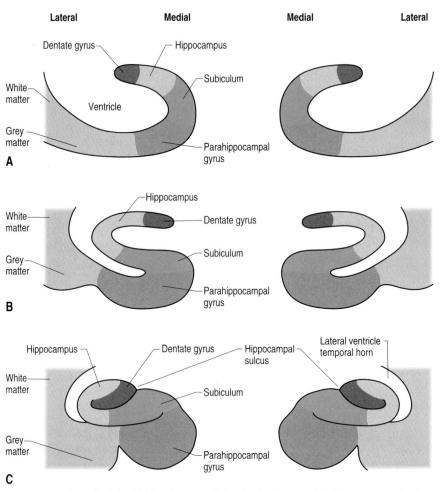

Fig.12.6 The complex embryological folding that occurs during the development of the hippocampus, subiculum, dentate gyrus, and parahippocampal gyrus.

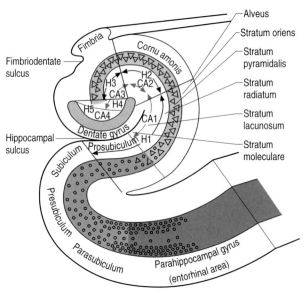

Fig.12.7 The components of the hippocampal formation includes the hippocampus proper, the subiculum, and the dentate gyrus.

cortical structure of the ancient cortices; the subiculum demonstrates a gradual shift from four layers to six layers through its length (Fig. 12.8). The hippocampal formation includes the following structures:

- The indusium griseum;
- The longitudinal stria;
- The dentate gyrus;
- The cornu ammonis (Ammon's horn);
- The subiculum; and
- Parts of the uncus.

The hippocampus consists of the complex interfolding of the dentate gyrus and the cornu ammonis and remains superior to the subiculum and the parahippocampal gyrus throughout its length.

Afferent projections received by the hippocampus include (Fig. 12.9):

- Cingulate gyrus;
- Septal nuclei;

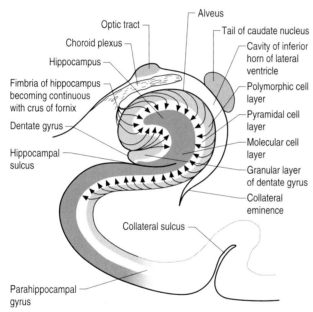

Fig. 12.8 The components of the hippocampal formation.

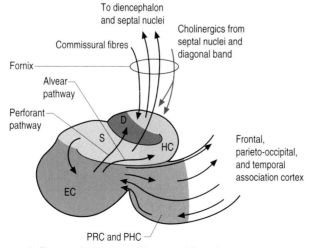

Fig. 12.9 The afferent and efferent projections to the hippocampal formation.

- Entorhinal cortex;
- Indusium griseum;
- Commissural fibres from the opposite hippocampal formation; and
- Aminergic fibres from the brainstem reticular formation.

The efferent outflow from the hippocampus courses through the fornix, which is mainly composed of the axons from pyramidal neurons in Ammon's horn and the dentate gyrus. These fibres terminate in the following structures:

- The cingulate gyrus;
- The septum pellucidum;
- Preoptic and anterior hypothalamic nuclei;
- Anterior thalamus;
- Mammillary nucleus;
- Reticular formation of the brainstem; and
- Tegmentum of the mesencephalon.

The hippocampus has several important functions including a primary role in the acquisition of associative behaviour. It is also is involved in the identification of contiguity between spatial and temporal events through memory recall mechanisms (McIntosh & Gonzalez-Lima 1998).

Functions of the Limbic System

The limbic system is involved in the complex integration of multimodal information concerning olfactory, visceral, and somatic input that emerges in the form of emotional and behavioural responses. This involves such behaviours as seeking and capturing prey, courtship, mating, raising children, the socialization of aggression, and the maintenance of human relationships. The limbic system also plays a role in the development of emotional drives and the establishment of memory. In the process of integrating the perceptions generated by the sensory systems, the amygdala is recruited to colour those perceptions with emotion. The hippocampus is called upon to store aspects of those perceptions in long-term memory.

The medial circuit or archicortical division of the temporolimbic system mediates important aspects of learning, memory, and attentional control, as well as information related to internal states. The lateral or basolateral circuit, which has extensive connections with dorsolateral prefrontal cortex and posterior parietal association cortex, processes information concerning the external world, the implicit integration of affect, drives, and social-personal interactions.

Disorders of Temporolimbic Function

Disorders of the limbic system produce a wide variety of bizarre behavioural syndromes, disorders of memory, and aggressive behaviours.

The hypothalamus, amygdala, and prefrontal cortex are the critical neural structures implicated in the expression of aggression (Weiger & Bear 1988). The ventromedial hypothalamic area, in particular, mediated primarily via cholinergic neurotransmission, has been associated with predatory-type aggression. Bilateral lesions in this area may lead to aggressive outbursts referred to as hypothalamic rage that are provoked by frustrated attempts to satisfy basic drives such as hunger, thirst, and sexual need. Hypothalamic rage typically involves outbursts of simple behaviours such as kicking, biting, scratching, or throwing objects and is usually a wild, lashing out response not directed against specific targets (Reeves & Plum 1969). After the event, patients may express remorse and exhibit some insight about their uncontrolled impulses. Aggressive behaviour is also the hallmark of intermittent explosive disorder, which likely involves frontotemporolimbic circuitry.

Patients with this disorder present with impulsive loss of behavioural control episodes, in response to minimal provocation which often leads to serious violence. The prefrontal cortex is intimately connected with the hypothalamus and the amygdala and is essential in the hierarchy of aggression control. Orbitofrontal lesions frequently lead to affective disinhibition, most commonly irritability with angry outbursts but also including silliness, euphoria, loud behaviour, and interpersonal and social disinhibition (Lichter & Cummings 2001). The actions of individuals that exhibit aggressive behaviour and violent criminal activity resulting from disinhibited frontal lobe syndromes are usually impulsive, and lack elaborate planning and consideration of consequences. The actions are usually simple in nature and committed without remorse. Abnormalities in prefrontal and subcortical circuitry may also underlie the aggressive and violent acts seen in patients with antisocial personality disorder. Aggressive behaviour has also been linked to disturbed neurotransmission involving specific neural circuitry in the limbic system. Serotonergic, noradrenergic, dopaminergic, and GABA-ergic circuits have all been identified as playing a role in modulating behaviours including aggressive behaviour. The most consistent findings relate to the serotonergic system. Both high and low concentrations of serotonin levels have been implicated in abnormal behaviours For example, low serotonin levels have been found in the cerebrospinal fluid of people who have attempted suicide and of those who have successfully completed suicide (Virkkunen et al 1995).

As outlined above, the amygdala receives sensory input from various cortical areas and projects to the hypothalamus and temporolimbic cortex via the ventral amygdalofugal pathway and stria terminalis (Othmer et al 1998). This connectivity provides a neural mechanism, whereby external stimuli receive emotional colouring. Hence, a limbic hyperconnection syndrome may account for the heightened emotional responsivity that is part of the rare and controversial behavioural syndrome, the *Gastaut-Geschwind syndrome*, which is characterized by dysfunction in three distinct areas of psychosocial interactions including heightened emotional responses, exaggerated behaviours, and lability in physiological drives. The altered emotional responses include periods of intense metaphysical preoccupation with hyperreligiosity, and exaggerated philosophic or moral concerns. They may also experience changes in affect such as depression, paranoia, or irritability. Their behavioural 'viscosity' manifests as exaggerated verbal, motor, and writing behaviours, nonrational adherence to ideas, interpersonal adhesiveness with prolonged encounters, obsessive preoccupation with detail, excessive need to collect background information, and copious description of thoughts and feelings with a moral or religious twang (Trimble et al 1997).

Finally, they experience prolonged and powerful alterations of physiological drives resulting in hyposexuality, aggression, and fear responses (Lichter & Cummings 2001).

Damage or dysfunction of the amygdala may result in alterations of perception of various learned emotional states. Sensory inflow for various learned emotional states, especially fear and anxiety, projects to the amygdala via the basolateral complex. Recall that this group of nuclei receives information directly from the thalamus and the cortex. Lesions of the lateral basal complex often result in placid, satiated, and neglectful responses to somatic, visual, and olfactory stimuli with no regard to the significance of the behaviour actually performed and the stimulus for performing it. It appears that lesions of the basolateral complex leave intact the learned association between conditional stimuli and non-rewarding aspects of the unconditional stimulus, but abolish the association between the conditional stimuli and rewarding aspects of the unconditional stimulus. This mechanism may explain the bizarre behaviour exhibited in the *Kluver-Bucy syndrome*. Classically, the person will try to put anything in their hand into their mouths. They often make attempts to have sexual intercourse with inappropriate species or objects. A classic example is of the unfortunate chap arrested whilst attempting to have sex with the pavement. Effectively, it is the 'what is this' pathway that is damaged with regard to foodstuff and choice of sexual partners. Monkeys with surgically modified temporal lobes have great difficulty in knowing what prey is, what a mate is, what food is, and in general what the significance of any object might be.

Other symptoms of temporolimbic dysfunction may include inability to visually recognize objects, which is referred to as visual agnosia, the loss of normal fear and anger responses, memory loss, distractibility, seizures, and dementia. The disorder may be associated with other diseases or conditions that can result in brain damage such as herpes encephalitis or trauma. Similar symptomatology can be seen with lesions of the hypothalamus as previously discussed.

The Amygdala Theory of Autism

It has been proposed that in humans a network of neural regions may comprise the 'social brain'; this network includes the amygdala. Since the childhood psychiatric condition of autism involves deficits in 'social intelligence', it has been proposed that autism may be caused by an amygdala dysfunction that results in deficits in social behaviour in these individuals. Recent studies involving the use of functional magnetic resonance imaging (fMRI) found that patients with autism did not activate the amygdala when making mentalistic inferences from the eyes, whilst people without autism did show amygdala activity. The amygdala is therefore proposed to be one of several neural regions that are abnormal in autism (Baron-Cohen et al 2000).

Learning and Memory

The hippocampus and various other areas of the limbic system are known to play a role in the establishment of memory and learning. The memory process will be explored in an overview fashion here since memory problems are frequently observed in patients with other neurological dysfunctions, and a rudimentary understanding of memory is clinically relevant to their treatment.

Implicit memory, which is the memory we use to perform a previously learned task and does not require conscious recall, and includes various types of memory such as procedural, priming, associative, and nonassociative. *Procedural* memory is involved with recall of how to perform previously learned skills or habits. It is thought to rely heavily on areas of the striatum. *Priming* is a type of memory in which the recall of words or objects is enhanced with prior exposure to the words or objects. This type of memory utilizes neocortical circuits. *Associative learning or memory* involves the association of two or more stimuli and includes classical conditioning and operant conditioning (Kandel et al 2000).

Classical conditioning involves the presynaptic facilitation of synaptic transmission that is dependent on activity in both pre- and postsynaptic cells. The neuron circuit learns to associate one type of stimulus with another. When stimuli are paired in this manner the result is a greater and longer lasting enhancement. For this form of activity-dependent facilitation to occur, the conditioned and unconditional stimuli must occur at closely spaced intervals in time. Influx of calcium in response to action potentials in the conditional stimulus pathway leads to potentiation of the stimulus by binding of activated calcium/calmodulin to adenylyl cyclase. This occurs in a fashion similar to sensitization due to serotonin release described above. Adenylyl cyclase acts as coincidence detector, recognizing molecular response to both a conditioned stimulus and an unconditional stimulus present simultaneously or within a required space of time. The postsynaptic component of classical conditioning is a retrograde signal to the sensory neurons that potentiation of the stimulus has indeed occurred.

In a simple circuit subjected to classical conditioning, the neuron has both the NMDA type and non-NMDA receptors. Only non-NMDA receptors are activated in habituation and sensitization due to a magnesium plug in the NMDA receptor channel. In classical conditioning, as a result of pairing of stimuli the magnesium plug is expelled, opening the NMDA channel, which results in the influx of calcium, thereby activating signalling pathways in the neuron. This gives rise to activation of a variety of retrograde messenger systems that enhance the amount of neurotransmitter released.

Therefore, in classical conditioning three signals need to converge within a specific period of time for learning to occur. These signals include:

1. Activation of adenylyl cyclase by calcium influx (conditioned);

2. Activation of serotonergic receptors coupled to adenylyl cyclase (unconditioned); and

3. Retrograde signal indicating that the postsynaptic cell has been adequately activated by the unconditioned stimulus.

Long-term storage of implicit memory involving both sensitization and classical conditioning involves the cyclic AMP (cAMP)–protein kinase A (PKA)–mitogen-activated protein kinase (MAPK)–cAMP response element-binding protein (CREB) pathway (see Chapter 3).

Operant conditioning involves the association of a stimulus to a behaviour utilizing rewards and punishments as reinforcement for the desired behaviour. Operant conditioning probably utilizes a similar neurophysiological mechanism as described above for classical conditioning.

Nonassociative learning or memory occurs when a person or neuron is exposed to a novel stimulus either once or repeatedly. This type of learning or memory involves the neurophysiological processes of habituation and sensitization of synaptic function, which are important processes in nonassociative learning and memory (Kandel et al 2000).

The process of *habituation* involves the presynaptic depression of synaptic transmission that is dependent on the frequency of activation of the circuit. In the presence of certain types of long-term inactivation or long-term activation of synaptic transmission, the structure of the sensory neuron will adapt to the stimulus. This process predominantly occurs at sites in the neuraxis specific for learning and memory storage. If habituating stimuli are presented one after the other without rest between sessions, a robust short-term memory can be formed, but long-term memory is seriously compromised. Therefore, the main principle for stimulating long-term memory is that frequent but well-spaced training is usually much more effective than massed training. To say this in another way, 'cramming' for an exam may work in the short term but for long-term memory retention frequent, spaced study sessions are much better.

The process of *sensitization* involves presynaptic facilitation of synaptic transmission. This process is particularly effective when a stimulus is harmful to the neuron or perceived as harmful to the person. Sensitization involves axoaxonic, serotonergic connections which activate the G protein, adenylyl cyclase, cAMP, PKA/PKC pathway, which increases release of transmitter from neurons through phosphorylation of several substrate proteins. The process of sensitization can occur in a direct fashion which only involves the pre- and postsynaptic neurons, or in an indirect fashion which involves the participation of interneurons.

Memory can be classified into two distinct, but functionally related systems, based on how the information contained in the memory is stored and retrieved. These classifications include implicit and explicit memory.

Explicit memory, which is the factual recall of persons, places, and things and the understanding of the significance of these things, is more flexible than implicit memory and includes various classifications of memory which include:

1. Episodic memory, which involves the recall of events in time and space; and

2. Semantic memory, which involves the recall of facts, words, names, and meanings.

For example, the statement 'Last year I attended the Rolling Stones concert with my sister' is utilizing episodic memory and the statement 'Mercury is the planet closest to the sun' is utilizing semantic memory.

Explicit memory involves the process of long-term potentiation of synapses in the hippocampus. The entorhinal cortex acts as both the primary input and primary output of the hippocampus in this process. The unimodal and polymodal areas of association cortex project to the parahippocampal gyrus and the perirhinal cortex, which both project to the entorhinal cortex. Information then flows from the entorhinal cortex to the hippocampus in three possible pathways including the perforant, the mossy fibre, and the Schaffer collateral pathways (Kandel et al 2000).

The perforant pathway projects from entorhinal cortex to granular cells of the dentate gyrus. This is the primary conduit for polymodal information from the association cortices to the hippocampus. The mossy fibre pathway, which contains axons of the granule cells and runs to the pyramidal cells in the CA3 region of hippocampus, is dependent on noradrenergic activation of beta-adrenergic receptors, which activate adenylyl cyclase. This pathway is nonassociative in nature and can be modified by serotonin. The Schaffer collateral pathway consists of excitatory collaterals of the pyramidal cells in the CA3 region and ends on the pyramidal cells in the CA1 region. Long-term potentiation in the Schaffer collateral and perforant pathways is associative in nature (Fig. 12.10).

Long term memory of explicit nature occurs through multiple sensory components being processed separately in unimodal and multimodal association cortices of the parietal, temporal, and frontal lobes. This information then passes simultaneously to the parahippocampal and perirhinal cortices. The information then projects to the entorhinal cortex and via the perforant pathway to the dentate gyrus and the hippocampus. From the hippocampus, information flows back to the entorhinal cortices

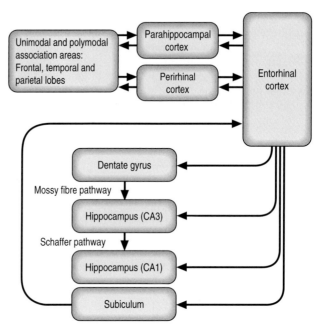

Fig.12.10 Input and output pathways of the hippocampal formation.

via the subiculum, then perirhinal and parahippocampal cortices, then polymodal association areas of the neocortex. The elements involved in long-term memory occur in the cortical association areas and appear to have an unlimited capacity for storage of memories.

The entorhinal cortex is the first site of pathological changes in Alzheimer's disease; therefore, the first sign would be loss of or defective explicit memory.

Memory processing can be divided into four processes which include:

1. *Encoding*—the process in which new material is attended to. The degree to which attention is allotted to the new information is directly related to the strength of the memory.

2. *Consolidation*—processes that make the memory more stable; includes expression of genes and synthesis of proteins in the neuron. Loss of consolidation of a memory occurs because of inhibition of mRNA or protein synthesis to block long-term memory selectively. Consolidation involves three processes which include:

    *   Gene expression;
    *   New protein synthesis; and
    *   Growth (or protein) of synaptic connections.

    Repeated application of serotonin causes the catalytic subunits of PKA to recruit another second messenger kinase: the mitogen-activated protein kinase (MAPK), which is commonly associated with cellular growth. PKA and MAPK translocate to the nucleus of the sensory neurons where they activate a genetic switch.

3. *Storage*—the process of solidifying the memory into long-term memory which seems to have unlimited storage capacity.

4. *Retrieval*—the process in which the memory is brought back to conscious awareness and is dependent to some extent on a working short-term memory circuit called the attentional control system.

The prefrontal cortex is the *attentional control system*, also referred to as the central executive centre. The attentional control system regulates information flow to two rehearsal systems, *the articulatory loop*, which is involved with language, words, and numbers processing, and the *visuospatial sketch pad*, which is involved with vision and actions such as memorizing data or recognizing the face of a friend at a party. This system is important for both establishing new memories and recalling long-term memories.

References

Baron-Cohen S, Ring HA, Bullmore ET et al 2000 The amygdala theory of autism. Neuroscience and Biobehavioral Reviews 24:(3):355–364.

Kandel ER, Kupfermann I, Iversen S 2000 Learning and memory. In: Kandel ER, Schwartz JH, Jessell TM (eds) Principles of neural science, 4th edn. McGraw-Hill, New York.

Lichter DG, Cummings JL 2001 Frontal-subcortical circuits in psychiatric and neurological disorders. Gulford Press, New York.

McIntosh AR, Gonzalez-Lima F 1998 Large-scale functional connectivity in associative learning: interrelations of the rat auditory, visual, and limbic systems. Journal of Neurophysiology 80:3148–3162.

Othmer JP, Othmer SC, Othmer E 1998 Brain functions and psychiatric disorders. A clinical view. Psychiatric Clinics of North America 21(3):517–566.

Reeves AG, Plum F 1969 Hyperphagia, rage and dementia accompanying a ventromedial hypothalamic neoplasm. Archives of Neurology 20:616–624.

Trimble MR, Mendez MF, Cummings JL 1997 Neuropsychiatric symptoms from the temporolimbic lobes. Journal of Neuropsychiatry and Clinical Neurosciences 9:429–438.

Virkkunen M, Goldman D, Nielsen DA 1995 Low brain serotonin turnover rate (low CSF 5-HIAA) and impulsive violence. Journal of Psychiatry and Neuroscience 20(4):271–275.

Weiger WA, Bear DM 1988 An approach to the neurology of aggression. Journal of Psychiatric Research 22(2):85–98.

Williams PL, Warwick R 1984 Gray's anatomy. Churchill Livingston, Edinburgh.

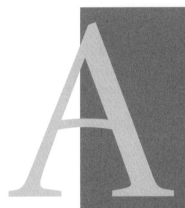

Clinical Case Answers

Case 12.1

12.1.1
Long-term memory of explicit nature occurs through multiple sensory components being processed separately in unimodal and multimodal association cortices of the parietal, temporal and frontal lobes. This information then passes simultaneously to the parahippocampal and perirhinal cortices. The information then projects to the entorhinal cortex and via the perforant pathway to the dentate gyrus and the hippocampus. From the hippocampus, information flows back to the entorhinal cortices via the subiculum, then perirhinal and parahippocampal cortices, then polymodal association areas of the neocortex. The elements involved in long term memory occur in the cortical association areas and appear to have an unlimited capacity for storage of memories. Short-term memory is established in the same pathways as above but does not project to the cortical areas and is sensitive to the process of habituation. The process of **habituation** involves the presynaptic depression of synaptic transmission that is dependent on the frequency of activation of the circuit. In the presence of certain types of long-term inactivation or long-term activation of synaptic transmission, the structure of the sensory neuron will adapt to the stimulus. This process predominantly occurs at sites in the neuraxis specific for learning and memory storage. If habituating stimuli are presented one after the other without rest between sessions, a robust short-term memory can be formed, but long-term memory is seriously compromised. Therefore, the main principle for stimulating long-term memory is that frequent but well spaced training is usually much more effective than massed training. To say this in another way, 'cramming' for an exam may work in the short term but for long-term memory retention frequent, spaced study sessions are much better.

12.1.2
The components of the limbic system include;

- the cingulate gyrus
- the septum pellucidum
- anterior thalamus
- mammillary nucleus
- reticular formation of the brainstem
- tegmentum of the mesencephalon
- the indusium griseum
- the longitudinal stria
- the cornu ammonis (Ammon's horn)
- the subiculum
- parts of the uncus

Disorders of the limbic system produce a wide variety of bizarre behavioral syndromes, disorders of memory and aggressive behaviours.

The hypothalamus, amygdala and prefrontal cortex are the critical neural structures implicated in the expression aggression (Weiger & Bear 1988). The ventromedial hypothalamic area, in particular, mediated primarily via cholinergic neurotransmission, has been associated with predatory-type aggression. Bilateral lesions in this area may lead to aggressive outbursts referred to as hypothalamic rage, that are provoked by frustrated attempts to satisfy basic drives such as hunger, thirst and sexual need. Hypothalamic rage, typically involves outbursts of simple behaviours such as kicking, biting, scratching or throwing objects and is usually a wild, lashing out, response not directed against specific targets (Reeves & Plum 1969). After the event, patients may express remorse and exhibit some insight about their uncontrolled impulses. Aggressive behaviour is also the hallmark of intermittent explosive disorder, which likely involves frontotemporolimbic circuitry.

Chapter

13

The Brainstem and Reticular Formation

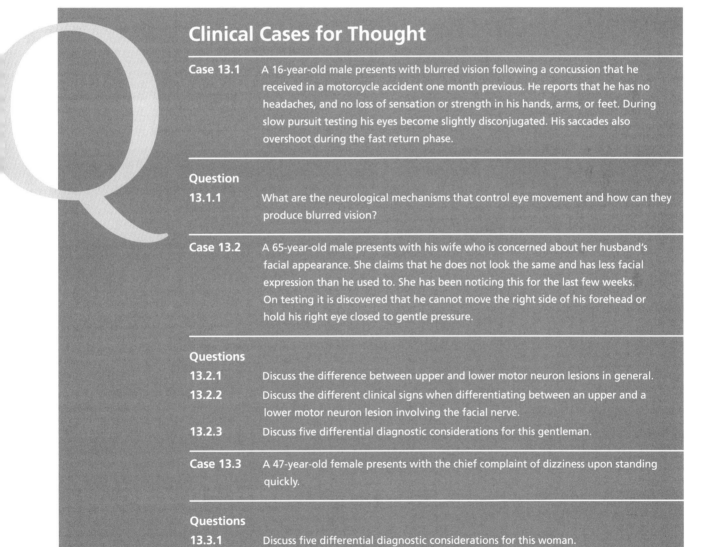

Clinical Cases for Thought

Case 13.1 A 16-year-old male presents with blurred vision following a concussion that he received in a motorcycle accident one month previous. He reports that he has no headaches, and no loss of sensation or strength in his hands, arms, or feet. During slow pursuit testing his eyes become slightly disconjugated. His saccades also overshoot during the fast return phase.

Question

13.1.1 What are the neurological mechanisms that control eye movement and how can they produce blurred vision?

Case 13.2 A 65-year-old male presents with his wife who is concerned about her husband's facial appearance. She claims that he does not look the same and has less facial expression than he used to. She has been noticing this for the last few weeks. On testing it is discovered that he cannot move the right side of his forehead or hold his right eye closed to gentle pressure.

Questions

13.2.1 Discuss the difference between upper and lower motor neuron lesions in general.

13.2.2 Discuss the different clinical signs when differentiating between an upper and a lower motor neuron lesion involving the facial nerve.

13.2.3 Discuss five differential diagnostic considerations for this gentleman.

Case 13.3 A 47-year-old female presents with the chief complaint of dizziness upon standing quickly.

Questions

13.3.1 Discuss five differential diagnostic considerations for this woman.

13.3.2 Discuss the physiological and neurological mechanisms and pathways involved in the control of blood pressure during quick posture changes.

Introduction

There is probably no more complicated area to study anatomically than the brainstem. Understanding the anatomy in a three-dimensional perspective is crucial for the application of clinical neurology. The reticular formation receives little attention in traditional neurology textbooks. It is an area that spans all levels of the brainstem, from the thalamus to the spinal cord, and is responsible for integrating information from the brain and periphery and linking sensory, motor, and autonomic nuclei of the brainstem. The reticular formation therefore mediates complex reflexes and functions such as eye movements, posture, feeding, breathing, homeostasis, arousal, sleep, control of vasomotor tone and cardiac output, and pain. The cranial nerves are very important as clinical windows into the functional state of various levels of the brainstem. The brainstem is also responsible for the control of vital functions like heart rate and respiration. This area, although complicated, promises access to a great amount of clinical information to those who spend the necessary investments of time and energy to thoroughly grasp the structure and functional relationships that compose the brainstem.

Anatomy of the Brainstem

The brainstem is composed of the following anatomical areas (Figs. 13.1, 13.2, and 13.3):

QUICK FACTS 1	Input from Primary Afferents and Their Collaterals Results in the Following

1. Monosynaptic reflex involving the alpha motor neurons
2. Inhibition of antagonist
3. Excitation of synergists
4. Inhibition of contralateral homologues
5. Excitation of antagonist of contralateral homologues
6. Excitation of IML neurons
7. Excitation of granular layer of the cerebellum, which leads to increased contralateral cortical integration via excitation of contralateral thalamus.

1. *Midbrain* or *mesencephalon* is contained between the cerebrum and the pons in an area which measures approximately 2.5 cm long;
2. *Pons* is contained between the midbrain and the medulla;
3. *Medulla oblongata*, which extends from the base of the pons to the first pair of cervical nerves. Caudally the medulla is continuous with the medulla spinalis or the spinal cord.

We will approach the description of the brainstem by outlining the structures observed at various levels in cross-sectional dissections.

Mesencephalon

The structures of the mesencephalon can be observed in a cross section of midbrain at the superior colliculus and the inferior colliculus (Figs 13.4 and 13.5).

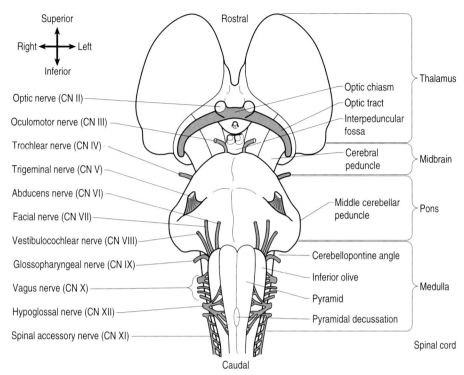

Superior
Right ◄──► Left
Inferior

Rostral

Optic nerve (CN II)
Oculomotor nerve (CN III)
Trochlear nerve (CN IV)
Trigeminal nerve (CN V)
Abducens nerve (CN VI)
Facial nerve (CN VII)
Vestibulocochlear nerve (CN VIII)
Glossopharyngeal nerve (CN IX)
Vagus nerve (CN X)
Hypoglossal nerve (CN XII)
Spinal accessory nerve (CN XI)

Optic chiasm
Optic tract
Interpeduncular fossa
Cerebral peduncle
Middle cerebellar peduncle
Cerebellopontine angle
Inferior olive
Pyramid
Pyramidal decussation

Thalamus
Midbrain
Pons
Medulla
Spinal cord

Caudal

Fig. 13.1 An anterior view of the anatomical structures of the brainstem.

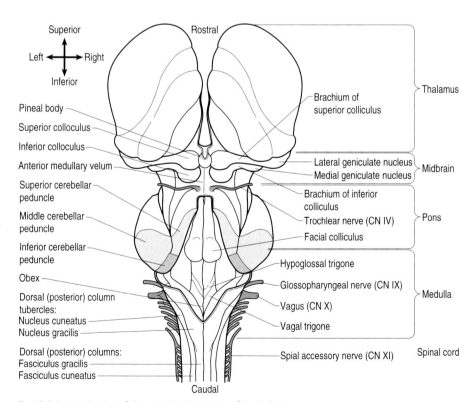

Superior
Left ◄──► Right
Inferior

Rostral

Pineal body
Superior colloculus
Inferior colloculus
Anterior medullary velum
Superior cerebellar peduncle
Middle cerebellar peduncle
Inferior cerebellar peduncle
Obex
Dorsal (posterior) column tubercles:
Nucleus cuneatus
Nucleus gracilis
Dorsal (posterior) columns:
Fasciculus gracilis
Fasciculus cuneatus

Brachium of superior colliculus
Lateral geniculate nucleus
Medial geniculate nucleus
Brachium of inferior colliculus
Trochlear nerve (CN IV)
Facial colliculus
Hypoglossal trigone
Glossopharyngeal nerve (CN IX)
Vagus (CN X)
Vagal trigone
Spial accessory nerve (CN XI)

Thalamus
Midbrain
Pons
Medulla
Spinal cord

Caudal

Fig. 13.2 A posterior view of the anatomical structures of the brainstem.

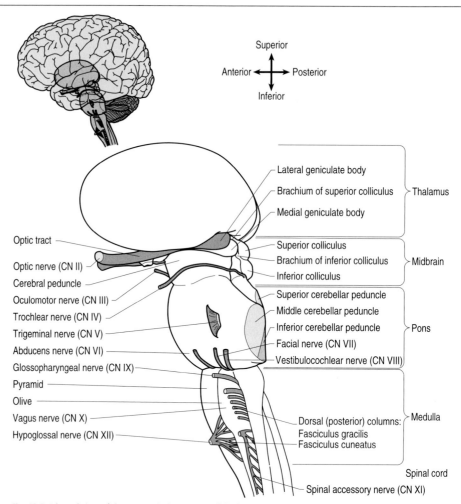

Superior

Anterior ← → Posterior

Inferior

Lateral geniculate body
Brachium of superior colliculus   Thalamus
Medial geniculate body

Optic tract
Superior colliculus
Optic nerve (CN II)   Brachium of inferior colliculus   Midbrain
Cerebral peduncle   Inferior colliculus
Oculomotor nerve (CN III)   Superior cerebellar peduncle
Trochlear nerve (CN IV)   Middle cerebellar peduncle
Trigeminal nerve (CN V)   Inferior cerebellar peduncle   Pons
Abducens nerve (CN VI)   Facial nerve (CN VII)
Glossopharyngeal nerve (CN IX)   Vestibulocochlear nerve (CN VIII)
Pyramid
Olive
Vagus nerve (CN X)   Dorsal (posterior) columns: Medulla
Hypoglossal nerve (CN XII)   Fasciculus gracilis
                                         Fasciculus cuneatus

                                         Spinal cord
                                   Spinal accessory nerve (CN XI)

Fig. 13.3 A lateral view of the anatomical structures of the brainstem.

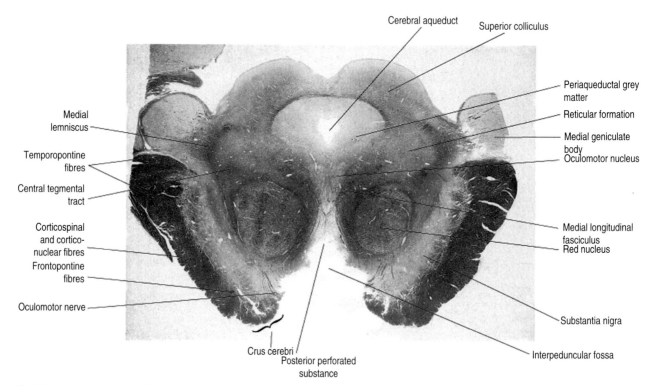

Cerebral aqueduct   Superior colliculus

Periaqueductal grey matter

Reticular formation

Medial lemniscus

Temporopontine fibres

Medial geniculate body
Oculomotor nucleus

Central tegmental tract

Corticospinal and cortico-nuclear fibres
Frontopontine fibres

Medial longitudinal fasciculus
Red nucleus

Oculomotor nerve

Substantia nigra

Crus cerebri
Posterior perforated substance

Interpeduncular fossa

Fig. 13.4 A cross-sectional view of the mesencephalon at the superior colliculus. (From Standring; Gray's Anatomy 39e. Elsevier Ltd 2005).

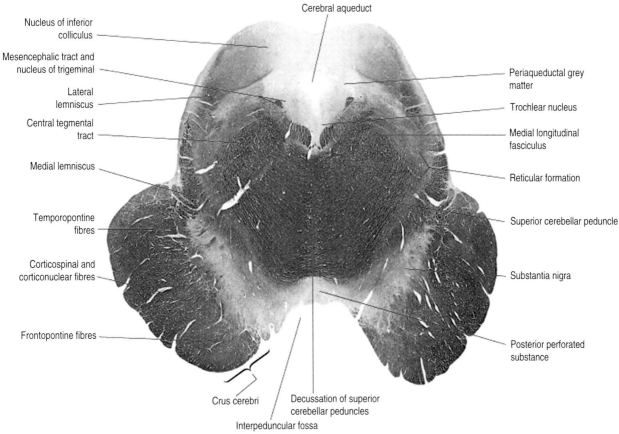

Fig. 13.5 A cross-sectional view of the mesencephalon at the inferior colliculus. (From Standring; Gray's Anatomy 39e. Elsevier Ltd 2005).

Periaqueductal Grey Area

The periaqueductal grey area is an area of neuron cell bodies that surrounds the cerebral aqueduct. It is continuous with the grey substance of the third ventricle.

What is the Extrapyramidal System? | QUICK FACTS 2

The extrapyramidal system is used to denote all areas and tracts of the brain and brainstem involved with motor control that are not part of the direct pyramidal or corticospinal projection system. The extrapyramidal system includes:

1. The basal ganglia
2. The reticular formation of the brain stem
3. Vestibular nuclei
4. The red nucleus

Tectum

The tectum comprises the 'roof' or dorsal portion of the midbrain and contains the corpora quadrigemina, which includes the superior and inferior colliculi and all the substances that lie dorsal to the cerebral aqueduct in the midbrain area of the neuraxis. The superior colliculi are involved with visual reflexes and project to the lateral geniculate bodies of the thalamus. The inferior colliculi are involved with reflexes associated with sound, and project to the medial geniculate bodies of the thalamus.

Tegmentum

The tegmentum consists of the bulk of the matter of the brainstem and comprises the area ventral to the cerebral aqueduct and fourth ventricle. It contains the bulk of the brainstem nuclei and the reticular formation of the midbrain, pons, and medulla.

Substantia Nigra

The substantia nigra is a broad layer of pigmented neurons that separates the basis from the tegmentum. It extends from the upper surface of the pons to the hypothalamus. It projects to and receives projections from the neostriatum, thalamus, subthalamic nucleus, superior colliculi, and the reticular system of the brainstem. The neuron of this region utilize dopamine as a neurotransmitter.

Oculomotor Nuclei

The oculomotor nuclei are the motor nuclei of the superior rectus, inferior rectus, and medial rectus muscles of the eye.

Red Nucleus

These bilateral structures are ovoid groups of nuclei composed of two different cell types, the magnocellular and parvocellular groups of neurons. The magnocellular neurons are large, multipolar cells located in the caudal area of the red nuclear mass. These neurons receive bilateral projections both from sensorimotor cortical areas via the corticorubral tracts and from collaterals via the corticospinal tracts. The cortical projections and their target neurons in the red nucleus are somatotopically organized. Axon projections from the magnocellular neurons form the rubrospinal tracts, which cross in the brainstem and project in a somatotopically organized fashion, mainly to the interneurons of the intermediate grey areas of the spinal cord. Some rubrospinal fibres terminate directly on ventral horn motor neurons as well. Some axons that form the rubrospinal tracts terminate on neurons in the pontomedullary reticular formation and the motor nuclei of various cranial nerves, forming the rubroreticular system and the rubrobulbar tracts respectively (Brown 1974). Reciprocal, bilateral projections to the superior colliculi are also present and form the rubrotectal tracts (Fig. 13.6). The rubrospinal and corticospinal

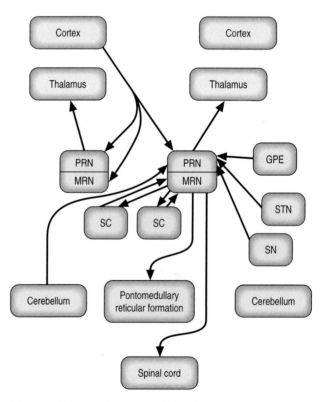

PRN — Parvocellular red nucleus   GPE — Globus pallidus pars externa
MRN — Magnocellular red nucleus   STN — Subthalamic nucleus
SC — Superior colliculus   SN — Substantia nigra

Fig. 13.6 Afferent and efferent projections of the red nucleus.

tracts form the lateral motor system of the spinal cord. The medial motor system is composed of the reticulospinal and vestibulospinal tracts.

The Parvocellular neurons of the red nucleus are small pyramidal- and spherical-shaped neurons, mostly located in the rostral areas of the red nuclear mass. These neurons receive projections from the dentate nucleus of the contralateral cerebellum, and from the ipsilateral globus pallidus pars externa, substantia nigra, and subthalamic nuclei. These neuron project to the ipsilateral thalamus (Fig. 13.6).

Medial Longitudinal Fasciculus (MLF)

This structure is a highly myelinated axon tract that descends from the interstitial nucleus of Cajal in the lateral wall of third ventricle through the midbrain, pons, and medulla to the spinal cord where it becomes continuous with the anterior intersegmental fasciculus. The MLF acts as a major communications conduit between all of the cranial nerve nuclei and all related structures including the reticular formations of the mesencephalon, pons, and medulla. The medial vestibulospinal tract axons project with the MLF to the spinal cord (Brodal et al 1962). Other axons from the vestibular nuclei ascend in the MLF to more rostral structures including the extraocular cranial nuclei. The MLF is the first fibre tract in the developing embryo to become myelinated and probably acts as a major pathway providing stimulus to developing neurons in the early stages of embryonic development.

Medial Lemnisci

The medial lemniscus is a bundle of axons that forms a triangular structure medial to the spinothalamic tract. The bundles are formed from axons of the contralateral dorsal column nuclei, the nucleus gracilis and cuneatus, which have decussated and formed the internal arcuate fibres which become continuous with the medial lemnisci. The fibres are joined by axons of the trigeminal sensory nucleus to project to the ipsilateral thalamus. Axons from the dorsal column nuclei terminate on neurons in the ventral posterior lateral nucleus of the thalamus, whereas axons from the trigeminal sensory nucleus terminate on neurons in the ventral posterior medial nucleus of the thalamus (Guyton & Hall 1996).

Crus Cerebri

This semilunar structure, also referred to as the basis, is located anterior to the substantia nigra and is composed of the corticospinal, corticonuclear, and corticopontine fibre tracts. The corticospinal fibres terminate on the ventral horn neurons of the contralateral spinal cord. The corticonuclear fibres terminate mainly on contralateral cranial nerve nuclei throughout the brainstem. The corticopontine fibres are composed of projections from the frontal and temporal cortical areas and terminate on the interneurons of the nuclei pontis. These nuclei then project mostly to the contralateral cerebellum.

Pons

The structures of the pons can be observed through a cross section at the level of the trigeminal nerves (Fig. 13.7), just superior to the cerebral peduncles.

Superior Cerebellar Peduncle

This structure, which is also referred to as the brachium conjunctivum, proceeds from the upper white substance of the cerebellar hemisphere to the tegmentum where it completely decussates at the level of the inferior colliculus. It is composed of:

Wallenberg's Syndrome	**QUICK FACTS 3**

This syndrome of symptoms can occur with damage or dysfunction to the posterior lateral medullary region from ischaemia or ablative stroke:

1. Ipsilateral Horner's syndrome
2. Contralateral loss of pain and temperature
3. Ipsilateral facial numbness
4. Nausea, vertigo, vomiting, and nystagmus
5. Ipsilateral cerebellar signs
6. Difficulty swallowing + hiccups

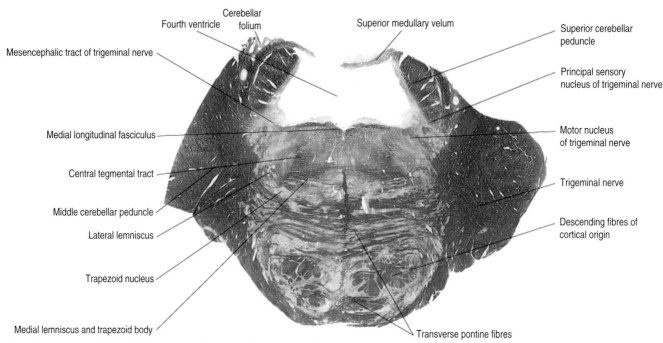

Fig. 13.7 A cross-sectional view of the pons at the level of the trigeminal nerves. (From Standring; Gray's Anatomy 39e. Elsevier Ltd 2005).

1. Dentatorubral and dentatothalamic fibres, both of which terminate contralaterally in the red nucleus and the thalamus, respectively;

2. Fibres of the ventral or anterior spinocerebellar tra ct projecting to the cerebellum from the spinal cord; and

3. Fibres of the uncinate fasciculus that contains fibres from the fastigial nucleus that will terminate in the lateral vestibular nucleus (Chusid 1982).

Anterior (Ventral) Spinocerebellar Tract

These tracts form bilateral structures that ascend in the spinal cord in the ventral lateral fasciculi. They terminate in the vermis and intermediate zones of the ipsilateral cerebellum. These tracts relay information to the cerebellum about what information or commands have arrived at the ventral horn cells. These pathways are part of the efference copy mechanism of the cerebellar motor system.

Lateral Lemnisci

This tract carries fibres from the contralateral dorsal cochlear nucleus to the inferior colliculus.

Middle Cerebellar Peduncle

These bilateral structures, which are also referred to as the brachium ponti, are the largest of the cerebellar peduncles. They carry fibres from the pontine nuclei to the contralateral neocerebellum. They are a component of the corticopontocerebellar pathways.

Reticular Formation

The reticular formation of the pons is continuous with the reticular formations of the medulla and the mesencephalon. This area receives input from virtually all areas of the neuraxis and projects widely throughout the neuraxis. (See below for more detail.)

Medial and Trigeminal Lemnisci

These structures were discussed earlier; see above.

Fourth Ventricle

This cavity is bounded by the pons and medulla ventrally and by the cerebellum dorsally. It is continuous with the cerebral aqueduct above and the central canal of the medulla below and has a capacity for cerebrospinal fluid (CSF) of about 20 ml. The floor of the fourth ventricle, which is also referred to as the rhomboid fossa, is formed by the dorsal surfaces of the pons and medulla. The fourth ventricle acts as a component of the CSF system (Chusid 1982).

Medulla

Structures of the medulla can be viewed by cross sections at:

1. Inferior olivary nuclei;
2. The lemniscal decussation; and
3. The pyramidal decussation.

Structures Found at a Cross Section at the Inferior Olive (Fig. 13.8)

Choroid Plexus of 4th

This structure is also referred to as the tela choroidea of the fourth ventricle and is composed of a layer of pia matter that has become highly vascularized. The choroid plexus produces CSF.

Nucleus Tractus Solitarius *CELLS OF* **QUICK FACTS 4**

The single most important component of the autonomic nervous system from a manipulatory point of view is the nucleus tractus solitarius (NTS, or solitary nucleus). The NTS receives afferent inputs from the viscera in addition to somatic and limbic structures and very heavy projections from the vestibular system. It mediates supraspinal visceral reflexes and contains a map of the viscera including the gastrointestinal system, cardiorespiratory system, and taste sensation.

Inferior Cerebellar Peduncle

These bilateral structures, which are also referred to as the restiform bodies, ascend laterally from the walls of the fourth ventricles to enter the cerebellum between the superior and middle cerebellar peduncles. They carry fibres of the following tracts:

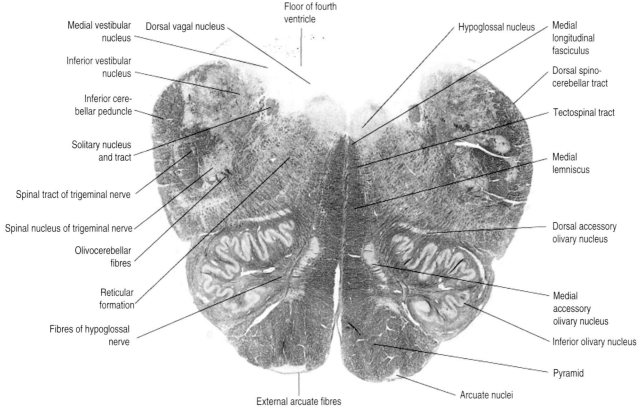

Fig. 13.8 A cross-sectional view of the medulla at the level of the inferior olive. (From Standring; Gray's Anatomy 39e. Elsevier Ltd 2005).

1. Olivocerebellar tract, which arises from neurons of the contralateral superior olivary nucleus and projects to the cerebellar hemispheres and vermis;

2. Dorsal spinocerebellar tract, which arises from neurons in the area of Clark's column of the spinal cord to project to the interpositus nuclear region and the palaeocerebellar cortex;

3. Dorsal external arcuate fibres from the nuclei gracilis and cuneatus;

4. Ventral external arcuate fibres from the lateral reticular nuclei of the medulla; and

5. Vestibulocerebellar tract, which arises from the vestibular nuclei and projects to the flocculonodular lobe of the cerebellum.

Cuneate Nucleus

These structures are located bilaterally, lateral and superior to the nuclei gracilis. They are composed of neurons that receive proprioceptive information from the arms and shoulders. Axons from these nuclei project via the internal arcuate fibres where they decussate to form the medial lemnisci projecting ultimately to the contralateral thalamus.

Lateral Spinothalamic Tract

These tracts are located medial and anterior to the ventral spinocerebellar tracts in the ventral lateral fasciculus of the spinal cord. They are formed by axons projecting from neurons located in the contralateral dorsal horn area. These neurons project their axons via the anterior white commissure to the opposite lateral spinothalamic tract where they terminate on the ipsilateral thalamus to the tract in which they ascend.

Inferior Olivary Nucleus

These bilateral groups of nuclei are located within the olive of the medulla. They receive projections from the cortex, from other brainstem nuclei, from the ipsilateral parvocellular red nucleus, and from the ipsilateral spinal cord. These neurons project axons, referred to as climbing fibres, via the inferior cerebellar peduncles to all areas of the cerebellar cortex. These structures are part of a group of projections and nuclei referred to as the inferior olivary nuclear complex, which forms a complicated loop from the cerebellar cortex to the dentate nucleus to the contralateral red nucleus to the inferior olivary nucleus and back to the contralateral cerebellar cortex (Fig. 13.9)

Dorsal Motor Nucleus of the Vagus Nerve (DMN)

These nuclei are located bilaterally, dorsal and lateral to the hypoglossal nuclei. These nuclei supply the preganglionic parasympathetic axons of the vagus and spinal accessory nerves.

Solitary Tract Nucleus

These nuclei are also referred to as the nuclei of the tractus solitarius (NTS). These nuclei are located ventrolaterally to the motor nuclei of the vagus nerve and run the full length of the medulla. All cranial visceral afferent nerves project to the NTS. The rostral portion of

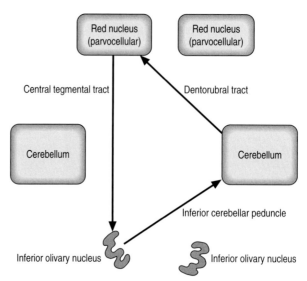

Fig. 13.9 The functional loop of the inferior olivary complex.

the NTS, which is referred to as the gustatory nucleus, receives projections from the special visceral afferent nerves (CN VII, CN IX, CN X) for taste. The caudal portion of the NTS, which is referred to as the cardiorespiratory nucleus, receives projections from the general visceral afferent fibres of CN IX and CN X.

Nucleus Ambiguus
These bilateral nuclei are located ventromedially to the spinal nucleus of the trigeminal nerve and run longitudinally throughout the medulla. The neurons of these nuclei supply the branchial motor output of the glossopharyngeal (CN IX), the vagus (CN X), and the spinal accessory (CN XI) nerves.

Vagus Nerve
These nerves exit the rostral medulla ventrolaterally from the pontomedullary junction as several rootlets between the inferior olive and the inferior cerebellar peduncle. The nerves exit the skull via the jugular foramen. The nerves supply the preganglionic parasympathetic output to all structures below the neck including the heart, lungs, pancreas, liver, kidneys, and gastrointestinal tract, and the branchial motor supply to the pharyngeal muscles and the muscles of the larynx.

Pyramids
These bilateral structures are found on the ventral surface of the medulla from the pontomedullary junction to the pyramidal decussation. They are formed by the axons of the motor output neurons of the cortex that largely involve the pyramidal neurons. These axons will form the corticospinal tracts of the spinal cord.

Hypoglossal Nerve
These nerves exit the medulla ventromedially between the pyramids and inferior olivary nuclei. The hypoglossal nerve exits the skull via the hypoglossal canal and supplies the motor axons to the tongue.

Hypoglossal Nucleus
These nuclei are located bilaterally near the ventral lateral portion of the central canal in the lower half of the medulla.

Structures Found in a Cross Section at the Lemniscal Decussation (Fig. 13.10)
Fasciculus Gracilis
These bilateral tracts run dorsally in the medulla medial to the cuneate fasciculi. They are formed by the axons of the dorsal root ganglion cells that detect proprioception and touch in the lower limbs and trunk usually below the T6 level. The axons enter the spinal cord via the dorsal root and ascend ipsilaterally in the fasciculus gracilis to the gracile nucleus.

Gracile Nucleus
These bilateral nuclei are located caudally and medially to the cuneate nuclei. These nuclei receive the axons of the fasciculus gracilis, which have arisen from the dorsal root ganglion cells detecting proprioception and touch in the lower limbs and trunk. The neurons project their axons via the internal arcuate fibres where they decussate and terminate in the contralateral ventral posterior lateral nucleus of the thalamus.

Fasciculus Cuneatus
These bilateral structures are located dorsally in the medulla, lateral to the fasciculus gracilis. They are formed by the axons of the dorsal root ganglion cells that detect proprioception and touch in the upper limbs and trunk usually above the T6 level. The axons enter the spinal cord via the dorsal root and ascend ipsilaterally in the fasciculus cuneatus to the cuneate nucleus.

Cuneate Nucleus
This structures was discussed earlier; see above.

Decussation of Lemnisci
Axons from the nucleus cuneatus and nucleus gracilis form the internal arcuate fibres that cross in the decussation and continue from there as the medial lemniscus.

Pyramid
This structure was discussed earlier; see above.

Medial Lemniscus
This structure was discussed earlier; see above.

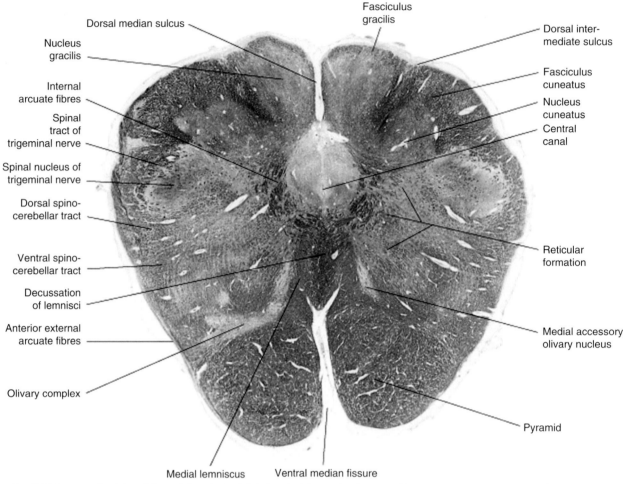

Fig. 13.10 A cross-sectional view of the medulla at the level of the lemniscal decussation. (From Standring; Gray's Anatomy 39e. Elsevier Ltd 2005).

Spinothalamic Tract
This structure was discussed earlier; see above.

Hypoglossal Nucleus
This structure was discussed earlier; see above.

Posterior and Anterior Spinocerebellar Tracts
These structures were discussed earlier; see above.

Structures Found at a Cross Section through Pyramidal Decussation (Fig. 13.11)

QUICK FACTS 5	The Parabrachial Nucleus

The parabrachial nucleus maintains reciprocal connections with the following systems:

- Vestibular system and midline cerebellum
- Cortical and subcortical visceral and limbic centres, including amygdala
- Somatic nuclei

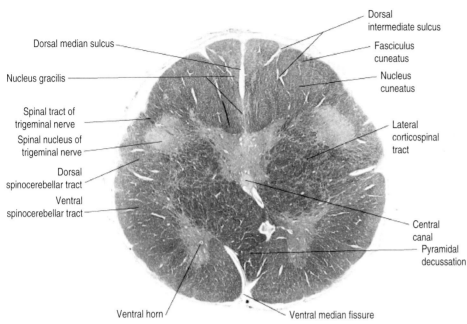

Fig. 13.11 A cross-sectional view of the medulla through pyramidal decussation. (From Standring; Gray's Anatomy 39e. Elsevier Ltd 2005).

Fasciculus Gracilis and Cuneatus
This structure was discussed earlier; see above.

Lateral Corticospinal Tract
This structure was discussed earlier; see above.

Pyramid
This structure was discussed earlier; see above.

Anterior Corticospinal Tracts
These bilateral tracts are contained in the pyramids of the medulla until the decussation of the pyramids where they do not decussate but continue ipsilaterally in the ventral medial portion of the ventral fasciculus of the spinal cord. These tracts relay motor information to the muscles of the trunk, spine, and proximal limbs.

Spinothalamic Tract
This structure was discussed earlier; see above.

Anterior and Posterior Spinocerebellar Tracts
These structures were discussed earlier; see above.

The Reticular Formation (RF)

The reticular formation receives little attention in traditional neurology textbooks. It is an area that spans all levels of the brainstem, from the thalamus to the spinal cord, and is responsible for integrating information from the brain and periphery and linking sensory, motor, and autonomic nuclei of the brainstem. The reticular formation therefore mediates complex reflexes and functions such as eye movements, posture, feeding, breathing, homeostasis, arousal, sleep, control of vasomotor tone and cardiac output, and pain. The reticular formation is composed of continuous groups of neurons interconnected via polysynaptic pathways that can be both crossed and uncrossed in nature. The RF receives projections from virtually all sensory modalities and projects to all areas of the neuraxis including direct projections to the cortex (Webster 1978).

The Cerebellopontine Angle

The cerebellopontine angle forms a triangle between the lateral aspect of the pons, the cerebellum, and the inner third of the petrous ridge of the temporal bone.

Cranial nerve (CN) V (motor) is at the rostral border while CN IX is at the caudal border. CN VI ascends at its medial edge, and CN VII and VIII traverse it before entering the internal auditory meatus.

Afferent projections to the RF include:

- Spinoreticular tracts;
- Spinothalamic tracts;
- Medial lemniscus;
- All cranial nerve nuclei;
- Cerebelloreticular tracts;
- Thalamoreticular tracts;
- Hypothalamoreticular tracts;
- Subthalamoreticular tracts;
- Corticoreticular tracts from frontal and parietal cortex; and
- Limboreticular projections.

Efferent projections from the RF include:

- Reticulobulbar tracts;
- Reticulospinal tracts;
- Projections to autonomic nuclei and intermediolateral (IML) column;
- Reticulocerebellar tracts;
- Reticulostriatal tracts;
- Reticulorubral tracts;
- Direct projections to the thalamus and cortex; and
- Direct projections to other areas of the reticular system.

Anatomy of the Reticular Formation

The neurons of the reticular formation form multiple interconnecting patterns that resemble a fish net; hence the name reticular, which means net-like. The neurons are located centrally in the neuraxis. The neurons can be roughly grouped into three columns

QUICK FACTS 7 **Pontomedullary Reticular Formation Functional Aspects**

There are four particular functions of the pontomedullary reticular formation (PMRF) that have particularly strong clinical relevance in practice:

1. Inhibits ipsilateral IML (sympathetic) output
2. Inhibits pain ipsilaterally
3. Inhibits the inhibition of all ventral horn cells (VHCs) ipsilaterally (facilitates muscle tone)
4. Inhibits ipsilateral anterior muscles above T6 and posterior muscles below T6

based on their size. The median column is located most centrally and is composed of intermediate-sized neurons. The medial column, which is just lateral to the median column, contains relatively large neurons. The lateral column is located most laterally and contains relatively small neurons (Fig. 13.12).

The neurons of the RF columns can be grouped into various nuclei which include the following (Fig. 13.12):

Median Column Nuclei

- Dorsal raphe nucleus;
- Superior central nucleus;
- Pontine raphe nucleus;
- Nucleus raphe magnus; and
- Nucleus obscures and pallidus.

Medial Column Nuclei

- Cuneiform and subcuneiform nuclei;
- Oral pontine reticular nucleus;
- Pontine tegmental reticular nucleus; and
- Nucleus gigantocellularis (magnocellularis).

Lateral Column Nuclei

- Pedunclulopontine tegmental nucleus pars compacta;
- Lateral parabrachial nucleus;
- Medial parabrachial nucleus;
- Central pontine nucleus; and
- Central medullary nucleus.

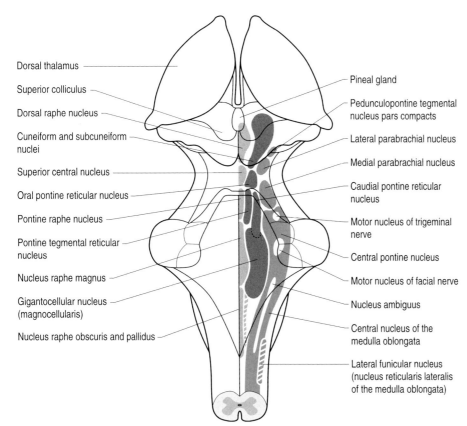

Fig. 13.12 The columnar structure of the reticular formation (RF) in the brainstem.

Reticular Neurons Projection Systems Utilize Different Neurotransmitters

Nuclear groups can also be identified based on the neurotransmitter that they release. Several projection systems have been discussed in detail in Chapter 9. Only those related to the reticular formation will be described here.

Cholinergic projection axons arise from neurons located in two areas of the pontomesencephalic region of the brainstem. The first group of neurons are located in the lateral portion of the reticular formation and periaqueductal grey areas in a nuclear group of neurons referred to as the pedunculopontine tegmental nuclei. The second group of neurons are located at the junction between the midbrain and pons referred to as the laterodorsal tegmental nuclei. Projection axons from both of these nuclear groups terminate in various nuclei, including the intralaminar nuclei of the thalamus.

Dopaminergic projection neurons arise from two pathways in the reticular nuclei. The mesolimbic projection pathway arises from neurons in the ventral tegmentum of the midbrain and projects to the medial temporal cortex, the amygdala, the cingulate gyrus, and the nucleus accumbens, all areas associated with the limbic system. Lesions or dysfunction of these projections are thought to contribute to the positive symptoms of schizophrenia such as hallucinations.

The mesocortical projection pathway arises from neurons in the ventral tegmental and substantia nigral areas of the midbrain and terminates in widespread areas of prefrontal cortex. The projections seem to favour motor cortex and association cortical areas over sensory and primary motor areas (Fallon & Loughlin, 1987).

The *noradrenergic projection system* consists of neurons in two different locations in the rostral pons and the lateral tegmental area of the pons and medulla. The neurons in the rostral pons area are referred to as the locus ceruleus and together with the neurons in the lateral tegmental area of the pons and medulla project to all areas of the entire forebrain including the limbic areas as well as to the cerebellum, brainstem, and spinal cord.

The *serotonergic projection system* consists of a group of nuclei in the midbrain pons and medulla referred to as the raphe nuclei and additional groups of neurons in the area postrema and caudal locus ceruleus. These nuclei can be divided into rostral and caudal groups. The rostral raphe nuclei project ipsilaterally via the median forebrain bundle to the entire forebrain where serotonin can act as either excitatory or inhibitory in nature, depending on the situation (Fallon & Loughlin 1987). The caudal raphe nuclei project to the cerebellum, medulla, and spinal cord.

The *histaminergic projection system* has only recently been identified. It consists of scattered neurons in the area of the midbrain reticular formation as well as a more defined group of neurons in the tuberomammillary nucleus of the hypothalamus.

Functions of the Reticular Formation

Functions of the reticular formation include the following:

1. *Modulation of motor control*—The RF can modulate the activation levels of both alpha and gamma motor neurons, and thus alter the tone and reflex activity of muscle. The RF is particularly involved with reciprocal inhibition of antagonist muscles and in the maintenance of muscle tone in antigravity muscles. Motor activity of the facial muscles associated with an emotional response is mediated by the RF. These pathways are independent of the corticobulbar tracts to the cranial nerve nuclei, and thus a person with a corticobulbar stroke can still smile symmetrically when stimulated emotionally.

    The *mesencephalic reticular formation* (MRF) is responsible for increasing flexor tone on the contralateral side. The *pontomedullary reticular formation* (PMRF) is responsible for the inhibition of ipsilateral anterior (flexor) muscles above T6, and the inhibition of ipsilateral posterior (flexor) muscles below T6.

2. *Modulation of somatic and visceral sensations*—The RF has the capacity to modulate all somatic and visceral sensations including pain. The PMRF in particular modulates the inhibition of pain.

3. *Modulation of the autonomic nervous system*—The RF is also involved with modulation of the activity of both sympathetic and parasympathetic functions of the autonomic nervous system. Activation of the MRF results in excitation of

the preganglionic sympathetic neurons of the IML bilaterally. Activation of the PMRF results in inhibition of the ipsilateral preganglionic neurons of the IML.

4. *Modulation of pituitary hormones*—The RF, through both direct and indirect pathways, modulates the output of releasing factors from the hypothalamus, thus modulating the release of pituitary hormones. The RF also influences the hypothalamic circadian and biological rhythm patterns.

5. *Modulation of reticular activation system*—The RF is also involved in the maintenance and level of consciousness through direct projections to wide areas of cortex. This projection system is referred to as the reticular activation system.

As an example of the complexity of the reticular formation, feeding reflexes such as chewing, sucking, salivating, swallowing, and licking are mediated via the pontomedullary reticular formation in conjunction with cranial nerves (CN) V, VII, IX, X, and XII. However, feeding behaviour can also be influenced by CN I, II, III, IV, VI, VIII, and XI as well as the MRF and mesolimbic reward centres—e.g. an infant responds to the stroke of a cheek by turning its head (CN IX, VIII and mesencephalic reticular formation) and performing sucking movements. Like animals, humans can respond to certain spatial characteristics such as the location of a stimulus such as food in the visual field. The odour and appearance of food and our satisfaction will be mediated by the reward centres. Respiratory reflexes such as phonation, sneezing, coughing, sighing, vomiting, and hiccupping are also mediated in the reticular formation.

Importantly, the relationship between the spine, vestibular system, midline cerebellum, cortex, limbic system, and the autonomic nervous system can be seen intimately in this region and may influence immune function and behavioural characteristics such as fear, anxiety, panic, mood, disinhibition, sleep, arousal, and risk taking.

Functional Systems and Clinical Implications of the Reticular System Dysfunction

The cortex projects to excite the MRF bilaterally and the PMRF ipsilaterally. The MRF then projects as described above to excite the IML and the flexor muscle groups bilaterally. Loss of functional integrity of the MRF would result in a decreased activation of the sympathetic nervous system bilaterally and decreased flexor tone bilaterally (Fig. 13.13).

The PMRF projects to inhibit the IML and flexor groups ipsilaterally (Fig. 13.14). Decreased PMRF integrity may therefore result in the following clinically relevant signs:

- Increased blood pressure;
- Increased V:A ratio;
- Increased sweating;
- Decreased skin temperature;
- Arrhythmia (L) or tachycardia (R);

Decreased PMRF Activation May Result in the Following Functional Affects — QUICK FACTS 8

- Increased blood pressure
- Increased V:A ratio
- Increased sweating
- Decreased skin temperature
- Arrhythmia (L) or tachycardia (R)
- Large pupil (also due to decreased mesencephalic integration)
- Ipsilateral pain syndromes
- Global decrease in muscle tone ipsilaterally
- Flexor angulation of the upper limb ipsilaterally
- Extensor angulation of the lower limb ipsilaterally

QUICK FACTS 9   **Cerebropontocerebellar Pathways**

These pathways constitute enormous axon projections of over 20 million fibres between the cerebral cortex and the cerebellum. Neurons synapse in the pontine nuclei before decussation. Signals from all areas of the cerebral cortex therefore reach the cerebellum via the pons and the contralateral middle cerebellar peduncle. The afferent (incoming) to efferent (outgoing) ratio in the cerebellum is approximately 40:1, making the cerebellum a major site of integration for the control of mental, motor, sensory, and autonomic functions.

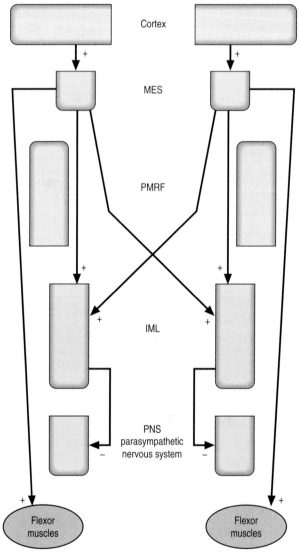

Fig. 13.13 Functional projections of the MRF and PMRF.

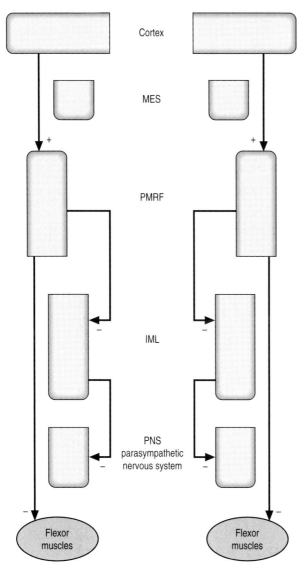

Fig. 13.14 Functional projections of the PMRF.

- Large pupil (also due to decreased mesencephalic integration);
- Ipsilateral pain syndromes;
- Global decrease in muscle tone ipsilaterally;
- Flexor angulation of the upper limb ipsilaterally;
- Extensor angulation of the lower limb ipsilaterally.

Cranial Nerves

The cranial nerves, with the exception of the olfactory (CN I) and optic (CN II), all arise from nuclei in the brainstem (Figs 13.15 and 13.16).

Olfactory Nerve (CN I)

Olfactory epithelium is bathed in lipid substance produced by Bowman's glands. Primary afferents synapse with mitral cells of the olfactory glomerulus after passing through the cribriform plate unmyelinated. Axons of mitral cells make up the olfactory nerve (Fig. 13.17).

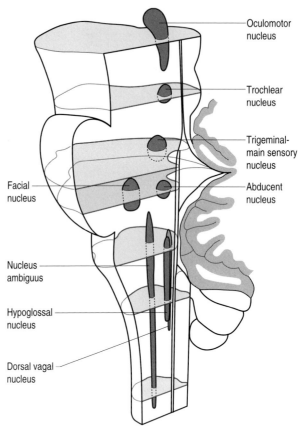

Fig. 13.15 A lateral view of the anatomical position and relationships of the cranial nerve nuclei.

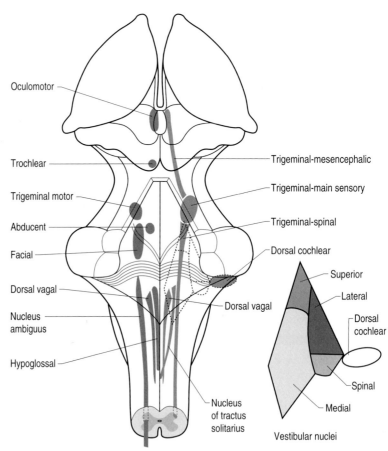

Fig. 13.16 A posterior view of the anatomical position and relationships of the cranial nerve nuclei.

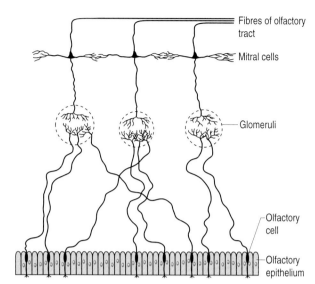

Fig. 13.17 The anatomy of the olfactory apparatus.

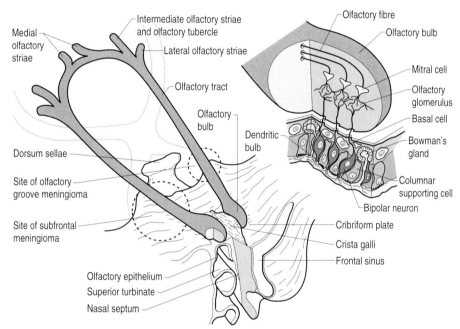

Fig. 13.18 The olfactory pathways and olfactory bulb.

The main tract has both centrifugal and centripetal fibres that help modulate receptor activity and enhance variety of perceived odours. The tract passes above the optic nerve and chiasm below the frontal lobes.

The tract terminates in three striae which synapse with neurons of the olfactory tubercle and gyrus, medial amygdaloid nucleus, and other limbic regions. The secondary olfactory cortex mediates along with the hypothalamus emotional and autonomic reflexes associated with smell (Moore 1980; Wilson-Pauwels et al 1988) (Fig. 13.18).

Optic Nerve (CN II)

Structurally the optic nerve is not a true nerve but a series of fibre projection tracts from the retina to the occipital cortex. The optic nerve proper is formed by the axons of the retinal ganglion cells. These axons then exit the retina via a nonreceptive area referred to as the optic disc to the optic chiasm where they are segregated into axons from right and left visual fields and become the optic tracts. The optic disc is located about 15° medially or towards the nose on each retina.

The optic tracts project to the lateral geniculate nucleus of the thalamus where they synapse. The projections of the axons from the thalamic neurons are referred to as the optic radiations. These axons terminate on the neurons in the visual cortex.

The visual image inverts and reverses as it passes through the lens of the eye and forms an image on the retina. Image from the upper visual field is projected on the lower retina and the lower visual field on the upper retina. The left visual field is projected to the right hemiretina of each eye in such a fashion that the right nasal hemiretina of the left eye and the temporal hemiretina of the right eye receive the image. The central image or focal point of the visual field falls on the fovea of the retina, which is the portion of the retina with the highest density of retinal cells and as such produces the highest visual acuity. The fovea receives the corresponding image of the central 1°–2° of the total visual field but represents about 50% of the axons in the optic nerve and projects to about 50% of the neurons in the visual cortex. The macula comprises the space surrounding the fovea and also has a relatively high visual acuity (Fig. 13.19).

The rods and cones are the primary receptors of light stimulation and are located at the deepest point on the retina adjacent to the pigment epithelial cells. They synapse with bipolar cells, which in turn synapse with the ganglion cells. The ganglion cells can be further classified as M cells, which have large receptive fields and respond best to movement, or P cells, which have small receptive fields and respond best to fine detail and colour (Fig. 13.20). Injury or dysfunction at any point along the optic nerves, tracts, or radiations can produce characteristic clinical visual field deficits (Fig. 13.21). Clinical testing of the optic nerve includes visual acuity and visual field testing (Moore 1980; Wilson-Pauwels et al 1988).

Oculomotor Nerve (CN III)

These nerves arise from the oculomotor nuclei of the midbrain and course through the red nucleus, exiting the skull through the superior orbit fissure to supply motor innervation of the superior rectus, inferior rectus, and medial rectus muscles of the eye. Parasympathetic fibres from the Edinger-Westphal nucleus also accompany the axons of these nerves to supply the parasympathetic component (Moore 1980, Wilson-Pauwels et al 1988) (Fig. 13.22).

Trochlear Nerve (CN IV)

These nerves arise from the trochlear nuclei located just caudal from the oculomotor nuclei at the level of the inferior colliculi. The axons exit posteriorly and cross in the anterior medullary velum and wind around the cerebral peduncles to exit the skull through the superior orbital fissure and innervate the superior oblique muscles of the eye (Moore 1980; Wilson-Pauwels et al 1988).

Normal Fundus

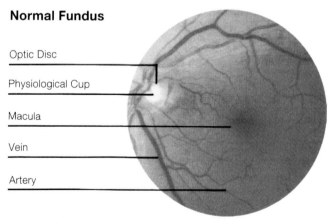

Optic Disc

Physiological Cup

Macula

Vein

Artery

Fig. 13.19 The appearance of a normal fundus.

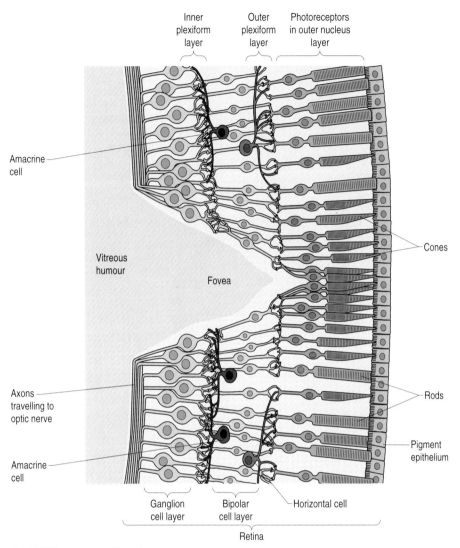

Fig. 13.20 The anatomy of the retina.

Abducens Nerve (CN VI)

These axons arise from nuclei in the floor of the fourth ventricle in the caudal portion of the pons. The axons course through the pons and exit anteriorly to run along the petrous portion of the temporal bone to the outer wall of the cavernous sinus, where the nerve exits the skull through the superior orbital fissure to supply motor innervation to the lateral rectus muscle (Moore 1980; Wilson-Pauwels et al 1988).

Control of Eye Movement

In order to understand oculomotor control it is necessary to remember that all eye movements are designed to keep a desired object centred on the fovea, which allows for the greatest visual acuity. In order for the desired object to be clearly visualized, it must be held relatively steady on the fovea, and the two eyes must be simultaneously aligned to within a few minutes of arc (Leigh & Zee 1992). Understanding normal function allows us to have a better understanding of when and why abnormal eye movements occur. The normal tendency of the eyeball is to return to primary position. To hold the eyeball in any other position requires constant contraction of the extraocular muscles in exactly the right proportions.

When the eye moves to a new target it does so by a movement called a saccade, which is a fast, burst-like movement. Saccades can reach velocities of 700° per second and vision is transiently suppressed during saccadic movements. The saccade is programmed with two distinct components, a pulse phase and a step phase. The pulse

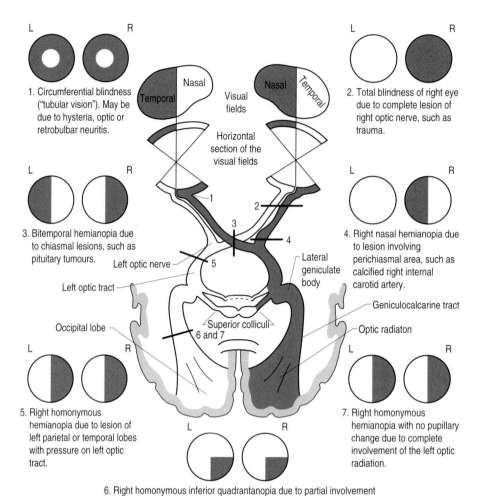

1. Circumferential blindness ("tubular vision"). May be due to hysteria, optic or retrobulbar neuritis.

2. Total blindness of right eye due to complete lesion of right optic nerve, such as trauma.

3. Bitemporal hemianopia due to chiasmal lesions, such as pituitary tumours.

4. Right nasal hemianopia due to lesion involving perichiasmal area, such as calcified right internal carotid artery.

5. Right homonymous hemianopia due to lesion of left parietal or temporal lobes with pressure on left optic tract.

7. Right homonymous hemianopia with no pupillary change due to complete involvement of the left optic radiation.

6. Right homonymous inferior quadrantanopia due to partial involvement of optic radiations (upper portion of left optic radiation in this case).

Nasal
Visual fields
Temporal
Horizontal section of the visual fields
Left optic nerve
Left optic tract
Occipital lobe
Lateral geniculate body
Geniculocalcarine tract
Superior colliculi
Optic radiaton

Fig. 13.21 Visual field defects associated with lesions of visual system.

phase is the burst of action potential activity to move the eye to the new target. The step phase is the new action potential firing rate to maintain the eye in the new position (Fig. 13.23).

Saccades can be horizontal or vertical in nature. The burst phase of activity for a *horizontal saccade* is generated by burst neurons in the pontine paramedian reticular formation. The duration of firing of a burst neuron begins just before the saccade and ends exactly when the saccade enters the step phase. In between burst outputs, the burst neurons are tonically inhibited by omnipause neurons in the nucleus raphe interpositus (Buttner-Ennever et al 1988). The omnipause neurons continuously discharge, inhibiting the burst neurons until they enter a pause cycle in which the burst neurons become disinhibited and fire a burst of action potentials that results in a saccade motion of the eye until the pause neurons resume their firing and inhibit the burst neurons. The step phase of the horizontal saccade is thought to be created by a neural gaze maintenance network or neural integrator that calculates the saccadic velocity to produce the appropriate position and to produce the appropriate contraction in the extraocular muscles to maintain the gaze at a specific point. The medial vestibular nucleus, the flocculus of the cerebellum, and the nucleus prepositus hypoglossi are important components of the neural integration system of horizontal movements (Zee et al 1981; Cannon & Robinson 1987) (Fig. 13.24).

The burst phase of activity for a *vertical saccade* is generated by burst neurons in the rostral interstitial nucleus of the medial longitudinal fasciculus (riMLF) (Buttner-Ennever et al 1988). This nucleus is located ventral to the aqueduct of Sylvius in the prerubral fields at the junction of the mesencephalon and the thalamus. The activity in this nucleus is dependent on ascending projections from the pontine paramedian reticular formation,

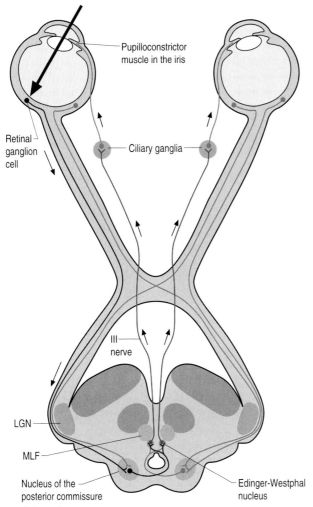

Fig. 13.22 The course of the oculomotor nerves.

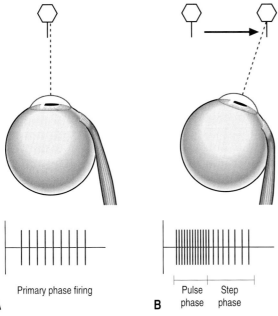

Fig. 13.23 Nerve activation phases of eye movements.

347

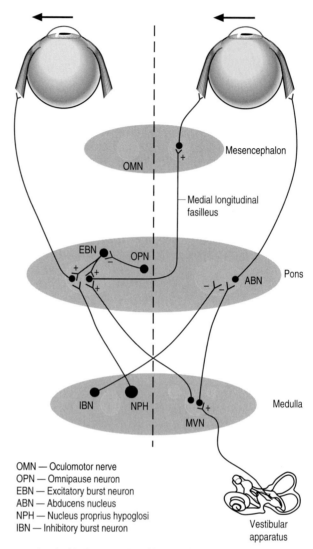

OMN — Oculomotor nerve
OPN — Omnipause neuron
EBN — Excitatory burst neuron
ABN — Abducens nucleus
NPH — Nucleus proprius hypoglosi
IBN — Inhibitory burst neuron

Fig. 13.24 The components involved in the generation of horizontal eye movements.

omnipause neurons in the nucleus raphe interpositus, and inputs from the contralateral vestibular nuclei. The riMLF projects to the ipsilateral oculomotor (CN III) and trochlear (CN IV) nuclei. Reciprocal connections occur between the right and left riMLF through the posterior and anterior commissures of the midbrain. The fibres of the elevator nuclei which innervate the superior rectus and the inferior oblique muscles pass through the posterior commissural pathways, and the projections to the depressor nuclei innervating the inferior rectus and superior oblique muscles pass through the anterior commissural pathways. The velocity commands of vertical saccadic movements are integrated by the interstitial nucleus of Cajal (Fukushima et al 1990) (Fig. 13.25).

Cortical Modulation of Saccadic Eye Movements
Cortical modulation of saccadic eye movements is also a necessary component for normal vision. The frontal lobe contains three areas that contribute to saccadic control; these are the frontal eye fields (FEF), the supplementary eye fields, and the dorsal lateral prefrontal cortex. The FEF are composed of a group of neurons in the posterior areas of Broadmann area 8 that discharge prior to saccadic movement and are thought to play a part in the initiation of saccades to previously seen or remembered targets (Bruce & Goldberg 1985). Excitation of these neurons results in contralateral saccades. Neurons in the supplementary FEF which are located in the dorsomedial frontal lobes are involved in programming saccades as part of complex learned behaviours (Mann et al 1988). The dorsal lateral prefrontal cortex is involved with programming saccades to remembered target locations (Boch & Goldberg 1989).

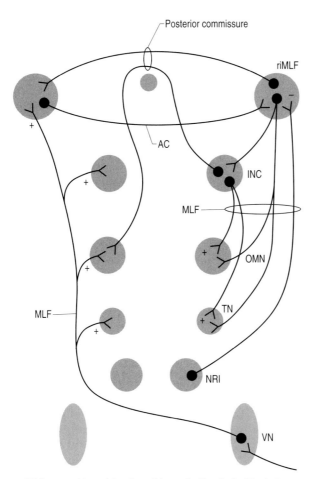

riMLF — rostral interstial nucleus of the medical longitudinal fasciculus
INC — interstitial nucleus of cajal
MLF — medial longitudinal fasciculus
OMN — oculomotor nucleus
NRI — Nucleus raphe interpositus
AC — anterior commissure
TN — trochlear nucleus

Fig. 13.25 The components involved in the generation of vertical eye movements.

Control of Smooth Pursuit

Smooth pursuit movements allow viewing of moving objects. They are much slower than saccades and can reach a maximum velocity of only 100° per second. They are not under voluntary control. Smooth pursuit activities seem to be modulated in the middle and superior medial temporal visual areas. These areas of cortex project to the dorsal lateral median pontine nuclei (Suzuki et al 1990). The dorsal lateral median pontine nuclei project to the flocculus, uvula, and dorsal of the cerebellum where the smoothness of the motion is calculated and adjusted.

Cerebellar Influences on Eye Movements

The cerebellum is involved in two basic operations involving eye control. The first involves its role in both real time positional eye control with respect to visual acquisition, and the second involves long-term adaptive control mechanisms regulating the oculomotor system (Leigh & Zee 1991).

The cerebellum functions to ensure that the movements of the eyes are appropriate for the stimulation that they are receiving. The flocculus of the vestibulocerebellum contains Purkinje cells that discharge in relation to the velocity of eye movements during smooth pursuit tracking, with the head either stationary or moving. For example, you can keep your head still and fixate your gaze on a moving object; in which case your eyes should smoothly follow the object across your visual field. Or you could keep your eyes fixed on a stationary object and rotate your head; in which case your eyes should still smoothly track in the opposite direction and at the same speed as the rotation of your head to maintain the target in focus (Zee et al 1981). Other neurons discharge during saccadic eye movement in relation to the position of the eye in the orbit. Individual control of eye movement is accomplished for the most part by the contralateral cerebellum although intimate bilateral integration is also important. For example the smoothness of pursuit activity and the return to centre function of saccadic movement of the right eye are under left cerebellar modulatory control.

Disorders of Saccadic Eye Movement
Disorders of saccadic eye movements can involve the accuracy, velocity, latency, and stability of the eye movements.

QUICK FACTS 10	The Corneal Reflex

Fig. 13.26 The corneal reflex.

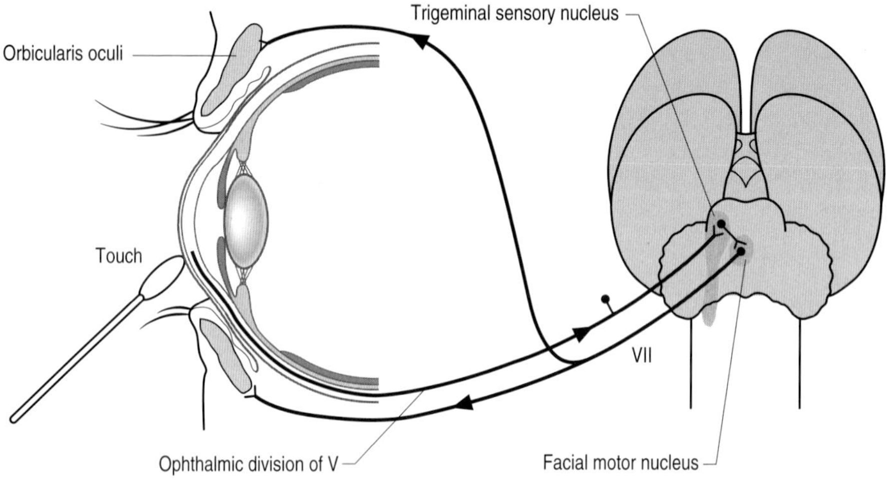

1. Saccadic dysmetria occurs when the saccade over- or undershoots the target. This type of lesion is characteristic of lesions of the dorsal vermis or fastigial nuclei of the cerebellum. In Wallenburg's syndrome a specific dysmetric pattern that involves overshooting saccades to the side of the lesion and undershooting saccades to the contralateral side occurs. When pure vertical saccades are attempted there is an inappropriate horizontal component to the saccade that results in the eye drifting towards the side of the lesion (Ranalli & Sharpe 1986).

2. Decreases in velocity of the saccade are usually related to dysfunction of the burst neurons. Slow horizontal saccades involve the horizontal burst neurons in the pons, and slow vertical saccades involve the vertical burst neurons in the midbrain. Diseases such as olivopontocerebellar atrophy and progressive supranuclear palsy can affect these neurons respectively.

3. A mismatch between the pulse phase and the step phase of saccadic movement can result in postsaccadic drift of the eyes or glissades. This condition occurs with dysfunction of the vestibulocerebellar inputs.

4. A combination of slow, hypometric saccades and glissades can occur with disorders such as ocular nerve palsies, myasthenia gravis, and ocular myopathies.

5. Saccades that exhibit an increased latency of action may be caused by dysfunction of the frontal or parietal lobes. They have been reported in Huntington's disease, supranuclear palsies, and Alzheimer's disease.

6. Saccadic oscillations are referred to as ocular flutter when they are limited to the horizontal plane and opsoclonus when they are multidirectional in nature such as vertical and/or torsional. These lesions have been reported with various types of encephalitis and neuroblastomas and in association with certain toxins.

Disorders of Smooth Pursuit

Disorders of smooth pursuit are often associated with dysfunction of the cerebellum or brainstem. Slow jerky pursuit motion can be associated with physiological decreases in activation due to medication or decreased cerebellar stimulation.

Nystagmus is a repetitive to and fro movement of the eyes that can be generated by watching moving targets such as occurs when looking out the window of a moving car or by moving an object such as an opticokinetic tape past an individuals eye. When nystagmus occurs inappropriately it reflects dysfunction in the mechanisms that hold targets steady on the fovea of the retina. These mechanisms involve areas of the vestibular system, the neural integrator, and pursuit control systems. A variety of nystagmic patterns can be observed and related to specific dysfunctional areas.

1. Lesions or dysfunction of the peripheral vestibular apparatus usually produce horizontal nystagmus with the slow phase towards the side of the lesion.

2. Up-beating nystagmus usually represents a lesion or dysfunction in pontomedullary or pontomesencephalic junction or areas surrounding the forth ventricle.

3. Down-beating nystagmus usually reflects disease or dysfunction of areas around the craniocervical junction such as Arnold-Chiari malformations or degenerative lesions of the cerebellum.

Trigeminal Nerve (CN V)

Trigeminal nerve has three projection divisions that supply different areas of the head and face. The ophthalmic division supplies sensation from the midpoint of the eyes to the apex of the frontal skull at the level of the ears. The maxillary division supplies the nasal mucosa and the skin from the upper lip to the inferior halve of the eye. The mandibular division supplies the internal mouth, tongue, teeth, skin of lower jaw, and part of the external ear and auditory meatus and meninges. The sensory neurons are located in the semilunar or Gasserian ganglion. Motor neurons in the motor nucleus of the trigeminal nerve, which is located in the mid-pons area, supply motor innervation to the muscles of mastication, which include the masseter, temporal, internal, and external pterygoid muscles. Neurons in the otic ganglion supply motor fibres to the tensor tympani and tensor veli palatine. Fibres of the trigeminal nerve also supply motor to the mylohyoid muscle and the anterior belly of the digastric muscle via the mylohyoid nerve (Moore 1980; Wilson-Pauwels et al 1988). Fibres of the ophthalmic division relay sensation of the cornea and are involved in the afferent loop of the corneal reflex (see Chapter 4) (Fig. 13.27).

Facial Nerve (CN VII)

The facial nerve supplies motor innervation to the muscles of facial expression. The neurons of the facial nerve are located in the facial nerve nuclei in the caudal pons. The facial nerve exits the brainstem ventrolaterally at the pontomedullary junction; it then travels along the subarachnoid space until it enters the internal auditory meatus and travels via the auditory canal to the facial canal where it then exits the skull via the stylomastoid foramen. The facial nerve acts as the efferent arm of the corneal reflex by supplying the muscles around the eye. The geniculate ganglion lies in the genu of the facial nerve and houses the neurons that receive taste sensation from the anterior two-thirds of the ipsilateral tongue.

The parasympathetic efferent projections of the facial nerve arise from the nervous intermedius and involve motor axons to the submandibular gland and the lacrimal gland. The motor fibres project in two different pathways and to two different ganglia. The motor projections to the *submandibular gland* arise from neurons in the superior salivatory nucleus in the medulla. The axons of these neurons emerge from the brainstem in the nervous intermedius and join the facial nerve until the stylomastoid foramen where they separate as the chorda tympani, which traverse the tympanic cavity until they reach and join with the lingual nerve. They travel with the lingual nerve until they reach and synapse on the postganglionic neurons of the submandibular ganglion. The axons from these neurons project to the submandibular glands via the lingual nerve supplying the secretomotor fibres to the gland. Activation of the postganglionic neurons results in dilatation of the arterioles of the gland and increased production of saliva (Moore 1980; Wilson-Pauwels et al 1988) (Fig. 13.28).

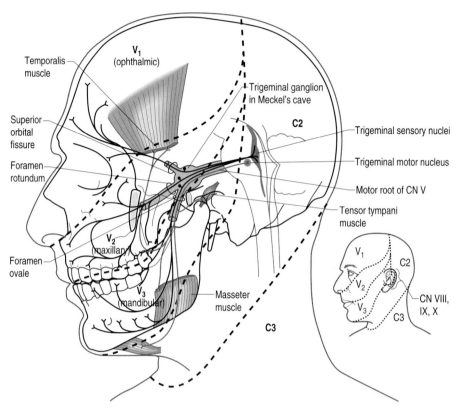

Fig. 13.27 Distribution of the trigeminal nerve (CN V).

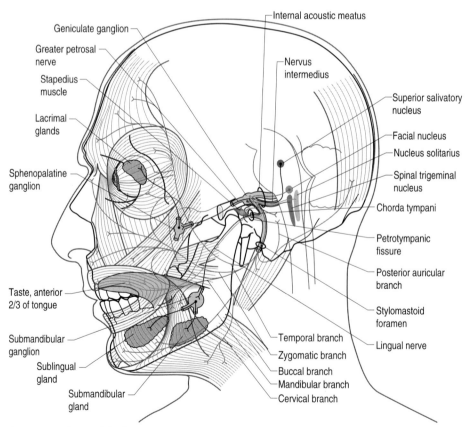

Fig. 13.28 Distribution of the facial nerve (CN VII) sensory and motor pathways.

Vestibulocochlear Nerve (CN VIII)

The vestibulocochlear nerve as the name implies is composed of two separate nerve supplies, the vestibular portion and the cochlear portion.

The axons from the hair cells of the utricle synapse in the superior vestibular ganglion. The axons of the neurons in the superior vestibular ganglion then form the superior vestibular nerve. These axons contribute along with the axons of the inferior vestibular nerve from the saccule and the cochlear nerve to form the ipsilateral vestibulocochlear nerve (see Chapter 14).

The cochlear nerves arise from the axons of the bipolar cells of the spiral ganglion which terminate in the ventral or dorsal cochlear nucleus (Moore 1980; Wilson-Pauwels et al 1988).

The Cochlea

The Cochlea consists of three fluid-filled tubes in helical arrangement called the scala media, scala tympani, and scala vestibuli. The conduction of sound pressure waves occurs as the stapes, which acts as a piston on the round window, depresses the cochlear partition, which increases pressure in scala tympani. This increase in pressure results in an outward bowing of the round window. Any up and down motion of fluid is detected by the basilar membrane between the scala tympani and media.

Organ Of Corti

The organ of Corti contains 16,000 hairs cells in four rows arranged as one inner row and three outer rows. The hair cells project into the gelatinous tectorial membrane and together support approximately 30,000 afferent nerve fibres and numerous efferent fibre terminals. Movement of the hair cells towards the tall edge results in excitation, whereas movement away from the tall edge or downward deflection results in inhibition.

Mechanical Transduction

The stapes footplate acts as a piston that pushes and pulls, causing a conduction of pressure waves through the fluid of the scala vestibuli. The pressure waves depress the cochlear partition, causing increase in pressure in the scala tympani and outward bowing of the round window. Up and down motion of the fluid is transmitted to the basilar membrane, resulting in deflection of the stereocilia on hair cells. Ca^{++} and K^+ enter through channels at the tips of stereocilia ('gating springs' or 'tip links'), resulting in a receptor potential. Hair cells of vestibular and cochlear apparatus transduce sound and accelerations into electrical responses. They act as synaptic terminals by releasing chemical neurotransmitters to activate nerve fibre terminals when ion channels are opened by mechanical bending of stereocilia. The afferent fibres encode intensity, time course, and frequency.

The Ventral Cochlear Nucleus (VCN)

The ventral cochlear nucleus is composed of two main cell types, the stellate cells, which are also known as chopper cells and give a steady regular rhythm of impulses denoting stimulus frequency, and the bushy cells, which generate only one action potential and signify the onset of sound. Therefore, they provide accurate information about the timing of acoustic stimuli and are involved in locating sound stimuli along the horizontal axis (azimuthal).

The various cell types of the cochlear nuclei project along parallel pathways to specific relay nuclei that serve a common purpose. The VCN comprises two main divisions which include:

1. *Anteroventral cochlear nucleus*—This division has the most prominent output and projects via the ventral acoustical stria and the trapezoid body to the superior olivary complex (medial and lateral divisions). The anteroventral cochlear nucleus receives input from the ascending branch of the cochlear nerve.

2. *Posteroventral cochlear nucleus*—This division contributes axons to the trapezoid body and to the lateral superior olive via the intermediate acoustical stria.

The Dorsal Cochlear Nucleus (DCN)

The DCN may be an important site of early auditory processing implicated in the physiology of tinnitus. In laboratory animals, the DCN has been found to comprise the following three layers that are parallel to the free surface of the brainstem:

1. Molecular layer;

2. Fusiform cell layer; and

3. Deep DCN layer.

The first and second layers are sometimes referred to as the superficial layers of the DCN. The molecular layer consists predominately of parallel fibres formed by the axons of granule cells and inhibitory interneurons including cartwheel and stellate cells. The anatomic organization of the superficial layers of the DCN is therefore considered to be similar in many ways to that of the cerebellar folium.

The superficial layers of the DCN receive both auditory and nonauditory information including vestibular afferents, which are primarily from the saccule and somatosensory inputs. Within the superficial layer, the granule cells form excitatory connections with type IV units and inhibitory interneurons (especially cartwheel cells). In turn, the cartwheel cells form inhibitory connections on the type IV units. Type IV units are the output cells of the DCN and project to other components of the extralemniscal pathway as well as some neurons within the lemniscal pathway. Increased FOF of type IV units has been associated with the expression of tinnitus episodes and these neurons are exquisitely sensitive to sound. In the deeper layers of the DCN there are two inhibitory interneuronal circuits that have been identified:

1. Type II units (thought to arise from vertical cells in the deep DCN region); and
2. Wideband inhibitors with evidence pointing to cells in the posteroventral cochlear nucleus (PVCN) region.

Type II units have very low spontaneous rates of firing and give weak responses to broadband noise. They primarily respond to best frequency tones and provide inhibition to type IV units of the DCN. They are also thought to form inhibitory connections with bushy and multipolar cells of the VCN.

Medial Superior Olive (MSO)

This nuclear area localizes sound sources along the horizontal axis by distinguishing interaural time delays as small as $10\,\mu s$, and hence location to a few degrees.

A source in the midsagittal plane should excite two ears at the same time. Axon terminals from the contralateral anterior ventral cochlear nucleus (AVCN) excite successive neurons throughout the medial superior olive. Input from one ear is insufficient to bring an MSO neuron to threshold, so the interaural time difference is exactly counterbalanced by delay in conduction from the opposite ear.

Therefore, the simultaneous excitatory sound potential brings an MSO neuron to threshold and a map of sound source location along the horizontal axis is formed over an array of MSO neurons.

Lateral Superior Olive (LSO)

This area is also involved in localization of sound but employs intensity cues rather than interaural time differences to calculate where a sound originated.

The LSO receives input from both cochlear nuclei such that ipsilateral inputs are direct and contralateral inputs from the sound source are via the nucleus of the trapezoid body. These inputs are antagonistic.

A given neuron in the LSO responds best when the intensity of a stimulus reaching one ear exceeds that on the opposite ear by a particular amount. The lateral olive is more efficient at processing high-frequency sounds because the head absorbs short wavelengths better than long wavelengths. This allows for clearer interaural intensity differences. Low-frequency sounds are processed more efficiently by the medial olive.

Inferior Colliculus

The lateral lemniscus includes axons from the superior olivary nucleus and the contralateral DCN via the dorsal acoustic stria. It provides passage for neurons to the inferior colliculus. The inferior colliculus consists of a dorsal region that receives both auditory and somatosensory inputs, and a central nucleus that comprises several layers forming a tonotopic map.

The multimodal division is sometimes referred to as the external nucleus of the inferior colliculus in research papers and forms part of the extralemniscal pathway.

Medial Geniculate Nucleus (MGN)

The central nucleus of the inferior colliculus projects by way of the brachium of the inferior colliculus to the principal nucleus of the MGN. The principal nucleus of the MGN projects its neurons to the primary auditory area (A1 or 41, 42) on the transverse gyri of Heschl. The remaining components of the MGN are multimodal and form part of the extralemniscal pathway.

Plasticity in the Auditory Cortex

Consider the role of either hemisphere in the processing of auditory inputs from either field of space. This is analogous to the independent ocular dominance columns of the visual system.

Tinnitus has been referred to as a phantom auditory sensation that may occur because of reorganization of the auditory cortex following some degree of deafferentation from the cochlear of the inner ear. Cochlear lesions resulting in loss of a specific range of frequencies can lead to reorganization of the auditory cortex due to replacement of the corresponding cortical areas with neighbouring areas of sound representation (McIntosh & Gonzalez-Lima, 1998).

Glossopharyngeal Nerve (CN IX)

These nerves exit the brainstem as several rootlets along the upper ventrolateral medulla, just below the exiting rootlets of the vestibulocochlear nerves, inferior to the pontomedullary junction. The nerves then course through the subarachnoid space to exit the skull via the jugular foramen. The nerves subserve a variety of functions including (Moore 1980; Wilson-Pauwels et al 1988) (Fig. 13.29):

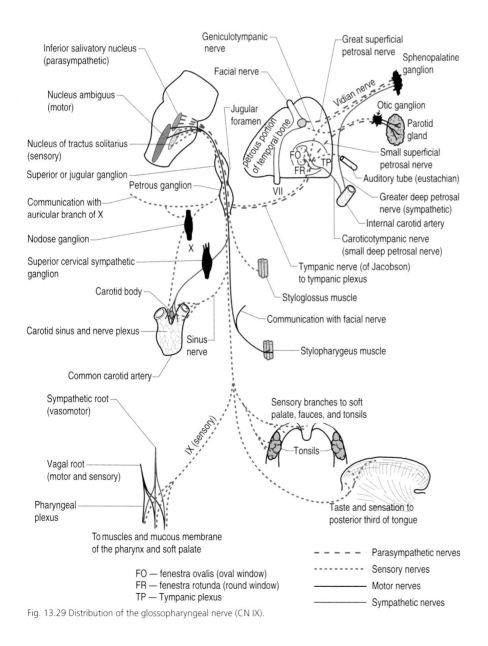

Fig. 13.29 Distribution of the glossopharyngeal nerve (CN IX).

1. The sensation of taste from the posterior third of the tongue via the rostral nucleus solitarius or the gustatory nucleus;

2. Information concerning blood pressure and blood gases via baroreceptors and chemoreceptors in the carotid body via the caudal nucleus solitarius or the cardiorespiratory nucleus;

3. The sensations relating to touch, pain, and temperature from the middle ear, external auditory meatus, pharynx, and posterior third of the tongue via the inferior and superior glossopharyngeal ganglia;

4. Parasympathetic supply to the parotid glands via the inferior salivatory nucleus, the lesser petrosal nerve, and the otic ganglia; and

5. Motor supply to the stylopharyngeus muscle via the nucleus ambiguus of the medulla.

Vagus Nerve (CN X)

The vagus nerves exit the ventral lateral medulla between the inferior olives and the inferior cerebellar peduncles. These nerves then course through the subarachnoid space to exit the skull via the jugular foramen.

QUICK FACTS 11   **Control of Blood Pressure during a Change in Posture**

Fig. 13.30 Control of blood pressure during a change in posture.

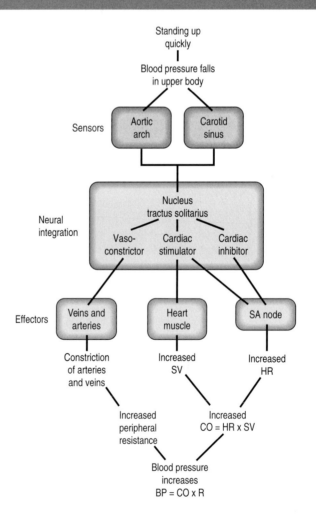

The *branchial motor projections*, which include motor supply to the muscles of the pharynx and larynx, arise from the nucleus ambiguous of the medulla. The branchial motor component includes the pharyngeal muscles responsible for the gag reflex and swallowing, and the laryngeal muscles that control the vocal cords. The laryngeal muscles are innervated by two branches of the vagus nerve, the recurrent laryngeal nerve, and the superior laryngeal nerve. The recurrent larngeal nerve is clinically important because it loops down around the aorta before ascending to the larynx and may be affected by cardiac or aortic involvement leading to a change or harshness in voice tone (Figs 13.31 and 13.32).

The *parasympathetic motor projections* of the vagus nerve arise from the neurons of the dorsal motor nucleus. The *cardiac branches* are inhibitory, and in the heart they act to slow the rate of the heartbeat. The *pulmonary branch* is excitatory and in the lungs they act as a broncho constrictor as they cause the contraction of the nonstriate muscles of the bronchi. The *gastric branch* is excitatory to the glands and muscles of the stomach but inhibitory to the pyloric sphincter. The *intestinal branches*, which arise from the postsynaptic neurons of the mesenteric plexus or Auerbach's plexus and the plexus of the submucosa or Meissner's plexus, are excitatory to the glands and muscles of the intestine, caecum, vermiform appendix, ascending colon, right colic flexure, and most of the transverse colon but inhibitory to the ileocaecal sphincter (Fig. 13.31). The ganglia for most of the vagal distribution occur in close association to the effector organs and are referred to as terminal ganglia.

The *general somatic sensory projections* of the vagus detect pain, temperature, and touch sensations in the pharynx, infratentorial meninges, and a small region of the external auditory meatus. The neuron cell bodies are located in the inferior or nodose ganglion and the superior or jugular ganglion. These ganglia are comparable to the dorsal root ganglion of the spinal cord (Fig. 13.31).

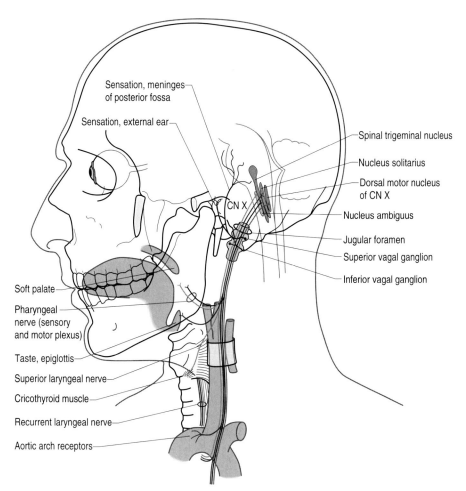

Fig. 13.31 The branchial motor projections of the vagus nerve (CN X).

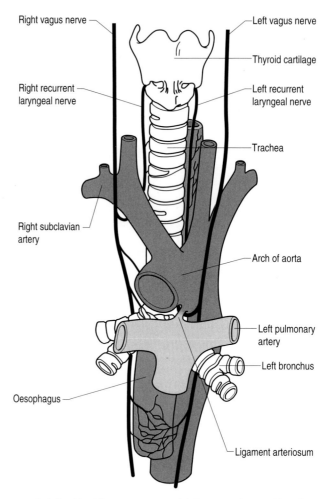

Fig. 13.32 The course and relationship of the vagus nerves and their recurrent laryngeal branches.

The *visceral sensory projections* of the vagus carry taste sensations from the epiglottis and pharynx to the rostral nucleus solitarius (gustatory centre), and chemo- and baroreceptor input from the aortic arch receptors to the caudal nucleus solitarius (cardiorespiratory centre). The neuron cell bodies are located mainly in the inferior or nodose ganglia (Moore 1980; Wilson-Pauwels et al 1988) (Fig. 13.31).

Accessory Nerve (CN XI)

These nerves are sometimes referred to as the spinal accessory nerves because some the projection fibres arise in the cervical spine and ascend to exit the skull via the jugular foramen in association with the cranial branches, which are accessory to the vagus nerves. The accessory nerves are formed by the union of the cranial and spinal projection axons but they are associated for only a very brief portion of their course. The cranial portion of the nerve arises in the caudal nucleus ambiguus and exits the lateral surface of the medulla to course via the jugular foramen, where it joins the vagus nerve on exiting. The cranial portion of the nerve supplies motor innervation to the wall of the larynx and pharynx. The spinal portion of the nerves arises in a column of neurons located in the anterior horn of the first five or six cervical segments referred to as the spinal accessory nuclei. The spinal roots exit the spinal cord laterally between the dorsal and ventral roots of the spinal cord to form a trunk that ascends in the subarachnoid space of the spinal canal, through the foramen magnum to exit the skull through the jugular foramen. The spinal portion of the nerve supplies two superficial muscles of the neck, the sternocleidomastoid and trapezius muscles (Fig. 13.33) (Moore 1980; Wilson-Pauwels et al 1988). The sternocleidomastoid muscles turn the head in the opposite direction.

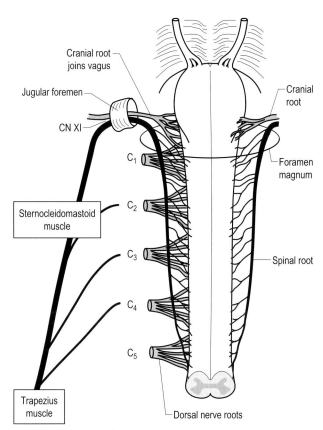

Fig. 13.33 Distribution of the spinal root of the accessory nerve (CN XI).

So the right sternocleidomastoid muscle turns the head to the left. This is important clinically because a lower motor neuron lesion of the CN XI nerve will result in an ipsilateral shoulder shrug weakness and a weakness in turning the head to the side opposite the shoulder shrug weakness. The upper motor neuron projections are thought to project to the ipsilateral spinal accessory nuclei, which would also result in weakness of ipsilateral shoulder shrug and turning the head away from the side of the lesion (Blumenfeld 2002).

The Hypoglossal Nerve (CN XII)

The hypoglossal nerves arise from the hypoglossal nuclei posterior part of the floor of the fourth ventricle in the medulla. These nerves exit the medulla between the olive and the pyramid and course through the subarachnoid space to exit the skull via the hypoglossal canal of the occipital bone. The many rootlets that have exited the medulla unite as they emerge from the hypoglossal canal and then course posterior to the vagus nerve, where they pick up fibres from the cervical roots of C1 and C2 spinal levels. The hypoglossal nerves supply the motor innervation to the tongue, and send collateral branches to the sympathetic trunk and the lingual nerves (Moore 1980; Wilson-Pauwels et al 1988) (Fig. 13.34).

Clinical Testing of Cranial Nerves

Clinical testing of cranial nerves is covered in detail in Chapter 4. I will include a brief overview here for completeness.

When performing the neurological examination it is most important to remember the functional relationships between the cranial nerves and the various levels of the neuraxis, including the reticular formation and lobes of the brain and cerebellum (Table 13.1).

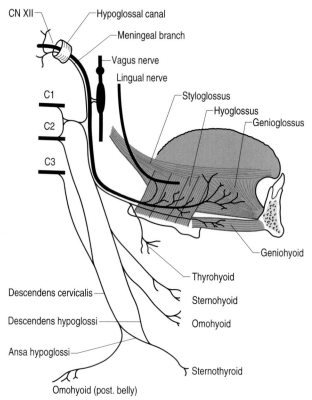

Fig. 13.34 Distribution of the hypoglossal nerve (CN XII).

Brainstem Respiratory Control Centres

Medullary respiratory centre is the primary centre for control of respiration. Output from the medullary respiratory centre is modulated by two higher centers in the pons, which are referred to as the apneustic centre and the pneumotaxic centre. The pneumotaxic centre appears to exert the 'brakes' on inspiration, while the apneustic centre enhances inspiratory 'drive'.

Quiet breathing involves alternating contraction and relaxation of the inspiratory muscles, which includes the diaphragm and external intercostal muscles. This is dependent on cyclical firing of a part of the medullar control centre called the dorsal respiratory group. The ventral respiratory group comprises both inspiratory and expiratory neurons, which are activated most during forced breathing when demands for ventilation are greatest. Forced expiration involves activation of the abdominal muscles and internal intercostals.

Hering-Breuer Reflex

When the tidal volume is large as during exercise, this reflex is triggered to prevent overinflation of the lungs. Stretch receptors in the smooth muscle of the airways are activated and trigger inhibition of inspiration via the medullary centres.

Regulation of Ventilation

Decreased arterial partial pressure of oxygen (PO_2) is detected by peripheral chemoreceptors located in the carotid and aortic bodies. These receptors are not dependent on total blood O_2 concentration; therefore severe anaemia may not trigger this reflex. These receptors are not sensitive to small changes in PO_2. In fact a change in PO_2 must be greater than a 40% reduction or it must drop below 60 mmHg due to the characteristics of oxygen interaction with haemoglobin (Hb). The reactivity forms a 'safety net' plateau on the O_2-Hb curve. For example, Hb is still 90% saturated at an arterial PO_2 of 60 mmHg, but drops dramatically below this.

Table 13.1 Cranial Nerve Function Tests

No.	Name	Entry Level	Functions and Tests
1	Olfactory	Forebrain	Smell
2	Optic	Thalamus (LGN) Midbrain	Vision Visual fields Pupil light reflexes (afferent CN II, efferent CN III)
3	Oculomotor	Midbrain	Corneal reflection test Six positions of gaze Pupil light reflexes (afferent CN II, efferent CN III)
4	Trochlear	Midbrain	Corneal reflection test Six positions of gaze—superior oblique muscle
5	Trigeminal	Midbrain Pons Medulla	Sensation on skin and mucous membranes of face/head Corneal reflex (V and VII) Muscles of mastication
6	Abducens	Pons (caud.)	Corneal reflection test Six positions of gaze—lateral rectus muscle
7	Facial	Pons (caud.)	Muscles of facial expression Corneal reflex (V and VII) Speech (labial sounds) Taste Salivation and lacrimation
8	Vestibular	Pontomedullary junction	Balance and posture, Spatial awareness Binocular movement control, OKN and OTR Autonomic function tests
	Cochlear	Pontomedullary junction	Hearing (through bone and air)
9	Glossopharyngeal	Medulla	Swallowing (sensory), Salivation (parotid) Taste (posterior), Gag reflex (sensory) Baroreceptor reflex (carotid sinus)
10	Vagus	Medulla	Palate elevation, swallowing, gag reflex (efferent limb) Speech (plosive sounds) Baroreceptor reflex (efferent limb) Digestion
11	Cranial accessory Spinal accessory	Medulla Medulla C1–C6	Swallowing Neck movement—SCM and superior trapezius fibres for orientation of head in space
12	Hypoglossal	Medulla	Tongue protrusion and other movements Observation for deviation, atrophy, and fasciculations Speech (lingual sounds)

The Affect of Increased Partial Pressure of Carbon Dioxide (PCO_2) on Neuron Function

Increased arterial PCO_2 exerts its effect via corresponding changes in brain extracellular fluid (ECF) H^+ ion concentrations. Carbon dioxide combines with water to eventually produce hydrogen ions (H^+) and bicarbonate ions (HCO_3^-). The following reaction outlines the chemical process involved.

$$CO_2 + H_2O \rightleftharpoons H_2CO_3 \rightleftharpoons H^+ + HCO_3^-$$

Changes in the H^+ concentration in the ECF stimulate the chemoreceptors in the vicinity of the medullary respiratory centres. In other words, the brain ECF H^+ concentration is a direct reflection of PCO_2 (Champe & Harvey 1994).

When you hold your breath, what do you think happens to PCO_2 and brain ECF H^+ ion concentration? Holding your breath results in an increase in PCO_2, which results in an increase in H^+ ions. Peripheral chemoreceptors are far more sensitive to $[H^+]$ than CO_2 or O_2, but less important in normal circumstances compared to PCO_2-induced changes in brain ECF H^+. Other causes of increased $[H^+]$ can be buffered by this pathway via the production of bicarbonate ions.

Regulation of Blood Pressure

Sympathetic imbalances may also arise because of altered integration in the brainstem reticular formation or the IML cell column of the spinal cord due to peripheral or descending central influences on the reticular neurons. Visceral afferents or ascending spinoreticular projections from somatic $A\delta$ and C fibres promote activation of the rostral ventrolateral medulla, which increases vasomotor tone (Holt et al 2006). This alters the systemic vascular resistance and modulates the systemic blood pressure.

References

Blumenfeld H 2002 Brainstem I: surface anatomy and cranial nerves. In: Neuroanatomy through clinical cases. Sinauer Associates, Sunderland, MA.

Boch RA, Goldberg ME 1989 Participation of prefrontal neurons in the preparation of visually guided eye movements in the rhesus monkey. Journal of Neurophysiology 61: 1064–1084.

Brodal A, Pompeiano O, Walberg F 1962 The vestibular nuclei and their connections, anatomical and functional correlations. Oliver and Boyd, Edinburgh.

Brown LT 1974 Corticorubral projections in the rat. Journal of Comparative Neurology 154:149–168.

Bruce CJ, Goldberg M 1985 Primate frontal eyefields, single neurons discharging before saccades. Journal of Neurophysiology 53:603–635.

Buttner-Ennever JA, Buttner U 1988 The Reticular formation. In: Buttner JA (ed) Review of oculomotor research, vol 2. Neuroanatomy of the oculomotor System. Elsevier, Amsterdam.

Cannon SC, Robinson DA 1987 Loss of the neural integrator of the oculomotor system from brainstem lesions in monkeys. Journal of Neurophysiology 57:1383–1409.

Champe P, Harvey R 1994 Lippincott's illustrated reviews: biochemistry, 2nd edn. JB Lippincott, Philadelphia, p 61–74.

Chusid JG 1982 Correlative neuroanatomy and functional neurology, 2nd edn. Lange Medical, Los Altos, CA.

Fallon JH, Loughlin SE 1987 Monoamine innervation of cerebral cortex and a theory of the role of monoamines in cerebral cortex and basal ganglia. In: Peters A, Jones JG (eds) Cerebral cortex. Plenium Press, New York, p 41–127.

Fukushima K, Fukushima J, Harada C et al 1990 Neuronal activity related to vertical eye movement in the region of the interstitial nucleus of Cajal in alert rats. Experimental Brain Research 79:43–64.

Guyton AC, Hall JE 1996 Textbook of medical physiology, 9th edn. WB Saunders, Philadelphia.

Holt K, Beck RW, Sexton SG Reflex effects of a spinal adjustment on blood pressure. In Association of Chiropractic Colleges (ACC) Conference Proceedings, Washington, DC. March: 16–18.

Leigh RJ, Zee DS 1991 The neurology of eye movements, 2nd edn. Davis, Philadelphia.

Leigh RJ, Zee D 1992 Oculomotor control: normal and abnormal. In: Asbury A, McKhann G, MacDonald W (eds) Diseases of the nervous system: clinical neurobiology. WB Saunders, Philadelphia.

McIntosh AR, Gonzalez-Lima F 1998 Large-scale functional connectivity in associative learning: interrelations of the rat auditory, visual, and limbic systems. Journal of Neurophysiology 80:3148–3162.

Mann SE, Thau R, Schiller PH 1988 Conditional task related responses in monkey dorsal medial frontal cortex. Experimental Brain Research 69:460–468.

Moore KL 1980 Clinically orientated anatomy. Williams and Wilkins, Baltimore.

Ranalli PJ, Sharpe JA 1986 Contrapulsion of saccades and ipsilateral ataxia: a unilateral disorder of the rostral cerebellum. Annals of Neurology 20:311–316.

Suzuki DA, May JG, Keller EL et al 1990 Visual motion response properties of neurons in dorsal lateral pontine nucleus of alert monkeys. Journal of Neurophysiology 63:37–59.

Webster KE 1978 The brainstem reticular formation. In: Hennings G, Hemmings WA (eds) The biological basis of schizophrenia. MTP Press, Lancaster.

Wilson-Pauwels L, Akesson EJ, Stewart PA 1988 Cranial nerves: anatomy and clinical comments. BC Decker, Toronto.

Zee DS, Yamazaki A, Butler PH et al 1981 Effects of the ablation of flocculus and paraflocculus on eye movements in primates. Journal of Neurophysiology 46:878–899.

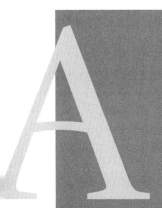

Clinical Case Answers

Case 13.1

13.1.1

When the eye moves to a new target it does so by a movement called a saccade, which is a fast, burst-like movement. Saccades can reach velocities of 700° per second and vision is transiently suppressed during saccadic movements. The saccade is programmed with two distinct components, a pulse phase and a step phase. The pulse phase is the burst of action potential activity to move the eye to the new target. The step phase is the new action potential firing rate to maintain the eye in the new position.

Saccades can be horizontal or vertical in nature. The burst phase of activity for a *horizontal saccade* is generated by burst neurons in the pontine paramedian reticular formation. The duration of firing of a burst neuron begins just before the saccade and ends exactly when the saccade enters the step phase. In between burst outputs, the burst neurons are tonically inhibited by omnipause neurons in the nucleus raphe interpositus. The omnipause neurons continuously discharge, inhibiting the burst neurons until they enter a pause cycle in which the burst neurons become disinhibited and fire a burst of action potentials that results in a saccade motion of the eye until the pause neurons resume their firing and inhibit the burst neurons. The step phase of the horizontal saccade is thought to be created by a neural gaze maintenance network or neural integrator that calculates the saccadic velocity to produce the appropriate position and to produce the appropriate contraction in the extraocular muscles to maintain the gaze at a specific point. The medial vestibular nucleus, the flocculus of the cerebellum, and the nucleus prepositus hypoglossi are important components of the neural integration system of horizontal movements.

The burst phase of activity for a *vertical saccade* is generated by burst neurons in the rostral interstitial nucleus of the medial longitudinal fasciculus (riMLF). This nucleus is located ventral to the aqueduct of Sylvius in the prerubral fields at the junction of the mesencephalon and the thalamus. The activity in this nucleus is dependent on ascending projections from the pontine paramedian reticular formation, omnipause neurons in the nucleus raphe interpositus, and inputs from the contralateral vestibular nuclei. The riMLF projects to the ipsilateral oculomotor (CN III) and trochlear (CN IV) nuclei. Reciprocal connections occur between the right and left riMLF through the posterior and anterior commissures of the midbrain. The fibres of the elevator nuclei which innervate the superior rectus and the inferior oblique muscles pass through the posterior commissural pathways, and the projections to the depressor nuclei innervating the inferior rectus and superior oblique muscles pass through the anterior commissural pathways. The velocity commands of vertical saccadic movements are integrated by the interstitial nucleus of Cajal.

Case 13.2

13.2.1   In the motor systems, including the cranial and spinal motor systems, a two-neuron chain is usually involved in motor activation. The upper motor neurons of the spinal motor system are usually neurons located in various supraspinal nuclei of the brainstem or cortex. One common pathway supplying upper motor neuron modulation to the spinal motor neurons in the ventral horn of the spinal cord is the corticospinal tract, which arises from various areas of cortex specifically focused on movement commands. Upper motor neurons in the cranial system also arise in the cortical areas specifically focused on movement commands and terminate on the neurons of the cranial nerve nuclei in the brainstem and are referred to as the corticobulbar projections or tracts. Usually an upper motor neuron lesion will initially produce a spastic paralysis, hyperactive reflex, and when involving the corticospinal tracts a pathological reflex referred to as the Babinski sign when the plantar surface of the foot is stroked. Lower motor neuron lesions usually initially produce a flaccid paralysis, hypoactive reflex activity, and muscle atrophy over time.

13.2.2   Lower motor neuron lesions of the facial nerve result in complete ipsilateral facial paralysis. Lesions of the upper motor neurons produce paralysis of the contralateral forehead and superior external facial muscles around the eye.

13.2.3
1. Stroke involving the facial motor neurons of the cortex;
2. Brain tumour;
3. Head trauma;
4. Incomplete Bell's palsy;
5. Acute suppurative ear disease including mastoiditis; and
6. Lyme disease in oedemic areas.

Case 13.3

13.3.1
1. Orthostatic hypotension related to sympathetic hypoactivation;
2. Orthostatic hypotension due to low blood volume;
3. Vestibular neuritis;
4. Benign paroxysmal positional vertigo; and
5. Cerebellar degeneration.

13.3.2   Initially upon standing the blood pressure in the upper body will drop instantaneously. This will result in an increased activation of the aortic arch and carotid sinus baroreceptors. This will result in an increased activation of the neurons in the cardiorespiratory nucleus of the nucleus tractus solitarius. These neurons will then excite neurons located in the IML of the spinal cord, which will result in an increased activation of the sympathetic nervous system. Increases in this system result in increases in both constriction of arterioles and rate and contraction of the heart. These actions will tend to increase the blood pressure via increased total peripheral resistance and increased cardiac output respectively. See Quick Facts.

The Vestibulocerebellar System

Clinic Cases for Thought

Case 14.1 A 44-year-old woman presents with severe dizziness and nausea. She reports that she felt slightly dizzy when she woke up but the dizziness and the nausea have increasingly worsened throughout the day. She also complains of double vision and vertical displacement of objects. She reports there is no hearing loss or other symptoms involving her ears.

Questions

14.1.1 Discuss five possible differential considerations in this case.

14.1.2 How can a central cause of her dizziness be differentiated from a peripheral cause in this case?

Case 14.2 A 78-year-old man presents with a chief complaint of headache and loss of balance. He is accompanied by his son who also states that he has been dropping things and knocking things over as he moves around the house. Rhomberg's test is positive and he falls to the right. He has also been repeatedly ill with a flu-like condition for several months.

Questions

14.2.1 Discuss five differential considerations in this case.

14.2.2 What anatomical pathways are involved in the maintenance of posture and balance?

14.2.3 How could his cerebellar dysfunction contribute to his decreased immune function?

Introduction

The cerebellum has traditionally been considered as a sensory motor integration centre involved in monitoring and modulating motor function in the spine, head, and limbs. The cerebellum receives afferent input from sensory receptors via the spinocerebellar tracts as well as from the brainstem and from the cerebral cortex.

The input and output connections flow through the superior, inferior, and middle cerebellar peduncles which connect the cerebellum to the brainstem The flocculonodular lobe is involved in the control of posture, eye movement, and certain autonomic responses via its connections with vestibular nuclei. The anterior lobe and posterior parts of the vermis receive input from the axial regions of the body and project to medial descending pathways. The lateral parts of the cerebellum and the central vermis are considered the 'neocerebellum' and are thought to play a role in the planning of movement rather than the execution of movement.

It is now widely accepted that the cerebellum also plays a part in controlling affect, emotion, and cognition, especially the lateral component of the cerebellum, which is referred to as the neocerebellum or cerebrocerebellum.

The prefix 'neo' indicates that this component of the cerebellum is the newest region to develop in human evolution. It is therefore the most advanced region of the cerebellum and its development parallels the growth of the lateral aspects of the cerebral hemispheres, the association cortices, and those areas associated with advanced communication, higher consciousness, and skilled use of the digits.

It is now clear that the cerebellum and vestibular systems also play a role in the integration of sensory information that is essential for generating appropriate responses to environmental stimuli and for a variety of other functions including constructing a perception of ourselves in the universe; controlling muscle movement; maintaining balance; maintaining internal organ and blood flow functionality; maintaining cortical arousal; and developing active plasticity in neural networks which allows environmental conditioning to occur. The importance of the cerebellum in the overall function of the neuraxis is demonstrated by the fact that there are approximately 20 million corticopontocerebellar fibres projecting between the cerebellum and the cortex, compared to only about 1 million corticospinal fibres supplying the cortical output to the voluntary muscles of the body. The integration function of the cerebellum is evident as the input-to-output or afferent-to-efferent ratio in the cerebellum is approximately 40:1.

Anatomy of the Cerebellum

The cerebellum is composed of an outer covering of grey matter, the cerebellar cortex, the internal white matter, and three pairs of deep cerebellar nuclei arranged on either side of the midline. The deep nuclei are the fastigial, interposed, and the dentate nuclei. The bulk of the output of the cerebellum emerges from these three nuclei.

QUICK FACTS 1	Removal of the Cerebellum

1. Does not alter sensory thresholds
2. Does not alter the strength of muscle contraction

Thus the cerebellum is not necessary in the perception or performance of movement.

The cerebellum lies behind the pons and medulla in the posterior cranial fossa (Fig. 14.1). It is separated from the cerebrum by an extension of dura mater, the tentorium cerebelli, and from the pons and medulla by the fourth ventricle (Fig. 14.2). It is somewhat smaller than the cerebrum but this difference varies with age, being 1/8 the size of the adult cortex but only 1/20 the size of the infant cortex.

The cerebellum is derived from the rhombencephalon, along with its homologues the pons and medulla, and is connected to the brainstem via three peduncles. These peduncles, together with the anterior and posterior medullary velum, are the main routes of entry or exit from the cerebellum. The *inferior cerebellar peduncle*, also known as the *restiform body*, conveys a number of axon projections into the cerebellum including (Figs 14.3 and 14.4):

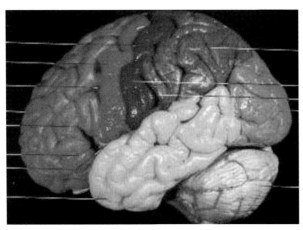

Fig. 14.1 The location of the cerebellum. The cerebellum lies behind the pons and medulla in the posterior cranial fossa. Frontal lobe, parietal lobe, occipital lobe, temporal lobe, cerebellum.

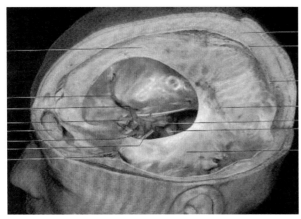

Fig. 14.2 The relationship of the cerebellum to the cortex.

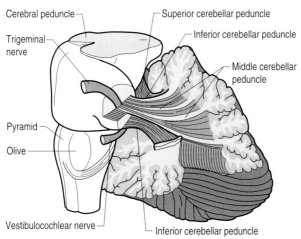

Fig. 14.3 The anatomical relationships of the inferior, middle, and superior cerebellar peduncles.

1. The posterior spinocerebellar tract, which contains mossy fibres from the spinal cord that project to the cortex of the spinocerebellum;

2. The accessory cuneocerebellar tract, arising from the dorsal external arcuate fibres from the accessory cuneate nucleus;

3. The olivocerebellar tract, which contains climbing fibres of the contralateral inferior olivary nucleus;

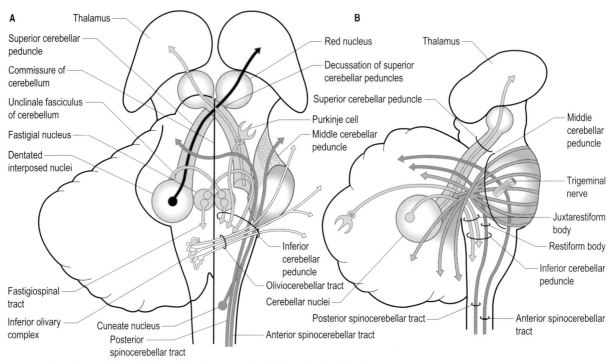

Fig. 14.4 The pathways of the cerebellar peduncles from a superior (left) and lateral (right) view.

4. The reticular cerebellar tract, which is formed from the ventral external arcuate fibres carrying projections from the arcuate and lateral reticular nucleus of the medulla; and

5. The vestibulocerebellar tract, which is formed from the projection fibres of the vestibular nuclei.

The *middle cerebellar peduncle* or *brachium pontis* is the largest of the cerebellar peduncles, and contains the massive afferent corticopontocerebellar pathways. The middle

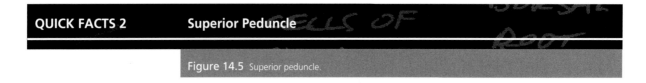

QUICK FACTS 2   **Superior Peduncle**

Figure 14.5 Superior peduncle.

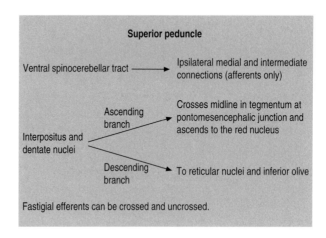

peduncle is composed of axon projection fibres from the pontine nuclei to the contralateral cerebellum (Figs. 14.3 and 14.4). The primary projections from the cerebral cortex to the cerebellum include premotor and supplementary motor areas (area 6), primary motor areas (area 4), primary sensory areas (areas 3, 1, and 2), and association and limbic cortices.

The *superior peduncle* or *brachium conjunctivum* supports both afferent and efferent fibres. The efferent fibres compose the following tracts:

1. The dentatorubral tract, which projects from the dentate nucleus of the cerebellum to the opposite red nucleus in the mesencephalon;

2. The dentatothalamic tract, which projects to the contralateral thalamus;

3. The uncinate fasciculus, which contains fibres from the fastigial nucleus enroute to the lateral vestibular nuclei in the medulla (Figs. 14.3 and 14.4); and

4. Aminergic afferent projections, including noradrenergic, dopaminergic, and serotonergic afferents projecting to all areas of the cerebellum.

Noradrenergic neurons in the locus ceruleus project to Purkinje dendrites in the molecular layer and with granule cells in the granular layer (Bloom et al 1971; Kimoto et al 1981). Dopaminergic fibres arising from the neurons in the ventral mesencephalic tegmentum project to the Purkinje and granule neurons of interposed and lateral cerebellar nuclei (Simon et al 1979). Serotonergic afferent fibres arise from the raphe nuclei of the brainstem and terminate in both the molecular and granule layers (Takeuchi et al 1982).

The anterior and posterior medullary velum also supports some decussating fibres of the superior cerebellar peduncles and trochlear nerve. The velum also supports fibres originating in the peduncles of the flocculus.

The cerebellar surface is a striking example of natural economics, in that it contains parallel convolutions or folia running in a transverse direction on the surface of the cerebellum that increase the surface area of the cerebellar cortex and give the cerebellum a tree-like appearance (Fig. 14.6). There are three primary lobes, anterior, posterior, and flocculonodular, on the cerebellar surface which are further dived into ten lobules. The cerebellum can be divided into nine regions along the vermis, which is a small unpaired structure in the median portion of the cerebellum separating the two large lateral masses. These nine regions are listed in Table 14.1 from anterior to posterior (see also Fig. 14.7). There are two major fissures that divide the cerebellum into three main lobes, and a number of other fissures that divide each lobe into its respective lobules.

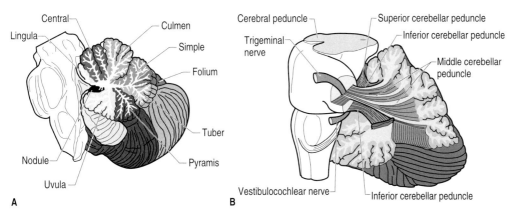

Fig. 14.6 (A) A midline section through the vermis leaving the right cerebellar hemisphere intact. Note the components of the lobes including the central lobule, culmen, declive, tuber, pyramid, uvula, and nodule. (B) Note the superior, middle and inferior peduncles.

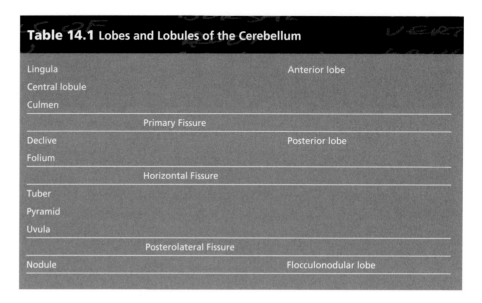

Table 14.1 Lobes and Lobules of the Cerebellum

Lingula	Anterior lobe
Central lobule	
Culmen	
Primary Fissure	
Declive	Posterior lobe
Folium	
Horizontal Fissure	
Tuber	
Pyramid	
Uvula	
Posterolateral Fissure	
Nodule	Flocculonodular lobe

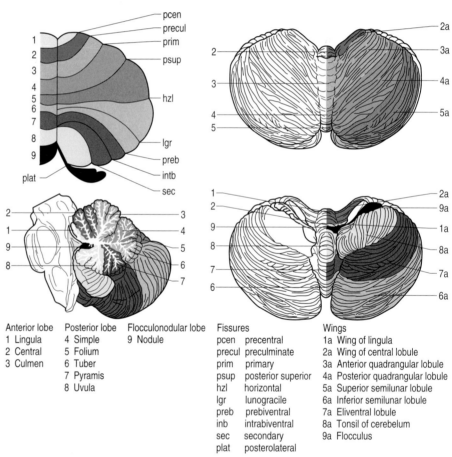

Anterior lobe	Posterior lobe	Flocculonodular lobe	Fissures		Wings	
1 Lingula	4 Simple	9 Nodule	pcen	precentral	1a	Wing of lingula
2 Central	5 Folium		precul	preculminate	2a	Wing of central lobule
3 Culmen	6 Tuber		prim	primary	3a	Anterior quadrangular lobule
	7 Pyramis		psup	posterior superior	4a	Posterior quadrangular lobule
	8 Uvula		hzl	horizontal	5a	Superior semilunar lobule
			lgr	lunogracile	6a	Inferior semilunar lobule
			preb	prebiventral	7a	Eliventral lobule
			inb	intrabiventral	8a	Tonsil of cerebelum
			sec	secondary	9a	Flocculus
			plat	posterolateral		

Fig. 14.7 The anatomical relationships of the different phylogenic areas of the cerebellum.

Embryological development of the cerebellum

Early in the third month of development, the cerebellum appears as a dumbbell-shaped mass on the roof of the hindbrain vesicle. A number of transverse grooves representing the fissures begin to appear on the dorsal surface of the cerebellum. Later in the third month the posterolateral fissure becomes the first landmark to demarcate its adjacent

---

Damage to Cerebellar Function Results in Dysfunction of the Following

QUICK FACTS 3

1. Spatial accuracy
2. Temporal coordination
3. Balance
4. Muscle tone
5. Motor learning
6. Certain cognitive functions

lobes from one another and results in the separation of the flocculonodular lobe from the remainder of the cerebellum.

At the same time, the primary fissure begins to cut into the surface of the cerebellum, separating the anterior from the posterior lobe and other smaller fissures develop on the inferior surface.

The cerebellum expands dorsally and the inferior aspects of the hemispheres undergo the greatest increase in size, causing the inferior vermis to be buried between them, thus forming the vallecula, which is a deep groove on the inferior surface.

From a functional point of view, we need to consider three main regions within the cerebellum. These three regions are derived from the archicerebellum, palaeocerebellum, and neocerebellum based on their time of appearance through evolutionary history (phylogeny).

The *archicerebellum* is the first region to appear in phylogeny and comprises the flocculi, their peduncles, the nodulus, and the lingula. The archicerebellum is the oldest and most medial portion of the cerebellum. In humans, archicerebellum contributes to the *vestibulocerebellum*, which comprises the flocculonodular lobe and the lingula (Fig. 14.7) (Brodal 1981). As its new name would indicate, the vestibulocerebellum is the region of the cerebellum that communicates most intimately with the vestibular system. In fact, the vestibular nuclei of the brainstem share similar relationships with the cortex of the archicerebellum as the deep cerebellar nuclei share with the cortex of the palaeo- and neocerebellum. They therefore serve functionally as a cerebellar nuclear complex. The vestibulocerebellum also contains the only cerebellar cortical cells that leave the body of the cerebellum before synapsing. In the other regions of the cerebellum, the output cells of the cerebellar cortex synapse on neurons of the deep cerebellar nuclei. The stimuli from these neurons evoke inhibitory post-synaptic potentials (IPSPs) in the deep cerebellar nuclei.

Phylogenically, the *palaeocerebellum* is next to develop. Apart from the lingula, it comprises the anterior lobe, the pyramid, and uvula of the posterior vermis. This separated the archicerebellum into two parts, the lingula anteriorly and the flocculonodulus posteriorly (Brodal 1981). The palaeocerebellum contributes to the *spinocerebellum*, which is involved in a variety of parameters associated with movement.

The *neocerebellum* was the most recent component to arise in phylogeny and comprises the posterior lobes apart from the pyramid and uvula. This developed in parallel with the expansion of the neopallium and neocortex of the brain and the posterior aspects of the thalamus, which reflects the extent of the association cortices of the brain. Both anterior and posterior lobes of the cerebellum have sensory motor maps of the complete body surface, which overlap each other exactly. The neocerebellum contributes to the *cerebrocerebellum*, which is thought to be involved in a wide range of activities including memory and learning.

The cerebellum was traditionally seen as a sensory motor integration centre involved in monitoring and modulating motor function in the spine, head, and limbs. It is now widely accepted that the cerebellum also plays a part in controlling affect, emotion, and cognition—especially the lateral component of the cerebellum, which is referred to as the neocerebellum or cerebrocerebellum.

The prefix 'neo' indicates that this component of the cerebellum is the newest region to develop in human evolution. It is therefore the most advanced region of the cerebellum and its development parallels the growth of the lateral aspect of the cerebral hemispheres (the association cortices) and those areas associated with advanced communication, higher consciousness, and skilled use of the digits.

371

Figure 14.8 Spinocerebellum.

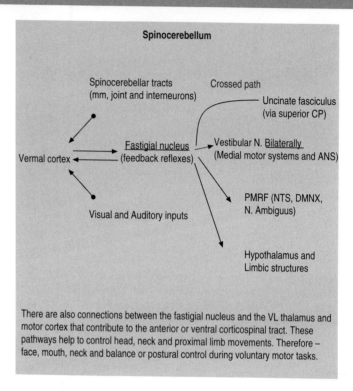

There are also connections between the fastigial nucleus and the VL thalamus and motor cortex that contribute to the anterior or ventral corticospinal tract. These pathways help to control head, neck and proximal limb movements. Therefore – face, mouth, neck and balance or postural control during voluntary motor tasks.

Figure 14.9 Spinocerebellum.

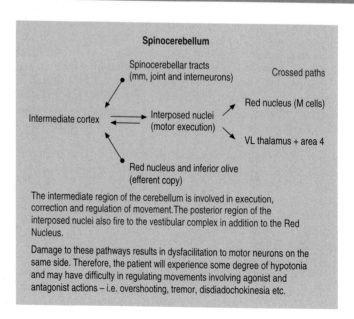

The intermediate region of the cerebellum is involved in execution, correction and regulation of movement. The posterior region of the interposed nuclei also fire to the vestibular complex in addition to the Red Nucleus.

Damage to these pathways results in dysfacilitation to motor neurons on the same side. Therefore, the patient will experience some degree of hypotonia and may have difficulty in regulating movements involving agonist and antagonist actions – i.e. overshooting, tremor, disdiadochokinesis etc.

Cerebrocerebellum

QUICK FACTS 6

Figure 14.10 Cerebrocerebellum

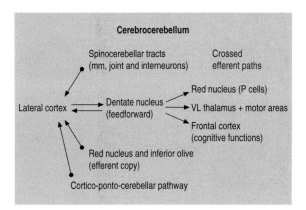

The Layers of the cerebellar Cortex

The cerebellar cortex is divided into three distinct layers: the molecular, Purkinje, and granule layers. The *molecular layer* is composed of axons of granule cells, known as parallel fibres running parallel to long axis of the folia, Purkinje dendrites, basket cell interneurons, and stellate cell interneurons, both of which are inhibitory interneurons. The basket cells have long axons that run perpendicular to parallel fibres and synapse with

Cerebellar Cortex Is Composed of 3 Layers and 5 Cell Types

QUICK FACTS 7

1. Molecular layer
   - Dendrites of Golgi cells
   - Contains parallel fibres (granule cell axons) running parallel to long axis of folia
   - Purkinje dendrites
   - Basket and stellate cells (inhibitory interneurons)
2. Purkinje cell layer
   - Single-cell layer containing the bodies of Purkinje cells.
   - The dendrites of Purkinje cells project outward to the molecular layer and form recurrent collaterals that inhibit adjacent Purkinje cells and Golgi type II neurons.
3. Granule cell layer
   - Granule cell bodies form the core of the cerebellar glomeruli and receive axodendritic synapses from Golgi cells.
   - Golgi cells promote inhibition of up to 10,000 granule cells and are also activated by mossy and climbing fibres in the granule cell layer. This promotes the sharpening of inputs in the cerebellar cortex by suppressing weak excitatory post-synaptic potentials (EPSPs)

Figure 14.11 Five cell types.

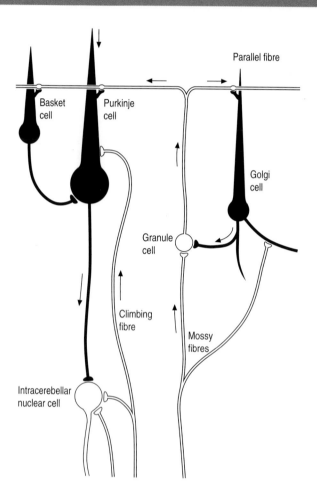

Purkinje dendrites. They also synapse directly to some Purkinje cell bodies. The basket cells form synapses anterior and posterior to the parallel fibre beams, therefore resulting in disinhibition of neighbouring parallel fibres. This is thought to produce a type of centre-surround antagonism. Stellate cells have smaller axons that inhibit local Purkinje cells and synapse on the distal aspect of their dendrites. Both basket cells and stellate cells are excited by parallel fibres.

The next layer, the *Purkinje layer*, consists of the only output fibres of the cerebellar cortex, the Purkinje cells. The dendrites of Purkinje cells project outwards to the molecular layer and form recurrent collaterals that inhibit adjacent Purkinje cells and Golgi type II neurons.

The *granule layer* consists of Golgi neurons and granule cells. Granule cell bodies form the core of the cerebellar glomeruli and receive axodendritic synapses from Golgi cells. Golgi cells promote inhibition of up to 10,000 granule cells and are also activated by mossy and climbing fibres in the granule cell layer. This promotes the sharpening of inputs in the cerebellar cortex by suppressing weak excitatory post-synaptic potentials (EPSPs).

The actual cellular interactions of the cortical cells consists of one inhibitory output tract, consisting of Purkinje cells which synapse on intracerebellar and vestibular nuclei, and two input tracts, each of which is excitatory. The two input tracts consist of climbing fibres, which are actually the axons of neurons which live in the contralateral inferior olive and the mossy fibres, which are axons of neurons of a variety of pontomedullary reticular nuclei and axons of neurons living in laminae VI and VII of the spinal cord (Ito 1984). As discussed earlier, aminergic neurons in the brainstem also project to the cerebellum. The climbing fibres first give off collateral projections to the deep cerebellar nuclei before synapsing on granule, Golgi, basket, and Purkinje cells in the cerebellar cortex (Gilman et al 1981; Van der Want et al 1989). Only one synapse per Purkinje cell occurs; however, many Purkinje cells are innervated by a single climbing fibre so that a single climbing fibre spike produces a burst of Purkinje cell activity. The mossy fibres influence the Purkinje activity indirectly via synapses on granule cells, which then synapse on Purkinje cells and Golgi cells, which then synapse on parallel fibres, which in turn synapse on the Purkinje cells directly or via basket or stellate interneurons. Each parallel fibre excites a long array of about 500 Purkinje neurons, whereas each Purkinje neuron receives input from approximately 200,000 parallel fibres (Gilman 1992) (Fig. 14.12).

All of the cerebellar neurons of the cortex are inhibitory except the granule cells. The Purkinje inhibitory output is exerted on the spontaneously active nuclear cells. Thus, the nuclear cells must have a strong 'pacemaker' potential or a powerful excitatory input to match the inhibition resulting from the Purkinje cells. The latter excitatory input may be manifested in excitatory impulses from axon collaterals of mossy and climbing fibres that each give off before synapsing in the cerebellar cortex.

The cerebellum receives information about all commands originating in the motor and association areas of the brain via the climbing fibres of the inferior olive. These olivary neurons also receive input from descending midbrain and telencephalic structures. Climbing fibres detect differences between actual and expected sensory inputs rather than simply monitoring afferent information. Neurons in the inferior olive are electronically coupled through dendrodendritic synapses and therefore can fire in synchrony. The synchronous inputs produce complex spikes in multiple Purkinje cells. In turn, the electrotonic coupling is under efferent control by GABA-ergic fibres from the deep cerebellar nuclei so that they can be functionally disconnected. This results in the selection of specific combinations of Purkinje cells. Climbing fibres modulate synaptic efficacy of parallel fibres by reducing strength of EPSPs of parallel fibres and by inducing selective long-term depression in synaptic strength of parallel fibres active concurrently (within 100–200 ms). Long-term depression depends on prolonged voltage-gated calcium influx.

Damage to the cerebellar cortex or inferior olive leads to inability to adapt. The largest input to the cerebellum is from the cerebral cortex contralaterally. This is known as the corticopontocerebellar pathway. There are approximately 20 million neurons in this pathway compared to only 1 million neurons in the corticospinal pathway of the spinal cord.

The axons of the Purkinje cells project to the deep cerebellar nuclei as well as to the vestibular nuclei. The cerebellum via these output nuclei is able to exert descending

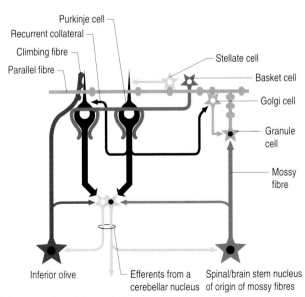

Fig. 14.12 The cellular connections of the cerebellar cortex.

influences on the spinal cord as well as ascending influences on the cerebral cortex. These outputs can be separated into three components:

The first component originates in the cortex of the vermis and flocculonodular lobes and acts on the fastigial and vestibular nuclei. The fastigial nucleus and its efferent targets, the vestibular nuclei, are often referred to as the vestibulocerebellum and are involved in limb extension and muscle tone in the neck and trunk to maintain posture. Being the earliest to arise in evolutionary history and embryological development, the vestibulocerebellum serves the most primitive function of the cerebellum. It receives extensive inputs from sensory receptors throughout the head and body that provide us with spatial coordinates for the purpose of spatial orientation and self-awareness.

This includes information from the retina and advanced visual processing systems of the brain, auditory and vestibular neurons including mono- and polysynaptic connections from the inner ear, and muscle and joint receptors particularly from the spine via the vestibular nuclei.

Fastigial efferent fibres can be crossed and uncrossed. The crossed fibres project via the uncinate fasciculus of the superior cerebellar peduncle to the super colliculus bilaterally, and to the interstitial nucleus of Cajal (Ito 1984). Some fibres also project to the ventral lateral and ventral posterior lateral nuclei of the thalamus via the superior cerebellar peduncle. The uncrossed fibres form the fastigiobulbar projections whose bulk form the smaller juxtarestiform body. These fibres project to all four of the ipsilateral vestibular nuclei and the ipsilateral reticular formation (Batton et al 1977). The fastigial nuclei fire after the commencement of movement. This nucleus receives large inputs from the periphery and sends few projections to the motor cortex. The fastigial nucleus is involved in the feedback mechanisms of the cerebellum.

The second component originates in the intermediate areas of the cerebellar hemispheres and projects to the interposed nuclei. Some neurons from the interpositus nuclei project through the superior peduncles to synapse on magnocellular neurons of the contralateral red nucleus (Asanuma et al 1983). The majority, however synapse on neurons of the contralateral thalamic nuclei of the ventral lateral pars caudalis and ventral posterolateral pars oralis. These thalamic neurons fire almost simultaneously to the primary motor cortex and are involved in efferent copy mechanisms. Efferent copy mechanism compares the intended programme from the cortex to the cerebellum's knowledge of the state of the organism. Corrections are sent to the brain prior to the movement being carried out. This minimizes the time delay in regulating evolving movements in a changing environment.

The inability to carry out a motor programme because of apparent weakness in muscles may in fact be due to a disturbance in midline cerebellar function. An example can illustrate the concept. As an arm or leg is raised or moved away from the body a greater demand is placed on postural mechanisms, which then fail because of poor reinforcement by medial descending motor pathways from the brainstem and cerebellum.

The third component originates in the lateral cortical areas and projects to the dentate nuclei. The axons of neurons of the dentate nucleus project through the brachium conjunctivum to the contralateral red nucleus where they terminate on the parvocellular neurons in the rostral third of the nucleus (Gilman 1992). The dentate nucleus is more heavily activated in tasks requiring the conscious evaluation of sensory information, for example, tasks requiring processing of sensory input to solve or programme complex spatial and temporal motor programmes. The dentate nucleus receives little input from the periphery and is involved in feedforward responses. The feedforward mechanisms are important for fast movements.

The lateral cerebellum is involved in preprogramming of learned volitional movements. It regulates tone and movement of the ipsilateral limbs and is also important in cognition. Stimulation results in facilitation of ipsilateral flexor tone. When an action is carried out without the need for prior sensory guidance, the lateral component of the cerebellum becomes more active in readiness for delivering a self-motivated plan of action to the cerebral cortex.

The fastigial and vestibular projections control the proximal limb muscles mostly through an excitatory action on proximal extensor muscles. The interposed nuclei control limb movements of the upper and lower extremities via the rubrospinal tract and through ascending fibres that project to motor cortex via the ventral posterior lateral nucleus of the thalamus. The dentate nuclei mainly project to the motor cortex via the ventral lateral and ventral anterior nuclei of the thalamus (Figs 14.14 and 14.15).

Figure 14.13 The canalith repositioning manoeuvre (Epley's manoeuvre).

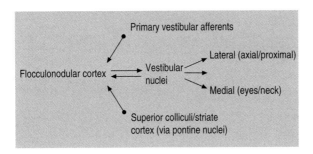

Fig. 14.14 The efferent (input) projections to the cerebellum.

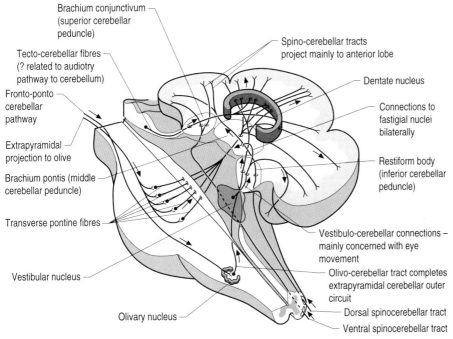

Various *functions of the cerebellum* have been described simply as a 'damping, clamping' system that smooths out irregularities from start and braking movements. Other possible functions proposed include the initiation of movements, both simple and compound, the correction of movement trajectory after perturbation, the control of the vestibulo-ocular reflex, and the stopping or braking of movements.

The function of the cerebellum may best be described if the various interacting components are considered as a circuit. The cerebellar circuit consists of a system of interconnecting brain parts that transform and combine messages on intent and the results of those actions into an optional set of instructions for motor execution appropriate at that time. Thus the cerebellum may be described as an implementer of higher brain functions which detects the variation between the programme demands and the actual muscular actions. In order to accomplish this the cerebellum requires a feedforward projection map of the intended actions which emanates from association cortex or other higher centres. This feedback most probably arises via coactivation of descending pathways to alpha motor neurons, and through conventional feedback mechanisms.

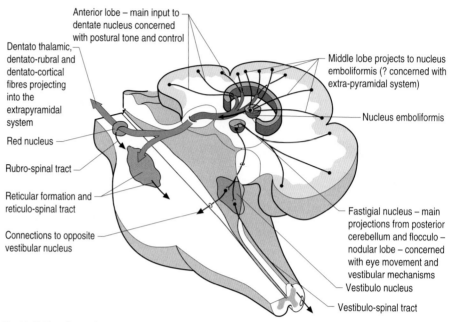

Fig. 14.15 The afferent (output) projections of the cerebellum.

Feedforward mechanisms are carried out through the dentato-rubro-thalamocortical pathway, which conveys a motor or cognitive plan from the cerebellum to the cerebral cortex, allowing the cerebral cortex to carry out a precise action. This is referred to as the 'feedforward' pathway of the cerebellum. Feedforward processes are anticipatory movement plans such as contraction of triceps after biceps reflex contraction. The feedforward pathway is not feedback and is necessary during anticipatory and ballistic movements where feedback mechanisms either are not available or are too slow to evoke an appropriate response. Damage of these processes therefore leads to defective anticipatory control of limb motion.

The actions of the fastigial nucleus, which increase sympathetic activity as a result of input from the labyrinthine systems via the vestibular apparatus in posture writing movements, and the actions of the cerebellum on the vasomotor centres, which alter blood flows to limb muscle before initiation of movement of those muscles, are also important aspects of cerebellar function.

Efference copy mechanisms integrate the sensory information concerning real-time status of the individual and the anticipated or programmed information from lateral brain and cerebellar regions in order to minimize error as the movement is evolving—or, as the environment in which the individual is performing the movement is changing.

The interposed nuclei and the intermediate zone of the cerebellar cortex serve as a key link between areas of the cerebellum involved in motor planning and those areas that respond reflexively to sensory inputs from the spine and midline structures. Consider a basketball player shooting for goal from outside the 3-point line. Just before the player extends his elbows and flexes his wrists to shoot the ball, an opponent nudges him from the side. If the player did not react and change the motor programme initially set before shooting for goal, he would more than likely miss the goal because his body was pushed off line. However, because of the feedback of sensory information from the spine, limbs, and the vestibular system, the player is able to alter the original motor programme sent from the lateral hemisphere of the cerebellum and cortex of the brain.

The fastigial nucleus and the vermis of the cerebellum are chiefly involved in *feedback mechanisms* of sensorimotor programming. This means that these areas receive large inputs from muscles, joints, and connective tissue, particularly from midline structures. For example, alterations in an individual's centre of mass leads to reflex changes in muscle tone that compensate for the anticipated perturbation in stability. Therefore, sensory inputs largely determine the output from the midline cerebellar nuclei and fastigial nuclei.

During learning of new tasks, feedback input is utilized first until the dentate and lateral cerebellum can begin firing to promote feedforward processes. In other words, we learn by trial and error. The cerebellum provides a signal to the brain that promotes the closest learned response and this is constantly updated based on judgment of degree of error and evolving changes in the environment, posture, etc. (Fig. 14.16).

Embryological Homologue—What Does It Mean? **QUICK FACTS 10**

During embryologic development neurons undergo migration and in so doing they maintain their connections with their embryologic homologues. Embryological homologues are those neurons that share common precursor cells or are related through their connectivity within a common axis. They tend to share a similar function or purpose within the nervous system albeit in a different location. Usually their activity is interdependent so that excitation/inhibition of one area will result in excitation/inhibition of the homologue as well.

Lesions of the cerebellum can result in a multitude of symptoms based on the area of involvement within the cerebellum. There are, however, some general signs and symptoms of cerebellar damage that can be detected through a thorough history and examination. The following are clinical pearls that signal cerebellar involvement:

1. Muscles that normally act together lose the capacity to do so, with muscles contracting out of sequence to perform the desired movement.

2. There are new errors in force, velocity and timing with loss of the ability to hit a target without several attempts.

3. There are disturbances in weight discrimination, which is thought to be the only sensory disturbance in cerebellar disease; however, it is now understood that cerebellar deficits can result in global sensory processing disturbances or distortions in sensory awareness because of alterations in cerebellar projections to the central lateral nuclei and other non-specific nuclei of the thalamus.

4. Cerebellar lesions may also clearly result in disturbances of spatial orientation and sensory perception of motion because of intimate connections with the vestibular system.

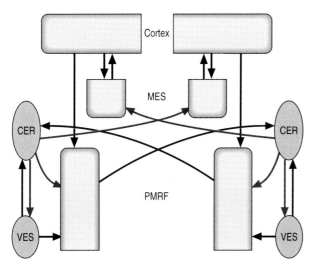

Fig. 14.16 Cerebellar functional systems The functional projections between the cerebellum, vestibular nuclei, pontomedullary reticular formation (PMRF), the mesencephalic reticular formation (MES), and the cortex. The cerebellum receives input through the PMRF via the pontine projections from the contralateral cortex. The cerebellum projects back to the contralateral cortex via the red nuclear projections in the MES. Reciprocal projections exist between the ipsilateral vestibular nuclei and the cerebellum.

Dysfunction in the lateral cerebellum also leads to delayed initiation and timing of movement (decomposition) and poor coordination between distal and proximal joints and independent finger manipulation. The lateral cerebellum is also heavily involved in verb association tasks, especially the right side of the cerebellum, which shares reciprocal communication with Broca's speech area.

Medial cerebellar lesions interfere only with accurate execution of a response, whereas lateral cerebellar lesions interfere with the timing of serial events. This applies not only to motor tasks but also judgment of elapsed time in mental or cognitive tasks. For example, a patient may have decreased ability to judge the difference between the length of two tones. This could result in poor judgment of prosodic speech or keeping time to music. A patient may have difficulty in detecting or responding to differences in speed of moving objects, such as optokinetic stimuli or judging the speed of oncoming traffic while crossing the road.

The Cerebellum is also involved in Learning

The cerebellum is active during all forms of learning including those associated with motor and cognitive function. It is particularly active during the early stages of learning when the individual is exposed to a novel stimulus. The cerebellum assumes increasing responsibility during learning until it gains essentially complete control of the motor tasks. The cerebellum becomes less active once the acquisition of the skill or task has been completed.

QUICK FACTS 11	An Evolutionary Theory of Thought

It has previously been proposed that the cerebellum grew larger in humans as we began to stand upright, which increased the exposure of our spinal muscles and joints to the forces of gravity. Mellilo and Leismann outlined this hypothesis with reference to the role of natural selection in the evolution of the human frame and posture. They also referred to Llinas' theory that cognition represents the internalization of motor function. This means that as motor function became more advanced and therefore more purposeful, there was a greater advantage in being able to predict what would happen in the future so that appropriate adjustments to motor strategies could be made to enhance the outcome of an individual's action (Mellilo & Leisman 2004).

The cerebellum is responsible for recognizing the context for action and automatically triggering an appropriate response to the stimulus. This also occurs in word association tasks. From a cognitive point of view, the cerebellum is involved in cognitive planning, associative learning, classical conditioning, instrumental learning, and voluntary shifts of selective attention between sensory modalities.

Cerebellar Influences on Eye Movements

The cerebellum is involved in two basic operations involving eye control. The first involves its role in both real-time positional eye control with respect to visual acquisition and the second involves long-term adaptive control mechanisms regulating the oculomotor system (Leigh & Zee 1991). The cerebellum functions to ensure that the movements of the eye are appropriate for the stimulation that they are receiving.

The flocculus of the vestibulocerebellum contains Purkinje cells that discharge in relation to the velocity of eye movements during smooth pursuit tracking, with the head either stationary or moving. For example, you can keep your head still and fixate your gaze on a moving object, in which case your eyes should smoothly follow the object across your visual field, or you could keep your eyes fixed on a stationary object and rotate your head, in which case your eyes should still smoothly track in the opposite direction and at the same speed as the rotation of your head to maintain the target in focus (Zee et al 1981). Other neurons discharge during saccadic eye movement in relation to the position of the eye in the orbit. Individual control of eye movement is accomplished for the most part by the contralateral cerebellum although intimate bilateral integration is also important. For example the smoothness of pursuit activity and the return to centre function of saccadic movement of the right eye are under left cerebellar modulatory control.

Lesions of the dorsal vermis and fastigial nucleus of the cerebellum result in saccadic dysmetria, especially hypermetria of centripetal saccades (Optican & Robinson 1980). Lesions of the flocculus result in a variety of eye movement dysfunctions including (Berthoz & Melvil-Jones 1985; Optican et al 1986):

1. Impairment of smooth visual tracking;
2. Horizontal gaze-evoked nystagmus;
3. Postsaccadic drift or glissades (see Chapter 13);
4. Downbeat and rebound nystagmus;
5. Decreased accuracy of vestibular ocular reflexes; and
6. Decreased ability to adapt to changing environmental inputs.

The vestibular system

The vestibular system is composed of three basic functional components; the peripheral afferent input network, an integration system that analyses the input, and an output mechanism that allows a motor response to the input received (Hain et al 1999).

Flocculonodular lesions	**QUICK FACTS 12**

- Stance and gait abnormalities
- Multidirectional nystagmus
- Head rotation
- Eye movement abnormalities

Afferent Projections into the Vestibular System

The input network is composed of afferent information from a variety of sources (Melillo & Leisman 2004) including:

1. The vestibular apparatus, which includes the semicircular canals and otolithic organs and vestibular nuclei;

Midline Cerebellar Lesions	**QUICK FACTS 13**

- Disordered stance and gait
- Truncal titubation
- Rotated postures of the head
- Disturbed extraocular movements
- Normal limb movements with isolated testing

QUICK FACTS 14

Paraverbal Lesions

Paraverbal lesions usually presents with a combination of medial and lateral cerebellar signs.

QUICK FACTS 15

Lateral Cerebellar Lesions

- Abnormalities of stance and gait (except if it is an isolated lesion)
- Disturbed extraocular movements
- Decomposition of limb movements
- Dysmetria
- Dysdiadochokinesia/dysrhythmokinesis
- Appendicular ataxia
- Impaired check and excessive rebound
- Kinetic and static tremor
- Dysarthria and hypotonia
- Cognitive disturbances

2. Proprioceptive information, which is relayed to the cerebellum via the climbing fibres which arise in Clark's column of the spinal cord;

3. Visual information from the striate cortex, the superior colliculus, and lateral geniculate nucleus of the thalamus;

4. Tactile information, which projects from the thalamus and somatosensory cortex; and

5. Auditory information from the inferior colliculus and medial geniculate body of the thalamus.

The Vestibular Apparatus

The vestibular apparatus contains the *semicircular canals* and the *otolithic* organs. The semicircular canals are a bilateral system of interconnected tube-like structures composed of three tubes on each side of the head orientated to different aspects of motion as depicted in Fig. 14.17. These structures detect angular velocity and angular tilt of the head. The canals are surrounded by a thin layer of fluid called *perilymph*, which is essentially the same composition as cerebrospinal fluid that cushions them from the surrounding bony labyrinth. They are filled with another fluid referred to as *endolymph*, which is very high in protein. The lateral canal is orientated 30° from the horizontal in the neutral position and is thus in the vertical plane when the head is tilted backwards by about 60°. Each canal is joined to a central structure called the *utricle*. As each canal joins the utricle the canal expands to form the ampulla, which contains a specialized structure called the cupola and hair cells. The receptors on the hair cells are polarized to respond to movement in one direction only, with respect to a single kinocilium also present on the hair cell (Fig. 14.18). The axons from the hair cells of the utricle synapse in the superior vestibular ganglion. The axons of the neurons in the superior vestibular ganglion then form the superior vestibular nerve. These axons contribute along with the axons of the inferior vestibular nerve from the saccule and the cochlear nerve to form the ipsilateral vestibulocochlear nerve (CN VIII). Most of these axons synapse in the vestibular nuclei but some of the axons continue without synapsing via the inferior cerebellar peduncle to synapse in the cerebellum.

The otolithic organs are contained in two specialized structures, the utricle and the saccule, which together form the vestibule. The otolithic organs of the utricle sense

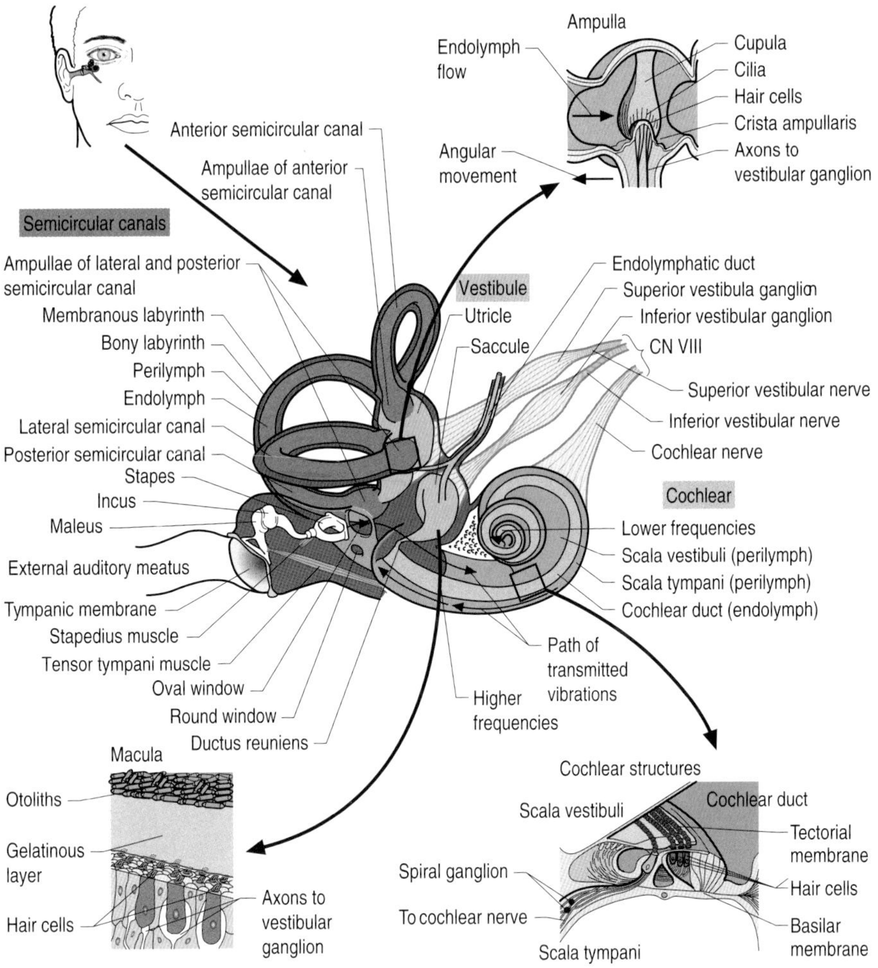

Fig. 14.17 Summary of vestibular and cochlear structures.

acceleration in the vertical (up/down) plane and those of the saccule linear acceleration in the horizontal (back and forth) plane. Both the semicircular canals and the otolithic organs are involved in controlling eye movements and vestibulo-ocular reflexes. Lesions in the semicircular canals usually result in nystagmus, whereas lesions in the otolithic organs usually result in slight static displacements of the eye such as exotropias that result in double vision. An important clinical feature of nystagmus is that nystagmus caused by peripheral lesions tend to disappear or diminish in amplitude when the patient is asked to fixate on a target. This does not occur when the nystagmus are centrally located. Peripheral lesions refer to lesions of the inner ear or vestibular nerves until they enter the brainstem. Central lesions refer to lesions involving the brainstem, and all other supraspinal structures.

The Vestibular Nuclear Complex

The vestibular nuclear complex is composed of two sets of four nuclei located bilaterally just inferior and medial to the inferior cerebellar peduncles (Fig. 14.19). Each set of nuclei contains:

1. Medial vestibular nucleus;
2. Lateral vestibular nucleus;
3. Inferior vestibular nucleus (Deiter's nucleus); and
4. Superior vestibular nucleus.

All of the vestibular nuclei receive projection axons from the vestibular nerve. All of the vestibular nuclei form reciprocal projections with the flocculus and nodule of the

QUICK FACTS 16   Blepharospasm

- Is spasms of the muscles around the eye so that the eye remains in a constant state of partial closure for prolonged periods.
- Presents with other cranial dystonias
- Spasmodic dysphonia
- Meige's syndrome
- Frequently observed in patients with chronic vestibulocerebellar disorders

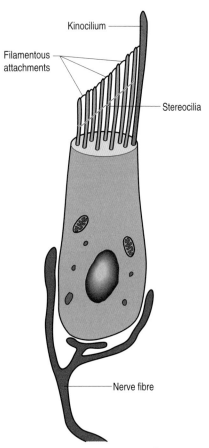

Fig. 14.18 The receptors on the hair cells are polarized to respond to movement in one direction only, with respect to a single kinocilium also present on the hair cell.

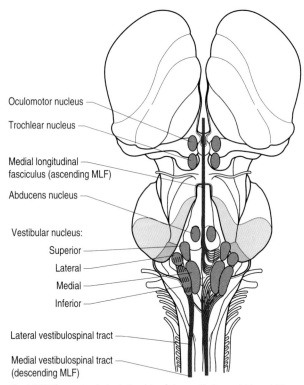

Fig. 14.19 The anatomical relationship of the vestibular nuclei (purple) in the brainstem.

posterior lobe of the cerebellum. These reciprocal projections form the cerebellovestibular fibres.

Projections from the medial vestibular nucleus ascend in the medial longitudinal fasciculus to synapse in the abducent, trochlear, and oculomotor nuclei. The majority of these axons project ipsilaterally but some are crossed and project to the contralateral extraocular nuclei. Descending projections from the medial vestibular nucleus form the medial vestibulospinal tract, which descends in the medial longitudinal fasciculus and synapses on ventral horn neurons in the cervical and thoracic spinal cord areas. These projections probably do not reach the lumbar areas of the cord and thus are involved with the postural corrections of neck and upper limb muscles exclusively (Fig. 14.20).

Projections from the lateral vestibular nuclei descend in the lateral vestibulospinal tracts to all levels of the cord (Fig. 14.20).

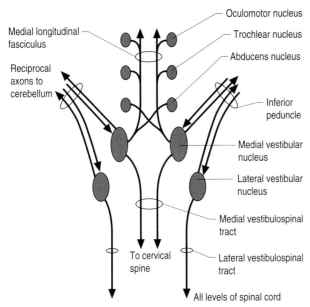

Oculomotor nucleus

Trochlear nucleus

Abducens nucleus

Medial longitudinal fasciculus

Reciprocal axons to cerebellum

Inferior peduncle

Medial vestibular nucleus

Lateral vestibular nucleus

Medial vestibulospinal tract

To cervical spine

Lateral vestibulospinal tract

All levels of spinal cord

Fig. 14.20 The functional projections between the vestibular nuclei and other structures of the brainstem and cerebellum.

The Integration System of the Vestibular System

The integration system is composed of a complex array of projection systems involving (Fig. 14.19):

1. The vestibular nuclei;
2. Areas of the brainstem reticular formation;
3. Areas of the mesencephalic reticular system;
4. All functional areas of the cerebellum (Shimazu & Smith 1971; Horak & Diener 1994);
5. Various nuclei of the thalamus;
6. Multiple areas of the cerebral cortex (Uemura et al 1977: Tomasch 1969).

Diaschisis   **QUICK FACTS 17**

- This occurs when there is remote pathology that leads to secondary cerebellar dysfunction.
- It is potentially reversible functional hypometabolism.
- Broca's aphasia nearly always creates right cerebellar diaschisis.

The Output Projections of the Vestibular System

The output mechanisms are also complex and wide ranging and may include:

1. Ocular movements controlled through areas of the brainstem and cortex;
2. Control of axial musculature via the lateral vestibular nucleus, the descending medial longitudinal fasciculus, and the reticulospinal tract (these tracts combine to provide the appropriate amount of inhibition and excitation to ventral horn neurons to provide postural stability);

Cause	Duration
Benign paroxysmal positional vertigo	Seconds
Vertebrobasilar insufficiency	Minutes
Menière's disease	Hours
Vestibular neuritis	Days
Labyrinth infarction	Days

3. Autonomic nervous system via fastigial nuclear and vestibular nuclear projections to the pontomedullary reticular nuclei including the nucleus tractus solitarius, which controls vagus nerve activity; and

4. Emotional components mediated via cerebellar-limbic projections (Brodal 1981; Robinson et al 1994; Wessel et al 1998).

The Functions of the Vestibular System

The functions of the vestibular system include:

1. The sensation and perception of position and motion—The vestibular system detects the position of the head only. In order to function appropriately, this information must also be integrated with information depicting the orientation of the head to the rest of the body. This is accomplished by the vestibulo-cervical reflexes, which integrate the information transmitted by the joint receptors, tendon organs, and muscle spindles of the muscles and joints of the neck in relation to vestibular activation. For example, when you bend your head and neck to the left, the semicircular canals and the proprioceptors of the neck both fire, giving you the perception that you are bending your neck to the left but the rest of your body is stationary. However, if your entire body falls to the left, only your semicircular canals would fire, giving you the perception that your whole body is falling to the left.

2. Orientation of the head and body to the vertical via the eye righting reflexes—The eyes maintain a parallel with the horizon despite deviations of the head. Visual clues are also important in postural and balance control. People with severe lesions to their vestibular systems can still maintain very good balance and posture until they close their eyes. When the visual cues are absent they become disoriented and fall almost immediately.

3. Dynamic and static positioning of the body's centre of mass—For example, if you are suddenly and unexpectedly pushed to the right, your right leg extensor muscles and left paraspinal muscles will contract so you do not fall to the right. All this happens before you perceive that you have been pushed.

4. Head stabilization during body movements (Horak & Shupert 1999)—The head is a relatively heavy object supported by a flexible narrow structure. The position of the head during movement is reflexively controlled to support the changing centre of gravity of the body.

5. Stabilization of the eyes while the head is moving—In order to focus on a target while the head is in motion a reflex feedback mechanism is necessary. The vestibulo-ocular reflex sends information to the extraocular muscles that cause them to move the eyes in an equal and opposite direction to that of the head.

Afferent Stimulus to the Vestibular System Can Be Accomplished through a Variety of Mechanisms

Several means of applying afferent input to stimulate a response of the vestibular system have been utilized including:

1. Large moving visual scenes (Lestienne et al 1977);
2. Electrical stimulation of the vestibular nerve (Nashner & Wolfson 1974);
3. Vibrations of tendons and muscles in the extremities (Lackner 1978);
4. Altering support surfaces and environmental stimuli (Shumway-Cook & Horak 1986);
5. Translating or rotating platforms (Nashner 1973; Keshner 1999); and
6. Vertically dropping subjects (Greenwood & Hopkins 1976; Melvill-Jones & Watt 1971).

Evaluation of the Vestibular Output

Several mechanisms have been used to evaluate the output of the vestibulocerebellar system in the clinical setting including:

1. Postural kinematics with extensive use of electromyographic (EMG) responses from various skeletal muscles (Keshner et al 1988);
2. Self-localization tests such as static and tandem Romberg's tests (Romberg 1853; Xerri et al 1988);
3. Stabilometry with destabilization and altered visual cues (Kapteyn et al 1983; Norre & Forrez 1986);
4. Stepping test of Fakuda (Fukuda 1983),
5. Tilt reactions generated via tilt boards (Martin 1965);
6. Angular velocity measures of torque about various joints following a challenge (Allum et al 1988; Horak et al 1990), and
7. Vestibulo-ocular and visuo-occular responses to perturbation (Paige 1989; Borello-France et al 1999).

Vestibulo-autonomic Reflexes

The vestibulo-autonomic reflexes are modulated throughout widespread areas of the neuraxis by the vestibulocerebellar system. Regions of the neuraxis known to mediate autonomic function and receive inputs from the vestibulocerebellar system include:

- Nucleus tractus solitarius (NTS);
- Parabrachial nuclei of the pons and midbrain;
- Hypothalamic nuclei;
- Rostral and caudal ventrolateral medulla (RVLM and CVLM);
- Dorsal motor nucleus (DMN) of the Vagus nerve;
- Nucleus ambiguus;
- Locus coeruleus;
- Superior salivatory nucleus (SSN) of the pons; and
- Edinger-Westphal nucleus of the midbrain.

Tremor often occurs with vestibulocerebellar dysfunction. There are various types and causes of tremor. *Terminal tremor* occurs because of errors in direction and extent of movement. *Cerebellar tremor* involves irregular oscillations with correcting jerks and is accentuated when greater accuracy is most essential. For example, when the patient is asked to touch an object such as their nose, the tremor will worsen the closer they get to the target. The worsening tremor results as the cerebellum tries to fine tune the action and fails. It primarily involves the proximal aspects of the limbs and the head and trunk. *Parkinsonian tremor* occurs at 4–6 Hz, whereas *physiological tremor* occurs at 8–12 Hz and is accentuated by fear, anxiety, and fatigue.

Toxic tremor can be caused by any of the following:

- Thyrotoxicosis;
- Uraemia;
- Lithium;

- Bronchodilators;
- Tricyclic antidepressants;
- Mercury, arsenic, and lead poisoning; and
- CO poisoning, alcohol withdrawal, and sedative drugs

Advanced Functions of the Vestibulocerebellar System

Being the earliest to arise in evolutionary history and embryological development, the vestibulocerebellum serves the most primitive function of the cerebellum. It receives extensive inputs from sensory receptors throughout the head and body that provide us with spatial coordinates for the purpose of spatial orientation and self-awareness. This includes:

1. Information from the retina and advanced visual-processing systems of the brain;
2. Information from auditory and vestibular neurons via monosynaptic and polysynaptic connections;
3. Information from the inner ear; and
4. Muscle and joint receptors particularly from the spine via the vestibular nuclei.

QUICK FACTS 19	The Canalith Repositioning Manoeuvre (Epley's Manoeuvre)

Epley's manoeuvre is a simple and long-lasting treatment for benign paroxysmal positional vertigo (BPPV).

Figure 14.21

Patient is supine with their head hanging over the edge of the table with the effected side down. In this position the patient will usually experience vertigo and nystagmus for the few seconds. Once the vertigo and nystagmus stops, the head is kept extended and rolled away from the effected side until the patient is facing the opposite direction. The head and body are then rolled as a unit to the unaffected side. A neck brace or collar is then applied and the patient told not to move their head or neck vigorously for 1 or 2 days. During this period they should also sleep sitting up in a chair. This manoeuvre is effective in as many as 90–95% of cases of BPPV.

In humans, the most classic signs associated with damage or disease of the vestibulocerebellum is an inability to maintain posture and balance, control eye and head movements, and respond to spatial cues in the surrounding environment. These functions are clearly essential for basic life functions such as responding to threat in the environment, finding food, finding a mate, and moving purposefully through the environment despite the forces of gravity.

Another key function of the vestibulocerebellum is the control of fuel supply to the head and body. The vestibular nuclei and older regions of the cerebellum are also important for adaptive cardiovascular and respiratory responses to changes in posture. Without these reflexes, we would be unable to maintain a constant adequate fuel supply to the nervous and muscular systems during movement or in various postures. These areas help to shift the blood volume or maintain resistance to passive shifts in blood volume during linear acceleration as that occurs while rising from a supine or seated position. This is achieved through the recruitment of neurons in the rostral medulla that form the descending limb of the excitatory vestibulosympathetic reflex.

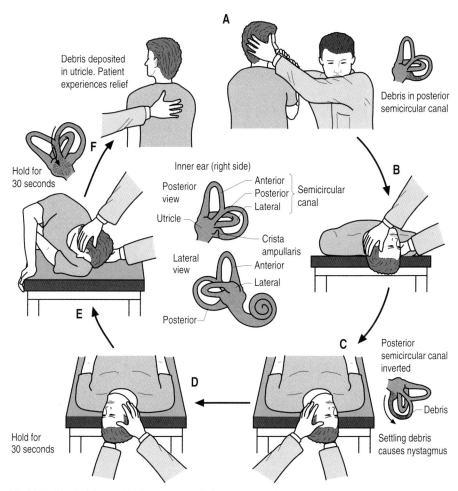

Fig. 14.21 The canalith repositioning manoeuvre (Epley's manoeuvre).

From an evolutionary and physiological perspective, normal spinal motion and stability is clearly important for optimal integrity of the vestibulocerebellum and spinocerebellum and therefore the neurological control over multiple organ systems and complex aspects of human expression.

Vestibulocerebellar Dysfunction and Asymmetry

There is substantial integration of spine, ear, and eye afferents at numerous levels of the neuraxis. The four major areas involved in this multimodal integration include the following:

- Vestibulocerebellar system;
- Mesencephalon;
- Pulvinar and posterior thalamic nuclei; and
- Parietotemporal association cortex.

The following aspects need to be considered when determining the presence of vestibulocerebellar dysfunction:

1. Vestibulosympathetic reflexes;
2. Vestibular/fastigial connections to the pontomedullary reticular formation (PMRF);
3. Motor consequences;
4. Sensory consequences; and
5. Mental consequences.

Testing for Cerebellar Dysfunction

A variety of tests have been developed to test vestibulocerebellar function (also see chapter 4). A selection of these tests include the following:

1. Walk in tandem, on heels, on toes; and backwards.
2. Accentuate dysmetria by increasing inertial load of limb, which may result in overshooting and undershooting of targets.
3. Rapidly alternating finger opposition, pronation, and supination of the elbow, and heel/toe floor tapping are all tests designed to expose dysdiadochokinesia, which is the inability to perform rapidly alternating movements with consistency and coordination.
4. The performance of finger to nose, toe to finger, heel to shin, figure of 8 with the foot are all tests to disclose kinetic tremor and dysmetria.

The cerebellum and vestibular system are also involved in the accurate and coordinated movement of the eyes. The cerebellum and vestibular system may be involved with all of the following dysmetric movements of the eyes:

- Saccadic dysmetria (hypermetric) and macrosaccadic oscillations;
- Pursuit;
- Saccadic lateropulsion;
- Gaze-evoked nystagmus;
- Rebound nystagmus;
- Downbeat nystagmus;
- Smooth tracking;
- Glissadic, postsaccadic drift;
- Disturbance in adjusting the gain of the VOR;
- Increase in duration of vestibular response; and
- Periodic alternating nystagmus.

Many patients who have undergone manipulation to the spine have reported improvements in their vision, balance, hearing, digestion, blood pressure, headaches, fertility, spinal pain, and other health complaints. While these improvements have traditionally been thought to occur because of segmental effects of restoring spinal movement and reducing noxious afferentiation, there is increasing evidence to suggest that such changes may be achieved because of supraspinal influences.

Diagnosis of Vestibular Dysfunction

The most common symptoms of vestibular dysfunction are dizziness and vertigo. Some of the more common conditions that involve dizziness or vertigo are describe below.

Menière's Disease
Patients will usually present with hearing loss, tinnitus, and dizziness. This condition is caused by decreased reabsorption of endolymphatic fluid in the inner ear, which results in dilatation and eventual perforation of the endolymphatic system. The term hydrops is sometimes used when the cause for the decreased reabsorption is known. The term Menière's disease is used when the cause of the decreased reabsorption is unknown. The cause is controversial but most probably immunological in nature. The treatment involves the dietary intake of 2 g of sodium per day and avoidance of caffeine and alcohol.

Benign Paroxysmal Positional Vertigo
This condition and migraine are the most commonly associated with patients presenting with dizziness. Each has an incidence of about two cases per thousand of population per year. The patient will report periods of vertigo lasting usually no more then a few seconds to a minute following head movements or changes in head position.

BPPV is caused by debris, usually a calcium carbonate derivative material from the utricle, in one or both semicircular canals. The most common location of the debris is in the posterior canal. Debris in the posterior canal usually produces vertigo and up-beating, torsional, nystagmus when the Hallpike-Dix manoeuvre is performed. Debris in the canals can be free floating, canalithiasis, or attached to the cupula, which is referred to as cupulolithiasis. The Hallpike-Dix manoeuvre is a very successful treatment in most cases.

Vestibular Neuritis

This condition is caused by inflammation of the vestibular nerve. The presentation usually involves sudden, severe prolonged vertigo lasting for days with no hearing impairment. The onset may be associated with a recent upper respiratory infection. The cause is thought to be viral in nature but this is controversial.

Migraine

Migraine-associated dizziness occurs with a prevalence of 6.5%, and can occur in conjunction with a headache or in isolation (not associated with a headache) (Furman & Whitney 2000). Diagnosis of this condition may be difficult because it is still largely a diagnosis of exclusion. This should be considered in all cases of dizziness associated with headache and without hearing loss. Other causes of dizziness or vertigo can include:

- Labyrinthitis;
- Anaemia;
- Carotid sinus hypersensitivity; and
- Vasovagal syncope.

References

Allum JH, Keshner EA, Honegger F et al 1988 Organization of leg–trunk–head coordination in normals and patients with peripheral vestibular defects. Progress in Brain Research 76:277–290.

Asanuma C, Thach WT, Jones EG 1983 Brainstem and spinal projections of the deep cerebellar nuclei in the monkey, with observations on the brainstem projections of the dorsal column nuclei. Brain Research Review 5:299–322.

Batton RR III, Jayaraman A, Ruggiero D et al 1977 Fastigial efferent projections in the monkey: an autoradiographic study. Journal of Comparative Neurology 174:280–305.

Berthoz A, Melvill Jones G (eds) 1985 Reviews of oculomotor research, vol 1: Adaptive mechanisms in visual-vestibular interactions. Elsevier, Amsterdam.

Bloom FE, Hoffer BJ, Siggins GR 1971 Studies on norepinephrive containing afferents to Purkinje cells of rat cerebellum. I. Localization of the fibers and their synapses. Brain Research 25:501–521.

Borello-France DF, Whitney SL, Herdman SJ 1999 Assessment of vestibular hypofunction. In: Herdman SJ (ed) Vestibular rehabilitation, 2nd edn. FA Davis, Philadelphia, p 247–286.

Brodal A 1981 Neurological anatomy in relation to clinical medicine, 3rd edn. Oxford University Press, New York.

Chusid JG 1982 Correlative neuroanatomy and functional neurology, 19th edn. Lange Medical, Los Altos, CA.

Fukuda T 1983 Statokinetic reflexes in equilibrium and movement. Tokyo University Press, Tokyo.

Furman JM, Whitney SL 2000 Central causes of dizziness. Physical Therapy 80(2):179–187.

Gilman S 1992 Cerebellum and motor dysfunction. In: Asbury AK, McKhann GM, McDonald WI (eds) Diseases of the nervous system: clinical neurobiology, 2nd edn. WB Saunders, Philadelphia, p 368–389.

Gilman S, Bloedel J, Lechtenberg R 1981 Disorders of the cerebellum. Davis, Philadelphia, PA.

Greenwood R, Hopkins AL 1976 Muscle responses during sudden falls in man. Journal of Physiology 254:507–518.

Hain TC, Ramaswamy TS, Hillman MA 1999 Anatomy and physiology of the normal vestibular system. In: Herdman SJ (ed) Vestibular rehabilitation, 2nd edn. FA Davis, Philadelphia, p 3–25.

Horak FB, Nashner LM, Diener HC 1990 Postural strategies associated with somatosensory and vestibular loss. Experimental Brain Research 82:167–177.

Horak FB, Diener HC 1994 Cerebellar control of postural scaling and central set in stance. Journal of Neurophysiology 72:479–493.

Horak FB, Shupert C 1999 Role of the vestibular system in postural control. In: Herdman SJ (ed) Vestibular rehabilitation, 2nd edn. FA Davis, Philadelphia, p 25–51.

Ito M 1984 The cerebellum and neural control. Raven Press, New York.

Kapteyn TS, Bles W, Njiokiktjien CJ et al 1983 Standardization in platform stabilometry being a part of posturography. Agressologie 24:321–326.

Keshner EA 1999 Postural abnormalities in vestibular disorders. In: Herdman SJ (ed) Vestibular rehabilitation, 2nd edn. FA Davis, Philadelphia, p 52–76.

Keshner EA, Woollacott MH, Debu B 1988 Neck and trunk muscle responses during postural perturbations in humans. Experimental Brain Research 71:455–466.

Kimoto Y, Tohyama M, Satoh K et al 1981 Fine structure of rat cerebellar noradrenaline terminals as visualized by potassium permanganate 'in situ perfusion' fixation method. Neuroscience 6:47–58.

Lackner JR 1978 Some mechanisms underlying sensory and postural stability in man. In: Held R et al (eds) Handbook of sensory physiology. Spinger-Verlag, New York, p 808

Leigh RJ, Zee DS 1991 The neurology of eye movements, 2nd edn. Davis, Philadelphia.

Lestienne F, Soechting J, Berthoz A 1977 Postural readjustments induced by linear motion of visual scenes. Experimental Brain Research 28:363–384.

Martin JP 1965 Tilting reactions and disorders of the basal ganglia. Brain 88:855–874.

Melillo R, Leisman G 2004 The cerebellum and basal ganglia. In: Neurobehavioral disorders of childhood: an evolutionary perspective. Kluwer Academic/Plenum, New York, p 47–69

Melvill-Jones G, Watt DG 1971 Observations on the control of stepping and hopping movements in man. Journal of Physiology 219:709–727.

Nashner LM 1977 Fixed patterns of rapid postural responses among leg muscles during stance. Experimental Brain Research 30:13–24.

Nashner L, Wolfson P 1974 Influence of head position and proprioceptive cues on short latency postural reflexes evoked by galvanic stimulation of the human labyrinth. Brain Research 67:255–268.

Norre ME, Forrez G 1986 Posture testing (posturography) in the diagnosis of peripheral vestibular pathology. Archives of Otorhinolaryngology 243:186–189.

Optican LM, Robinson DA 1980 Cerebellar-dependent adaptive control of the primate saccadic system. Journal of Neurophysiology 44:1058–1076.

Optican LM, Zee DS, Miles FA 1986 Floccular lesions abolish adaptive control of post saccadic ocular drift in primates. Experimental Brain Research 64:596–598.

Paige GD 1989 Nonlinearity and asymmetry in the human vestibulo-ocular reflex. Acta Otolaryngologica 108:1–8.

Robinson FR, Phillips JO, Fuchs AF 1994 Coordination of gaze shifts in primates: Brainstem inputs to neck and extraocular motor neuron pools. Journal of Comparative Neurology 346:43–62.

Romberg MH 1853 Manual of nervous diseases of man. Sydenham Society, London, p 395

Shimazu H, Smith CM 1971 Cerebellar and labyrinthine influences on single vestibular neurons identified by natural stimuli. Journal of Neurophysiology 34:493–508.

Shumway-Cook A, Horak FB 1986 Assessing the influence of sensory interaction on balance. Suggestion from the field. Physical Therapy 66:1548–1550.

Simon H, Le Moal M, Stinus L, Calas A 1979 Anatomical relationships between the ventral mesencephalic tegmentum—a 10 region and the locus coeruleus as demonstrated by anterograde and retrograde tracing techniques. Journal of Neural Transmitters 44:77–86.

Takeuchi Y, Kimura H, Sano Y 1982 Immunohistochemical demonstration of serotonin-containing nerve fibers in the cerebellum. Cell and Tissue Research 226:1–12.

Tomasch J 1969 The numerical capacity of the human cortico-ponto-cerebellar system. Brain Research 13:476–484.

Uemura T, Suzuki J, Hozawa J et al 1977 Neuro-otological examination. University Park Press, Baltimore.

Van der Want JJ, Wiklund L, Guegan M et al 1989 Anterograde tracing of the rat olivocerebellar system with Phaseolus vulgaris leucoagglutinin (PHA-L). Demonstration of climbing fiber collateral innervation of the cerebellar nuclei. Journal Comparative Neurology 288:1–18.

Wessel K, Moschner C, Wandinger KP et al 1998 Oculomotor testing is differential diagnosis of degenerative ataxic disorders. Archives of Neurology 55:949–956.

Xerri C, Borel L, Barthelemy J et al 1988 Synergistic interactions and functional working range of the visual and vestibular systems in postural control: normal correlates. Progress in Brain Research 76:193–203.

Zee DS, Yamazaki A, Butler PH et al 1981 Effects of the ablation of flocculus and paraflocculus on eye movement in primate. Journal of Neurophysiology 46:878–899.

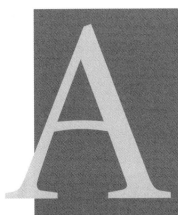

Clinical Case Answers

Case 14.1

14.1.1

1. Stroke;
2. Infection; meningitis/encephalitis;
3. Menière's disease;
4. Benign paroxysmal positional vertigo;
5. Vetsibular neuritis; and
6. Atypical migraine.

14.1.2 The critical decision in this case is to determine whether the dizziness has been caused by a central or peripheral cause. Peripheral causes include the inner ear and the vestibular nerve to its entry point in the brainstem. Central refers to the involvement of the CNS and brain. Most central dysfunctions present with other neurological finds, with the exception of cerebellar infarction or haemorrhage, which can present as only vertigo or dizziness. Most patients can be distinguished from this occurrence by their history. Do they have any of the risk factors associated with stroke, such as high blood pressure, smoking, old age, or obesity? The double vision in this case is worrisome because that is often a sign of central involvement but vestibular disorders can present with intermittent bouts of dizziness. The next step is to ask about hearing loss and examine hearing acuity. Any loss of hearing would be a strong sign that the cause is peripheral. The next clue is the degree of severity of her dizziness. Most patients with vestibular dysfunction can get up and walk if asked to; however, patients with cerebellar involvement can usually not even stand for any length of time unaided. Finally, you could check for the presence of nystagmus and if present how do they react to changes in the gaze directions of the eyes and on fixation. Peripheral nystagmus will usually disappear with fixation, whereas centrally caused nystagmus will not. Peripheral nystagmus will usually subside within a week or two of the onset of the dizziness, so if a patient has spontaneous nystagmus and the dizziness occurred greater than 2 weeks ago they probably are central in origin.

Case 14.2

14.2.1

1. Cerebellar degeneration;
2. Vestibular neuritis;
3. Alcohol intoxication;
4. Encephalitis; and
5. Brain tumour.

14.2.2

1. Vestibulospinal tracts;
2. Spinocerebellar tracts;
3. Reticulospinal tracts;
4. Spinoreticular tracts;
5. Rubrospinal tracts; and
6. Corticospinal tracts.

14.2.3   His decreased cerebellar activation can result in diaschisis of areas of his cortex that depend on the huge cerebellocortical input to maintain their level of activation. Cortical activation has been linked to immune function, and thus the reduced activation of his cortex could result in an inappropriate immune response.

Neuroimmune Functional Interactions

Clinical Cases for Thought

Case 15.1   A 56-year-old woman is referred to you by her general practitioner with medication-resistant depression of 2 years duration. She first experienced the depression when her son and daughter were killed in a plane crash 2 years previous. She also reports frequent viral infections for the past year.

Question 15.1.1   Describe a possible physiological connection between her depression and her frequent viral infections.

Case 15.2   A 34-year-old woman presents with the chief complaint of rheumatoid arthritis. She has been told that the disease she has is an autoimmune dysfunction.

Question 15.2.1   Describe to this patient how our immune system determines self from non-self.

Introduction

The connection between the nervous system and the immune system has been postulated seriously for the past century, and in the past two decades in particular we have experienced an explosion in the amount of interest and research into the neuroimmune communication and integration systems. Experimental evidence from the fields of psychology, immunology, and neurology has demonstrated that the immune system is not an autonomously regulated system but is influenced and modulated by bidirectional communication with the central nervous system. In fact it is getting very difficult to separate what constitutes psychology, neurology, and immunology when we talk about the functions of the big three supersystems. The key role of the immune system is the defence against antigens and pathogens that attempt to enter our bodies. Allergic hypersensitivity and autoimmunity are two situations where the immune system for some reason reacts inappropriately against a certain antigen or starts attacking the components of our own bodies, respectively. Understanding how and why this happens may lead us to a way of manipulating the activity of the immune system in order to relieve suffering in our fellow man. We are learning more and more everyday and the exciting discovery of cortical asymmetry and its influence on immune function has given us another virtually uncharted avenue of exploration. Brain asymmetry is associated with different patterns of immune reactivity. Left brain deficits have been associated with a decline in NK and T-cell activity and IL-2 production, suggesting a dominance of the left side of the brain in immunomodulation.

Overview of the Immune System

The immune system is a complex system of interacting components including physical barriers, bone marrow, lymphoid tissues, leukocytes, and soluble mediators. These elements function together to recognize, engulf, and destroy invading microbes, tumour cells, and any substance recognized as non-self. For the immune system to mount an effective response to invading antigens an intricate series of cellular events must occur. The antigen must be recognized and if deemed necessary bound and processed by antigen-presenting cells, which must then communicate with activated T and B cells. The T-helper cells must then assist in the activation and formation of B cells and cytotoxic T cells. Activated cells must then undergo a series of proliferative steps that involve activation of second and third messengers and selective genetic proliferation that result in an adequate response to the antigen presenting. Once an antigen has presented, a memory cell must be produced to enable a more efficient and deadly defence should the antigen present again in the future (Roitt 1994). To further complicate matters all of these complex activities must be accomplished in a controlled and selective manner so as not to destroy cells or tissues not contaminated or of use to the host.

Barriers Resisting Infection

Our bodies are constantly exposed to bacteria, fungus, and parasites. Many of these organisms are capable of causing severe disease should they be allowed access to the deeper tissues.

The simplest way for an organism to avoid infection or invasion by a foreign antigen is to prevent entry being gained into their body in the first place. Humans are no exception. In humans, the major physical barrier of defence is the skin, which, when intact, is virtually impermeable to most infectious agents (Roitt 1994). In addition, a large variety of micro-organisms cannot survive long on the skin due to the low pH which results from the presence of lactic acid, and fatty acids in the sweat (Abbas et al 1997).

Mucous secreted by the membranes lining the inner surfaces of the body acts as a protective barrier that blocks the adhesion of bacteria to epithelial cells. Other microbes become trapped in the mucous and are removed via the mechanical action of coughing, sneezing, or swallowing (Roitt 1994).

Many secreted body fluids contain bactericidal components such as acid in gastric juice, spermine and zinc in semen, and lactoperoxide in milk. The washing action of tears and saliva which both contain lysozyme is also a barrier to microbial invasion (Youmans 1980). Finally, the normal bacterial flora of the body acts as a form of microbial antagonism, which is effective in suppressing the growth of many pathologic bacteria and fungi (Sommers 1980).

Cells of the Immune System

Although all of the components of the immune system must function in a multifactorial interactive process in order to function effectively, the most crucial cell types involved are the leukocytes or white blood cells (WBC), which form the mobile foot soldiers of the immune system (Fig. 15.1). Leukocytes normally account for about 1% of total blood volume. In normal circumstances the WBC number between 4,000 and 11,000 per cubic millimetre of blood, with an average of 7,000 (Marieb 1995; Guyton & Hall 1996).

Leukocytes are grouped into two major categories, granulocytes and agranulocytes, based on their structural and chemical properties. Granulocytes contain highly specialized cytoplasmic granules. Agranulocytes lack any obvious intercellular granules. Granulocytes include neutrophils, basophils, and eosinophils. Agranulocytes include the T and B lymphocytes and non-T and non-B lymphocytes.

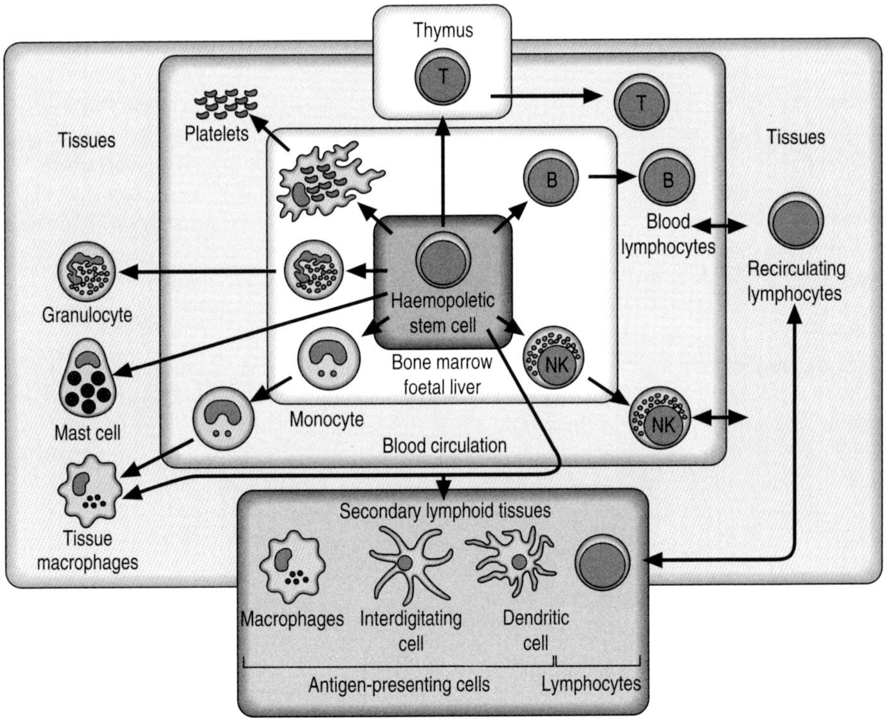

Fig. 15.1 The different types of white blood cells or leukocytes.

Immunology Definitions   QUICK FACTS 1

Neutrophils—are mobile phagocytic cells that engulf and destroy unwanted matter.

Eosinophils—secrete chemicals that destroy parasites and are involved in allergic reactions.

Basophils—are also involved in allergic reactions.

B lymphocytes—transform into plasma cells to secrete antibodies and prepare foreign matter for destruction indirectly.

T lymphocytes—are involved in cell-mediated immunity to directly destroy cells by non-phagocytic means that have been damaged by viruses or mutations.

Macrophages—are derived from circulating monocytes and become localized phagocytic specialists.

Non-specific immune responses—include inflammation, interferon, NK cells, and the complement system. These operate even when there has been no previous exposure to an offending material.

Specific immune responses—include antibody-mediated immunity by B-cells and cell-mediated immunity by T-cells.

Neutrophils, or *polymorphonuclear leukocytes*, are derived from pleuripotent haematopoietic stem cells and eventually differentiate from myeloid cells in the bone marrow. Neutrophils are short-lived cells with a life span of hours to days, but are present in large numbers in the bone marrow, peripheral blood, and marginal pool, which is a reserve of cells adherent to the walls of postcapillary venules. These cells are crucial to the host defence against bacteria and some fungi. Neutrophils and monocytes can move from the bloodstream into the tissues by a process called *diapedesis*. In this process the leukocytes squeeze through tiny pores in the vessel walls by assuming the size and shape of the pores. Once in the tissues the cells move around by amoeboid-like motion (Guyton & Hall 1996).

Neutrophils become phagocytic upon encountering bacteria and bacterial killing is promoted by a process called respiratory burst, in which oxygen is metabolized to produce hydrogen peroxide, an oxidizing, bleach-like substance which kills bacteria. Neutrophils can become actively phagocytic immediately upon confrontation with an antigen and do not have to experience a period of maturation as do other cells like monocytes which need to undergo activation processes to eventually mature into macrophages.

Eosinophils are filled with large, course granules that contain a variety of unique digestive enzymes. These cells exhibit chemotaxis to the sites of basophil and mast cell activation but are weak phagocytes for pathogens. These cells are mainly involved in attacking parasitic organisms too large to be phagocytized and are also probably involved in the deactivation of inflammatory substances released by mast cells and basophils to prevent widespread activity of these agents to other tissues not involved.

Basophils are the rarest white blood cells. They are morphologically very similar to the large mast cells that inhabit tissues exposed to the outside environment such as nasal passages and the lungs. Their cytoplasm contains large cytoplasmic granules containing histamine, heparin, bradykinin, slow-reacting substance of anaphylaxis, and serotonin. Histamine is an inflammatory chemical that acts as a vasodilator, which makes blood vessels 'leaky' and also attracts other WBC to the site of injury or inflammation. Heparin is a substance that reduces the ability of blood to clot.

The *agranulocytes*, as stated above, include lymphocytes and monocytes. Monocytes are only agranulocytic before they mature to macrophages and become granulocytic in nature.

Monocytes are derived from myeloid precursor cells in the bone marrow, which migrate through the circulation to the tissues where they mature as macrophages. Monocytes have very little contribution to immunity until they have matured into macrophages. Often in people who are actively fighting a serious infection, the numbers of monocytes in the blood will increase but have little involvement in the immunological processes until they are activated and mature into macrophages. *Macrophages* are highly mobile and are actively phagocytic. These cells have life spans ranging from months to years depending on how often and to what severity they are called upon to fight antigens (Guyton & Hall 1996). These cells have three important immunological roles:

1. They process antigens and present the essential cell membrane fragments of partially digested antigens, called epitopes, to lymphocytes which then initiate the process of cell-mediated immunity against the antigen.
2. They secrete many immunologically active substances such as cytokines, complement, and prostaglandins.
3. They are themselves activated by T-lymphocytes to phagocytose bacteria and intercellular parasites.

The macrophages are particularly concentrated in the lung and the liver where they are referred to as Kupffer cells, and the lining of the spleen sinusoids and lymph node medullary sinuses. They also occur in large concentrations in the glomerulus of the kidney where they are referred to as mesangial cells, in the brain where they are known as the microglial cells, and in bone where they form the class of cells called osteoclasts which engulf components of bone in the remodelling process.

When neutrophils and macrophages attack pathogens a number of them are also killed in the battle. The resulting necrotic tissue, dead macrophages, dead neutrophils, and tissue-fluid accumulation due to the process of inflammation, results in an interesting mixture referred to as *pus*. Generally after a few days the pus is reabsorbed by the surrounding tissues and most of the evidence that it ever existed disappears. Occasionally this process does not occur, and a pus-filled cavity called an abscess may form that needs to be mechanically drained before healing can occur.

Lymphocytes are the primary cells of the cellular immune response. These cells originally derive from pluripotent stem cells in the bone marrow and eventually differentiate into T cells, B cells, non-T cells, and non-B cells in the various lymphoid tissues of the body. Lymphocytes develop in the thymus and populate the germinal centres in the lymph nodes and spleen. Although there are large numbers of lymphocytes in the body very few are present normally in the peripheral blood. Usually the only lymphocytes present in the blood are those travelling to a specific lymphoid tissue or those travelling to the site of an infection. About 80% of the lymphocytes present in peripheral blood are T cells, which have many important functions including (Simon 1991):

1. The regulation of the immune response;
2. The production of lymphokines;
3. The initiation of cell-medicated immunity; and
4. The induction of B cells to produce antibody.

There are three major populations of T cells that are antigen-bearing: *helper T-cells, cytotoxic T cells*, and *suppressor T cells*. Both the helper and suppressor T cells are involved in the regulation aspect of the immune response, mainly the initiation and termination, respectively. Recent understanding of the structural differences in the membrane glycoproteins of these cells has lead to a new classification system. CD4 or T4 cells express a specific glycoprotein structural receptor on their membranes specific for primary helper T cells. Two classes of helper T cells have also been distinguished and are referred to as T_h1 and T_h2 classes. These cells show different levels of activation and cytokine production that regulates the shift between cellular and humeral immunity processes (see below). The CD4 receptor moiety is the suspected attachment site for the HIV virus, which exclusively targets helper T cells. CD8 or T8 cells express a specific glycoprotein structural receptor on their membranes specific for both cytotoxic and suppresser T cells populations (Marieb 1995).

B lymphocytes develop in the bone marrow and undergo a secondary differentiation when exposed to an antigen to become non-dividing plasma cells which secrete immunoglobulins or antibodies. *Plasma cells* develop an elaborate intercellular rough endoplasmic reticulum which is capable of secreting huge amounts of antibody. Non-T, non-B cells do not carry the surface marker glycoproteins of either T or B cells. The major cell type of this class is the *natural killer cells*, which are capable of killing a large variety of non-specific targets without the presence of antibody or without the prior sensitization of antibodies present (Simon 1991). These cells are augmented by *interferons*, which are a family of broad spectrum antiviral agents synthesized by cells when they become infected with a viral agent (Heaney & Golde 1998).

Innate and Specific Immunity

The characteristics of *innate immunity* or *non-specific immunity* include its limited capacity to distinguishing one microbe from another, and it is a system that functions in much the same way against most infectious agents. The principle components of innate immunity are:

1. Physical and chemical barriers; and
2. Blood proteins including compliment and mediators of inflammatory neutrophils, macrophages, and natural killer cells (Abbas et al 1997).

The *complement system* is a collection of a variety of proteins (approximately 20) present in the plasma and paracapillary tissue spaces. Many of these proteins exist in the form of precursors that can activate a cascade of reactions that terminate in the death or destruction of a target pathogen (Fig. 15.2). In normal circumstances the precursors remain inactive in the plasma unless they are activated in one of two ways:

1. *The classical activation pathway*—initiated by antigen antibody binding. When the antibody binds an antigen it undergoes a change in its structure that results in the activation of the C1 precursor protein of complement. C1 activation results in a feedforward cascade that amplifies as it progresses so that a small initial stimulus results in a much larger reaction with the formation of multiple end products (Fig. 15.3).
2. *The alternative activation pathway*—initiated by the activation of precursor proteins B and D, which enter the previous cascade at the C3 precursor level. The activation of B and D precursors is achieved when they come into contact with large polysaccharide molecules usually present on the membranes of pathogens and no antibody formation is necessary for this activation to occur. The end result is the same as the classical activation pathway (Fig. 15.4).

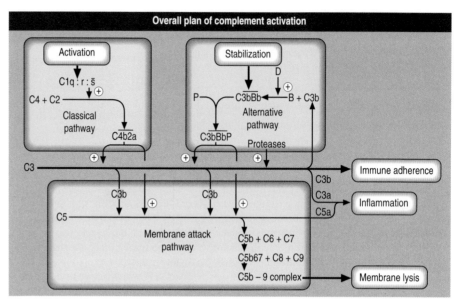

Fig. 15.2 Overall plan of the *classical*, *alternative*, and *membrane attack pathways* of complement activation. Individual components have numbers or capital letters, e.g. C4 or P. Lower-case letters indicates complement fragments, e.g. $\overline{C3b}$. A horizontal bar above a component indicates that it has become activated, $\overline{C3b}$ e.g. ⊕ indicates enzymatic activity.

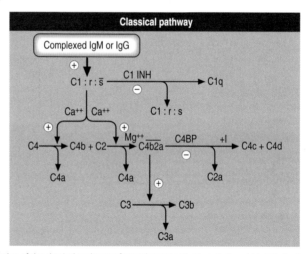

Fig. 15.3 Detailed plan of the classical pathway of complement activation. Ca⁺⁺ and Mg⁺⁺ indicate a requirement for divalent calcium and magnesium ions. ⊕ indicates enzymatic acitivity; ⊖ indicates the action of inhibitory proteins.

Innate immunity provides the early line of defence against microbes. In contrast to innate immunity, *specific immunity* involves more highly evolved defence mechanisms stimulated by exposure to infectious agents and have the ability to increase the magnitude of response with each successive exposure to a particular antigen.

The characteristics of adaptive or specific immunity are specificity for distinct molecules, specialization, and 'memory' capability that allows a more vigorous response to repeated exposure to the same microbe. The components of specific immunity are the lymphocytes and their products. Foreign substances that induce specific responses such as the production of antibodies are called *antigens*. These two systems do not function in isolation but act in an integrated fashion. Innate immunity not only provides early defence against microbes, but also plays an important role in the induction of specific immune responses. One mechanism that illustrates this cooperative effort occurs when a macrophage is exposed to an inflammatory stimulus; it secretes protein hormones called cytokines that promote activation of the lymphocytes specific for the microbial antigens. Another mechanism of interaction occurs when macrophages that have ingested microbes secrete a particular cytokine which stimulates development of T lymphocytes particularly effective at activating macrophage activity. Thus, the interactions between innate specific immunity are bidirectional (Roitt 1994).

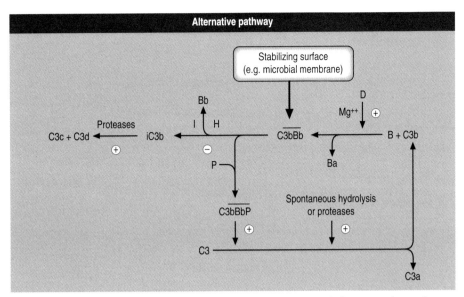

Fig. 15.4 Detailed plan of the alternative pathway of complement activation. Mg++ indicates a requirement for divalent magnesium ions. ⊕ indicates enzymatic activity; ⊖ indicates the action of inhibitory proteins.

Specific immune responses are able to combat microbes that have evolved to successfully resist innate immunity. The specific responses may also function by enhancing the activities of the innate system such as in the binding of antibodies (produced by the specific system) to bacteria, which markedly enhances complement activation (innate system). Specific immune responses are classified into two types based on the components of the system that mediate these responses: humoral and cell-mediated immunity. Both types of immunity are initiated by exposure to an antigen.

Humoral Response

The primary humoral responses occur when an antigen binds to the surface receptors of a B-lymphocytic cell, causing activation of a variety of second and third messengers that eventually result in the activation and replication of cellular DNA to initiate synthesis of antibodies or immunoglobulins (Ig's). The activation of surface receptors causes the B-lymphocyte to multiply into a series of clones that mature into plasma cells capable of secreting antibodies (Ig's) against the antigen (Fig. 15.5). Some of these B lymphocytes become memory cells, which are capable of storing the memory of the assaulting antigen in case re-exposure occurs in the future. This results in the secondary humoral response, which involves the IgM antibodies and is much more vigorous and rapid than the primary response. The antibodies

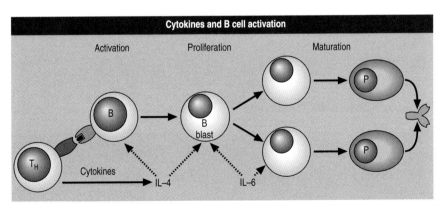

Fig. 15.5 The role of cytokines in B cell activation. The differentiation of a B cell (following interaction with a T$_h$ cell via presentation of antigen associated with HLA class II) involves an increase with metabolic activity and size, giving rise to a lymphoblast which undergoes mitosis and finally matures into an antibody-secreting plasma cell (P). Cytokines secreted by T$_h$ cells (and other cells) act on the B cell at different stages of differentiation. This is illustrated with IL-4 and IL-6, but other cytokines may also be involved: e.g. IL-1 and BCGF-I (B cell growth factor) promote early activation; IL-2, BCGF-II, and IFN-γ stimulate replication; IL-2 and IFN-α promote maturation to plasma cells.

produced combine with the specific antigen that stimulated their production and form an antigen–antibody complex that allows other cells such as macrophages, natural killer cells, and neutrophils to recognize and destroy the antigen-bearing complex.

Antigens

The antibody molecule or immunoglobulin (Ig) is composed of two identical heavy and two identical light chain peptides held together by interchain disulfide bonds (Figs 15.6 and 15.7). Five classes of antibody have been identified, each with a variety of subgroups also identified. These classes of antibody are IgG, IgA, IgM, IgE, and IgD.

IgG

This immunoglobulin is the most abundant immunoglobulin of the internal body fluids especially in extravascular fluid where it combats micro-organisms and their toxins. When

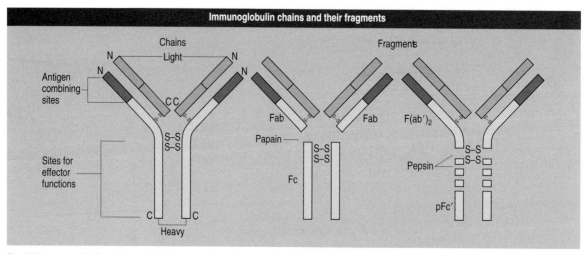

Fig. 15.6 Immunoglobulin chains and the fragments formed by proteolytic digestion. N, amino terminus; C, carboxy terminus.

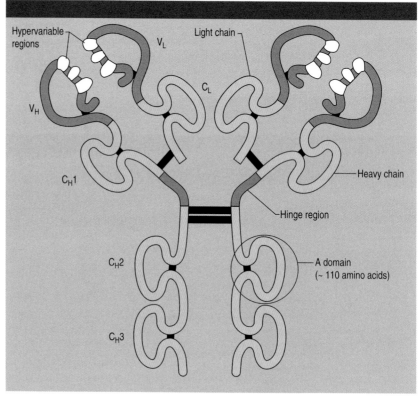

Fig. 15.7 The basic components of an immunoglobulin molecule.

IgG complexes with a bacteria or antigen the classical complement cascade is triggered, which results in chemotactic attraction of polymorphonuclear (PMN) cells, which then can adhere to the bacteria or antigen through surface receptors that recognize segments of the IgG antibody called constant regions and stimulate the PMN cell to ingest the bacteria through the process of phagocytosis.

Receptors for IgG constant regions are present on monocytes, neutrophils, eosinophils, platelets, and B lymphocytes. When IgG antibody binds to the B cells, receptor down-regulation of cellular responsiveness occurs, which leads to the decrease production of antibody in a negative feedback fashion.

IgG is the only antibody that can cross the human placenta such that it provides a major line of defence for the first few weeks of the baby's life (Fig. 15.8).

IgA
This antibody only appears in the seromucous secretions such as saliva, tears, nasal fluids, sweat, colostrum, and secretions of the lung, gastrointestinal, and genitourinary tracts, where it has the job of defending the body against attack by micro-organisms. IgA is synthesized by plasma cells, and functions by inhibiting the adherence of coated micro-organisms to the surface of mucosal cells, thereby preventing entry into the body tissues. IgA can also activate the alternative (not classical) complement pathway (Fig.15.8).

IgM
This antibody is formed as a pentamer of IgG molecules and is the largest of all the immunoglobulins. For this reason it is very effective at agglutinating bacteria and initiating the classical complement pathway (Fig. 15.9).

IgD
This antibody is mostly present on the lymphocyte cell surface and may be involved in the control of lymphocyte activation and suppression (Fig. 15.8).

IgE
This antibody is largely responsible for the protection of external body surfaces. It is also effective in parasitic infections and is responsible for the symptoms of atopic allergy, due to the stimulation of degranulation of mast cells it causes (Fig. 15.8).

Cell-Mediated Immune Response

Cell-mediated immunity involves the T-lymphocyte cell series, which unlike B lymphocytes are unable to recognize free antigens but can only respond to processed fragments of protein antigens displayed on the surfaces of the body's own cells. The T-lymphocyte attack is directed against body cells infected with viruses, bacteria or intracellular parasites, and cells recognized as non-self such as transplanted or infused tissue (Marieb 1995).

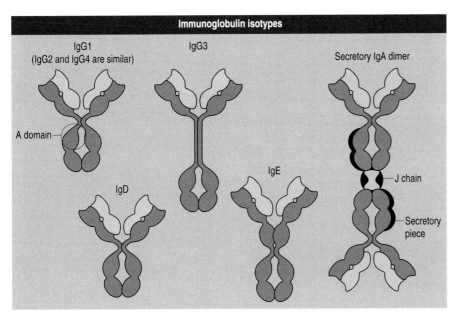

Fig. 15.8 The structure of immunoglobulins IgG, IgD, IgA, and IgE.

Discrimination of self from non-self is one of the most remarkable properties of every normal individual's immune system. This ability is called self-tolerance. Self-tolerance is maintained partly by the elimination of lymphocytes that may express receptor specific for self-antigens and partly by functional inactivation of self-reactive lymphocytes after their encounter with self-antigens. The T lymphocyte recognizes 'self' and 'non-self' by proteins on the cell membrane called major histocompatibility complex (MHC).

The MHC is a region of highly polymorphic genes whose product proteins are expressed on the surfaces of a variety of cells. This allows T lymphocytes the ability to survey the body for the presence of peptides derived from foreign proteins. There are two different types of MHC gene products called class I and class II MHC molecules. Any given T lymphocyte recognizes foreign peptides bound to only one class I or one class II MHC molecule (Fig. 15.10) (Abbas et al 1997).

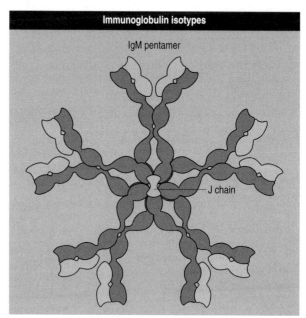

Fig. 15.9 The structure of the immunoglobulin IgM.

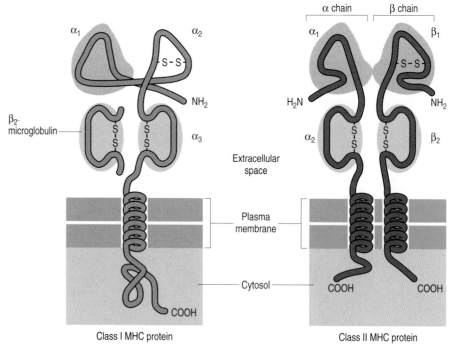

Fig. 15.10 The structure of the major histocompatibility complexes (MHC) type I and type II.

Class I MHC proteins are present on all cells of the body except red blood cells. These allow the T cells to recognize 'self'. Class II MHC proteins are present only on B cells, some T cells, and antigen-presenting cells such as macrophages. The proteins of class II MHC are composed of pieces of foreign antigen that have been phagocytosed and broken down by intracellular mechanisms and recycled back to the plasma membrane. The role of MHC proteins in the immune response is extremely important because they provide the means for signalling the immune system cells that infected or cancerous cells are present but camouflaged inside our own cells (Roitt 1994).

One Form of Communication Between the Brain and the Immune System Probably Occurs via the Autonomic Nervous System

Anatomically, the autonomic outflow of the autonomic nervous system occurs through a neuron chain consisting of a pre- and postganglionic component. The autonomic system can be divided into three functionally and histologically distinct components: the parasympathetic, sympathetic, and enteric systems.

Functions of Catecholamines	**QUICK FACTS 2**

When the body is in a neutral environment, catecholamines contribute to the maintenance of homeostasis by regulating a variety of functions:

- Cellular fuel metabolism
- Heart rate
- Blood vessel tone
- Blood pressure and flow dynamics
- Thermogenesis
- Certain aspects of immune function

The *parasympathetic system* communicates via several cranial nerves including the oculomotor (CN III) nerve, the trigeminal (CN V) nerve, the facial (CN VII) nerve, and the vagus (CN X) nerve. The vagus nerve and sacral nerve roots compose the major output route of parasympathetic enteric system control (Furness & Costa 1980). The neurotransmitter released both pre- and post-synaptically is acetylcholine. Functionally, the neurological output from the parasympathetic system is the integrated end product of a complex interactive network of neurons spread throughout the mesencephalon, pons, and medulla. This complex interactive network receives modulatory input from wide areas of the neuraxis including all areas of cortex, limbic system, hypothalamus, cerebellum, thalamus, vestibular nuclei, basal ganglia, and spinal cord (Walberg 1960; Angaut & Brodal 1967; Brodal 1969; Brown 1974; Webster 1978). The relationship of the parasympathetic outflow to the immune system has received very little study to date and as a consequence very little is known about the influence of parasympathetic or the enteric system on immune function.

The *sympathetic system* enjoys a wide-ranging distribution to virtually every tissue of the body. The presynaptic neurons live in a region of the grey matter of the spinal cord called the intermediomedial and intermediolateral cell columns. The output of the preganglionic neurons of the sympathetic system is the summation of a complex interactive process involving segmental afferent input from dorsal root ganglion and suprasegmental input from the hypothalamus, limbic system, and all areas of cortex via the mesencephalic and pontomedullary reticular formations (Donovan 1970; Webster 1978; Williams & Warwick 1984). Most postganglionic fibres of the sympathetic nervous system release norepinephrine as their neurotransmitter. The chromaffin cells of the adrenal medulla, which are embryological homologues of the paravertebral ganglion cells, are also innervated by preganglionic sympathetic fibres which fail to synapse in the paravertebral ganglia. When stimulated these cells release a neurotransmitter/neurohormone that is a mixture of epinephrine and norepinephrine with a 4:1 predominance of epinephrine (Elenkov et al 2000).

Both epinephrine and norepinephrine are manufactured via the tyrosine–dihydroxyphenylalanine (DOPA)–dopamine pathway and are called catecholamines. When the body is in a neutral environment, catecholamines contribute to the maintenance of homeostasis by regulating a variety of functions such as cellular fuel metabolism, heart rate, blood vessel tone, blood pressure and flow dynamics, thermogenesis and as explained below, certain aspects of immune function. When a disturbance in the homeostatic state is detected, both the sympathetic nervous system and the hypothalamus–pituitary–adrenal axial system become activated in the attempt to restore homeostasis via the resulting increase in both systemic (adrenal) and peripheral (postganglionic activation) levels of catecholamines and glucocorticoids. In the1930s Hans Selye described this series of events or reactions as the general adaptation syndrome or generalized stress response (Selye 1936). Centrally, two principal mechanisms are involved in this general stress response; these are the production and release of corticotrophin-releasing hormone produced in the paraventricular nucleus of the hypothalamus and increased norepinephrine release from the locus ceruleus norepinephrine-releasing system in the brainstem. Functionally, these two systems cause mutual activation of each other through reciprocal innervation pathways (Chrousos & Gold 1992). Activation of the locus ceruleus results in an increase release of catecholamines, of which the majority is norepinephrine, to wide areas of cerebral cortex, subthalamic, and hypothalamic areas. The activation of these areas results in an increased release of catecholamines from the postganglionic sympathetic fibres as well as from the adrenal medulla (Fig. 15.11).

QUICK FACTS 3	Integration of Catecholamine Release

When a disturbance in the homeostatic state is detected, both the sympathetic nervous system and the hypothalamus–pituitary–adrenal axial system become activated in the attempt to restore homeostasis via the resulting increase in both systemic (adrenal) and peripheral (postganglionic activation) levels of catecholamines and glucocorticoids.

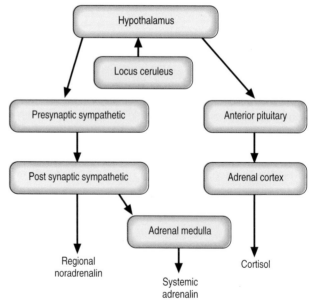

Fig. 15.11 Integration of catecholamine and cortisol releases. The interactions between the activation of the locus ceruleus and the release of catecholamines from the adrenal glands are shown.

Catecholamine-releasing nerve fibres have been found in a wide range of cells and tissues including thymus, spleen, lymph nodes, tonsils, bone marrow, mucosa-associated lymphoid tissue (MALT), gut-associated lymphoid tissue (GALT), and the parenchyma of lymphoid tissues not associated with blood vessels. Generally, these areas of adrenogenic innervation appear to be in areas with high concentrations of T lymphocytes, macrophages, and plasma cells. This is in contrast to areas of high concentrations of developing B lymphocytes, which seem to be poorly innervated by these fibres (Felton et al 1985). The appearance of these fibres occurs early in the development of these cell types, suggesting a possible role in the maturation and development process of these cell types and in immune system maturation (Elenkov et al 2000). Current understanding of synaptic transmission processes suggests that the majority of the interactions between the above described cell types and the nerve fibres in the lymphoid tissues occur via an alternate form of synaptic transmission recently termed 'non-synaptic transmission' (Vizi & Labos 1991; Vizi 2000). In this alternate form of neurotransmission, neurotransmitters are released from postsynaptic sympathetic neurons and diffuse over relatively large distances before interacting with receptors on the various cell types previously described. Thus three main classes of neurochemical interactions in sympathetic/immune communication may be identified. These include fast synaptic transmission; moderately fast nonsynaptic transmission, and slow neurohormonal transmission. Nonsynaptic transmission may also play a role in the norepinephrine regulation of blood flow in various tissues and also in modulating lymphocyte trafficking through the body (Villaro et al 1987).

Neuroimmune Interactions

Our understanding of the bidirectional communication between the nervous and the immune system has developed over the past 25 or so years to the point that it is clear that these two systems have a well-developed bidirectional communications system, involving neurotransmitters and cytokines (Besedovsky et al 1981; Ader & Cohen 1982). Cytokines are a group of chemical mediators utilized by cells as a form of communication. A vast number of cytokines have been identified to date (Tables 15.1 and 15.2)

How Do the Immune System and Nervous Systems Communicate?   QUICK FACTS 4

- Glucocorticoids (cortisol) secreted from the adrenal cortex
- Catecholamines (noradrenalin) secreted from the sympathetic nerve terminals
- Catecholamines (adrenalin) secreted from the adrenal medulla
- Hormones (ACTH) secreted from the pituitary gland
- Cytokines, lymphokines, interleukins, interferons, anti-necrosis factors produced by immune cells.

Communication between Sympathetic Neurons and Immune Cells   QUICK FACTS 5

Communications between sympathetic neurons and other cells is mediated by two principal types of receptors. These principal types of receptors have been classified as alpha (α) and beta (β) adrenergic receptors. Both classes have subsequently been subclassified to include beta 1, 2, and 3 and alpha 1 and 2 subtypes, with even more subtypes in each class known to exist.

Table 15.1 Cytokines: Sources and Functions

Cytokine	Immune Cells	Other Cells	Immunological Effects
IL-1α,β	Monocytes/ macrophages	Endothelial, epithelial, and neuronal cells, fibroblasts	Activation of T and B cells, macrophages and endothelium. Stimulation of acute phase responses.
IL-2	T cells		Proliferation and/or activation of T, B, and LGL.
IL-3	T cells, mast cells, thymic epithelium	Keratinocytes, neuronal cells	Proliferation of pluripotent stem cells. Production of various blood cell types.
IL-4	T and B cells, macrophages, mast cells and basophils, bone marrow stroma		Activation of B cells. Differentiation of T_h2 cells and suppression of T_h1 cells.
IL-5	T cells, mast cells		Development, activation and chemoattraction of eosinophils.
IL-6	T cells, monocytes or macrophages	Fibroblasts, hepatocytes, endothelial and neuronal cells	Activation of haemopoietic stem cells. Differentiation of B and T cells. Production of acute phase proteins.
IL-7	Bone marrow stroma		Growth of B cell precursors. Proliferation and cytotoxic activity of T cells.
IL-8	T cells, monocytes, neutrophils	Endothelial and epithelial cells, fibroblasts	Chemoattraction of neutrophils, T cells, basophils. Activation of neutrophils.
IL-9	T cells		Development of erythroid precursors.
IL-10	T and B cells, macrophages	Keratinocytes	Suppression of macrophage functions and T_h1 cells. Activation of LGL and T cells.
IL-11	Bone marrow stroma	Trophoblasts	Stimulation of haemopoietic precursors. Production of acute phase proteins.
IL-12	B cells, macrophages		Differentiation of T_h1 cells. Activation of LGL and T cells.
IL-13	T cells		Activation of B cells. Inhibition of monocytes or macrophages.
IL-14	T cells		Proliferation of activated B cells but inhibition of immunoglobulin secretion.

Reeves G, Todd I, 1996 Lecture notes on immunology. Blackwell Science, London.

Cytokines such as interleukin-1 (IL-1), interleukin-6 (IL-6), and tumour necrosis factor-alpha (TNF-α) can signal the brain via a complex pathway involving the activation of both the sympathetic nervous system and the hypothalamic–pituitary–adrenal axis. The involvement of both fast-acting and slow-acting mechanisms suggests that both acute and chronic types of interactions are possible and in fact occur functionally (Berkenbosch et al 1989; Elenkov et al 1996).

Communication between sympathetic neurons and other cells is mediated by two principal types of receptors. These principal types of receptors have been classified as alpha (α) and beta (β) adrenergic receptors. Both classes have subsequently been subclassified to include beta 1, 2, and 3 and alpha 1 and 2 subtypes, with even more subtypes in each class known to exist. A crucial discovery in relating the nervous system to the immune system occurred when it was observed that beta adrenergic receptors are found on all types of lymphoid cells. The quantity across various cell types seems to vary with natural killer cells having the greatest density and helper T-lymphocytes having the lowest density (Khan et al 1986; Maisel et al 1990). Recent investigations have

Table 15.2 Cytokines: Sources and Functions

Cytokine	Immune Cells	Other Cells	Immunological Effects
IL-15	T cells		Proliferation of T cells
TNF-α	Macrophages, lymphocytes, neutrophils	Astrocytes, endothelium, smooth muscle	Activation of macrophages, granulocytes, cytotoxic cells, and endothelium. Enhanced HLA class I expression. Stimulation of acute phase response. Antitumour effects.
TNF-β	T cells		Similar to TNF-α
ITN-α, -β	T and B cells monocyte or macrophages	Fibroblasts	Antiviral activity. Stimulation of macrophages and LGL. Enhanced HLA class I expression.
IFN-γ	T and LGL		Antiviral activity. Stimulation of macrophages and endothelium. Enhanced HLA class I and class II expression. Suppression of T_h2 cells.
G-CSF	T cells, macrophages, neutrophils	Fibroblasts, endothelium	Development and activation of neutrophils.
M-CSF	T cells, macrophages, neutrophils	Fibroblasts, endothelium	Development and activation of neutrophils.
GM-CSF	T cells, macrophages, mast cells, neutrophils, eosinophils	Fibroblasts, endothelium	Differentiation of pluripotent stem cells. Development of neutrophils, eosinophils, and macrophages.
TGF-β	T cells, monocytes	Chondrocytes, osteoblasts, osteoclasts, platelets, fibroblasts	Inhibition of T and B cell proliferation and LGL activity.

IL, interleukin; TNF, tumour necrosis factor; IFN, interferon; CSF, colony stimulating factor; TGF, transforming growth factor.
Reeves G, Todd I, 1996 Lecture notes on immunology. Blackwell Science, London.

demonstrated that two subclasses of helper T-lymphocytes show different receptor characteristics with the helper type-1 lymphocytes expressing beta-2 adrenergic receptors on their membrane but these same receptors are not expressed on type-2 helper lymphocyte membranes (Sanders 1998). As we shall discuss later this receptor variation may play an important part in the different functional reactions of these two lymphocyte subclasses.

Once activated, the beta adrenergic receptors activate a chain of G-proteins that act as intracellular effectors, which in turn stimulate the activation of a series of successive enzymes such as adenylate cyclase, cyclic adenosine monophosphate (cAMP), inositol-1,4,5-triposphate (IP3), and diacylglycerol (DAG) (see Chapter 3). Variations in the intracellular concentrations of these various 'second messenger' enzymes result in different functional outcomes. Activity of different receptors can also alter the production and activation thresholds of second messengers within the cell. For example, the activation of adrenergic–G-protein complexes usually results in inhibition of adenylate cyclase and a subsequent decrease in the production of cAMP in the cell. cAMP has been shown to modulate a variety of transcription factors important in the expression of various genes, including those genes involved in the production of a variety of cytokines produced in lymphocytes. Thus activation of beta-2 adrenergic receptors by catecholamines usually results in a decreased transcription rate of genes responsible for the production of TNF-α and IL-12. The same receptor activation pathway also stimulates the activation of genes that transcribe the production enzymes for IL-10 (Elenkov et al 1995; Hasko et al 1998). This series of events is important in the activation shift between cellular and humoral immunity as outlined below.

The T-lymphocyte subclasses, T-helper type 1 (T_h1) and T-helper type 2 (T_h2), are both components of the cellular or acquired immunity response but may activate or inhibit activity of other immune responses via cytokine mechanisms. T_h1 lymphocytes primarily produce and release interferon gamma (IFN-γ), IL-2, and TNF-α, which promote cellular immunity processes, whereas T_h2 lymphocytes produce and release a different set of cytokines, namely IL-1, IL-4, IL-10, and IL-13, which promote humoral immunity processes (Abbas et al 1996; Grohmann et al 2000). Unactivated CD4$^+$ lymphocytes (T_h0) are lymphocytes that have not been exposed to an antigen and are referred to as antigen inexperienced or naïve. These cells are bipotential and have the capability to develop into either T_h1 or T_h2 lymphocytes. Which development pathway these cells follow will depend to a large extent on the cytokines released by the antigen-presenting cells that initially induce their activation. For instance, IL-12 produced by a macrophage presenting an antigen acts in concert with other signalling mechanisms to induce the development of T_h1-type lymphocytes. Because T_h1 lymphocytes are involved in the production of IL-12, TNF-α, and IFN-γ these lymphocytes are considered to promote the process of inflammation and are classed functionally as proinflammatory lymphocytes. In contrast the T_h2 lymphocytes promote anti-inflammatory processes and are termed as such (Trinchieri 1995; Mosmann & Sad 1996).

The cytokines produced in T_h1-type lymphocytes inhibit the response and activation of T_h2-type lymphocytes and vice versa. Thus IL-4 and IL-10 inhibit T_h1 responses and IL-12 inhibits T_h2 responses. The T_h2 production of IL-10 promotes the stimulation of humoral immunity by stimulating both the growth and activation of mast cells and eosinophils and the activation and maturation of B lymphocytes to plasma cells. This cytokine also stimulates the plasma cell into the process of immunoglobulin switching from IgG to IgE, all of which inhibit the production of T_h1 proinflammatory cytokines and promote anti-inflammatory states in the region. The activation of catecholamine receptors on T-helper cells seems to inhibit type-1 activities and favour type-2 activities. This results in a functional shift from cellular immunity towards humoral immunity. The major mechanism involved in this shift is the inhibition of IL-12 via stimulation of beta-2 adrenergic receptors. Activation of these same receptors also results in the inhibition of TNF-α, another proinflammatory cytokine, while at the same time promoting the production of IL-10, one of the most potent anti-inflammatory cytokines (Suberville et al 1996) (Fig. 15.12).

The discussion thus far has focused on the systemic effects of catecholamine release on the balance between cellular and humoral immunity in T-helper lymphocytes. Locally these responses may be different to that discussed earlier. In local responses in specific tissue areas release of catecholamines may result in predominately alpha receptor

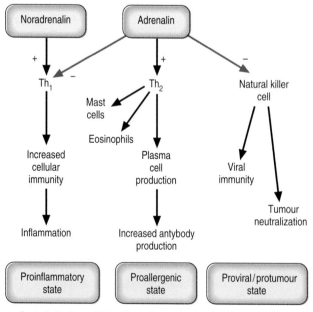

Fig. 15.12 Summary of catecholamine activities. The pathways that may be responsible for the development of proinflammatory, proallergy, and protumour states are shown.

stimulation, which promotes the activation of inflammatory responses through the stimulation and recruitment of polymorphonuclear leukocytes in the regions involved. This proinflammatory process occurs through a complex series of interactions involving chemotactic cytokines called chemokines. Other components of the immune system seem to be modulated by the activity of catecholamines. Natural killer cells seem to be inhibited by catecholamine release and in fact may be the most sensitive cell type to the circulating concentration of catecholamines due to the large number of beta-2 adrenergic receptors on their membranes (Irwin 1994). The effect of catecholamines on macrophage function is complex and appears to be somewhat dependent on the state of activation of the macrophage at the time of interaction. Some evidence suggests that naïve or non-antigen challenged macrophages may respond more aggressively to alpha adrenergic receptor stimulation, which results in increased activation of the macrophage. Activated macrophages show increased receptiveness to beta-adrenergic receptor stimulation, which results in a reduction in activation or an inhibition of activity. The final activation state of a macrophage may also depend on the presence of other cytokines or proinflammatory mediators in the immediate environment of the cell (Baker & Fuller 1995). The effect of catecholamines on cytotoxic (CD8$^+$) lymphocytes is sketchy at best. Some indication that catecholamines may stimulate the development of CD8$^+$ lymphocytes but inhibit their functional activity at the same time has been postulated (Benschop et al 1996). Neutrophil function appears to be inhibited by catecholamines over a wide range of activities including phagocytosis, chemotaxis, release of lysosomal enzymes, and superoxide formation (Zurier et al 1974; Gibson-Berry et al 1993).

Can Immune Function be Modulated by Different Areas of Cortex?

There is widespread evidence that asymmetric lateralization of cortical functioning does occur. Several of the lateralized functions are also known to be involved in brain neuroimmune modulation such as emotional arousal, sympathetic innervation, neurotransmitter concentrations, and neuroendocrine activity (Wittling 1998). It would seem from the widespread evidence of cortical functional hemispheric dominance in other systems that modulation of the immune system would also fall under asymmetric cortical control.

A growing body of evidence indicates that immune system function is modulated by different areas of the cortex in an asymmetrical fashion. For instance, a variety of studies have demonstrated that the rostral portions of the frontal cortical areas are differentially activated when the individual is exposed to different emotional stimulus and that the activation state experienced altered the immune response of the individual (Kang et al 1991). The left frontal cortex appears to be activated during the expression or experience

T-Lymphocytes Have Two Major Classes of Cells   QUICK FACTS 6

The T-lymphocyte subclasses, *T-helper type 1* (T$_h$1) and *T-helper type 2* (T$_h$2), are both components of the immunity response but may activate or inhibit activity of cellular or humeral immunity via cytokine mechanisms.

Activation of T cells May Shift Immunity Processes   QUICK FACTS 7

T$_h$1 lymphocytes primarily produce and release interferon gamma (IFN-γ), IL-12, and TNF-α, which promote cellular immunity processes.

T$_h$2 lymphocytes produce and release a different set of cytokines, namely IL-1, IL-4, IL-10, and IL-13, which promote humoral immunity processes.

of positive emotional states, whereas the right frontal cortex seems to be activated during the expression or experience of negative emotional states (Davidson 1984; Davidson & Tomarken 1989; Leventhal & Tomaren 1986; Silberman & Weingartner 1986). One of the difficulties in this type of research is the huge individual variability of immune responses in individuals that occurs to a variety of cognitive stimulus. A few studies have tried to specifically address this problem and the results indicate that individual responses can be significantly correlated to immunological change. For instance, individuals with depression seem to show a range of immune activation, which is dependent on the severity of the depressive symptoms (Irwin et al 1990). The severity of symptoms in depression has been linked to the activation levels in the left frontal cortex (Robinson et al 1984). Those patients with left frontal cortex lesions but sparing of the right frontal cortex showed the most severe depressive symptoms, which suggests that the asymmetrical activation levels between the right and left cortical areas may also be important in the modulation of immune response (Davidson et al 1990). Another study showed that individual personality traits were predictive of natural killer cell activity both before and after a stressful event (Kiecolt-Glaser et al 1984). Another study found that natural killer cell activity was significantly increased in human females with extreme left frontal cortical activation when compared to females with extreme right cortical frontal activation (Kang et al 1991). The level of hemispheric activation in these women was determined by electroencephalographic (EEG) determinants of regional alpha power density. This measurement has been shown to be inversely related to emotional or cognitive brain activation (Davidson 1988).

QUICK FACTS 8	Inflammatory Processes May Be Modulated by T Cells

T_h1 lymphocytes are considered to promote the process of inflammation and are classed functionally as proinflammatory lymphocytes.

T_h2 lymphocytes promote anti-inflammatory processes.

A variety of animal studies have also provided direct evidence of the relationship between cerebral asymmetry and immune system function (Barneoud et al 1987; Neveu 1988). Partial ablation of the left frontoparietal cortex in mice, which results functionally in relative right cortical activation, resulted in decreased immune responses and partial right cortical ablation, which would result functionally in a left cortical activation showed no change or a reduced immune response (Renoux et al 1983; Neveu et al 1986).

A variety of further studies have found several consistent findings relating to ablation of cortical areas and resultant immune dysfunction (Renoux et al 1983; Biziere et al 1985; Renoux & Biziere 1986; Barneoud et al 1988). These finds show the following:

1. Development of the lymphoid organs including the spleen and thymus occurs with left cortical lesions, whereas increased development of the spleen and thymus occurs with right cortical lesions

2. Activation of T cells is significantly diminished in lesions involving the left cortex and elevated with lesions of the right cortex.

These findings indicate that T-cell-mediated immunity is modulated asymmetrically by both hemispheres, with each hemisphere acting in opposition to the other. Increased activity of the left cortex seems to enhance the responsiveness of a variety of T-cell-dependent immune parameters, whereas increased right cortical activity seems to be immunosuppressive. B-cell activity was found not to be affected by cortical activation asymmetry (LaHoste et al 1989; Neveu et al 1988).

In summary, most studies have shown that changes in hemispheric activation because of either ablation of cortical areas or modulation in physiological activation levels result in changes in immunological response activity. Both hemispheres seem to be active in the modulation of immune response, with the left hemisphere enhancing cellular immune responses and the right inhibiting those responses. Some evidence does suggest that the involvement of the right hemisphere may not act directly on immune components but may modulate the activity of the left hemisphere which does act directly to regulate immune function (Renoux et al 1983).

Hemispheric chemical dominance can also influence the nature of immune reactivity. Various studies have shown that right hemispheric chemical dominance was associated with up-regulation of the hypothalamic-mediated isoprenoid pathway and was more prevalent among individuals with various metabolic and immune disorders including a high body mass index, various lung diseases including asthma and chronic bronchitis, increased levels of lipid peroxidation products, decreased free radical scavenging enzymes, inflammatory bowel disease, systemic lupus erythematosus (SLE), osteoarthritis, and spondylosis. Left hemispheric chemical dominance was associated with a down-regulated isoprenoid pathway and was more prevalent among individuals with low body mass index, osteoporosis, and bulimia.

Cerebellar–Hypothalamic Communication may also be Important in Immune System Function

The posterior part of the dorsomedial hypothalamic nucleus and posterior hypothalamic nucleus receive direct distinct projections from the cerebellum, whereas the anterior part of the dorsomedial hypothalamic nucleus does not. These observations bring a new perspective on the question of how the cerebellum is involved in the regulation of visceromotor functions.

The hypothalamo-cerebellar projections arise primarily from the lateral, posterior, and dorsal hypothalamic area; the dorsomedial, ventromedial, supramammillary, tuberomammillary, and lateral mammillary nuclei; and the periventricular zone. Available evidence suggests that hypothalamo-cerebellar fibres terminate in the neurons of the layers of the cerebellar cortex and cerebellar nuclei.

Cerebello-hypothalamic projections arise from all four cerebellar nuclei, pass through the superior cerebellar peduncle, cross in its decussation, follow the trajectory of cerebellothalamic fibres, and then separate from that thalamic fasciculus to enter the hypothalamus. These fibres terminate primarily in the contralateral lateral, posterior, and dorsal hypothalamic areas including the dorsomedial and paraventricular nuclei. Of particular interest to functional neurological practitioners is the influence of midline areas of the cerebellum on hypothalamic function. Midline areas of the cerebellum including the vermis of the cerebellar cortex and the midline fastigial nuclei communicate extensively with spinal, vestibular, visual, and auditory afferents.

The hypothalamo-neurohypophyseal system as well as the autonomic nervous system is involved in homeostatic responses associated with changes in head position and orthostatic reflex. The responses induced by body tilt on earth are thought to be attributed to changes in inputs from baroreceptors, vestibular organs, and proprioreceptors normally required for postural control. The information from these organs is sent to the hypothalamus, which thereby influences both neuroendocrine and autonomic systems as well as various kinds of emotional behaviour. The fastigial input to the hypothalamus suggested that the fastigial nucleus plays a significant role in these homeostatic responses through its connections with the brainstem and the hypothalamus (Katafuci et al 1995).

Hypothalamic Modulation of Immune Function

The hypothalamic-mediated isoprenoid pathway produces four key metabolites including digoxin, dolichol, ubiquinone, and cholesterol. These metabolites can alter intracellular calcium/magnesium ratios, Na^+/K^+ ATPase activity, free radical scavenging and cellular respiration, and altered glycoconjugate metabolism. All of these factors are influential on immune function at the cellular level and can result in defective formation and transport of MHC–antigen complexes.

Does Immune Activity Equate to Appropriate Immune Function?

The complex nature of neuroimmune interactions has made interpreting the impact of these reactions on the health and well being of the person in question very difficult. For example, in some cases an increase in certain cytokines may be appropriate and in other cases cause the person great despair. If we are just measuring the concentration of that cytokine without regard to appropriateness of its action the true meaning of the increase may well be lost. It is also important to understand which aspects of immune function are being measured and if they are actually measuring immune function or just quantitative aspects of cell mobilization. For instance, an increase in total lymphocyte count may not indicate the actual activity of those cells, which must undergo a complex interactive process of activation in order to actually perform their immune functions. A simple measure of concentration may be misleading.

All immune responses are initiated by recognition of foreign antigens. This leads to activation of lymphocytes that specifically recognize the antigen and hopefully culminates in the elimination of the antigen. The specific immune response consists of the binding of foreign antigens to specific receptors on the mature lymphocytes, the B lymphocytes. The cells of humoral immunity express antibody molecules on their surfaces that can bind foreign proteins, polysaccharides, or cell-associated forms. T lymphocytes are responsible for cell-mediated immunity, and express receptors that only recognize short peptides sequences in protein antigens present on the surfaces of other cells. The activation phase of immune response is the sequence of events induced in lymphocytes as a consequence of specific antigen recognition. All lymphocytes undergo two major changes in this phase. First, they proliferate, leading to expansion of the clone population of antigen-specific lymphocytes. Second, the progeny of these antigen-specific lymphocytes differentiate into effector cells capable of antigen elimination. The effector phase of immune response entails the specific activation of functions that lead to the elimination of antigen.

Immune function can be affected at any phase just described, and the effectiveness of the system depends on the complete interactive process as well as the appropriateness of the response at any given time in the individual. The appropriateness of the response may be partially under the modulation of the nervous system and thus asymmetries in neural function may result in inappropriate immune responses. The appropriateness of the neuroimmune response of the individual should be constantly assessed if possible and always a concern in the clinical management of any patient.

Clinical Implications

It is clear from the previous discussion that the interactions between the nervous and immune systems are complicated and are multifactorial in nature. Inappropriate interaction via efferent or afferent loops of this communication system may result in dysfunction or disease (Fig. 15.13).

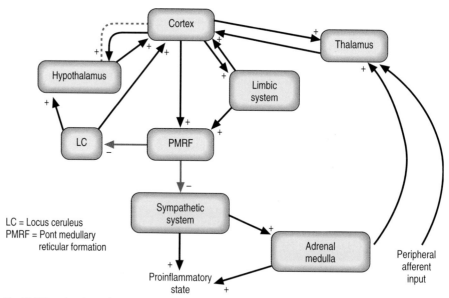

LC = Locus ceruleus
PMRF = Pont medullary
reticular formation

Fig. 15.13 Functional neuroimmune interactions.

Inappropriate levels of systemic catecholamines have been associated with a variety of clinical conditions associated with immune dysfunction including (Elam et al 1992; Jarek et al 1993; Abbas et al 1996; Li et al 1997):

1. Both onset and progression of a variety of infectious diseases;
2. *Helicobacter pylori*, both onset and progression;
3. Increased susceptibility to the common cold;
4. Increased complications following major trauma;
5. Rheumatoid arthritis;
6. Multiple sclerosis;
7. Type I diabetes mellitus;
8. Autoimmune thyroid disease;
9. Crohn's disease; fibromyalgia;
10. Increased rate of tumour growth; and
11. Systemic hypertension and cardiovascular disease.

Several studies have investigated the effect of changes in spinal afferentiation as a result of manipulation on the activity of the sympathetic nervous system (Korr 1979; Sato 1992; Chiu & Wright 1996). Suprasegmental changes, especially in brain function, have demonstrated the central influence of altered afferentiation of segmental spinal levels (Thomas & Wood 1992; Carrick 1997; Kelly et al 2000). Changes in immune system function can be mediated through spinal afferent mechanisms. These mechanisms may operate via suprasegmental or segmental levels by modulating the activity of the sympathetic nervous system (Beck 2003).

References

Abbas A, Lichtman A, Pober J 1997 Cellular and molecular immunology, 3rd edn. Saunders, Philadelphia.

Abbas AK, Murphy KM, Sher A 1996 Functional diversity of helper T lymphocytes. Nature 383:787–793.

Ader R, Cohen N 1982 Behaviorally conditioned immunosuppression and murine systemic lupus erythematosis. Science 215:1534–1536.

Angaut P, Brodal A 1967 The projection of the vestibulocerebellum onto the vestibular nuclei of the cat. Archives Italiennes de Biologie 105:441–479.

Baker AJ, Fuller RW 1995 Loss of responce to beta-adrenoreceptor agonists during the maturation of human monocytes to macrophages in vitro. Journal of Leukocyte Biology 57:395–400.

Barneoud P, Neveu PJ, Vitiello S et al 1987 Functional heterogeneity of the right and left cerebral neocortex in the modulation of the immune system. Physiology and Behaviour 41:525–530.

Barneoud P, Neveu PJ, Vitiello S et al 1988 Early effects of right or left cerebral cortex ablation on mitogen-induced speen lymphocyte DNA synthesis. Neuroscience Letters 90:302–307.

Beck RW 2003 Psychoneuroimmunology. In: Beirman R (ed) Handbook of clinical diagnosis. Sydney, p 27–35.

Benschop RJ, Rodriguez-Feuerhahn M, Schedlowski M 1996 Catecholamine-induced leukocytosis: early observations, current

research and future directions. Brain, Behavior, and Immunity 10:77–91.

Berkenbosch F, de Goeij D, Rey AD 1989 Neuroendrocrine sympathetic metabolic processes induced by interleukin-1. Neuroendocrinology 50:570–576.

Besedovsky HO, del Rey AE, Sorkin E 1981 Lymphokine containing supernatants from Con A-stimulated cells increase cortisone blood levels. Journal of Immunology 126:385–389.

Biziere K, Guillaumin JM, Degenne D et al 1985 Lateralized reocortical modulation of the T-cell lineage. In: Guillermin R, Cohn M, Melnechuk T (eds) Neural modulation of immunity. Raven Press, New York, pp 81–91.

Brodal A 1969 Neurological anatomy. Oxford University Press, London.

Brown LT 1974 Corticorubral projections in the rat. Journal of Comparative Neurology 154:149–168.

Carrick FR 1997 Changes in brain function after manipulation of the cervical spine. Journal of Manipulative and Physiological Therapeutics 20:(8):529–545.

Chiu T, Wright A 1996 To compare the effects of different rates of application of a cervical mobilisation technique on sympathetic outflow to the upper limb in normal subjects. Manual Therapy 1(4):198–203.

Chrousos GP, Gold PW 1992 The concepts of stress and stress system disorders: Overview of physical and behavioral homeostasis. Journal of American Medical Association 267:1244–1252.

Davidson RJ 1984 Affect, cognition, and hemispheric specialization. In: Izard CE, Kagan J, Zajonc R (eds), Emotion, cognition and behaviour. Cambridge University Press, New York, pp 320–365.

Davidson RJ 1988 EEG measures of cerebral asymmetry: conceptual and methodological issues. International Journal of neuroscience 39:71–89.

Davidson RJ, Ekman P, Saron CD et al 1990 Approach/withdrawal and cerebral asymmetry; emotional expression and brain physiology I. Journal of Personality and Social Psychology 58:330–341.

Davidson RJ, Tomarken AJ 1989 Laterality and emotion: and electrophysiological approach. In: Boller F, Grafman J (eds) Handbook of neuropsychology. Elsevier Science, New York, pp 419–441.

Donovan BT 1970 Mammillian neuroendocrinology. McGraw-Hill, New York.

Elam M, Johansson G, Wallin BG 1992 Do patients with primary fibromyalgia have an altered muscle sympathetic nerve activity? Pain 48:371–375.

Elenkov IJ, Hasko G, Kovacs KJ 1995 Modulation of lipopolysaccharides induced tumour necrosis factor-alpha production by selective alpha and beta adrenergic drugs in mice. Journal of Neuroimmunology 61:123–131.

Elenkov IJ, Papanicolaou DA, Wilder RL et al 1996 Modulatory effects of glucocorticoids and catecholamines on human interleukin-12 and interleukin-10 production: Clinical implications. Proceedings of the Association of American Physicians 108:374–381.

Elenkov IJ, Wilder RL, Chrousos GP et al 2000 The sympathetic nerve—an integrative interface between two supersystems: The brain and the immune system. Pharmacological Reviews 52(4):595–638.

Felten DL, Felten SY, Carlson SL et al 1985 Noradrenergic and peptidergic innervation of lymphoid tissue. Journal of Immunology 135(2 suppl):755s–765s.

Furness JB, Costa M 1980 Types of nerves in the enteric nervous system. Neuroscience 5:1–20.

Gibson-Berry KL, Whitin JC, Cohen HJ 1993 Modulation of the respiratory burst in human neutrophils by isoproterenol and dibutyryl cyclic AMP. Journal of Neuroimmunology 43:59–68.

Grohmann U, van Snick J, Campanile F et al 2000 IL-9 protects mice from gram –ve bacterial shock, suppression of TNF-α, IL-12, and INF-γ and induction of IL-10. Journal of Immunology 164:4197–4203.

Guyton A, Hall J 1996 Textbook of medical physiology, 9th edn. Saunders, Philadelphia.

Hasko G, Szabo C, Nemeth ZH et al 1998 Suppression of IL-12 production by phosphodiesterase inhibition in murine endotoxemia is IL-10 dependant. European Journal of Immunology 88:57–61.

Heaney M, Golde D 1998 Soluble receptors in human disease. Journal of Leukocyte Biology 64:135–146.

Irwin M 1994 Stress induced immune suppression: the role of brain corticotropin releasing hormone and autonomic nervous systems mechanisms. Advances in Neuroimmunology 4:29–47.

Irwin M, Patterson T, Smith TL et al 1990 Reduction of immune function in life stress and depression. Biological Psychiatry 27:22–30.

Jarek MJ, Legare EJ, McDermott MT et al 1993 Endocrine profiles for outcome prediction from the intensive care unit. Critical Care Medicine 21:543–550.

Kang DH, Davidson RJ, Coe CL et al 1991 Frontal brain asymmetry and immune function. Behavioural Neuroscience 105(6):860–869.

Katafuchi T, Hori T, Oomura Y et al 1995 Cerebellar afferents to neuroendocrine cells: implications for adaptive responses to simulated weightlessness. Endocrine Journal 42(6):729–737.

Kelly DD, Murphy BA, Backhouse DP 2000 Use of a mental rotation reaction-time paradigm to measure the effects of upper cervical adjustments on Cortical processing: A pilot study. Journal of Manipulative and Physiological Therapeutics 23(4):246–251.

Khan MM, Sansoni P, Silverman ED et al 1986 Beta adrenergic receptors on human suppressor, helper, and cytolytic lymphocytes. Biochemical Pharmacology 35:1137–1142.

Kiecolt-Glaser JK, Garner W, Speicher C et al 1984 Psychosocial modifiers of immunocompetence in medical students. Psychosomatic Medicine 46:7–13.

Korr IM 1979 The spinal cord as organiser of disease processes: III. Hyperactivity of sympathetic innervation as a common factor in disease. Journal of the American Osteopathic Association 79(4):232–237.

LaHoste GJ, Neveu PJ, Mormede P et al 1989 Hemispheric asymmetry in the effects of cerebral cortical ablations on mitogen-induced lymphoproliferation and plasma prolactin levels in female rats. Brain Research 483:123–129.

Leventhal H, Tomarken AJ 1986 Emotion: today's problems. Annual Review of Psychology 37:565–610.

Li T, Harada M, Tamada K et al 1997 Repeated restraint stress impairs the antitumour T cell response through its suppressive effect on Th1-type CD4+ T cells. Anticancer Research 17:4259–4268.

Maisel AS, Harris T, Rearden CA et al 1990 Beta adrenergic receptors in lymphocyte subsets after exercise. Alterations in normal individuals and patients with congestive heart failure. Circulation 82:2003–2010.

Marieb E 1995 Human anatomy and physiology, 3rd edn. Benjamen/Cummings, New York, pp 594–595

Mosmann TR, Sad S 1996 The expanding universe of T-cell subsets, Th1, Th2, and more. Immunology Today 17:138–146.

Neveu PJ 1988 Minireview: Cerebral neocortex modulation of immune functions. Life Sciences 42:1917–1923.

Neveu PJ, Barneoud P, Vitiello S et al 1988 Brain modulation of the immune system: Association between lymphocyte responsiveness and paw preference in mice. Brain Research 457:392–394.

Neveu PJ, Taghzouti K, Dantzer R et al 1986 Modulation of mitogen-induced lymphoproliferation by cerebral neocortex. Life Sciences 38:1907–1913.

Renoux G, Biziere K 1986 Brain neocortex lateralized control of immune recognition. Integrative Psychiatry 4:32–40.

Renoux G, Biziere K, Renoux M et al 1983 A balanced brain asymmetry modulates T cell-mediated events. Journal of Neuroimmunology 5:227–238.

Robinson RG, Kubos KL, Starr LB et al 1984 Mood disorders in stroke patients: Importance of location of lesion. Brain 107:81–93.

Roitt I 1994 Essential immunology, 8th edn. Blackwell Scientific, London.

Sanders VM 1998 The role of norepinephrine and beta-2-adrenergic receptor stimulation in the modulation of Th1, Th2, and B lymphocyte function. Advances in Experimental Medicine and Biology 437:269–278.

Sato A 1992 The reflex effects of spinal somatic nerve stimulation on visceral function. Journal of Manipulative and Physiological Therapeutics 15(1):57–61.

Selye H 1936 Thymus and the adrenals in the response of the organism to injuries and intoxications. British Journal of Experimental Pathology 17:234–238.

Silberman EK, Weingartner H 1986 Hemispheric lateralization of functions related to emotion. Brain and Cognition 5:322–353.

Simon HB 1991 Exercise and human immune function. Ader R, Felten DL, Cohen N (eds) Psychoneuroimmunology, 2nd edn. Academic Press, San Diego, CA, pp 869–895

Sommers H 1980 The indigenous microbiota of the human host. Youmans GP, Patterson PY, Sommers HM (eds) The biological and clinical basis of infectious diseases. WB Saunders, Philadelphia, pp 65–80.

Suberville S, Bellocq A, Fouqueray B et al 1996 Regulation of IL-10 production by beta adrenergic agonists. European Journal of Immunology 26:2601–2605.

Thomas MD, Wood J 1992 Upper cervical adjustments may improve mental function. Journal of Manipulative Medicine 6:215–216.

Trinchieri G 1995 Interleukin -12: A proinflammatory cytokine with immunoregulatory functions that bridge innate resistance and antigen specific adaptive immunity. Annual Review of Immunology 13:251–276.

Villaro AC, Sesma MP, Vazquez JJ 1987 Innervation of mouse lymph nodes: nerve endings on muscular vessels and reticular cells. American Journal of Anatomy 179:175–185.

Vizi ES 2000 Role of high-affinity receptors and membrane transporters in nonsynaptic communication and drug action in the CNS. Pharmacological Reviews 52:63–89.

Vizi ES, Labos E 1991 Nonsynaptic interactions at presynaptic level. Progress in Neurobiology 37:145–163.

Walberg F 1960 Further studies on the descending connections to the inferior olive. Reticulo-olivary fibers: an experimental study in the cat. Journal of Comparative Neurology 114:79–87.

Webster KE 1978 The brainstem reticular formation. In: Hennings G, Hemmings WA (eds) The biological basis of schizophrenia. MTP Press, Lancaster.

Williams PL Warwick R 1984 Gray's anatomy. Churchill Livingstone, Edinburgh.

Wittling W 1998 Brain asymmetry in the control of autonomic-physiologic activity. In: Davidson R, Hugdahl K (eds) Brain asymmetry. MIT Press, Cambridge, MA.

Youmans G 1980 Host bacterial interaction: external defense mechanisms. In: Youmans GP, Patterson PY, Sommers HM (eds) The biological and clinical basis of infectious diseases. WB Saunders, Philadelphia pp. 12–54.

Zurier RB, Weissmann G, Hoffstein S et al 1974 Mechanisms of lysosomal enzyme release from human leukocytes. II. Effects of cAMP and cGMP, autonomic agonists, and agents which affect microtubule function. Journal of Clinical Investigation 53:297–309.

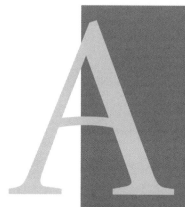

Clinical Case Answers

Case 15.1

15.1.1   There is widespread evidence that asymmetric lateralization of cortical functioning does occur. Several of the lateralized functions are also known to be involved in brain neuroimmuno modulation such as emotional arousal, sympathetic innervation, neurotransmitter concentrations, and neuroendocrine activity. It would seem from the widespread evidence of cortical functional hemispheric dominance in other systems that modulation of the immune system would also fall under asymmetric cortical control.

A growing body of evidence indicates that immune system function is modulated by different areas of the cortex in an asymmetrical fashion. For instance, a variety of studies have demonstrated that the rostral portions of the frontal cortical areas are differentially activated when the individual is exposed to different emotional stimulus and that the activation state experienced altered the immune response of the individual. The left frontal cortex appears to be activated during the expression or experience of positive emotional states, whereas the right frontal cortex seems to be activated during the expression or experience of negative emotional states. Asymmetric activation of the cortex could lead to asymmetric activation of the sympathetic nervous system and catecholamine release, which alters immune function. The cortex itself develops two-way communication with the immune system and a reduction in activation that has resulted in the cognitive expression of depression may also affect immune function.

Case 15.2

15.2.1   Discrimination of self from non-self is one of the most remarkable properties of every normal individual's immune system. This ability is called self-tolerance. Self-tolerance is maintained partly by the elimination of lymphocytes that may express receptor specific for self-antigens and partly by functional inactivation of self-reactive lymphocytes after their encounter with self-antigens. The T lymphocyte recognizes 'self' and 'non-self' by proteins on the cell membrane called major histocompatibility complex (MHC).

The MHC is a region of highly polymorphic genes whose product proteins are expressed on the surfaces of a variety of cells. This allows T lymphocytes the ability to survey the body for the presence of peptides derived from foreign proteins. There are two different types of MHC gene products called class I and class II MHC molecules. Any given T lymphocyte recognizes foreign peptides bound to only one class I or one class II MHC molecule.

Class I MHC proteins are present on all cells of the body except red blood cells. These allow the T cells to recognize 'self'. Class II MHC proteins are present only on B cells, some T cells, and antigen-presenting cells such as macrophages. The proteins of class II MHC are composed of pieces of foreign antigen that have been phagocytosed and broken down by intracellular mechanisms and recycled back to the plasma membrane. The role of MHC proteins in the immune response is extremely important because they provide the means for signalling the immune system cells that infected or cancerous cells are present but camouflaged inside our own cells.

Chapter 16

Psychoneurological Aspects of Functional Neurology

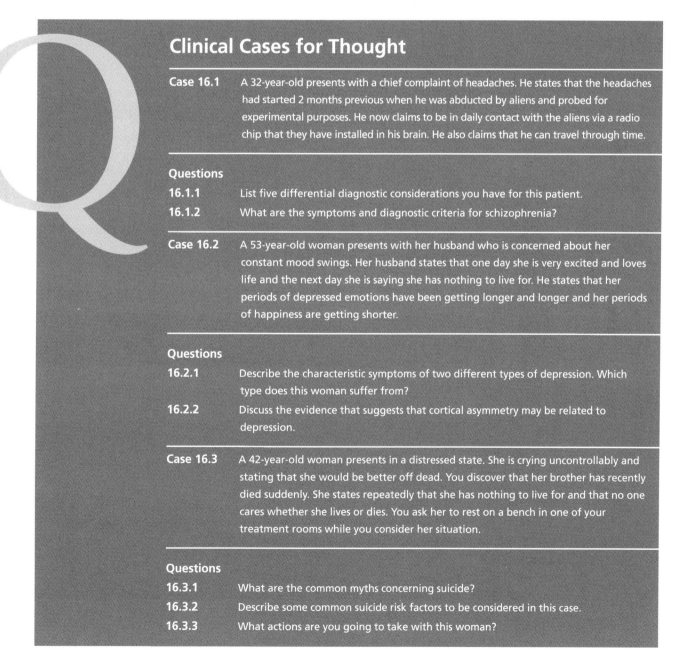

Clinical Cases for Thought

Case 16.1   A 32-year-old presents with a chief complaint of headaches. He states that the headaches had started 2 months previous when he was abducted by aliens and probed for experimental purposes. He now claims to be in daily contact with the aliens via a radio chip that they have installed in his brain. He also claims that he can travel through time.

Questions

16.1.1   List five differential diagnostic considerations you have for this patient.

16.1.2   What are the symptoms and diagnostic criteria for schizophrenia?

Case 16.2   A 53-year-old woman presents with her husband who is concerned about her constant mood swings. Her husband states that one day she is very excited and loves life and the next day she is saying she has nothing to live for. He states that her periods of depressed emotions have been getting longer and longer and her periods of happiness are getting shorter.

Questions

16.2.1   Describe the characteristic symptoms of two different types of depression. Which type does this woman suffer from?

16.2.2   Discuss the evidence that suggests that cortical asymmetry may be related to depression.

Case 16.3   A 42-year-old woman presents in a distressed state. She is crying uncontrollably and stating that she would be better off dead. You discover that her brother has recently died suddenly. She states repeatedly that she has nothing to live for and that no one cares whether she lives or dies. You ask her to rest on a bench in one of your treatment rooms while you consider her situation.

Questions

16.3.1   What are the common myths concerning suicide?

16.3.2   Describe some common suicide risk factors to be considered in this case.

16.3.3   What actions are you going to take with this woman?

Introduction

In order to understand the role and function of emotion and its relationship to the nervous and immune systems, consideration of the theoretical constructs upon which emotion is defined, described, and measured is necessary. To do this a consideration of the current popular theories and a brief historical overview of the development of these theories will be presented. What are emotions? Why do we have emotions? Why do they exist? What functions do they serve? These are questions that have challenged man since time began. From these basic questions several different views on the theory of emotions have developed.

These different theoretical approaches are sometimes difficult to classify, but may be broadly categorized into three classes: social learning theory, biological theory, and cognitive theory. 'Mood' can be defined as the way that we feel, while 'affect' can be defined as how we behave as a result of our mood. Neurologically, mood and affect depend on the complex interplay among diffuse networks of the frontal lobes and subcortical circuits. They can be influenced by genetic and environmental factors, similar to any form of activity in the nervous system. Overviews of a variety of clinically relevant psychological conditions are also supplied in the chapter.

Historical Development of Emotional Theories

Plato's model of emotion was essentially dualist in nature. The dualism involved the existence of a soul and an earthly body it inhabited. Plato placed the emotions as a direct function of the soul, which was composed of three forces: reason, desire, and appetite. Plato envisioned the emotions as wild uncontrollable forces in continual opposition to the controlling powers of reason. Two distinct ideas emerge from Plato's theory of emotion. Firstly, emotions are to be contrasted with that which is rational and secondly, that emotions play a role in psychological conflict. The second concept implies that there must also exist processes to defend against the powers of emotions.

The view that the emotions should be the slaves of reason and that reason dwelled in the divine soul made the 'feeling' or Platonic theory of emotion very popular among the Christian and Islamic scholars who dominated Western thinking until the late nineteenth century. René Descartes elaborated on the Platonic theory in a pamphlet entitled 'On the Passions of the Soul'. Descartes describes the soul as the 'switch master' or control that allows the movement of the spirits through the body via the pineal gland in the brain. The body then experiences these movements as emotions. Emotions to Descartes were simply the experience of awareness of the spirit movements through the body. Emotions had no function, but were simply a phenomenon that occurred in response to a stimuli. For example, the movement of bodily spirits may produce the experience of fear excited by the recognition of external danger, but cannot be influenced by a cognitive appraisal of the danger or produce an appropriate behavioural response. These are two of the major criticisms of the Platonic or 'feeling' theory: that it can give no explanation as to how emotions can result in behaviours, and it can give no explanation as to how cognitive processes can appraise the external stimuli to alter or modify the fear response (Lyons 1992).

Regardless of the criticisms of Descartes he was the first to suggest that some emotions might be more basic or primitive than others and listed six primary 'passions': wonder, joy, sadness, love, hatred, and desire. He was also the first to suggest that emotions may exist on more than one level at the same time, for example, fear and excitement (Powers & Dalgleish 1997).

William James added to the 'feeling' theory of emotion in his classic work *Principles of Psychology* in which he emphasized the physiological aspects of emotions and outlined the distinctions of each emotion which cleared the way for psychological experimentation. James was the last influential psychologist to present the feeling theory of emotion with such conviction, and with his death came the decline of the feeling theory in psychology (Powers & Dalgeish 1997).

With the decline of the dualist theory came the emergence of Darwin's 'survival of the fittest' concept outlined in his *Origin of Species* monograph in 1859. It was Darwin's view that emotions were a throwover from primitive man and were no longer of any use to modern man. This theory was not widely accepted as far as it applied to the emotions, but other parts of his theory shocked most of upper society and ironically stimulated a fury of investigation that renewed interest in the biological theory of emotion.

In contrast to Darwin's view that emotions were no longer of use but were vestigial like the appendix, and the Platonic or dualistic view that emotions were irrational, others such as Aristotle took the view that emotions have important short- and long-term functions that enable individuals to adapt to changes in their social and physical environment. Aristotle was probably the first to propose a functionalist model of emotional development. Aristotle's theory was not widely accepted in his day as it was overshadowed by his teacher Plato's theories, which were much more amenable to contemporary religious leaders.

Aristotle's most comprehensive discussion of the emotions occurs in *The Art of Rhetoric*. In this monograph, he outlines the relationship between an emotion and the behaviour that it produces. He also describes ten specific emotions: four positive (calm, friendship, favour, pity) and six negative (anger, fear, shame, indignation, envy, jealousy). Aristotle argued that for any emotion to arise it was necessary for three conditions to be satisfied. First, the individual must be in the appropriate 'state of mind' to experience the emotion; second, there must be a 'stimulus' to elicit the emotion; thirdly, there must be an 'object' for the emotion. For example, if an individual is in a state of mind that something dangerous may happen to them, and then he/she is confronted by an assailant they might evaluate the situation as one of impending danger. This evaluation may, in turn, result in a stimulus that produces fear. It is the evaluation of the situation and not the situation itself that stimulates the emotion. In the above example, if the assailant was not perceived as threatening to the individual, the resulting emotion may have been completely different, such as anger. Aristotle's theory laid the foundation for the functionalist's approach to emotions and their development.

Behavioural and Social Learning Theories

Social learning theory emphasizes the importance of modelling others' emotional reactions as a means of developing emotional patterns and responses. The behaviourists have developed a number of various classifications of behavioural theory, depending largely on the degree to which they refer to metaphysical or epistemological claims in their explanations of emotion. The two main categories of behaviour theory are psychological behaviourism and philosophical behaviourism. The psychological behaviourist approach to emotions can best be exemplified by the theories of James Watson and B. F. Skinner. Watson in 1919 described emotion as 'a hereditary pattern-reaction involving profound changes in bodily mechanisms as a whole, but particularly of the visceral and glandular systems'.

In Watson's model of emotion only three emotions can be distinguished: fear, rage, and love. He further states that these primary emotions can only by demonstrated in the newborn. Watson's major contribution was his finding that emotional reactions could be learned through classical conditioning (Watson & Raynor 1920).

In 1967, Etzel and Gewirtz demonstrated that operant conditioning could have an impact on emotional development. Skinner refined Etzel and Gerwirtz's work into a complex model where emotions evolve from an operant conditioning framework, where emotion is defined by the sets of operants and reinforcers that one optimizes in any given setting (Skinner 1974). One of the major criticisms of Skinner's theory is that some emotions exhibit little or no operant behaviour. For example, grief, especially when about a loss or death, does not result in any operant behaviour because no behaviour can bring about the desired results (Lyons 1992).

One of the most influential philosophical behaviourists was Gilbert Ryle. In 1949 his work *The Concept of Mind* outlined that emotion can be described in four different ways: inclination, moods, agitations, and feelings. Ryle viewed inclinations as the permanent disposition state of personality. Moods, agitations, and feelings were short-term displays overlying the main inclination theme. For example, if a person has the inclination to be kind, he may still experience short-term occurrences of irritability or cruelty, which would be attributed to his mood or feeling swings.

Further expansion of the social learning theory in recent years has been accomplished by Albert Bandura, who has added a cognitive component. According to Bandura, as a person's representational ability improves, he/she can engage in emotional self-arousal by thinking about their own emotionally charged past experiences or even by recalling the experiences of others (Bandura 1986, 1989, 1991).

One of the main criticisms of social learning/behavioural theory is that it cannot explain the emergence of emotions that have not been acquired through modelling or conditioning, but seem to appear spontaneously.

Biological Theories

The theory that emotions are nothing more than chemical reactions at synaptic connections has not been a popular theory among psychologists in the past. However, several recent findings and advancements in understanding of the neurochemical component of emotion have caused a wave of interest in the theories of biological emotion. Many neurochemical systems now appear necessary for the understanding and expression of emotions. Several areas of the brain have been implicated in the development, generation, and expression of emotions, particularly those regions known as the limbic system, which includes the hypothalamus, hypothalamus–pituitary axis, the anterior thalamus, the cingulated gyrus, the hippocampus, and amygdala (Rolls 1992; Halgren & LeDoux 1993). The importance of the amygdala in particular has emerged in its ability to determine the motivational significance of a stimuli (Gaffan et al 1988), in the assignment of reward value to a stimuli (LeDoux 1990), and in the stimulation of behavioural and autonomic responses.

Cognitive Theories

Instead of viewing emotions as central forces in the development of social interaction, cognitive psychologists view emotions as byproducts of cognitive processes (Berk 1994). Several examples of cognitive theories follow, including Hebb's discrepancy theory, Alder's style of life theory, Epsteins cognitive-experiential self theory, and Apler's reversal theory.

Donald Hebb (1947, 1949) explained in his discrepancy theory how distress reactions are elicited by novel stimuli. According to Hebb, when a person encounters a new stimulus, they compare it to a scheme or internal representation of a familiar object. The discrepancy between the stimulus and the internal representation determines the emotional response. Other researchers have modified Hebb's theory, suggesting that a wide variety of emotional reactions could be explained by Hebb's theory. For example, they argue that a positive emotion such as happiness could result from only moderate discrepancies between current stimuli and the internal scheme. Negative emotions, such as anxiety and fear, could result as the discrepancy between the present stimuli and the interval scheme widens (McCall & McGhee 1977; Kagan et al 1978). This theory falls short when it is observed that people sometimes seek out activities that are new and not in agreement with their internal scheme willingly.

Alfred Adler, in his 1954 work *Understanding Human Nature*, was probably the first to integrate emotions, motivations, and cognition into one theory (Epstein 1993). According to Adler, individuals construct a belief system and a way of relating to the world which he termed a 'style of life'. At the center of a person's style of life is a fictional goal which guides the individual in his attempts to overcome inferiority to gain social approval, a goal to which all humans strive. Emotions enter into Adler's theory in two ways. Firstly, the quest for overcoming the feelings of inferiority provides an incentive for developing a style of life. Secondly, once the style of life has been developed, the emotions corresponding to that style of life are encouraged to develop. In other words the style of life that one develops is a major determinant of the emotions that a person experiences, much like Aristotle's 'state of mind' (Epstein 1993).

In the cognitive experiential self theory (CEST), emotions are considered to be both influencing and being influenced by a person's implicit theory of reality. The theory considers the primary emotions to be anger, sadness, joy, and affection. Cognitive affective units are constructed around the nuclei of the primary emotions. These cognitive units direct the development of critical adaptive behaviour patterns such as fighting, withdrawing, exploring, and showing affection. The development of these behavioural patterns result in emotionally rewarding experiences when they are consistent with a beneficial outcome to the individual (Epstein et al 1992).

Apter's reversal theory is explained in some detail here because it is one of the few theories that has a theoretical construct for encompassing changes over time in the individual which are clinically relevant for the functional neurologist. The centrepiece of reversal theory is a typology of distinct psychological states of mind. When people are in one of these states they want to experience a particular kind of emotion. The states are meta-motivational because they determine what types of experiences people want. In different states, people may react to the same stimuli in different ways, and experience distinctly different emotions. This theory focuses on how a person differs over time rather than on differences between people. Reversal theory suggests that there are eight different meta-motivational states, four pairs of opposite states. The reversal from one state to its opposite is the key feature of the theory. The two states of a pair are mutually exclusive and exhaustive; for example a person is always in one state or the other, never both at the same time or neither state. The eight states of the reversal theory are serious–playful, compliant–defiant, power-oriented–affection-oriented, and self-oriented–other-oriented (Apter 1988). The first pair of meta-motivational states is composed of the telic and paratelic states. When in the telic state the person is primarily goal-oriented. Conversely, when a person is in the paratelic state they are best described as being playful. In this state the person does not attach much significance to what they are doing; they could care less. The lability of a person, how readily they reverse back and forth between opposite states, varies at different times. The actual reversal process is dependent on one of three reasons: contingency, satiation, and frustration. Contingency is any change in the environment that instigates or necessitates a reversal. Satiation occurs when in the absence of an environmental change a reversal will eventually occur. Frustration-motivated reversals occur when a person remains in a particular state too long without achieving satisfaction (Frey 1997).

Reversal theory takes the approach of starting with motivation and experience and then interpreting the behaviour generated in light of these. Reversal theory emphasizes that people are inconsistent and self-contradictory and goes as far to say that healthy people are characterized by instability not stability (Murgatroyd 1987).

Developing A Theoretical Construct for Emotion

How are changes in emotional states brought about by changes or alterations in neuraxial function in humans? Can how we feel influence the function of the neuroimmune system? Emotional factors have been linked to a variety of diseases including Grave's disease, rheumatoid arthritis, systemic lupus erythematosis (SLE), asthma, and diabetes (Koh 1998). Could these diseases be caused or precipitated by emotional factors? Several psychological states have been linked to alterations in neural activity in the limbic circuits of the brain involving the amygdala and hippocampus, which are areas historically associated with emotional response generation (Pribram & McGuinness 1975). Imbalances in emotional activation and reaction have been investigated in a number of studies (Sackeim et al 1982; Robinson et al 1984; Flor-Henry 1986). The advances made by these researchers have lead to the discovery that cells of the immune system (lymphocytes) produce stress-associated peptides thought to only be produced in the brain and pituitary. When this finding is coupled with the discovery of neurotransmitter receptors and hormone receptors on neurons and immune cells (Blalock 1984) the existence of a bidirectional communication relationship between emotion and neuroimmune systems seems unavoidable.

How do we define and measure emotional states or changes in those states? To what extent does the interaction determine health?

What Is the Connection between Emotion, Mood, Affect, and Neurological Function?

Campos et al (1994) define emotion as those processes which establish, maintain, change, or determine the relation between the person and the environment on matters of significance to the person. A person's mood may be determined by a complex interplay of the emotions that they are experiencing at any one time as per the reversal theory. 'Mood' therefore can be defined as the way that we feel, while 'affect' can be defined as how we behave as a result of our mood. Neurologically, mood and affect depend on the complex interplay among diffuse networks of the frontal lobes and subcortical circuits. They can be influenced by genetic and environmental factors, similar to any form of activity in the nervous system. Long-term changes in mood and behaviour may occur because of 'plastic' changes in these networks. This refers to the moulding of nerve excitability and interconnectivity referred to as neural plasticity that occurs following repeated or essential exposure to an environmental stimulus, and subsequent alteration of gene expression in the associated nerves.

Other, probably genetically determined neural systems seem primed to perform a variety of innate activities called 'fundamental functions' in the cortex. Fundamental functions comprise diffuse, overlapping, or parallel units that contribute to more complex interactions and multimodal processing in the nervous system. The more recent definition of fundamental functions applies to frontal-subcortical and limbic circuits, which are largely intact from birth. Executive/integrative functions apply to the prefrontal circuitry, which also comprise diffuse, overlapping, or parallel influences that contribute to more complex interactions and multimodal processing in the nervous system. Fundamental functions are generally less modularized than motor or sensory functions. In other words they are less dependent on one single area within the brain, and instead receive their input from multiple sources and generate an output that can influence the entire state of the individual. Dysfunction associated with these networks can therefore lead to so-called 'circuit-related disorders' affecting complex aspects of cognition or leading to mood and behavioural changes. Therefore, abnormalities associated with fundamental or executive regions of the brain may result in either 'negative' or 'positive' symptoms. Negative symptoms or deficits generally refer to decreased expression of a normal function, whereas positive symptoms refer to release of primitive functions or new behaviours. An example of a negative symptom is depression, where a patient may exhibit withdrawal from normal activities and social interaction and less expression in their face and body movements. An example of a positive symptom can be seen clinically in paranoid schizophrenia where environmental stimulus is amplified and taken out of context of reality. Positive symptoms may also be referred to as productive symptoms, release or escape phenomena. A classic example of 'escape' phenomena is the exaggerated autonomic reactivity that may be observed in patients with panic or anxiety disorders. Primitive areas of the brain and brainstem are allowed to summate or increase their firing more easily because of a loss of descending reticular inhibition from the more developed frontal areas of the brain. Obsessive compulsive disorder (OCD) can also be viewed as an example of a release phenomena. The patient develops an irresistible urge to perform a specific action that will bring about relief of tension. While not purely seen as a 'disinhibition' syndrome, the patient often feels compelled to carry out an action that interferes with their daily lives. Cortical and subcortical areas implicated in mood and behavioural functions receive tonic influences from a large array of different neuronal circuits, some of which involve parallel distributed processing circuits that utilize a wide variety of neurotransmitters including dopamine, serotonin, noradrenalin, and acetylcholine. Thus the cumulative activity of these various circuits results in a temporal variation in the relative concentrations of the neurotransmitters utilized in each circuit.

The concept of parallel distributed processing is essential for health care practitioners to gain an understanding of the link between psychological and somatic or visceral health complaints. Not only may somatic health complaints affect the ability of an individual to exercise their normal daily routines, thus leading to altered mood and behaviour, but direct physiological connections exist that involve somatic and visceral afferents and the limbic system or ascending reticular activating systems of the brainstem and hypothalamus. One example of parallel distributed processes is outlined below involving the rostral cingulate cortex as the limbic motor response area that responds to parallel afferent information also received by the sensory cortex. The rostral cingulate motor area (area 24) is responsible for primitive motor behaviours (fear, avoidance, etc.) mediated via the corticospinal and reticulospinal pathways. Activity in this region is also dependent on activation of the caudal cingulate motor area (area 25), which orientates the body in space. These cingulate motor areas and receptive regions of the cingulate and insular cortex that project to it are not only influenced presynaptically by subcortical and spinal neurons carrying sensory information, but they are also heavily modulated by monoaminergic neurons from the brainstem. The influence of dopamine, noradrenalin, and serotonin on sensory modulation, arousal, and orientation is complex in nature and discussed in further detail in Chapter 9.

Chronic Pain and Emotional Responses

Functional neuroimaging using quantitative EEG (qEEG) suggests similar mechanisms between chronic pain syndromes and mood disorders in that similar areas appear to be activated in these patients. A strong tendency for overactivation of the right hemisphere or decreased left hemisphere activation has been identified in patients who demonstrate negative behaviour or affect (Davidson 1992). Similar findings are often present in patients with chronic pain syndromes suggesting that pain, stress, and negative emotions may share common influences on association areas of the cortex concerned with contextual processing. Pain-related circuits in the brain, particularly those associated with 'older' pathways, tend to adapt and undergo plastic changes when closely associated with a behaviour or an emotion. Functional magnetic resonance imaging of the brain has been used to identify the neural networks involved in aversive conditioning, and anticipation of visceral pain. Actual and anticipated visceral pain elicited similar cortical responses. This demonstrates similarities with the principle that imagined movements through visual imagery can strengthen learning of new motor sequences. At some point in the sequencing of neural activity, motor execution is inhibited or restrained during motor imagery. However, actual, imagined, and perhaps anticipated movements or perceptions may share the same neural networks up until this point of restraint. With respect to mood and affective disorders the anticipation of negative consequences associated with illness, injury, or social and environmental stimuli may therefore induce a new 'virtual reality' that bears all the hallmarks of 'actual' disease and disability.

The amygdala receives direct synaptic connections from thalamic and spinal cord neurons that are involved in aversive conditioning and fear-potentiated behaviour. Approximately half of the neurons projecting to limbic or striatal regions terminate in the hypothalamus. This suggests that somatic and visceral afferents to the spinal cord are intrinsically linked to higher limbic centres and may profoundly affect behaviour. Since mood and behaviour are inextricably dependent on the central integrated state of both limbic and higher cortical centres, presynaptic influences on these areas may have a central role in the aetiology of mood and behavioural disorders. Increased activation of pain pathways has already been mentioned, particularly with respect to activation of the 'older' pain pathways. However, other sensory systems share similar relationships with the limbic system, including the visual, auditory, vestibular, olfactory, and gustatory systems. An overview of the relationship between the auditory system and mood and behaviour is detailed below.

Brain imaging studies have shown similar activation patterns in chronic tinnitus sufferers and chronic pain sufferers who also suffer from depression. Plastic changes in receptors associated with brain-derived neurotrophic factor and neurokinins have also been identified in the hippocampus of these patients.

Mood and behavioural problems may be associated with altered ascending inputs from various subcortical circuits such as those in the dorsal cochlear nucleus (DCN) and somatic or vestibular processing pathways. It has been postulated that the cause of tinnitus may represent a distributed phenomenon with the possibility of dysfunction in a variety of pathways individually or simultaneously rather than damage at one location. Thus, interactions between many brain regions may be the cause. The same principle is likely to apply to mood and behavioural problems. The auditory portions of the DCN and vestibular nucleus share some similarities with respect to their apparent influence on limbic/reticular nuclei and therefore mood. The output from both of these nuclei may be heavily influenced via interactions with cervical spine afferents. In a detailed review of the literature concerning the effect of rehabilitation exercises on vestibular adaptation, Black and Pesznecker (2003) found that vestibular rehabilitation outcome is negatively affected by anxiety, depression, and cognitive dysfunction, suggesting a role for mood, affect, and cognition in modulating balance and/or spatial processing. A number of mechanisms linking balance control and anxiety have been found:

- The parabrachial nucleus serves an important role in mediating interactions between somatic, vestibular, and visceral afferents and influencing avoidance conditioning, and anxiety-conditioned fear responses.
- Parallel connections pass from noradrenergic and serotonergic nuclei in the brainstem to both vestibular and limbic regions. Noradrenergic projections are likely to mediate effects of vigilance and alertness on the sensitivity of the vestibular system.

The most likely mechanism for these interactions is that the serotonergic pathways mediated by the raphe nuclei and receptors of targets of the parabrachial nucleus calibrate the sensitivity of affective responses to aversive aspects of motion.

When alterations in emotion are related to changes in the neuroimmune system, many variables arise. Researchers have attacked the problem by breaking the broad concept of emotion into smaller more manageable sections, mainly positive and negative emotional states. Knapp et al (1992) asked subjects to recall and relive maximally disturbing situations in their lives which he classified as negative emotions and maximally pleasurable situations in their lives which he classified as positive emotions. He found that negative emotional states promoted significant declines in mitogenic lymphocyte reactivity followed by a return to pre-emotional levels. They also found a similar decrease in cytotoxic T-cell function with negative emotional stimuli. Modulation of the immune system in these studies was thought to have occurred via nervous system function. Psychotic disorders such as schizophrenia have repeatedly been shown to have altered immune system function, and some investigators have suggested that immunological dysfunction may in fact contribute towards the multifactorial aetiology of schizophrenia via bidirectional parallel circuit feedback systems (Kirch 1993; Syvalahti 1994; Rothermundt et al 1998). Several clinical conditions are outlined below with some discussion of their neuroimmunological relationships.

Mania

Affect, which is another way to describe emotion, gives richness and meaning to our experience of the world around us and many would say is an indispensable dimension of our humanism. When the behaviours or feelings produced by emotions becomes inappropriate or extreme they can be the source of overwhelming psychological distress (Bootzin & Acocella 1984). Disturbances in mood which result in intense feelings of sadness or elation that are unrealistic and last over a prolonged period of time result in depression or mania, respectively.

The affective disorders or disorders of feeling have been recognized and written about since the history of medicine has been recorded. Melancholia, which is another term for depression, was noted by Hippocrates in the 4th century BC and has been found referenced as early as the 1st century AD. Some very famous people have fallen victim to depression including Abraham Lincoln and Winston Churchill. Even though these conditions have been investigated for centuries they still remain somewhat of a mystery. Some disturbances in affect can be caused by inappropriate responses to intense or chronic mental stress.

How do people usually respond to mental stress? Some of us try to distract our attention from the effects of the stress by becoming feverishly active and energetic; others accomplish the distraction by surrounding themselves with people or by constantly going out to parties or social events. Doing unusual amounts of work is another tactic. In short, many of us respond to stress in a way that resembles manic behaviour. When does this behaviour become pathological in nature?

Overactivity becomes manic when it becomes extreme, prolonged, and uncontrollable. Manic individuals are hyperactive, talkative, and endlessly energetic and usually perform these behaviours in bursts of activity that eventually result in a burnout period of exhaustion. They find great superficial pleasure in people and things that never interested them before until their attention is turned to another more interesting topic. In the process of these bursts of mania, their self-image becomes grossly inflated. They tend to ignore their limits, believing they can do anything. They love and admire themselves without reservation and ironically they are often irritable, unhappy, and reckless in their actions (Bootzin & Acocella 1984).

Depression

Most people report that they have gone through periods of depression or extreme dejection at some point in their lives. They admit to 'feeling sorry for themselves' and may report the following symptoms:

- Sleep disturbances;
- Loss of appetite;
- Reduced sex drive;
- Feelings of sadness, guilt, and futility;
- Difficulties in focusing their thoughts; and
- Recurrent thoughts of death or suicide.

These symptoms that most people have reported as experiencing are similar to the symptoms of pathological depression. It is essential to grasp the concept that most psychological dysfunctions, including pathological depression, are determined based on the degree of symptom expression. Pathologically depressed patients often show a degree of utter despair and hopelessness that is foreign to the experience of most people (Bootzin & Acocella 1984).

People with depression live in a state of sheer hopelessness, in which there exists no source of pleasure, and in some, no reason for living. Some people who are depressed do in fact kill themselves. They may experience delusions and hallucinations which do not occur in 'normal' periods of depression. For example, they fear the imminent destruction of the world, or that terrible tragedies are in store for them or their loved ones.

Persons who undergo one or more major depressive episodes with no intervening manic episodes are classified as major depressive in nature. In the United States the prevalence of major depression is about 3% for men and about 9% for women and the lifetime risk, which is defined as the chance of experiencing at least one episode of major depression, is 12% for men and 26% for women (Boyd & Weissman 1981). Depression is second only to schizophrenia as the primary condition for admissions to mental hospitals (Woodruff et al 1975).

Some groups of people, such as low socioeconomic classes, of both sexes, middle-aged and elderly, and women in general are more susceptible than others to developing depression. It is distressing to note that young people have recently started to increase their prevalence of depressive episodes. Even the incidence in infants has been reported to be on the increase.

In about 50% of the cases the first episode is also the last episode. They have no recurrence. However, for the remaining 50% the depression will come and go many times (Bootzin & Acocella 1984). The episodes may occur in clusters or be separated by many years of normal function. In most cases adjustment back to a normal life occurs relatively quickly. However, in about 20% of people, return to their normal premorbid state following a major depressive episode does not occur. Why these people do not return to their normal or premorbid state becomes understandable to a certain extent when consideration is given to the affects that a depressive episode can have on their lives. A major episode of depression often erodes self-confidence, disrupts family and marital relationships, interferes with progress at school or work, and alters other people's expectations of the depressed individual. Thus, the event itself sets up a vicious circle of reoccurrence by the state in which it leaves the individual.

Classification

Several classifications of depression have been developed. The following classification is based on the age or stage of development of the individual.

Infantile Depression

The infant expressed a number of symptoms ranging from excessive sleep to indifference to their environment. The major symptom reported by mothers of these infants is a disturbing and alarming disinterest in food.

Childhood Depression

This condition manifests as inactivity or apathy that may be linked to separation anxiety. The child clings frantically to the parents, refusing to leave them to attend school or other childhood functions. The child may report fears that the parent will die and leave them alone.

Adolescent Depression

The diagnosis of adolescent depression can be extremely difficult, because the symptoms are an exaggeration of normal adolescent behaviour. The problems that depressed adolescents claim as the cause of their depression are also the same or similar problems experienced by the majority of adolescents under normal conditions. Most prominent symptoms include:

- Sulkiness;
- Negativism;
- Withdrawal;
- Complaints of not being understood or appreciated; and
- Antisocial behaviour and drug abuse.

Depression in the Elderly

It is important to remember that like a variety of diseases, dysfunctional states, or in other psychological disorders, depression may manifest itself differently at different stages of life. In the elderly the major symptoms include:

- Apathy;
- Difficulties concentrating and thinking;
- Memory loss; and
- Mild disorientation.

Bipolar Disorder

This disorder involves both manic and depressive episodes. Usually, bipolar disorders will appear in the manic phase followed by a normal period then a depressed phase, although many different patterns have been identified. In rare instances the mood may alternate between manic and depressive states with no periods of normal functioning; this is referred to as the cycling type of bipolar disorder. Another rare form of bipolar disorder involves the appearance of manic and depressive episodes simultaneously, which is referred to as a mixed type of bipolar disorder. For example, the person may show manic hyperactivity but weep and threaten suicide at the same time.

Bipolar disorder is much less common than major depression, occurring in about 0.4–1.2% of the population (Hirschfeld & Cross 1982). Bipolar disorders occur in both sexes with equal frequency but in contrast to major depression is more prevalent in the upper classes (Bootzin & Acocella 1984). The premorbid history in bipolar disorder is usually normal with no warning symptoms and usually has its onset before age 30. The episodes of bipolar disorder are usually briefer and more frequent than major depression. Bipolar disorder is also more likely than major depression to have a familial connection.

Depression and Neuroimmune Function

Depression has been shown to be related to schizophrenia (Crow 1984), herpes simplex virus (Halonen et al 1974), Ebstein-Barr virus (Amsterdam et al 1986), human immunodeficiency virus (HIV) type I (Levy & Bredesen 1989), several autoimmune diseases (Johnstone & Whaley 1975), leukaemia (Greene 1954), and a variety of cancers (Persky et al 1987). These relationships suggests disorders of the neuroimmune system in some fashion or other.

The role of neuroimmune function in depression has attracted attention for many years (Calabrese et al 1987). Depressive illness poses a major public health problem with 2 to 3%

of the population hospitalized or seriously afflicted at any one time; in this light, many investigators have approached depression from a neuroimmunological prospective (Stein et al 1991). Many studies document that patients with depression show reduced immune function throughout a wide variety of immune function measures. Stein et al (1985) found that in-patients with depression have poorer blastogenic responses than non-depressed controls. Depressed patients have also been shown to have a lower percentage of helper T-lymphocytes than non-depressed controls (Krueger et al 1984). Irwin et al (1990) showed that when compared to normal controls, men with major depressive disorder were associated with a 50% reduction in T-cell cytotoxicity. Not all research supports the above findings. Stein et al (1991) reported in a comprehensive review that out of eight studies that they looked at only one found lymphopenia to be significant in depressive patients studied. Out of five additional studies examined by the same authors, again only one showed an alteration in neutrophil counts in depressed patients. Immune function studies in patients with depression have also been explored. Irwin et al (1987b) found a decrease in cytotoxicity of natural killer cells in depressed patients as compared to controls. Other studies relating to natural killer cell cytotoxicity did not find any significant difference between controls and depressed patients (Mohl et al 1987; Schleifer et al 1989). It is important to consider that depression is a diagnosis derived from a diagnostic criteria composed of many variables (DSM IV). It is also necessary to realize that a diagnosis of clinical depression does not preclude the coexistence of other dysphoric mood states including anxiety and/or hostility. Depressed patients may have different combinations of symptoms and still be diagnosed with depression. For example, a patient may have predominately psychological symptoms such as self-reproach, difficulty concentrating, loss of interest, and recurrent thoughts of death or suicide. In contrast, another patient may have predominately vegetative symptoms including poor appetite and weight loss, sleep disturbance, loss of energy, or psychomotor agitation. These two types of patients may have vastly different neuroimmunological alterations as a result of the same diagnosis. This heterogeneous population may in some way explain the inconsistent results obtained when populations are not controlled for variables such as those described.

The degree of immunosuppression may also be related to the severity of the depression studied (Stein et al 1985). Kemeny (1994) found that higher levels of a depressed mood were associated with lower numbers of cytotoxic T-cells. In both types of studies, functional and enumerative, no consistent results have been reported for any cell types or subtypes studied. This inconsistency as described above may be a result of both conceptual and methodological concerns that limit the interpretation and generalization of these study results. Few of the studies distinguished between any of the many recognized types of depression. As previously stated, the severity of depression may play a role in the cytological response and distinguishing between types may be necessary for more consistency in results. Small sample size and no controls for age, ethnic backgrounds, gender, and medication status may also have led to the inconsistent results reported in the above-mentioned studies.

Loneliness is a paradigm closely related to depression and several studies have found similar results of decreased immune response and function in lonely subject populations studied. A team led by Kiecolt-Glaser in 1984 found in separate studies that both medical students (Kiecolt-Glasser et al 1984a) and psychiatric patients (Kiecolt-Glasser et al 1984b) suffering from loneliness had lower cytotoxic killer cell activity and lymphocyte responses to mitogen stimulation. It is clear that more research into this area is necessary to determine the true effects and modulating variables of depression and loneliness on neuroimmune system function, especially studies controlling for degree of severity and types of symptoms expressed in study populations.

Is Depression Related to Cortical Asymmetries in Function?

Several studies have demonstrated increased prevalence of depressed mood in patients who have suffered damage to the left frontal region of the brain compared to patients with lesions on the right. In addition, it was noted that the more anterior the location of the lesion, the more likely the patient would experience depression (Davidson 1992). The left brain is thought to be responsible for brain functions assigned to the will to perform or act. Right-handed reaching and positive affect are taken to be the collective manifestation of an approach system centred in the left frontal region. Damage to the left frontal region results in behaviour and experience which might best be characterized as a deficit in approach. Therefore, patients with damage or dysfunction involving the left hemisphere may lose pleasure and interest in people or objects and have difficulty initiating voluntary action. During withdrawal-related emotional states such as fear and disgust, the right anterior regions of the brain are activated. PET brain imaging has identified hyper-responsive regions of the right hemisphere that project to the amygdala in panic-prone patients. In order for depression to manifest clinically more than just an injury to the left cortex is necessary. The person must also be exposed to the right set of environmental stimuli for the depression to be initiated. In a patient with left anterior cortical damage, depressive symptomatology would be expected only if that patient were exposed to the requisite environmental stresses. Left anterior damage is not in itself sufficient for the production of depressive symptomatology. We would therefore not expect all patients with left frontal damage to show depressive symptomatology. Only those exposed to an appropriate set of environmental stresses would be expected to show the hypothesized final state (Davidson 1992). Quantitative EEG studies have also proven to be effective in measuring changes in cortical activity associated with depression. Increases in left frontal alpha power are consistent with decreased activation of this area of the brain, along with frontal hypocoherence or decreased synchrony between the hemispheres.

Suicide

In any discussion on depressive disorders, some discussion on suicide must be included because of the strong association between suicide and affective disorders. In his work *The Savage God*, Alvarez states, 'The processes which lead a man to take his own life are at least as complex and difficult as those by which he continues to live.' Yet we know that a major factor in deciding whether to take one's own life is the feeling of hopelessness that occurs in depression. In a study of successful suicides, experimenters found that 94% of them had gone through episodes of serious depression (Robins et al 1959).

The statistics on suicide are difficult to obtain because some who commit suicide want it to look accidental for a variety of reasons, some of which include insurance claims, or to spare families the shame that suicide usually brings. Some researchers have estimated that as many as 15% of all traffic deaths were suicides (Finch et al 1970). Suicide is one of the top ten causes of death in the United States. About 1% of the population has attempted suicide at least once (Epstein 1974).

Among young people in New Zealand, between 15 and 24 years of age, it is considered the second leading cause of death. Three times as many women attempt suicide as men, but three times as many men than women actually succeed in killing themselves. Two times as many single people kill themselves as married people do. The most common profile to commit suicide is a native-born male, in his forties or older that is depressed or ill and kills himself by hanging, shooting, or poisoning by CO (Shneidman & Farberow 1970).

Is there a certain personality type more likely to kill themselves than another? Apparently not! Freud even had suicidal thoughts throughout his life (Jones 1963). There are, however, certain types of reasoning that can lead people to kill themselves (Shneidman & Mandelkorn 1970).

1. Catalogic thinking—This type of person is desperate and destructive, lonely, fearful, and pessimistic, and feels helpless.
2. Logical thinking—This type of person is at the other extreme from the catalogic type. Their thought processes are rational. These people seem to perceive great physical pain, due to a long-term illness, or have been recently widowed. Death offers release from psychological or physical burdens.
3. Contaminated thinking—Beliefs allow the view that death is a transition into a better life, or as a means to 'save face'.
4. Palaeologic thinking—These people are guided by delusions or hallucinations and may kill themselves because voices are telling them that they will be transformed into a supernatural being.

Common Stereotypical Beliefs about Suicide
1. *People who threaten to kill themselves will not carry it out, only the silent types will actually do it.* This is quite untrue. About 70% of those who threaten suicide

actually attempt it (Stengel 1964). In other words, when someone threatens to kill themselves it must be taken seriously.

2. *People who attempt suicide and fail were not serious about it in the first place.* This statement is also untrue. The statistics tell us 75% of all successful suicides have made a previous attempt (Cohen et al 1966). As many as 12% of those who experienced a failed attempt will make a second successful attempt within 3 months (Shochet 1970).

3. *People suffering from depression should not be questioned about suicidal thoughts.* Many people have held the view that depressed people should not be questioned about suicidal thought in the fear that this questioning will put the idea into their head, or it will reinforce it if it is already there. It is now believed that questioning these people directly can help them overcome their feelings and at the very least offer information to direct a therapeutic direction.

4. *When a person commits suicide often family and friends are astonished.* This statement is often true. Friends and family will often make statements such as 'He was in such good spirits'; 'She had so much to live for.' This highlights the fact that friends and relatives are often oblivious to the clues that most people contemplating suicide give out before they kill themselves.

Activities That May Indicate Suicidal Tendencies

The following activities may indicate suicidal tendencies:

- Sudden secretive behaviour;
- Direct verbal statements;
- Withdrawal into a contemplative state;
- Reduce food intake;
- Give away their valuable possessions;
- Implications in speech that will not be seeing you again;
- Rapid tranquillity in a previously agitated person; and
- Most associated with events like births, deaths, and family gatherings.

It may be that about 75% of all those who attempt suicide do not actually want to die. They are using the attempt as a cry for help.

The Humanistic–Existential Perspective on Life and Death

Existentialists place great emphasis on the individual's confrontation with death. Death in fact gives life absolute meaning or value (May 1958). The defining statement of the humanistic–existentialist perspective can be summarized into the following statement. 'I know only two things for sure. 1. I will die and 2. I am not dead now. The only question is what will I do between these two points.'

In other words knowledge of our inevitability of death allows us to take life in earnest and utilize it to pursue our greatest potential. In this perspective suicide is an act of waste and defeat, for it eliminates the possibility of reaching one's potential. The treatment approach under this perspective would try to focus the person on full realization of their human experience and current existence, in hopes that they would find meaning in their life again (Bootzin & Acocella 1984).

Psychotic Versus Neurotic

Psychological disorders can be distinguished based on severity as either neurotic or psychotic. This distinction has traditionally hinged on the matter of reality contact, which is the ability to perceive and interact in one's environment in a reasonable manner. Neurotics may be severely incapacitated but they can seldom be characterized as out of contact with reality. Psychotics, on the other hand, demonstrate a perception of reality that is grossly distorted. Many psychotics have hallucinations and delusions; others withdraw into themselves, creating their own private world (Bootzin & Acocella 1984). In psychosis their sense of reality is so severely impaired that they cannot achieve even the most marginal adaptive functioning. For this reason most psychotics are hospitalized.

Two further classifications of depression have been established based on whether the person expresses neurotic or psychotic tendencies. In neurotic depression, the person may experience extreme anguish but they still know what is going on around them. In psychotic depression, the person may experience hallucinations, delusions, or extreme withdrawal, which effectively cuts the tie between the individual and the environment precluding adaptive functioning. There are some psychologists who have expressed the opinion that neurosis and psychosis are not two different entities but rather two ends of the spectrum of the same disorder (Beck 1967).

Psychosis

The psychoses are usually divided into two broad categories:

1. Biogenic psychoses—associated with some physical cause; and
2. Functional psychoses—no physical basis and probably psychogenic in nature.

The functional psychoses are divided into three classes:

1. Major affective disorders, which involve mood disorders such as depression;
2. Schizophrenic disorders, which involve disorders of thought; and
3. Paranoid disorders, which involve delusional thinking.

Schizophrenia

Schizophrenia is marked by a variety of symptoms and actions including bizarre behaviour, social withdrawal, and severe distortion of thought, perception, and affect. Schizophrenia is probably not a single entity involving a single part of the brain. On the contrary, it is most likely a group of disorders which differ widely in aetiology and symptomatology. About 1 in every 100 people has had or will have a schizophrenic episode. There are about 1,000,000 active schizophrenics in the USA (Berger 1978). Half of all beds in mental hospitals are taken by schizophrenics. Half of all schizophrenics released from mental institutions will return within 2 years of release (Gunderson et al 1974).

The fundamental symptoms of schizophrenia can be remembered by the pneumonic of the four A's:

1. Association—the person shows evidence of a thought disorder by way of his/her use of language;
2. Affect—the person's emotional responses are blunted or inappropriate;
3. Ambivalence—the person is indecisive and unable to carry on normal goal-directed activities; and
4. Autism—the patient is withdrawn and self-absorbed.

QUICK FACTS 1	What Does It Mean?

Delusion: false beliefs

Hallucinations: false sensory perceptions

The secondary symptoms of schizophrenia may include:

1. Hallucinations;
2. Paranoid thinking;
3. Grandiosity;
4. Hostility and belligerence;
5. Delusions; and
6. Genetic link is now well established;

The development of schizophrenia may present in phases which include;

1. *The prodromal phase*—Onset usually occurs in adolescence or early adulthood. In some cases it is very sudden; in just a few days a normal person is transformed into

Examples of Delusional Thoughts	**QUICK FACTS 2**

1. 'My brain activity and thoughts are being controlled by radio waves from outer space.'
2. 'I'm a doctor you know, I just don't have a diploma, but I was in New York once by television and I am the personification of Casper the friendly ghost. I am now a week pregnant and my name is Jack Warden.'
3. 'I am 3 months pregnant with God's baby but Mick Jagger wants to marry me. When you have Jesus in your life you don't need a diet. I use Covergirl creamy natural make-up. I am the face of Covergirl so I get it free.'

a delusional psychotic. In other cases there is a slow insidious deterioration of function that may go on for years.

2. *The active phase*—The person starts showing prominent psychotic symptoms: hallucinations, delusions, disorganized speech, and severe withdrawal.
3. *The residual phase*—A remission phase where the behaviour returns to premorbid levels. Blunting or flat affect is common in this stage. Sometime the residual phase ends with the person regaining completely normal function. This unfortunately is rare.

There are five types of schizophrenia commonly recognized clinically:

1. Disorganized (hebephrenic)—Childish behaviour predominates: giggling, making funny faces, incoherence of speech;
2. Catatonic—Disturbed motor activity, either violently hyperactive or mute inactivity, or both;
3. Paranoid—Delusions of persecution or grandeur and/or hallucinations on the same theme;
4. Residual—Persons in the residual phase of schizophrenia; and
5. Undifferentiated—Miscellaneous category for patients that do not fit into the other categories, or who show symptoms of several subtypes.

Some Common, Firmly Held Beliefs That Have No Basis in Reality, Often Expressed by Schizophrenics	**QUICK FACTS 3**

1. Persecution (conspiracy plots, spied on)
2. Control (other beings are controlling them)
3. Reference (events in the news relate to them)
4. Sin and guilt (they have committed great sins)
5. Nihilistic (the world has come to an end)
6. Grandeur (I am Christ, I am Napoleon)
7. Thought broadcasting (one's thoughts are being broadcast over the TV)
8. Thought insertion (other people are inserting thoughts)
9. Thought withdrawal (other people are stealing thoughts)

The Dopamine Hypothesis
Schizophrenia has been associated with excessive activity of those parts of the brain that use dopamine as a neurotransmitter. The most effective drugs in use for treatment of schizophrenia are phenothiazines and butyrophenones, which exert their effects by

blocking the brain's receptor sites for dopamine. This leads to a decrease in activity of the areas of the brain that utilize dopamine.

Is Schizophrenia Linked to Cortical Asymmetrical Activation?

A number of laterality studies have used initial lateral eye movements as a measure of unbalanced frontal hemisphere activity. Several of these studies have demonstrated that schizophrenics look to their right more often than normals or depressives when thinking about spatial and/or emotional material. This increase in right gaze responses has been taken to represent increased left hemisphere responsiveness for spatial and emotional material (Schweitzer 1982). Schizophrenics may have a primary deficit in their right hemisphere, which affects visuospatial processing. It is suggested that the apparent left hemisphere increase in activity may be a compensatory mechanism for a primary failure of the schizophrenic's right hemisphere to maintain normal attention and vigilance (Schweitzer 1982).

Neurosis

Originally this term was thought to be an organic disorder involving a general affliction of the nervous system that produced various forms of bizarre nervous behaviour. Throughout the nineteenth century, those people who were demonstrably sane but nevertheless engaged in rigid and self-defeating behaviours were labelled neurotic and thought to be victims of some identified neurological dysfunction. Around the turn of the century this biogenic view of neurosis was gradually replaced by Freud's psychogenic view (Freud 1894). To Freud, neurosis was not due to organic causes, but rather to anxiety. As repressed memories and desires threatened to break through from the unconscious to the conscious mind, anxiety occurred as a danger signal to the ego. The neurotic behaviour that developed was either the expression of that anxiety or defence against it. This view has held until the past few decades where there has been a growing opposition to using the term neurosis to describe all of the anxiety disorders due to the fact that not all of the neuroses express anxiety directly.

Anxiety

Anxiety is a multistate phenomenon which involves subjective state changes, a state of physiological arousal and a state of cognitive disruption. For this reason, anxiety is difficult to measure accurately. Tests of these different dimensions of anxiety often disagree with one another because we have no reliable yardstick with which to measure anxiety. Without such a yardstick it is hard to use anxiety in making diagnostic distinctions. Anxiety is not limited to so-called neurotics; normal people feel it too, as do psychotics, depressives, and sexual deviants. Anxiety can be experienced in three basic patterns:

1. In generalized anxiety disorder and panic disorder, the anxiety is unfocused; either it is with the person continually or descends out of nowhere, unconnected to any special stimulus.
2. In phobic disorders on the other hand, the fear is aroused by one particular object or situation.
3. In obsessive–compulsive disorder, anxiety occurs if the person does not engage in some thought or behaviour that otherwise serves no purpose and in fact may be unpleasant and embarrassing.

Anxiety involves three basic components:

1. Subjective reports of tension, apprehension sense of impending danger; and expectations of an ability to cope;
2. Behavioural responses, such as avoidance of the situation at hand and paired speech and motor functioning and paired performance on cognitive tasks; and
3. Physiological responses, including muscle tension, increased heart rate, increased blood pressure, rapid breathing, dry mouth, nausea, diarrhoea, and frequent urination.

Anxiety disorders involve a state of fear and apprehension that affects many different areas of functioning. The anxiety disorders include the following:

1. Generalized anxiety disorder;
2. Panic disorder;
3. Phobic disorders;

4. Obsessive–compulsive disorders; and

5. Post-traumatic stress disorders.

Generalized Anxiety Disorders (GAD)

The main feature of this disorder is a chronic state of diffuse unfocused anxiety. People with this disorder cannot say what the cause of their anxiety is. All they know is that they feel a persistent sense of tension and dread (Bootzin & Acocella 1984). People with GAD are continually on edge, waiting for something dreadful to happen either to themselves or to those they care about. Eventually they may develop secondary anxiety, which involves a state of anxiety about their anxiety, fearing that their condition will cause them to develop health problems, lose their jobs, default on their mortgages, go crazy, and so forth.

The subjective feelings produced in these individuals spills over into their cognitive and physiological activities, in such a way as to disrupt their normal existence. The person finds it hard to concentrate, make decisions, and remember commitments (Bootzin & Acocella 1984). At the same time, chronic muscle tension and heighten arousal in the nervous system give rise to numerous physiological complaints such as:

- Muscular aches;
- Nervous twitches;
- Headaches;
- Breathing difficulties;
- Clammy hands;
- Racing pulse;
- Tingling feelings in their hands and feet.;
- Indigestion; and
- Insomnia.

The diagnosis of generalized anxiety disorders includes:

- Excessive anxiety and worry for at least 6 months duration about a number of events and activities that would not normally cause this heightened state of anxiety; and
- The person shows continuous and persistent difficulty in controlling their worry.

Three or more of the following six symptoms must also be present:

- Restlessness or feeling keyed up or on edge;
- Easy fatigability;
- Difficulty concentrating or mind going blank;
- Irritability;
- Muscle tension;
- Sleep disturbance; and
- Significant impairment in social, occupational, or other areas of functioning.

The Affects of Anxiety on Neuroimmune Function High levels of anxiety have been shown to occur concomitantly with blunted T-cell blastogenesis (Fawzy 1995) and inhibited lymphocyte response (Linn et al 1981). Koh and Lee (1998) found that untreated patients with anxiety disorders showed significantly reduced lymphocyte proliferative response and decreased interleukin-2 response when compared to normal controls. However, in the same study they could find no significant difference in T-cell cytotoxicity between groups. Another study by Surman et al (1986) found no significant difference in lymphocyte proliferative response between panic patients and control groups.

Although most studies have shown a decrease in immune function with high anxiety levels, some studies have found the opposite, that high levels of anxiety can be associated with increased immune function (Koh 1997). Koh found that students undergoing anxiety from highly competitive exams actually had enhanced lymphocyte proliferation. These finding may reflect the fact that anxiety is a very complex emotional state to measure. Izard (1972) using the differential emotions scale (DES) determined that anxiety is experienced as a variety of emotions including fear, guilt, sadness, and shame. The inconsistent findings relating the immune response to anxiety may be due to the fact that different anxiety characteristics are being measured, which results in different responses of the immune system.

QUICK FACTS 4   **Hysteria Has Played an Interesting Role in the History of Psychological Development**

Hippocrates believed that hysteria was confined to women, particularly childless women, and was due to the overactions of the uterus not being put to the proper use. Idle and frustrated the uterus would travel around inside the body creating havoc in different organ systems. The cure that Hippocrates prescribed was marriage. Freud's explanation of hysteria stressed sexual conflicts as the cause and this laid the foundation for the theory of the unconscious, which evolved into his psychodynamic theory.

Another explanation for the inconsistent findings described above, as outlined by Koh (1993); is that the different researchers were measuring different severities of anxiety, mainly acute anxiety and subacute anxiety. Koh suggests that subclinical anxiety may be associated with increased immune function, which may be a transient phenomenon occurring prior to any down-regulation of immune function shown to occur with clinical anxiety.

Is Anxiety Related to Asymmetrical Cortical Activation? In patients with anxiety, the predominant finding is an increase in activation of the right frontal regions, which in terms of brain asymmetry may be viewed as similar to those findings in depression, but representing different absolute intensities of activation.

Panic Disorder

In panic attacks, the feeling of anxiety mounts to an almost unbearable level. The person sweats, feels dizzy, trembles, shivers, and gasps for breath. Their pulse quickens and their heart pounds. Above all, there is a feeling of inescapable doom; the person may feel that he or she is about to die, go insane, or commit some horrible act (Bootzin & Acocella 1984). These attacks usually last several minutes, though they may continue for hours. When the attack subsides, the person often feels exhausted as if he or she has been involved in a traumatic experience. In cases where the panic attack is triggered by a phobia, it is referred to as a phobic attack. However, in instances where these attacks occur in the absence of any phobic stimulus, it is referred to as panic disorder.

Since the panic attacks are unpredictable, patients cannot go anywhere. The movies, the grocery store, a restaurant are all out of bounds because these people fear that they may have another attack in front of everyone. Consequently, victims of panic disorder may cease to go anywhere and develop the disorder known as *agoraphobia*. Agoraphobia is anxiety of being in places or situations from which escape might be difficult, or where help may not be available in the event of having an unexpected panic attack. Fears commonly involve clusters of situations, like being alone, being in a crowd, standing in a line, travelling on a bus, or sitting in a classroom (Bootzin & Acocella 1984).

The mnemonic for panic disorder is 'Students Fear the 3 C's':

S: sweating

T: trembling

U: unsteadiness

D: depersonalization, derealization

E: excess heart rate (palpitations)

N: nausea

T: tingling in the limbs (paraesthesia)

S: shortness of breath

FEAR: of dying, losing control, going crazy

3 C's: chest pain, chills, choking.

Diagnosis of Panic Disorder The American Psychiatric Association's (APA) *Diagnostic and Statistical Manual* (DSM-IV) classifies panic disorder as an abrupt onset of fear or discomfort that peaks in approximately 10 minutes and includes at least four of the following:

- Palpitations, pounding heart, or rapid heart rate;
- Sweating;
- Tremor;
- Sensations of smoothing or shortness of breath;
- Feeling of choking;
- Chest pain or discomfort;
- Nausea or abdominal distress;
- Dizziness, lightheadedness, or faint;
- Feelings of unreality;
- Fear of losing control or 'going crazy';
- Fear of dying;
- Paraesthesia; and
- Hot flashes.

Diagnosis also requires that the panic attacks recur every 2 weeks or that a single attack is accompanied by at least 1 month of persistent concern about future attacks, worry that the attacks will cause physical illness or insanity, or significant changes in behaviour related to the attacks.

There is no consensus about the initial appearance of panic. The commonplace description of panic patients is that attacks 'come out of the blue'. There are two professional views of how panic develops. The first, a biological view, is that panic initially appears almost fully fledged in its physical manifestations. It is recognized, however, that following the initial panic manifestations, cognitively driven elaborations, and amplifications may subsequently develop. The second view is that physical perturbations in combination with certain attitudes/cognitions which may or may not be fully conscious lead to the experience of panic.

The 'cognitions' in people experiencing panic attacks may be considered as triggers only, as the underlying mechanism of panic attacks may be related to a heightened sensitivity of limbic circuits that are 'wound up' by a loss of inhibition. This may occur due to metabolic or neurotransmitter imbalances, altered afferentiation from the periphery, or decreased effect of more central influences due to hemisphericity, diffuse axonal injury following concussion or whiplash, and environmental exposures such as chemical and emotional stressors.

Phobias

A phobia usually involves two distinct aspects:

1. An intense fear of some object or situation, which the individual realizes actually poses no major threat; and
2. Avoidance of the phobic stimulus.

Often the stimulus is one that carries a very slight suggestion of danger, for example, dogs, insects, snakes, or high places. It is important to understand that so-called 'normal' people may not prefer to step out onto the roof of a building or touch a wild animal either; the difference between these so-called normal reactions and a phobia is one of severity. Phobias, in severe cases, may actually stimulate a panic attack. People with phobias unlike 'normal' people must design their lives so that they avoid the thing they fear. Phobias are fairly common affecting up to 8% of the general population (Agras et al 1969).

The two types of phobias are general phobias and social phobias. Among the more frequently seen types of general phobias are:

Acrophobia—fear of heights;

Claustrophobia—fear of enclosed or crowded spaces; and

Agoraphobia—fear of open spaces or leaving home.

Social phobias occur when a person is afraid to perform certain actions when exposed to the scrutiny of others, for example, public speaking, eating in public, or using public bathrooms (Bootzin & Acocella 1984).

Obsessive–Compulsive Disorder

An obsession is a thought or an image that keeps recurring or returning to the mind. The individual may consider the thought or image a senseless activity and may even find the recurring nature or the thought itself extremely unpleasant in nature. A compulsion is an action that the individual feels compelled to repeat again and again, to reduce the level of anxiety that seems to continuously build up within them. Usually the person has no conscious desire to perform the act but does so anyway (Bootzin & Acocella 1984).

Mild obsessions strike many of us from time to time. We may dwell repeatedly on some song lyric or a thought may keep running through our mind. But these minor obsessions pass and do not prevent us from getting on with our normal lives. Pathological obsessions do not pass. They keep recurring and recurring day in and day out. Usually pathological obsessions take the form of a violent or demoralizing quality, such as a mother obsessing with the idea of drowning her baby in the bath or a man obsessed with the fear he will masturbate in public (Bootzin & Acocella 1984).

Compulsions tend to fall into two categories (Rachman & Hodgson 1980):

1. Checking rituals—people who are compelled to interrupt their activities again and again to go and make sure that they have done something that they were supposed to do, for example, locking and relocking doors; and

2. Cleaning rituals—compulsive hand-washers.

It is important to make the distinction between true obsessive–compulsive disorders and conditions such as compulsive gamblers or compulsive eaters. True obsession and compulsion does not bring pleasure to the victims. Compulsive gamblers or compulsive eaters may be deeply pained by the consequences of these excesses. Nevertheless, they take pleasure in eating and gambling so these are not true obsessive–compulsive behaviours (Bootzin & Acocella 1984).

Post-traumatic Stress Disorder

These disorders are acute psychological reactions to the person's exposure to an intensely traumatic event. For example, the person may be involved in or witness an assault, natural disaster, an airplane crash, a devastating fire, torture, and/or bombings. This condition differs from other anxiety disorders in that the source of the stress is an external event of an overwhelmingly painful nature, so to a certain extent it may seem justified or normal to feel this way. These disorders can be extremely debilitating. For example, victims may go on for days, weeks, or months re-experiencing the traumatic event in their minds. They may show a diminished responsiveness to their present surroundings, a sort of 'emotional anaesthesia'. They may find it difficult to respond to affection. They may develop insomnia, decreased sex drive, and heightened sensitivity to noise. They also have greater expression of depression.

The traumatic event is persistently re-experienced through one or more of the following:

- Recurrent distressing recollections involving images or thoughts;
- Recurrent distressing dreams;
- Acting or feeling as if the event is reoccurring through flashbacks, illusions, and hallucinations;
- Distress at exposure to cues that resemble events; and
- Psychological reactivity in response to cues.

Diagnosis of post-traumatic stress disorder requires that there be persistent avoidance of stimuli associated with trauma, as well as persistent symptoms of the following:

- Increased arousal;
- Insomnia;
- Irritability;
- Difficulty concentrating;

- Hypervigilance; and
- Exaggerated startle response.

Symptoms must be present for greater than 1 month for the diagnosis of post-traumatic stress disorder to apply.

Somatoform Disorders

The primary feature of somatoform disorders is that psychological conflicts take on a somatic or physical form. Some patients complain of physical discomfort, stomach pains, breathing problems, and so forth. Other patients show an actual loss or impairment of some normal physiological function; for instance they are suddenly unable to walk or swallow (Bootzin & Acocella 1984). In either case, there is no organic evidence to explain the symptom, while there is evidence that the symptom is linked to a psychological cause.

There are several types of somatoform disorders. We will look at three forms:

1. Hypochondriasis;
2. Somatization disorder; and
3. Conversion disorder.

Hypochondriasis

The primary feature of this condition is a continuous, inescapable fear of disease. The fear is maintained by constant misinterpretation of physical signs and sensations as abnormal and representing clinical signs or symptoms of a disease process. Hypochondriacs have no real physical disability or disease process that can be clinically proven to exist.

Often when hypochondriacs present at a health professional's office, they have already diagnosed their condition, for they are usually avid readers of medical textbooks, and have spent countless hours on the Internet searching their symptoms for the diseases that cause similar symptoms. When the healthcare professional tells them that they can find no physical cause for their symptoms and there is actually nothing wrong with them they are disappointed and will often change healthcare professionals until they find someone who at least agrees to perform more tests to prove that they do in fact have a disease or condition. Often these people go through several healthcare professionals per year.

It should be noted that hypochondriacs do not fake their symptoms. They truly feel the pains they report. They cannot be reassured by the medical evidence presented to them that their fears are irrational (Bootzin & Acocella 1984). However, these fears do not have the bizarre quality of the disease delusions experienced by psychotics, who will report that their feet are about to fall off or their brains are shrivelling. Instead hypochondriacs tend to confine their anxieties to more ordinary syndromes, such as heart disease or cancer. Eventually they generally focus on a single disorder.

Somatization Disorder

This disorder is also known as Briquet's syndrome (Bootzin & Acocella 1984). This condition is characterized by numerous and recurrent physical complaints which have persisted for several years and have caused the person to seek medical help, but for which no medical or scientific explanation can be given. This condition resembles hypochondriasis in that it involves symptoms with no demonstrable physical cause. Yet the two disorders differ in the focus of the patient's distress. What motivates the hypochondriac is the fear of disease, usually a specific disease. The symptoms are troubling only because they indicate the presence of that disease. In contrast, it is actually the symptoms themselves that concern the patient with somatization disorder.

The diagnosis of this condition can be extremely complicated and frustrating for a number of reasons. Firstly, the patient usually describes dramatic and exaggerated symptoms. Secondly, in the case of hypochondriac's, they often fear one particular disease, and therefore their complaints tend to be fairly limited. In someone with somatization disorder, on the other hand, the complaints are many and varied. In fact, this condition requires 12 to 14 different kinds of complaints for this diagnosis to be given. The occurrence is more common in females than males and 1% of women may develop some form of this disorder throughout their lives (Bootzin & Acocella 1984).

Conversion Disorder

In hypochondriasis and somatization disorder, there is no real physical disability, only a fear of, or complaints about, an illness or disability. In conversion disorder, there is an actual disability. The disability usually includes the loss or impairment of some motor or sensory function (Bootzin & Acocella 1984). Formerly known as hysteria, conversion disorder has played a central role in the history of psychology (see Quick Facts 4).

Like the symptoms in hypochondriasis and somatization disorder, conversion symptoms are not supported by medical evidence. But neither are they faked. The symptoms are involuntary responses, which are not under the person's conscious control. At the same time, they contradict the physiological facts; for instance, upon examination, the eyes will be found to be perfectly free from defect or damage and yet the person will not be able to see. Thus, conversion disorders differ from psychosomatic disorders such as ulcers in that in psychosomatic disorders there is an observable medical dysfunction.

Conversion symptoms vary considerably. Among the most common are:

- Blindness;
- Deafness;
- Paralysis; and
- Anaesthesia (partial or total).

Many patients with conversion disorder seem completely unperturbed by their symptoms. Whereas most people would react with horror to the discovery that they were suddenly blind or could no longer walk, the conversion patient is relatively unconcerned. This phenomenon is referred to as 'La belle indifference'. In fact, they are typically eager to discuss their symptoms and will describe them in the most full and vivid terms to anyone who will listen. They also do not seem particularly eager to part with their symptoms.

In conversion disorder patients the patient's body appears to be in good health. Biologically and physiologically conversion patients can do whatever it is they say they can not do. However, either by trickery or under hypnosis or the influence of drugs they can perform the task that they deny the ability to perform. Further evidence for their lack of organic pathology is that the symptoms are often selective. For example, conversion epileptics seldom injure themselves or lose bladder control during a seizure as do true epileptics. Likewise, in conversion blindness, patients rarely bump into things. It must be reinforced at this time that conversion patients by definition are not consciously refusing to use parts of their body. Their response is involuntary.

Diagnosis of this disorder is difficult. First, malingering, the conscious faking of a symptom in order to avoid some responsibility, must be ruled out. The second and much more difficult task is ruling out an actual organic disorder. Certain signs may suggest conversion disorder. These include:

1. Rapid appearance of symptoms, especially after some psychological trauma;
2. Le belle indifference; and
3. Selective symptoms such as paralysis. For example, if paralysed legs move during sleep, the paralysis is presumably not organic.

Stress

In 1936, Selye reported that laboratory animals presented a common reaction to exposure to noxious stimuli such as cold, heat, X-rays, adrenaline, insulin, or muscular exercise. Selye called this specific biological response stress and anything that induced this response a stressor. Since Selye first introduced his stress/stressor theory, this concept has undergone a progressive evolution from animal models consisting of only physical stressors to human models involving the distinction between physical stress and psychological stress. Studies carried out by Lazarus (1966) were instrumental in the evolution of the above concept by describing the fundamental role of the central nervous system, and of psychological factors in the response to stressors. The first scientist to investigate the role of the immune system to stress conditions appears to be Ishigami in 1919. While studying the effects of chronic tuberculosis he observed a decrease in the phagocytic activity of leukocytes during periods of the greatest psychological stress. Many studies have since shown the interconnection of the central nervous system and the immune system in response to stress (Kiecolt-Glaser & Glaser 1991; Plotnikoff et al 1991; Seymour 1993; Madden & Felten 1995; Bondi & Zannino 1997). Most authors today consider the neuromodulation of host immunocompetence the principal system involved in the mediation of pathogenic effects of psychosocial factors (Bondi & Zannino 1997), although modulation of anatomical microfunctional barriers and host modulation of the infectious agent may also play a less important role (Cohen et al 1991; Evans & Edgerton 1991). Human studies involving psychological stress have mostly focused on 'physical' stressors such as sleep deprivation and noise (Palmbald et al 1976, 1979; Weisse et al 1990; Hall et al 1998) and interestingly, space flights (Fischer et al 1972; Kimzey et al 1976). In these studies, strong associations between stress and impaired cytotoxic T-cell activity were found.

However, very few studies have focused on purely psychological experimental stressors. Some studies have utilized psychological stress in the form of confronting subjects with a short-term uncontrollable interpersonal situation and found resulting increases in suppressor T-lymphocyte concentrations and cytotoxic T-cell activity (Naliboff et al 1991; Brosschot et al 1991, 1992).

Esterling et al (1995) found a decrease in cytotoxic T-cell function in chronic caregivers as long as 3 years after the death of the care receiver, suggesting that the chronic stresses of caregiving may have far-reaching and potentially important physiological implications. They suggested that former caregivers are not reintegrated into society, which results in a persistent lack of social support which sustains the level of chronic stress even after the death of the care receiver. These results seem to indicate that the immune system response to a short-term psychological stress situation and a chronic stress situation are different and significant with regards to cytotoxic T-cell activity and function.

The cytotoxic T-cells play an important role in a variety of immune functions including defence against viral infections, surveillance of tumour cells, and most particularly the control of metastases (Herberman 1992). Some studies involving humans and their response to stress have focused on stressful life events and how the stress from these events affected the person's risk of contracting a given disease. Epidemiological studies have demonstrated clear differences between bereaved and non-bereaved controls in terms of cancer mortality (Verbrugge 1979) and lymphocyte proliferative response and mitogenitic activity (Schleifer et al 1983). Convergent data from several investigations suggest that bereavement may be associated with depression of some components of the immune system such as those suggested above (Kiecolt-Glaser & Glaser 1991). Irwin et al (1987a) and others (Bartrop et al 1977; Schleifer et al 1983; Calabrese et al 1987) have demonstrated an impaired T-lymphocyte proliferative response in bereaved spouses that may last for a period of several months. The exact stimuli and response mechanisms of this response remain unclear (Knapp et al 1992).

Epidemiological data also suggest that divorced individuals are at risk for both physical and mental illness (Verbrugge 1979). Evidence suggests that continued preoccupation with the ex-spouse (overattachment) leads to distress-related symptoms (Weiss 1975). Consistent with these results Kiecolt-Glaser et al (1988) found that divorced individuals who had been separated for shorter periods or who had stronger feelings of attachment had a decreased immune function.

It appears that consistent data seem to be emerging indicating a correlation between marital interruption and down-regulation of the immune system. Herbert and Cohen (1993) used meta-analytic procedures to evaluate the literature on stress and immunity in humans. In all, they examined and analysed 31 different studies and concluded that a substantial amount of evidence from both functional and enumerative measures links stress to immune function. In terms of cell numbers, they found stress is reliably associated with higher number of circulating white blood cells and lower numbers of circulating B cells, T cells, helper and suppressor T cells, and cytotoxic T cells. They found that stress is also reliably associated with decreases in total serum IgM and salivary IgA concentrations. Some limitations were evident with the study, namely that 11 of the 31 studies used were from the same investigators but, nevertheless, a strong correlation seemed to exist.

The effects of chronic stress were evaluated by Fiore et al (1983) and Kiecolt-Glaser and Glaser (1991). Both groups utilized caregivers of Alzheimer's patients as representatives of chronic stress recipients. They found that contrary to animal studies where acute stress appeared immunosuppressive and chronic stress immunoenhancing (Monjan & Collecter 1977), in humans chronic stress resulted in chronic down-regulation of the immune system. In contrast to the results obtained in studies of the effects of long-term or chronic stress, several recent studies have focused on the effects of relatively short-term stressful life events such as tandem jumps of first-time parachutists (Schedlowski et al 1993), waiting for notification of HIV-1 test results (Ironson et al 1990), and threatened missile attack at Israeli sites (Weiss et al 1996). The results of these studies found an elevation rather than reduction in the number and activity of cytotoxic T-cells, both immediately before and after the stressful event.

Behavioural Conditioning

The paper of Ader and Cohen (1975) demonstrating the classical conditioning of immune response sparked a renewed interest in the concept of psychoneuroimmune link. In their study Ader and Cohen used a distinctively flavoured drink, which they paired with an injection of immunosuppressive drug (cyclophosphamide) on a population of rats. When the rats, who had been conditioned to immunosuppression, stopped receiving the injection of cyclophosphamine but drank from the flavoured drink they still remained immunosuppressed. Ader and Cohen, through a series of further experiments (Ader & Cohen 1993) confirmed by other studies (Lysle et al 1988) showed that the rat's immune systems had been conditioned to respond through psychological conditioning.

The biological impact of such a discovery becomes evident when applications of the conditioning operation occur in tissue graph rejection experiments. In mice, re-exposure to a condition stimulus previously paired with an immunosuppressive drug treatment prolonged the survival of foreign tissue graphs on mice without further administration of the drug (Gorczynski 1990).

Further clinical implications for humans remain to be identified. However, at least one case study describes the successful application of conditioning in reducing the amount of Cytoxan therapy received by a child with lupus (Olness & Ader 1992). Another team of investigators used a different form of behavioural conditioning to investigate the effects of coping on immune system function. Laudenslager et al (1983) used a shocking mechanism on human subjects and found that inescapable shocks lead to a suppression of lymphocyte proliferation, whereas escapable shocks did not. They concluded that the degree of control that a subject had over the unpleasant stimuli determined the type of immune response to a large degree.

Humour and Happiness

The idea that humour and health may be related is not a new idea. In fact, it is an idea that has long enjoyed widespread support, both from the lay public and among professionals in the fields of psychology and medicine (Lefcourt & Martin 1986). It seems surprising that a relationship so widely held by society has not been investigated by more than a handful of researchers. Cousins (1979) in an autobiographical account describes the positive effect that humour had on his recovery from an extremely painful disease. He reported a decrease in pain perception and a drop in his sedimentation rate following exposure to humour. Several investigators have shown that mirthful laughter is accompanied by a widespread variety of psychobiological changes. These changes include respiratory changes, facial muscle contractions, circulatory changes, sympathetic activation (Lefcourt & Martin 1986; Fry 1980), and an increase in spontaneous lymphocyte blastogenesis and natural killer cell activity (Lefcourt & Thomas 1998). Dillon et al (1985) used a humourous videotape to induce humour, compared to a didactic videotape and found increases in salivary IgA concentration in subjects viewing the humourous videotape. Dillon and Totten (1989) expanded on Dillon's original work with a study involving breastfeeding mothers. The study found a positive correlation between ratings on the cognitive Humour Scale and a decreased incidence of respiratory infections in both mothers and their breastfed babies.

Futterman et al (1992) induced positive and negative mental states in actors and found that all experimentally induced mood states produced greater immunological fluctuations in natural-killer cells than a neutral state and that these effects were stronger for more 'aroused' moods such as happiness. If immune function can be experimentally conditioned in humans, then happiness may be one step on the voyage to understanding the relationship between a positive emotional state and healing.

Most theories of humour involve the concept of psychological arousal as a necessary component of humour elicitation; however, several fundamental issues remain unresolved when studying humour as an emotional concept. First, humour must be differentiated from other aesthetic qualities that may be associated with making one laugh, such as beauty, wit, nonsense, sarcasm, ridicule, satire, or irony. Confusion of results may occur when researchers consider humour as an umbrella term for all phenomena that makes one laugh. This terminology involves such diverse categories as aggressive humour, copying humour, mock humour, ridicule humour, and just plain humour. It is important to appreciate that these different forms of humour may be generated by different neuronal mechanisms which may result in different effects on the other systems of the body.

References

Ader R, Cohen N 1975 Behaviourally conditioned immunosuppression. Psychosomatic Medicine 37:333–340.

Ader R, Cohen N 1993 Psychoneuroimmunology: conditioning and stress. Annual Review of Psychology 44:53–58.

Agras S, Sylvester D, Oliveau D (1969) The epidemiology of common fears and phobias. Unpublished manuscript

Alvarez A 1971 The savage god: a study of suicide. Weidenfeld and Nicolson, London.

Amsterdam JD, Henle W, Winokur A et al 1986 Sermin antibodies to Ebstein-Barr virus in patients with major depressive disorder. American Journal of Psychiatry 143:1593–1596.

Apter MJ 1988 Reversal theory as a theory of the emotions. In: Apter MJ, Kerr JH, Cowles MP (eds) Progress in reversal theory. Elsevier, Amsterdam.

Bandura A 1986 Social foundations of thought and action: A social cognitive theory. Prentice-Hall, Englewood Cliffs, NJ.

Bandura A 1989 Social cognitive theory. In: Vasta R (ed) Annals of child development. JAI Press, Greenwich, CT, p 1–60

Bandura A 1991 Social cognitive theory of moral thought and action. In: Kirtines WM, Gewitz JL (eds) Handbook of moral behaviour and development. Lawrence Elbaum, Hillsdale, NJ, p 45–103

Bartrop RW, Lockhurst E, Lazarus L et al 1977 Depressed lymphocyte function after bereavement. Lancet 1:834–836.

Beck AT 1967 Depression: clinical, experimental, and theoretical aspects. Harper & Row, New York.

Berger PA 1978 Medical treatment of mental illness. Science 200:974–981.

Berk L 1994 Child development, 3rd edn. Allyn and Bacon, Boston.

Black FO, Pesznecker SC 2003 Vestibular adaptation and rehabilitation. Current Opinion in Otolaryngology and Head and Neck Surgery 11:(5)355–360.

Blalock JE 1984 The immune system as a sensory organ. Journal of Immunology 132:1067–1070.

Bondi M, Zannino L 1997 Psychological stress, neuromodulation and susceptibility to infectious diseases in animals and man: A review. Psychotherapy and Psychosomatics 66:3–26.

Bootzin RR, Acocella JR 1984 Abnormal psychology; current perspectives. Random House, New York.

Boyd JH, Weissman MM 1981 Epidemiology of affective disorders: A reexamination and future directions. Archives of General Psychiatry 38:1039–1045.

Brosschot J, Smelt D, DeSmet M et al 1991 Effects of experimental psychological stress of T-lymphocytes and NK cells in man: an exploratory study. Journal of Psychophysiology 5:59–67.

Brosschot J, Benschop R, Godaert G et al 1992 Effects of experimental psychological stress on distribution and function of peripheral blood cells. Psychosomatic Medicine 54:394–406.

Calabrese JR, Kling MA, Gold PW 1987 Alterations in immunocompetence during stress, bereavement, and depression: focus on neuroendocrine regulation. American Journal of Psychiatry 144:(9):1123–1134.

Campos JJ, Mumme DL, Kermoian R et al 1994 A functionalist perspective on the nature of emotion. In: Fox NA (ed) The development of emotion regulation. Monographs of the Society for Research in Child Development, 59(2 and 3):284–303.

Cohen E, Motto JA, Seiden RH 1966 An instrument for evaluating suicide potential: A preliminary study. American Journal of Psychiatry 122:886–891.

Cohen S, Tyrrel DAJ, Smith AP 1991 Psychological stress and susceptibility to the common cold. New England Journal of Medicine 325:606–612.

Cousins N 1979 Anatomy of an illness. Norton, New York.

Crow TJ 1984 A re-evaluation of the viral hypothesis: Is psychosis the result of retroviral integration at a site close to the cerebral dominance gene? British Journal of Psychiatry 145:243–253.

Davidson RJ 1992 Anterior cerebral asymmetry and the nature of emotion. Brain and Cognition 20:125–151.

Dillon KM, Minchoff B, Baker K 1985 Positive emotional state enhancement of the immune system. International Journal of Psychiatric Medicine 15:13–17.

Dillon KM, Totten MC 1989 Psychological factors immunocompetence and health of breast feeding mothers and their infants. Journal of Genetic Psychology 150:155–162.

Esterling B, Kiecolt-Glaser J, Glaser R 1996 Psychosocial modulation of cytokine induced natural killer cell activity in older adults. Psychosomatic Medicine 58:264–272.

Epstein H 1974 A sin or a right?. *The New York Times Magazine,* September 8, pp 91–94.

Epstein S 1993 Emotion and self theory. In: Lewis M, Haviland J (eds) Handbook of emotion. Gilford Press, New York,

Epstein S, Lipson A, Holstein C et al 1992 Irrational reactions to negative outcomes; Evidence for two conceptual systems. Journal of Personality and Social Psychology 62:328–338.

Etzel B, Gewirtz J 1967 Experimental modification of caretaker-maintained high rate operant crying with reinforcement of eye contact and smiling. Journal of Experimental Child Psychology 5:303–317.

Evans PD, Edgerton N 1991 Life events and moods as predictors of the common cold. British Journal of Medical Psychology 64:35–44.

Fawzy FI 1995 Behaviour and immunity: In: Kaplan HI, Socock BJ (eds) Comprehensive textbook of psychiatry. Williams & Wilkins, Baltimore, MD, p 1559–1570

Finch JR, Smith JP, Pokoray AD 1970 Vehicular studies. Paper presented at meetings of the American Psychiatric Association.

Fiore J, Becker J, Coppel DB 1983 Social network interactions: A buffer or a stress?. American Journal of Community Psychology 11:423–429.

Fischer CL, Daniels JC, Levin WC et al 1972 Effects of the space flight environment on man's immune system. II. Lymphocyte counts and reactivity. Aerospace Medicine 43:1122–1125.

Flor-Henry P 1986 Observations, reflections, and speculations on the cerebral determinants of mood and on the bilateral asymmetrical distribution of the major neurotransmitter systems. Acta Neurologica Scandinavica Supplementum 74:75–89.

Freud S 1953 The defense neuropsychoses (1894). In: Strachey J (ed) The standard edition of the complete psychological works of Sigmund Freud, vol 1. Hogarth Press, London.

Frey KP 1997 About reversal theory. In: Suebak S, Apter M (eds) Stress and Health: the reversal theory perspective. Taylor and Francis, London.

Fry WF Jr 1980 Humour and healing. University of California Press, San Francisco.

Futterman AD, Kemeny ME, Shapiro D et al 1992 Immunological variability associated with experimentally induced positive and negative states. Psychological Medicine 22:231–238.

Gaffan EA, Gaffan D, Harrison S 1988 Disconnection of the amygdala from visual association cortex impairs visual reward-association learning in monkeys. Journal of Neuroscience 8:(9):3144–3150.

Gorczynski RM 1990 Conditioned enhancement of skin allographs in mice. Brain, Behavior, and Immunity 4:85–92.

Greene WA 1954 Psychology factors and retiuloendothelial disease. Psychosomatic Medicine 16:220–230.

Gunderson JG, Autry JH, Mosher LR et al 1974 Special report: schizophrenia, 1973. Schizophrenia Bulletin 2:15–54.

Halgren E, LeDoux JE 1993 Emotional networks in the brain. In: Lewis M, Haviland J (eds) Handbook of emotion. Gilford Press, New York,

Hall M, Baum A, Buysse D et al 1998 Sleep as a mediator of the stress-immune relationship. Psychosomatic Medicine 60:48–51.

Halonen PE, Rimon R, Arochouka K 1974 Antibody levels to herpes simplex type 1 measles and rubella viruses in psychiatric patients. British Journal of Psychiatry 125:461–465.

Hebb DO 1947 The effects of early experience on problem solving at maturity. American Psychologist 2:306–307.

Hebb DO 1949 The organisation of behaviour. Wiley, New York.

Herberman R 1992 Tumor immunology. Journal of American Medicine Association 268:2935–2939.

Herbert TB, Cohen S 1993 Stress and immunity in humans: a meta-analytic review. Psychosomatic Medicine 55:364–379.

Hirschfeld RMA, Cross CK 1982 Epidemiology of affective disorders: psychosocial risk factors. Archives of General Psychiatry 39:35–46.

Ironson G, LaPerriere AA, Antoni M et al 1990 Changes in immune and psychological measures as a function of anticipation and reaction to news of HIV-1 antibody testing. Psychosomatic Medicine 52:247–270.

Irwin M, Daniels M, Smith TL et al 1987a Impaired natural killer cell activity during bereavement. Brain, Behavior, and Immunity 1:98–104.

Irwin M, Smith TL, Gillin JC 1987b Low natural killer cytotoxicity in major depression. Life Sciences 41:2127–2133.

Irwin M, Caldwell CL, Smith TL et al 1990 Major depressive disorder, alcoholism, reduced natural killer cell cytotoxicity. Archives of General Psychiatry 47:713–718.

Ishigami T 1919 The influence of psychic acts on the progress of pulmonary tuberculosis. American Review of Tuberculosis 2:470–484.

Izard CE 1972 Patterns of emotions—a new analysis of anxiety and depression. Academic Press, New York.

Johnstone EC, Whaley K 1975 Antinuclear antibodies in psychiatric illness: Their relationships to diagnosis and drug treatment. British Medical Journal 2:724–725.

Jones E 1963 Rationalization in everyday life. In: Papers on Psychoanalysis. Wood, New York.

Kagan J, Kearsley RB, Zelazo PR 1978 Infancy: its place in human development. Harvard University Press, Cambridge, MA.

Kemeny ME 1994 Stressful events, psychological responses and progression of HIV infection. In: Glaser R, Kieholt-Glaser JK (eds) Handbook of human stress and immunity. Academic Press, San Diego, CA, pp 245–266.

Kiecolt-Glaser JK, Garner W, Speicher C et al 1984a Psychological modifiers of immunocompetence in medical students. Psychosomatic Medicine 46:7–14.

Kiecolt-Glaser JK, Ricker D, George J et al 1984b Urinary cortisol levels, cellular immunocompetency and loneliness in psychiatric patients. Psychosomatic Medicine 46:15–23.

Kiecolt-Glaser JK, Kennedy S, Malkoff S et al 1988 Marital discord and immunity in males. Psychosomatic Medicine 50:213–229.

Kiecolt-Glaser JK, Glaser R 1991 Stress and immune function in humans. In: Ader R, Felten DL, Cohen N (eds) Psychoneuroimmunology, 2nd edn. Academic Press, San Diego, CA.

Kimzey SL, Johnson PC, Ritzman SE et al 1976 Hematology and immunology studies the second manned Skylab mission. Aviation, Space, and Environmental Medicine 47:383–390.

Kirch DG 1993 Infection and autoimmunity as etiological factors in schizophrenia: A review and reappraisal. Schizophrenia Bulletin 19:355–370.

Knapp PH, Levy EM, Giorgi RG et al 1992 Short term immunological effects of induced emotion. Psychosomatic Medicine 54:133–148.

Koh KB 1993 The relationship between stress and natural killer-cell activity in medical college students. Korean Journal of Psychosomatic Medicine 3:3–10.

Koh KB 1997 Exam stress enhances lymphocyte proliferation. 14th World Congress of Psychosomatic Medicine.

Koh KB 1998 Emotion and immunity. Journal of Psychosomatic Research 45:107–115.

Koh KB, Lee BK 1998 Reduced lymphocyte proliferation and interleukin-2 production in anxiety disorders. Psychosomatic Medicine 60:479–483.

Krueger RB, Levy EM, Cathcart ES 1984 Lymphocyte subsets in patients with major depression: preliminary findings. Advances 1:5–9.

Laudenslager ML, Ryan SM, Drugan RC et al 1983. Coping and immunosuppression: Inescapable but not escapable shock suppresses lymphocyte proliferation. Science 221:568–570.

Lazarus RS 1966 Psychological stress and the coping process. McGraw-Hill, New York.

LeDoux JE 1990 Information flow from sensation to emotion: Plasticity in the neural computation of stimulus value. In: Gabriel M, Moore J (eds) Learning and computational neuroscience. MIT Press, Cambridge, MA.

Lefcourt HM, Martin RA 1986 Humour and life stress: antidote to adversity. Springer-Verlag, New York.

Lefcourt HM, Thomas S 1998 Humour and stress revisited. In: Ruch W (ed) The sense of Humour: explorations of a personality characteristic. Mouton de Gruyter, Berlin.

Levy RM, Bredesen DE 1989 Controversies in HIV-related central nervous system disease: Neuropsychological aspects of HIV-1 infections. In: Volberding P, Jacobson M (eds) AIDS clinical review. Dekker, New York.

Linn BS, Linn MW, Jensen J 1981 Anxiety and immune responsiveness. Psychological Reports 49:969–970.

Lyons W 1992 An introduction to the philosophy of emotions. In: Strongman KT (ed) International review of studies on emotion, vol 2 . Wiley, Chichester.

Lysle DT, Cunnick JE, Fowler H et al 1988 Pavlovian conditioning of shock induced suppression of lymphocyte reactivity, acquisition, extinction, and pre-exposure effects. Life Science 42:2185.

McCall R, McGhee P 1977 The discrepancy hypothesis of attention and affect. In: Weizmann F, Uzgiris I (eds) The structure of experience. Plenum Press, New York.

Madden KS, Felton DL 1995 Experimental basis for neural-immune interactions. Physiological Reviews 75:77–106.

May R 1958 Contributions of existential psychotherapy. In: May R, Angel E, Ellenberger HF (eds) Existence: a new dimension in psychiatry and psychology. Basic Books, New York.

Mohl PC, Huang L, Bowden C et al 1987 Natural killer cell activity in major depression. American Journal of Psychiatry 144:1619.

Monjan AA, Collecter MI 1977 Stress induced modulation of the immune response. Science 196:307–308.

Murgatroyd S 1987 Reversal theory and psychotherapy: A review. Counseling Psychology Quarterly 3:371–381.

Naliboff B, Benton D, Solomon G et al 1991 Immunological changes in young and old adults during brief laboratory stress. Psychosomatic Medicine 53:121–132.

Olness K, Ader R 1992 Conditioning as an adjunct in the pharmacotherapy of lupus erythemotosis. Journal of Developmental and Behavioral Pediatrics 13:124–125.

Palmbald J, Cantell K, Strander H et al 1976 Stressor exposure and immunological response in man: Interferon – producing capacity and phagocytosis. Journal of Psychosomatic Research 20:193–199.

Palmbald J, Bjorn P, Wasserman J et al 1979 Lymphocyte and granulocyte reaction during sleep deprivation. Psychosomatic Medicine 41:273–278.

Persky VM, Kempthorne-Rawson J, Shekelle RB 1987 Personality and risk of cancer. 20 year follow up the Western Electric Study. Psychosomatic Medicine 49:435–449.

Plotnikoff N, Margo A, Faith R et al (eds) 1991 Stress and immunity. CRC Press, Boca Raton, FL.

Powers M, Dalgleish T 1997 Cognition and emotion, from order to disorder. Psychology Press, Hove, UK.

Pribam K, McGuinness D 1975 Arousal, activation and effort in control of attention. Psychological Review 82:116–149.

Rachman SJ, Hodgson RR 1980 Obsessions and compulsions. Prentice-Hall, Englewood Cliffs, NJ.

Robins E, Gassner J, Kayes J et al 1959 The communication of suicidal intent: A study of 134 successful (completed) suicides. American Journal of Psychiatry 1156:724–733.

Robinson RG, Kubos KL, Starr L 1984 Mood disorders in stroke patients: importance of location of lesion. Brain 107:81–93.

Rolls ET 1992 Neurophysiology and functions of the primate amygdala. In: Aggleton JP (ed) The amygdala: neurobiological aspects of emotion, memory and mental dysfunction. Wiley–Liss, New York.

Rothermundt M, Arolt V, Weitzsch C et al 1998 Immunological dysfunction in schizophrenia: a systematic approach. Neuropsychobiology 37:186–193.

Ryle G 1949 The concept of mind. University of Chicago Press.

Sackeim H, Greenberg MS, Weiman AL 1982 Hemispheric asymmetry in the expression of positive and negative emotions: neurologic evidence. Archives in Neurology 39:210–218.

Schedlowski M, Jacobs R, Alkre J et al 1993 Psychophysiological, neuroendocrine and cellular immune reactions under psychological stress. Neuropsychobiology 28:87–90.

Schleifer SJ, Keller SE, Camerino M et al 1983 Suppression of lymphocyte stimulation following bereavement. Journal of American Medical Association 250:374–377.

Schleifer SJ, Keller SE, Bond RN et al 1989 Major depressive disorder: role of age, sex, severity and hospitalization. Archives in General Psychiatry 46:81–87.

Schweitzer L 1982 Evidence of right cerebral hemisphere dysfunction in schizophrenic patients with left hemisphere overactivation. Biological Psychiatry 17:(6):655–673.

Selye H 1936 A syndrome produced by diverse, nocuous agents. Nature 138:132.

Seymour R 1993 Neuroendocrine-immune interactions. New England Journal of Medicine 329:1246–1253.

Shneidman ES, Farberow NL 1970 Attempted and completed suicide. In: Shneidman ES, Farberow NL, Litman RE (eds) The psychology of suicide. Science House, New York.

Shneidman ES, Mandelkorn P 1970 How to prevent suicide. In: Shneidman ES, Farberow NL, Litman RE (eds) The psychology of suicide. Science House, New York.

Shochet BR 1970 Recognizing the suicidal patient. Modern Medicine 38:114–117,123.

Skinner BF 1974 About behaviourism. Alfred Knopf, New York.

Stein M, Keller SE, Schleifer SI 1985 Stress and immunomodulation: The role of depression and neuroendocrine function. Journal of Immunology 135:827–833.

Stein M, Miller AH, Trestman RL 1991 Depression and the immune system. In: Ader R, Felten DL, Cohen N (eds) Psychoneuroimmunology, 2nd edn. Academic Press, San Diego, CA.

Stengel E 1964 Suicide and attempted suicide. Penguin, Baltimore, MD.

Surman OS, Williams J, Sheehan DV et al 1986 Immunological response to stress in agoraphobia and panic attacks. Biological Psychiatry 21:768–774.

Syvalahti E 1994 Biological factors in schizophrenia. Structural and functional aspects. British Journal of Psychiatry 164:9–14.

Verbrugge LM 1979 Marital status and health. Journal of Marriage and Family 41:267–285.

Watson JB, Raynor R 1920 Conditioned emotional reactions. Journal of Experimental Psychology 3:1–14.

Weiss DW, Hirt R, Tarcic N et al 1996 Studies in psychoneuro-immunology (PNI): psychological immunological and neuroendocrinological parameters in Israeli civilians during and after a period of SCUD missile attacks. Behavioral Medicine 22:5–14.

Weiss RS 1975 Marital separation. Basic Books, New York.

Weisse CS, Pato CN, McAllister CG et al 1990 Differential effects of controllable and uncontrollable acute stress on lymphocyte proliferation and leukocyte percentages in humans. Brain, Behavior, and Immunity 4:339–351.

Woodruff RA, Clayton PJ, Guze SB 1975 Is everyone depressed?. American Journal of Psychiatry 132:627–628.

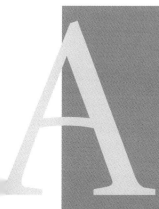

Clinical Case Answers

Case 16.1

16.1.1 Brain tumour, epilepsy, schizophrenia, head trauma, and delusions are caused by infection such as meningitis or encephalitis.

16.1.2 The diagnostic criteria must involve one of the major attributes and any of the secondary symptoms.

Major attributes include:

1. Association—the person shows evidence of a thought disorder by way of his/her use of language;
2. Affect—the person's emotional responses are blunted or inappropriate;
3. Ambivalence—the person is indecisive and unable to carry on normal goal-directed activities; and
4. Autism—the patient is withdrawn and self-absorbed.

The secondary symptoms of schizophrenia may include:

1. Hallucinations;
2. Paranoid thinking;
3. Grandiosity;
4. Hostility and belligerence;
5. Delusions; and
6. Genetic link, which is now well established.

Case 16.2

16.2.1 Major depression and bipolar depression. This woman is probably suffering from bipolar depression, which includes both manic and depressive episodes. Usually, bipolar disorders will appear in the manic phase followed by a normal period then a depressed phase, although many different patterns have been identified.

16.2.2 Several studies have demonstrated increased prevalence of depressed mood in patients who have suffered damage to the left frontal region of the brain compared to patients with lesions on the right. In addition, it was noted that the more anterior the location of the lesion, the more likely the patient would experience depression. In order for depression to manifest clinically more than just an injury to the left cortex is necessary. The person must also be exposed to the right set of environmental stimuli for the depression to be initiated. In a patient with left anterior cortical damage, depressive symptomatology would be expected only if that patient were exposed to the requisite environmental stresses. Left anterior damage is not in itself sufficient for the production of depressive symptomatology. We would therefore not expect all patients with left frontal damage to show depressive symptomatology. Only those exposed to an appropriate set of environmental stresses would be expected to show the hypothesized final state. Quantitative EEG studies have also proven to be effective in measuring changes in cortical activity associated with depression. Increases in left frontal alpha power are consistent with decreased activation of this area of the brain, along with frontal hypocoherence or decreased synchrony between the hemispheres.

Case 16.3

16.3.1

1.   *People who threaten to kill themselves will not carry it out; only the silent types will actually do it.* This is quite untrue. About 70% of those who threaten suicide actually attempt it. In other words when someone threatens to kill themselves it must be taken seriously.

2.   *People who attempt suicide and fail were not serious about it in the first place.* This statement is also untrue. The statistics tell us 75% of all successful suicides have made a previous attempt. As much as 12% of those who experienced a failed attempt will make a second successful attempt within 3 months.

3.   *People suffering from depression should not be questioned about suicidal thoughts.* Many people have held the view that depressed people should not be questioned about suicidal thoughts in the fear that this questioning will put the idea into their head, or it will reinforce it if it is already there. It is now believed that questioning these people directly can help them overcome their feelings and at the very least offer information to direct a therapeutic direction.

4.   *When a person commits suicide often family and friends are astonished.* This statement is often true. Friends and family will often make statements such as 'He was in such good spirits'; 'She had so much to live for.' This highlights the fact that friends and relatives are often oblivious to the clues that most people contemplating suicide give out before they kill themselves.

16.3.2

In this case all of the risk factors are important. These include:

*   Sudden secretive behaviour;
*   Direct verbal statements;
*   Withdrawal into a contemplative state;
*   Reduced food intake;
*   Giving away their valuable possessions;
*   Implications in speech that will not be seeing you again;
*   Rapid tranquillity in a previously agitated person; and
*   Most associated with events like births, deaths, family gatherings.

It may be that about 75% of all those who attempt suicide do not actually want to die. They are using the attempt as a cry for help.

16.3.3

In this case the woman needs to be watched closely. The husband needs to be informed of the possibility that his wife may attempt to harm herself. Counselling should be arranged for this woman. Attempts should be continued to correct any cortical asymmetric activation that may be present.

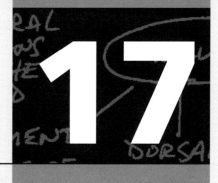
Functional Neurological Approaches to Treatment

Clinical Cases for Thought

Case 17.1   A 42-year-old woman presents with medication-resistant depression of 2 years duration. Following your physical examination you conclude that she has a left cortical decrease in activation (hemisphericity).

Question 17.1.1   Outline an approach to therapy that would address her left cortical hemisphericity.

Case 17.2   A 14-year-old boy presents with vertigo. He describes that he feels as though he is constantly spinning to the right. Following your physical exam you determine that he probably has a decreased activation of his left cerebellum.

Question 17.2.1   Outline an approach to therapy that would address his left cerebellar dysfunction.

Introduction

It is important for the clinician to understand the nervous system. It must be remembered, however, that each individual's nervous system is different based on the stimulation that it has been exposed to over the duration of the individual's lifetime. Anatomical pathways may differ from those physiologically or clinically expected. This is a key concept of functional neurology; we as clinicians are concerned with function. Where a dysfunction occurs its cause may be physiological or pathological or both and may occur at any point of the pathway from receptor to cortex. Often because of these individual factors the course of a treatment application cannot be predicted until a trial therapy and observation of the patient's response has been performed. There are a large variety of treatment modalities available today for the functional stimulation of various neural circuits. I have included manipulation as a major technique because of its widespread availability and relative safety of the application. Many other stimulus techniques have been listed in a chart fashion for ease of locating the techniques during the course of a busy clinic day.

General Concepts in Treatment Application

The general approach to different treatment applications in functional neurology can be summarized by the following three steps.

1. *Education*—The patient should be taught about their condition, the expected time course of treatment, and any side effects that they may also expect.

2. *Graded application of therapy*—All treatment modalities should be applied in a graded fashion, proceeding from low intensity to an intensity that produces the desired therapeutic effect.

3. *Monitor the affect of the treatment on the neuraxis*—Monitoring of each therapy should be conducted as soon as possible following the therapy and then at appropriate intervals such as hourly, daily, or weekly, depending on the intensity of the therapy. Monitoring the affect of the intervention can be accomplished by monitoring the changes in time to activation, and fatigue in a neural circuit before and after the intervention.

The *time to activation* (TTA) of a neuron is a measure of the time from which the neuron receives a stimulus to the time that an activation response can be detected. Obviously, in clinical practice the response of individual neurons cannot be measured but the response of neuron systems such as the pupil response to light can be. As a rule, the time to activation will be less in situations where the neuron system has maintained a high level of integration and activity, and greater in situations where the neuron has not maintained a high level of integration and activity or is in the late stages of transneural degeneration. Again an exception to this rule can occur in situations where the neuron system is in the early stages of transneural degeneration and is irritable to stimulus and responds quickly. This response will be of short duration and cannot be maintained for more than a short period of time.

The *time to fatigue* (TTF) in a neuron is the length of time that a response can be maintained during a continuous stimulus to the neuron. The TTF effectively measures the ability of the neuron to sustain activation under continuous stimuli, which is a good indicator of the adenosine triphosphate (ATP) and protein stores contained in the neuron. This in turn is a good indication of the state of health of the neuron. The TTF will be longer in neurons that have maintained high levels of integration and stimulus and shorter in neurons that have not maintained a high state of integration. TTF can be very useful in determining whether a fast *time to response* (TTR) is due to a highly integrated neuron system or a neuron system that is in the early stages of transneural degeneration.

For example, in clinical practice the response of one pupil to light can be compared to the other pupil's response. If both pupils respond very quickly to light stimulus (fast TTR), and they both maintain pupil contraction for 3–4 seconds (long TTF) this is a good indication that both neuronal circuits are in a good state of health. If, however, both pupils respond quickly (fast TTR) but the right pupil immediately dilates despite the continued presence of the light stimulus (short TTF), this may be an indication that the right neuronal system involved in pupil constriction may be in an early state of transneural degeneration and more detailed examination is necessary.

Treatment should be composed of a three-pronged approach:

1. Modulation of the central integrative state (CIS) of a system, to maximize function of the viable neurons within the dysfunctional system, to promote regeneration and decrease iatrogenic loss of neurons, and to stimulate a repair process in any injured neurons;

2. Assist oxygen delivery to the system; and

3. Ensure that adequate fuel and other physiologically necessary substrates are delivered to the system.

In some instances when the CIS of a system is so poor that any stimulus will cause injury, it may be necessary to avoid direct excitatory activation of the system. In these instances it may require the promotion of inhibition of the neuronal pool by excitation of an antagonist pool of neurons.

Treatment Approaches

Manipulation

Afferent Modulation of the Neuraxis via Manipulation of Spinal Joints

Vertebral joint manipulation has been reported to have an effect on numerous signs and symptoms related to central nervous system function including visual dysfunction (Carrick 1997; Stephens et al 1999), reaction time (Kelly et al 2000), central motor excitability, dizziness, tinnitus or hearing impairment, migraine, sleep bruxism (Knutson 2001), bipolar and sleep disorders, and cervical dystonia. There have also been reports that spinal joint manipulation may assist in the improvement of otitis media and asthma in addition to other non-musculoskeletal complaints. Ample evidence exists to suggest that noxious stimulation of spinal tissues can lead to autonomically mediated reflex responses, which may explain how spinal joint manipulation can relieve some of these non-musculoskeletal complaints.

Several studies have investigated the effect of changes in spinal afferentiation as a result of manipulation on the activity of the sympathetic nervous system (Korr 1979; Sato 1992; Chiu & Wright 1996). Suprasegmental changes, especially in brain function, have demonstrated the central influence of altered afferentiation of segmental spinal levels (Thomas & Wood 1992; Carrick 1997; Kelly et al 2000). Immune system function may be mediated through spinal afferent mechanisms that may operate via suprasegmental or segmental levels by modulating the activity of the sympathetic nervous system (Beck 2003).

Based on the above it is likely that spinal joint manipulation may influence the CIS of various neuronal pools through changes in afferent inputs from joint and muscle receptors. A few studies have reported that upper cervical spinal joint manipulations have asymmetrical affects on measures of central nervous system function (Carrick 1997). This may account, in part, for reduction of symptoms in migraine sufferers following spinal manipulation as asymmetry in blood flow to the head is thought to be a key feature in migraine and other headache types (Drummond et al 1984; Drummond, 1988, 1993).

Spinal afferents may also influence output from the locus coeruleus, which influences cortical and subcortical neuronal activity, including trigeminal and vestibular thresholds as shown in animal research. Locus coeruleus has widespread projections to all levels of the neuraxis, including the hypothalamus and to other monoaminergic nuclei.

A number of potential pathways exist that may explain why spinal manipulations have the potential to excite the rostral ventrolateral medulla (RVLM) and therefore result in modulatory affects on the neuraxis (Holt et al 2006). The pathways and mechanisms most likely involved include the following:

1. Cervical manipulations excite spinoreticular pathways or collaterals of dorsal column and spinocerebellar pathways. Spinoreticular fibres originate at all levels of the cord but particularly in the upper cervical segments. They synapse on many areas of the pontomedullary reticular formation (PMRF).

2. Cervical manipulations cause modulation of vestibulosympathetic pathways. This may involve the same pathways as above or could reflect modulation of vestibular neurons at the level of the vestibular nuclei.

3. Cervical manipulations cause vestibulocerebellar activation of the nucleus tractus solitarius (NTS), dorsal motor nucleus of vagus, and nucleus ambiguous.

4. Manipulations may result in brain hemisphere influences causing descending excitation of the PMRF, which will exert tonic inhibitory control of the intermediolateral (IML) cell column.

5. Lumbosacral manipulations may result in sympathetic modulation due to direct innervation of the RVLM via dorsal column nuclei or spinoreticular fibres that ascend within the ventrolateral funiculus of the cord.

6. Spinal manipulation may alter the expression of segmental somato-sympathetic reflexes by reducing small-diameter afferent input and enhancing large-diameter afferent input. This may influence sympathetic innervation of primary and secondary organs of the immune system.

7. Spinal manipulations may alter the expression of suprasegmental somato-sympathetic reflexes by reducing afferent inputs on second-order ascending

spinoreticular neurons. This may influence sympathetic innervation of immune system organs at a more global level.

8. Spinal manipulations may alter central integration of brainstem centres involved in descending modulation of somato-sympathetic reflexes. This may occur via spinoreticular projections or interactions between somatic and vestibular inputs in the reticular formation. Both somatic (high-threshold) and vestibular inputs have been shown to increase output from the RVLM, which provides tonic excitatory influences on the IML cell column of the spinal cord. Proprioceptive (low-threshold) inputs from the cervical spine have been shown to have an antagonistic effect on vestibular inputs to the RVLM. Neurons in the brainstem reticular formation also mediate tonic descending inhibition of segmental somato-sympathetic reflexes. Segmental somato-sympathetic reflexes appear to be most influential in the absence of descending inhibitory influences from the brainstem.

9. Spinal manipulations may alter central integration in the hypothalamus via spinoreticular and spinohypothalamic projections and the influence of spinal afferents on vestibular and midline cerebellar function. Direct connections have been found to exist between vestibular and cerebellar nuclei and the hypothalamus, nucleus tractus solitarius, and parabrachial nuclei. The latter two nuclei project to the hypothalamus, in addition to visceral and limbic areas of the medial temporal and insular regions of the cortex.

10. Spinal manipulations may influence brain asymmetry by enhancing summation of multi-modal neurons in the CNS, monoaminergic neurons in the brainstem or basal forebrain regions, or cerebral blood flow via autonomic influences, or by influencing the hypothalamic-mediated isoprenoid pathway.

A Variety of Manipulations Can Be Performed to Stimulate Afferent Systems
Many excellent textbooks and video programs exclusively describing how to perform manipulations of virtually every joint of the body have been written (Carrick 1991, 1994). I will simply provide an overview of some of the more common manipulations that I have found clinically effective.

1 POSITIONING THE PATIENT FOR LUMBAR AND PELVIC MANIPULATIONS

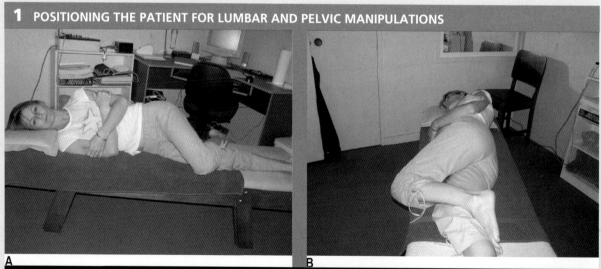

Fig. 17.1 Positioning the patient for lumbar and pelvic manipulations.(A) The patient lies comfortably on their side with the superior leg slightly bent at the knee and hip. The patient's arms are crossed loosely over their chest. (B) The patient should be stable and balanced while in this position and should not feel like they are going to roll off the table.

The standard position for position for lumbar and pelvic manipulations is referred to as the lateral recumbent position. The patient is lying comfortably on their side with the superior leg slightly bent at the knee and hip (Fig. 17.1A). The patient's arms are crossed loosely over their chest. The patient should be stable and balanced while in this position and should not feel like they are going to roll off the table (Fig. 17.1B).

2 **LUMBAR MAMMILLARY PUSH MANIPULATION**

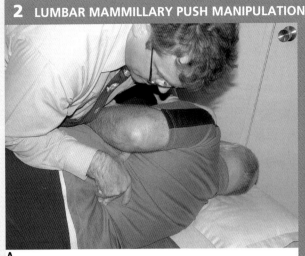 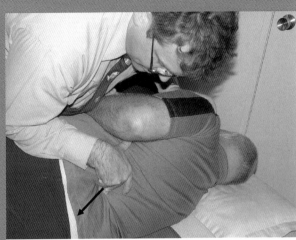

A B

Fig. 17.2 Lumbar mammillary push manipulation. (A) Roll the patient towards you and contact mammillary process of the lumbar vertebra in question with the tips of the second and third fingers reinforcing each other. Place the elbow of the thrust hand on the patient's hip for added support. (B) Thrust line of drive for a mammillary push lumbar manipulation.

Indication

This manipulation can be used to address any lumbar segment from L1 to L5 that has shifted posterior, or is not moving into rotation. This manipulation can also be used to stimulate the ipsilateral cerebellum or contralateral cortex in relation to the contact.

Contact

The contact hand is semi-flexed into an 'L' shape with the fingers reinforcing each other. The tips of the second and third fingers on the hand contacting the mammillary process vertebra of choice is the most efficient contact for this manipulation (Fig. 17.2A).

Patient Position

The patient should be comfortably lying on their side, with the involved side up; their arms should be crossed over their chest. The manipulating neurologist then rolls the patient towards them and establishes a contact with the mammillary process of the vertebra in question. When the manipulating neurologist has established his/her contact, the patient is further rolled towards the manipulator to remove any tissue slack. The patient is then asked to relax and take a deep breath in and out and allow their body to relax.

Adjuster's Position

The manipulating neurologist should be positioned standing but in a crouching position to the side of the patient; the contact arm is bent with the elbow contacting the patient's hip for added support and control. The non-contact hand maintains a gentle supporting pressure on the patient's shoulder. The contact hand maintains a gentle pressure on the contact (see Fig. 17.2B). The manipulating neurologist then centres his/her sternal area over the contact and pushes against the patient's shoulder and the patient's hip in opposing directions until mild pressure is established.

Thrust

The thrust is a body drop impulse along the facet joint line of the lumbar vertebra in question, usually about 45° inferior to superior and anterior to posterior, in such a way that the thrust on the lumbar vertebra causes the vertebra to rotate away from the contact (Fig 17.2B).

Clinical Comments

This manipulation must be performed with the patient relaxed. The support hand does not thrust or twist the body but simply stabilizes. The manipulating neurologist must concentrate the line of drive of the thrust through the contact. The contact is more focused and the adjustment easier to perform if a space is maintained between the manipulator's wrist and the patient. Asking the patient to exhale just before thrusting can also be helpful.

3 SACROILIAC MANIPULATION

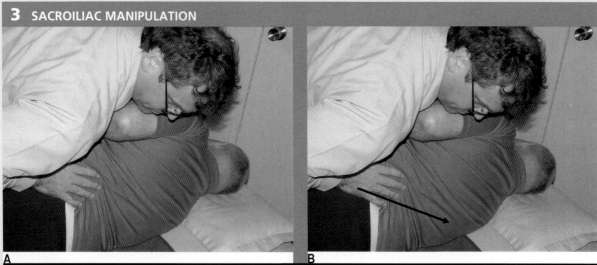

Fig. 17.3 Sacroiliac manipulation. (A) From a lateral recumbent position, roll the patient towards you and contact the sacral arch above the second sacral tubercle for ipsilateral joint manipulation and below the second sacral tubercle for contralateral joint manipulation. (B) Thrust line of drive for a sacroiliac ipsilateral 'upside' manipulation.

Indication

This manipulation can be used to address a sacroiliac joint that is not moving through its complete range of motion. This manipulation can also be used to stimulate the ipsilateral cerebellum or contralateral cortex in relation to the contact.

Contact

The pisiform of the contact hand establishes a contact on the sacral angle above the second sacral tubercle to manipulate the ipsilateral or 'upside' sacroiliac joint. A contact on the sacral arch below the second sacral tubercle can be used to manipulate the sacroiliac joint on the contralateral or 'down side' (Fig. 17.3A).

Patient Position

The patient should be comfortably lying on their side with their superior leg bent at the knee and hip to form a 45° angle, with their arms crossed over their chest. The manipulating neurologist then rolls the patient towards them and establishes a contact with the angle of the sacrum. When the manipulating neurologist has established his/her contact the patient is asked to relax and take a deep breath in and out and allow their body to relax.

Adjuster's Position

The manipulating neurologist should be positioned standing but in a crouching position to the side of the patient. The manipulating neurologist contacts the angle of the sacrum with the hand closest to the patient and stabilizes the patient's superior shoulder with the other hand. Maintain a gentle pressure on the contact so that the patient is locked against the neurologist and the table (see Fig. 17.3A). The manipulating neurologist then centres his/her sternal area over the contact, making sure that his/her shoulder is held as tightly to his/her body as possible.

Thrust

The thrust is a body drop impulse along the joint line of the sacroiliac joint, usually about 45° inferior to superior and posterior to anterior (Fig 17.3B).

Clinical Comments

This manipulation must be performed with the patient relaxed. The support hand does not thrust or twist the body but simply stabilizes. The manipulating neurologist must concentrate the line of drive of the thrust through the contact. Asking the patient to exhale just before thrusting can also be helpful. The two most common mistakes made when performing this adjustment are:

1. The line of drive of the thrust is aligned too much in the posterior to anterior plane, the thrust should be inferior to superior as well; and

2. The elbow of the contact arm is allowed to move away from the body of the neurologist (winging). This position puts a great amount of strain on the shoulder and results in shoulder problems down the line.

4 ILIUM FLEXION PUSH MANIPULATION

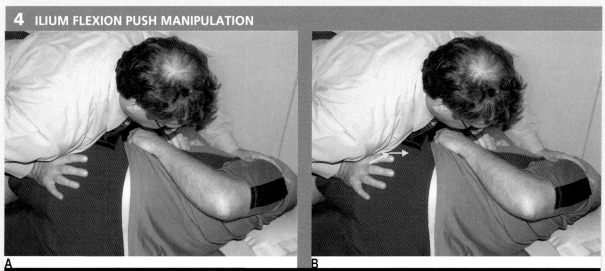

Fig. 17.4 Ilium flexion manipulation. (A) Roll the patient towards you and contact the ischium of the ilium in question with the heel of the contact hand. (B) Thrust line of drive for a left flexion ilium manipulation.

Indication

This manipulation can be used to address an ilium that has shifted into extension, or is not moving into flexion. This manipulation can also be used to stimulate the ipsilateral cerebellum or contralateral cortex in relation to the contact.

Contact

The ischium of the ilium is cupped into the contact hand with the heel of the hand establishing a firm contact (Fig. 17.4A).

Patient Position

The patient should be comfortably lying on their side, with the involved side up; their arms should be crossed over their chest. The superior leg is slightly flexed. The manipulating neurologist then rolls the patient towards them and establishes a contact with the ischium of the ilium in question. When the manipulating neurologist has established his/her contact, the patient is further rolled towards the manipulator to remove any tissue slack. The patient is then asked to relax and take a deep breath in and out and allow their body to relax.

Adjuster's Position

The manipulating neurologist should be positioned standing but in a crouching position slightly to the rear and side of the patient. The contact arm is bent so that the shoulder is firmly behind the contact. The non-contact hand maintains a gentle supporting pressure on the patient's shoulder. The contact hand maintains a gentle pressure on the contact (see Fig. 17.4B). The manipulating neurologist then centres his/her sternal area behind the contact and pushes against the patient's ischium until a mild pressure is established.

Thrust

The thrust is a body drop impulse with a scoop-like motion along the facet joint line of the ilium in question, in such a way that the thrust on the ilium causes the ilium into flexion (Fig. 17.4B).

Clinical Comments

This manipulation must be performed with the patient relaxed. The support hand does not thrust or twist the body but simply stabilizes. The manipulating neurologist must concentrate the line of drive of the thrust through the contact. The contact is more focused and the adjustment easier to perform if the manipulator positions their shoulder immediately behind the contact for maximum thrust power. Compared with other manipulations, this manipulation requires considerable power to accomplish properly. Asking the patient to exhale just before thrusting can also be helpful.

5 ANTERIOR COCCYX MANIPULATION

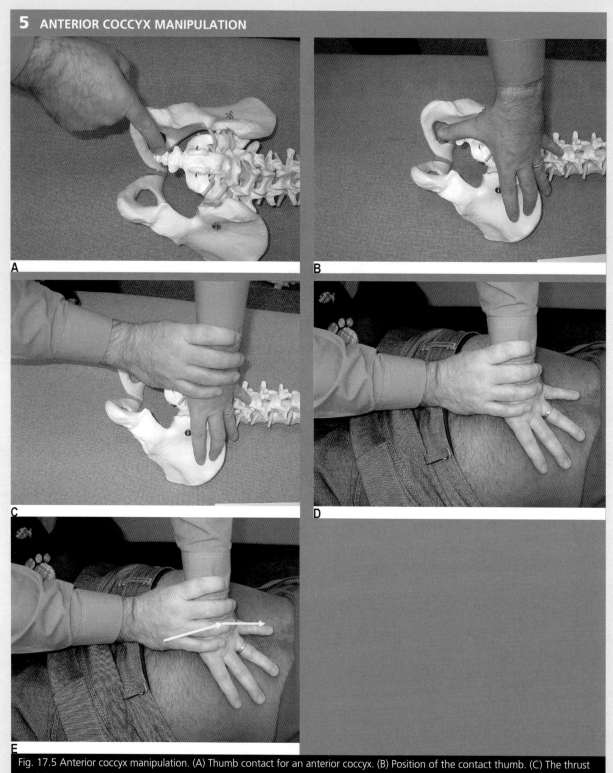

Fig. 17.5 Anterior coccyx manipulation. (A) Thumb contact for an anterior coccyx. (B) Position of the contact thumb. (C) The thrust hand contacts the thumb knuckle with the pisiform. (D) Position of the adjuster for an anterior coccyx. Note the thrust arm is directed upwards. (E) The thrust for an anterior coccyx. The pink thick arrow shows the resultant line of drive.

Indication

This adjustment can be used to address a coccyx that has shifted anterior, or is not moving into extension. This adjustment will most probably result in a stimulation of parasympathetic output from the coccygeal plexus.

Contact

A pisiform contact with the thrust hand contacting the knuckle of the thumb, which is in firm contact with the posterior inferior coccyx, is the most efficient contact for this adjustment (Figs 17.5A–C).

5 ANTERIOR COCCYX MANIPULATION continued

Patient Position

The patient should be comfortably prone with their arms at their sides. When the adjuster has established his/her contact, the patient is then asked to relax and take a deep breath in and out.

Adjuster's Position

The adjuster should be behind and centred to the patient with a gentle pressure on the contact (see Fig. 17.5D).

Thrust

The thrust is an impulse tangential to the coccyx in such a way that the pull on the thumb causes the coccyx to move posteriorly.

Clinical Comments

This adjustment must be performed skin on skin as we are relying on the skin tension to actually pull the coccyx anterior. This adjustment may cause the patient (and the adjuster) nervous embarrassment because of the location of the contact. It is advisable to have an assistant in the room when this adjustment is performed and also to make sure the patient understands how and why you are performing this adjustment prior to commencing the setup. This adjustment is often necessary after childbirth or following a fall on the buttocks.

6 BILATERAL THENAR THORACIC MANIPULATION

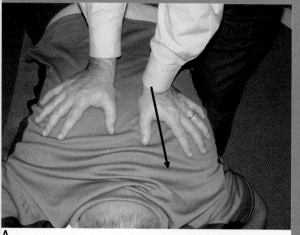 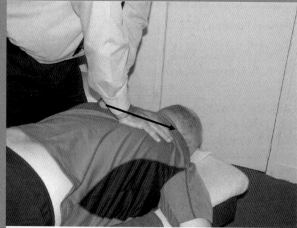

Fig. 17.6 Bilateral thenar thoracic manipulation. (A) From a position on the ipsilateral side of the involved segment, contact the transverse process of the thoracic vertebra in question with the pisiform of your contact hand. The non-contact hand contacts the contralateral transverse process to assist in stabilization. (B) The thrust is inferior to superior and posterior to anterior along a line of drive following the facet lines of the thoracic vertebra in question with the contact hand (black arrow). The non-contact hand supports the contralateral transverse processes for stability.

Indication

This manipulation can be used to address a thoracic vertebra that is fixed posteriorly or not moving into rotation. This manipulation can also be used to stimulate the ipsilateral cerebellum and contralateral cortex in relation to the contact.

Contact

The manipulating neurologist contacts the transverse process of the thoracic vertebra in question with the pisiform of their contact hand. The non-contact hand contacts the contralateral transverse process to aid in stabilization (Fig. 17.6A).

Patient Position

The patient should be comfortably prone, with their arms at their sides. The patient is then asked to relax and take a deep breath in and out and allow their body to relax.

Adjuster's Position

The manipulating neurologist should be positioned standing to the side the patient, with their contact hand contacting the transverse process of the thoracic vertebra in question (Fig. 17.6A).

Thrust

The thrust is inferior to superior and posterior to anterior along a line of drive following the facet lines of the thoracic vertebra in question with the contact hand. The non-contact hand supports the contralateral transverse process for stability (Figs. 17.6A and 17.6B).

Clinical Comments

This manipulation must be performed with the patient relaxed. The manipulating neurologist must concentrate the line of drive of the thrust through the contact. Asking the patient to exhale just before thrusting can also be helpful.

7 **ANTERIOR THORACIC MANIPULATION**

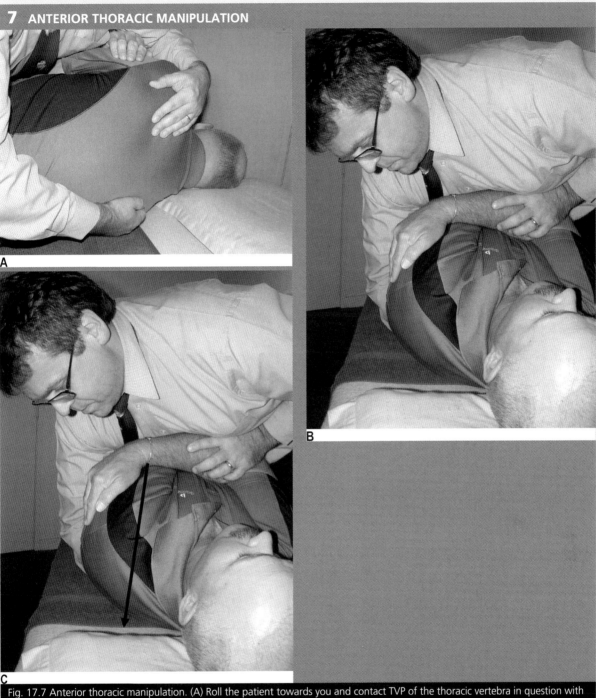

Fig. 17.7 Anterior thoracic manipulation. (A) Roll the patient towards you and contact TVP of the thoracic vertebra in question with the thenar aspect of the thumb with your hand maintained in a fist for the anterior thoracic manipulation. (B) Thrust line of drive for an anterior thoracic manipulation. (C) Line of drive for the anterior thoracic manipulation. The force of the thrust is focused over the contact and comes from a body drop impulse of the body of the manipulating neurologist.

Indication

This manipulation can be used to address any thoracic segment from T2 to T12 that has shifted posterior, or is not moving into rotation. This manipulation can also be used to stimulate the ipsilateral cerebellum or contralateral cortex in relation to the contact.

Contact

The contact hand is formed into a fist, and a contact established along the thenar eminence of the thumb on the hand contacting the transverse process (TVP) of the thoracic vertebra of choice is the most efficient contact for this manipulation (Fig. 17.7A).

7 ANTERIOR THORACIC MANIPULATION continued

Patient Position

The patient should be comfortably lying on their back with their arms crossed over their chest. The manipulating neurologist then rolls the patient towards them and establishes a contact with the TVP of the vertebra in question. When the manipulating neurologist has established his/her contact the patient is then rolled back onto their back and asked to relax and take a deep breath in and out and allow their body to relax.

Adjuster's Position

The manipulating neurologist should be positioned standing but in a crouching position to the side of the patient, with their arm encircling the patient to maintain a gentle pressure on the contact (see Fig. 17.7B). The manipulating neurologist then centres his/her sternal area over the contact and lowers their body onto the patient's chest until mild pressure is established.

Thrust

The thrust is a body drop impulse along the facet joint line of the thoracic vertebra in question, usually about 45° inferior to superior and anterior to posterior above T6 and 45° superior to inferior and anterior to posterior below T6, in such a way that the thrust on the thoracic vertebra causes the vertebra to rotate away from the contact (Fig. 17.7C).

Clinical Comments

This manipulation must be performed with the patient relaxed. The support hand does not thrust or twist the body but simply stabilizes. The manipulating neurologist must concentrate the line of drive of the thrust through the contact. Asking the patient to exhale just before thrusting can also be helpful.

8 CROSSED BILATERAL THORACIC MANIPULATION

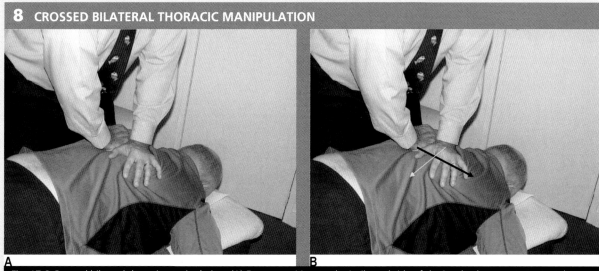

Fig. 17.8 Crossed bilateral thoracic manipulation. (A) From a position on the ipsilateral side of the involved segment, contact the transverse process of the thoracic vertebra in question with the pisiform of your contact hand. The non-contact hand contacts the contralateral transverse process to assist in the torque component of this manipulation. (B) The thrust is inferior to superior and posterior to anterior along a line of drive following the facet lines of the thoracic vertebra in question with the contact hand (black arrow). The non-contact hand thrusts in the opposite direction, producing a torque around the joint (green arrow).

Indication

This manipulation can be used to address a thoracic vertebra that is fixed posteriorly or not moving into rotation. This manipulation can also be used to stimulate the ipsilateral cerebellum and contralateral cortex in relation to the contact.

Contact

The manipulating neurologist contacts the transverse process of the thoracic vertebra in question with the pisiform of their contact hand. The non-contact hand contacts the contralateral transverse process to aid in the delivery of the torque component of this manipulation (Fig. 17.8A).

Patient Position

The patient should be comfortably prone, with their arms at their sides. The patient is then asked to relax and take a deep breath in and out and allow their body to relax.

Adjuster's Position

The manipulating neurologist should be positioned standing to the side of the patient, with their contact hand contacting the transverse process of the thoracic vertebra in question (Fig 17.8A).

Thrust

The thrust is inferior to superior and posterior to anterior along a line of drive following the facet lines of the thoracic vertebra in question with the contact hand. The non-contact hand thrusts in the opposite direction, producing a torque around the joint (Fig. 17.8B).

Clinical Comments

This manipulation must be performed with the patient relaxed. The manipulating neurologist must concentrate the line of drive of the thrust through the contact. The torque component of the manipulation allows for a greater speed of delivery and thus makes the manipulation easier to perform. Asking the patient to exhale just before thrusting can also be helpful.

9 STANDING THORACIC LONG-AXIS MANIPULATION

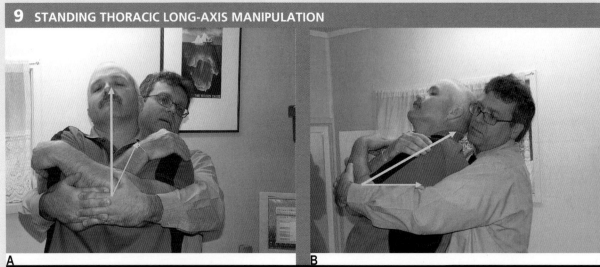

Fig. 17.9 Standing thoracic long-axis manipulation. (A) From behind the patient contact their thoracic spine area with your sternum. Pull the patient tightly against you by contacting both elbows with a reinforced palmer grip to establish a firm contact. (B) The position of both the patient and the manipulating neurologist for the performance of the standing thoracic long-axis manipulation.

Indication

This manipulation can be used to address generalized thoracic and rib fixations. This manipulation can also be used for bilateral stimulation of the cerebellum and cortex.

Contact

The manipulating neurologist contacts the patient's thoracic spine area with their sternum (Fig. 17.9A).

Patient Position

The patient should be comfortably standing, facing away from the manipulator; their arms should be crossed over their chest. The patient is asked to lie back onto the manipulating neurologist, who grasps the patient's elbows with their palms in a reinforced cupped contact. The patient is then asked to relax and take a deep breath in and out and allow their body to relax.

Adjuster's Position

The manipulating neurologist should be positioned standing behind the patient, with their arms around the patient and grasping the patient's elbows (see Fig. 17.9B). The manipulating neurologist then centres his/her sternal area behind the contact. With a mild pull on the patient's elbows and a push against the patient's back, a mild pressure is established to remove any slack between the patient and the manipulator.

Thrust

The thrust is an impulse generated by a quick contraction of the biceps. The line of drive should be inferior to superior and anterior to posterior in nature (Figs 17.9A and 17.9B).

Clinical Comments

This manipulation must be performed with the patient relaxed. The manipulating neurologist must concentrate the line of drive of the thrust through the contact. Compared with other manipulations, this manipulation requires considerable power to accomplish properly. Asking the patient to exhale just before thrusting can also be helpful.

10 SITTING ATLAS LATERAL FLEXION MANIPULATION

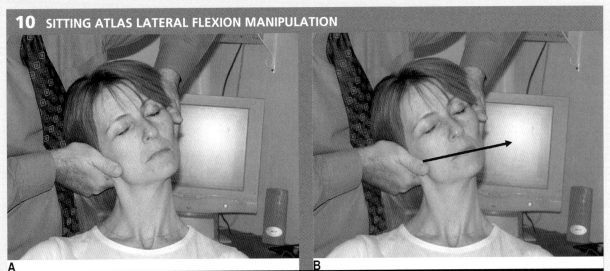

Fig. 17.10 Sitting atlas lateral flexion manipulation. (A) Contact the most lateral portion of the posterior arch of the atlas. The head is slightly laterally flexed to the side of contact. The stabilizing hand cups the contralateral ear and stabilizes the head. (B) Thrust line of drive for a sitting atlas lateral flexion manipulation.

Indication

This manipulation can be used to address the atlas (C1) that has shifted laterally, or is not moving into lateral flexion. This manipulation can also be used to stimulate the ipsilateral cerebellum or contralateral cortex in relation to the contact.

Contact

A contact along the medial aspect of the thumb of the thrust hand contacting the most lateral edge of the posterior arch of the atlas is the most efficient contact for this manipulation (Fig. 17.10A).

Patient Position

The patient should be sitting comfortably with their arms at their sides. When the manipulating neurologist has established his/her contact the patient is then asked to relax and take a deep breath in and out and allow their head to slowly be laterally flexed. Extension of the neck should be avoided.

Adjuster's Position

The manipulating neurologist should be positioned standing behind and slightly to the side of the patient. The patient's head should be at the level of the manipulator's mid-sternal area. The non-contact hand should be gently cupping the contralateral ear and supporting the head; the contact thumb should apply a gentle pressure on the contact (see Fig. 17.10A). The head is laterally flexed to the side of contact until a firm end feel is established. Extension of the neck should be avoided.

Thrust

The thrust is an impulse along the facet joint lines of the atlas in a lateral plane (Fig. 17.10B).

Clinical Comments

This manipulation must be performed with the patient relaxed. This adjustment usually produces two audible clicks in quick succession like snapping the fingers of both hands. The support hand does not thrust or twist the head but simply stabilizes the neck and head. It is important that the manipulating neurologist does not approach or contact the patient's eye with the thumb of the support hand.

11 SITTING 'CERVICAL PULL' MANIPULATION

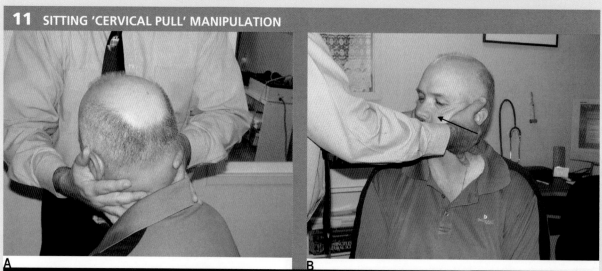

Fig. 17.11 Sitting cervical pull manipulation. (A) Contact posterior arch of the cervical vertebra in question with the palmer aspect of the third finger for the sitting cervical pull manipulation. (B) Thrust line of drive for a sitting cervical pull manipulation.

Indication

This manipulation can be used to address any cervical segment from C2 to C7 that has shifted posterior, or is not moving into rotation. This manipulation can also be used to stimulate the ipsilateral cerebellum or contralateral cortex in relation to the contact.

Contact

A contact along the palmer aspect of the third finger of the thrust hand contacting the posterior arch of the cervical vertebra of choice is the most efficient contact for this manipulation (Fig. 17.11A).

Patient Position

The patient should be comfortably sitting with their arms at their sides. When the manipulating neurologist has established his/her contact the patient is then asked to relax and take a deep breath in and out and allow their head to slowly be turned into a rotated and laterally flexed position.

Adjuster's Position

The manipulating neurologist should be positioned to the side opposite the contact, with a gentle pressure on the contact (see Fig. 17.11A). The head can be laterally flexed either to the side of contact or away from the contact. When laterally flexing away from the contact the manipulation takes advantage of the normal coupled motion of the cervical vertebral motion units and produces a greater stimulus.

Thrust

The thrust is an impulse along the facet joint line of the cervical vertebra in question, usually about 45° inferior to superior and posterior to anterior in such a way that the pull on the cervical vertebra causes the vertebra to rotate towards the manipulating neurologist (Fig. 17.11B).

Clinical Comments

This manipulation must be performed with the patient relaxed. The support hand does not thrust or twist the head but simply stabilizes the neck and head.

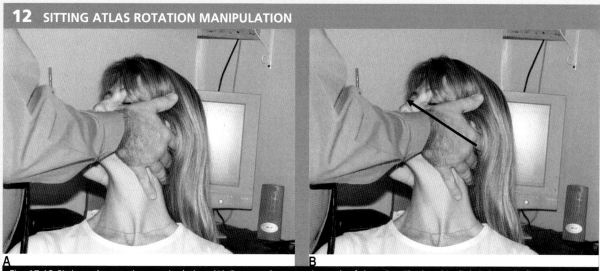

12 SITTING ATLAS ROTATION MANIPULATION

Fig. 17.12 Sitting atlas rotation manipulation. (A) Contact the posterior arch of the atlas. The head is slightly laterally flexed to the side of contact. The stabilizing hand cups the contralateral ear and stabilizes the head. (B) Thrust line of drive for a sitting atlas lateral flexion manipulation.

Indication

This manipulation can be used to address the atlas (C1) that has shifted posteriorly, or is not moving into rotation. This manipulation can also be used to stimulate the ipsilateral cerebellum or contralateral cortex in relation to the contact.

Contact

A contact along the medial aspect of the first finger of the thrust hand contacting the posterior arch of the atlas is the most efficient contact for this manipulation (Fig. 17.12A).

Patient Position

The patient should be sitting comfortably with their arms at their sides. When the manipulating neurologist has established his/her contact the patient is then asked to relax and take a deep breath in and out and allow their head to slowly be laterally flexed. Extension of the neck should be avoided.

Adjuster's Position

The manipulating neurologist should be positioned standing in front and slightly to the side of the patient. The patient's head should be at the level of the manipulator's mid-sternal area. The non-contact hand should be gently cupping the contralateral ear and supporting the head; the contact thumb should apply a gentle pressure on the contact (see Fig. 17.12A). The head is laterally flexed to the side of contact until a firm end feel is established. Extension of the neck should be avoided.

Thrust

The thrust is an impulse along the facet joint lines of the atlas in an inferior to superior plane (Fig. 17.12B).

Clinical Comments

This manipulation must be performed with the patient relaxed. The support hand does not thrust or twist the head but simply stabilizes the neck and head. It is important that the manipulating neurologist does not approach or contact the patient's eye with the thumb of the support hand.

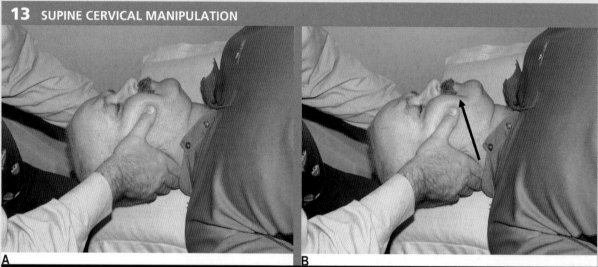

13 SUPINE CERVICAL MANIPULATION

Fig. 17.13 Supine cervical manipulation. (A) Contact posterior arch of the cervical vertebra in question with the palmer aspect of the first finger for the supine cervical manipulation. (B) Thrust line of drive for a supine cervical manipulation.

Indication

This manipulation can be used to address any cervical segment from C2 to C7 that has shifted posterior, or is not moving into rotation. This manipulation can also be used to stimulate the ipsilateral cerebellum or contralateral cortex in relation to the contact.

Contact

A contact along the palmer aspect of the first finger of the thrust hand contacting the posterior arch of the cervical vertebra of choice is the most efficient contact for this manipulation (Fig. 17.13A).

Patient Position

The patient should be comfortably lying on their back with their arms at their sides. When the manipulating neurologist has established his/her contact the patient is then asked to relax and take a deep breath in and out and allow their head to slowly be turned into a rotated and laterally flexed position.

Adjuster's Position

The manipulating neurologist should be positioned standing but in a crouching position to the head of the patient, with a gentle pressure on the contact (see Fig. 17.13A). The head can be laterally flexed to the side of contact until a firm end feel is established.

Thrust

The thrust is an impulse along the facet joint line of the cervical vertebra in question, usually about 45° inferior to superior and posterior to anterior in such a way that the thrust on the cervical vertebra causes the vertebra to rotate into the direction of thrust (Fig. 17.13B).

Clinical Comments

This manipulation must be performed with the patient relaxed. The support hand does not thrust or twist the head but simply stabilizes the neck and head. It is important that the manipulating neurologist does not approach or contact the patient's eye with their thumb.

14 SUPINE ATLAS ROTATION MANIPULATION

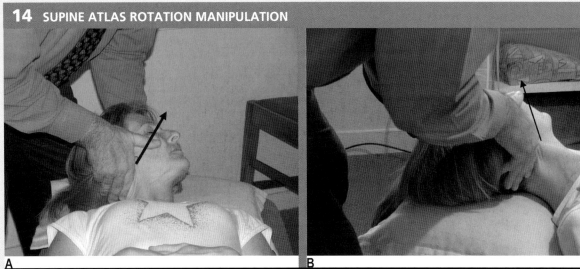

Fig. 17.14 Supine atlas rotation manipulation. (A) Contact posterior arch of the atlas. The second and third fingers reinforce the first finger contact. (B) Thrust line of drive for a supine atlas rotation manipulation.

Indication

This manipulation can be used to address the atlas (C1) that has shifted posterior, or is not moving into rotation. This manipulation can also be used to stimulate the ipsilateral cerebellum or contralateral cortex in relation to the contact.

Contact

A contact along the lateral aspect of the first finger of the thrust hand contacting the posterior arch of the atlas is the most efficient contact for this manipulation (Fig. 17.14A).

Patient Position

The patient should be comfortably lying on their back with their arms at their sides. When the manipulating neurologist has established his/her contact the patient is then asked to relax and take a deep breath in and out and allow their head to slowly be turned into a rotated and laterally flexed position.

Adjuster's Position

The manipulating neurologist should be positioned standing but in a crouching position to the head of the patient, with a gentle pressure on the contact (see Fig. 17.14A). The head can be laterally flexed to the side of contact and rotated away from the contact until a firm end feel is established.

Thrust

The thrust is an impulse along the facet joint lines of the atlas, usually about 45° inferior to superior and posterior to anterior in such a way that the thrust on the atlas causes the vertebra to rotate into the direction of thrust (Figs 17.14A and 17.14B).

Clinical Comments

This manipulation must be performed with the patient relaxed. The support hand does not thrust or twist the head but simply stabilizes the neck and head. It is important that the manipulating neurologist does not approach or contact the patient's eye with their thumb.

15 SUPINE ATLAS LATERAL FLEXION MANIPULATION

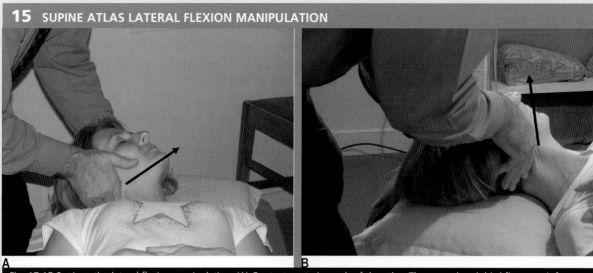

Fig. 17.15 Supine atlas lateral flexion manipulation. (A) Contact posterior arch of the atlas. The second and third fingers reinforce the first finger contact. The head is first rotated then laterally flexed. (B) Thrust line of drive for a supine atlas rotation manipulation.

Indication

This manipulation can be used to address the atlas (C1) that has shifted laterally, or is not moving into lateral flexion. This manipulation can also be used to stimulate the ipsilateral cerebellum or contralateral cortex in relation to the contact.

Contact

A contact along the lateral aspect of the first finger of the thrust hand contacting the posterior arch of the atlas is the most efficient contact for this manipulation (Fig. 17.15A).

Patient Position

The patient should be comfortably lying on their back with their arms at their sides. When the manipulating neurologist has established his/her contact the patient is then asked to relax and take a deep breath in and out and allow their head to slowly be turned into a rotated and laterally flexed position. Extension of the neck should be avoided.

Adjuster's Position

The manipulating neurologist should be positioned standing but in a crouching position to the head of the patient, with a gentle pressure on the contact (see Fig. 17.15A). The head can first be rotated away from the contact and then laterally flexed to the side of contact until a firm end feel is established. Extension of the neck should be avoided.

Thrust

The thrust is an impulse along the facet joint lines of the atlas in a lateral plane (Figs 17.15A and 17.15B).

Clinical Comments

This manipulation must be performed with the patient relaxed. This adjustment usually produces two audible clicks in quick succession like snapping the fingers of both hands. The support hand does not thrust or twist the head but simply stabilizes the neck and head. It is important that the manipulating neurologist does not approach or contact the patient's eye with their thumb.

16 SUPINE OCCIPUT MANIPULATION

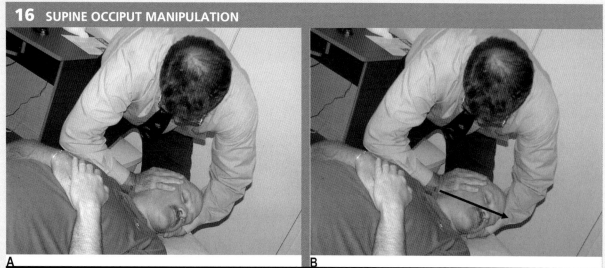

Fig. 17.16 Supine occiput manipulation. (A) From above the patient roll their head into full rotation, cup their head in your non-contact hand, and contact their superior occipital area with the pisiform of your contact hand. (B) The position of both the patient and the manipulating neurologist for the performance of the supine occiput manipulation. The thrust is inferior to superior and posterior to anterior along a line of drive following a path from the patient's occiput through the patient's nose.

Indication

This manipulation can be used to address an occiput that is fixed in flexion (posterior) or not moving into extension. This manipulation can also be used to stimulate the ipsilateral cerebellum and contralateral cortex in relation to the contact.

Contact

The manipulating neurologist contacts the patient's occiput in question with the pisiform of the contact hand (Fig. 17.16A).

Patient Position

The patient should be comfortably supine, with their arms crossed over their chest. Roll the patient's head into full rotation with the involved occiput superior. The patient is then asked to relax and take a deep breath in and out and allow their body to relax.

Adjuster's Position

The manipulating neurologist should be positioned standing above and to the side the patient,

Thrust

The thrust is an impulse along a line of drive that follows a path from the patient's occiput to their nose. The line of drive should be inferior to superior and posterior to anterior in nature (Fig. 17.16B).

Clinical Comments

This manipulation must be performed with the patient relaxed. The manipulating neurologist must concentrate the line of drive of the thrust through the contact. Asking the patient to exhale just before thrusting can also be helpful. This is a very powerful manipulation and patients should be advised to remain lying quietly for a few moments before attempting to sit up following the adjustment.

17 COMBINATION CERVICAL/THORACIC MANIPULATION

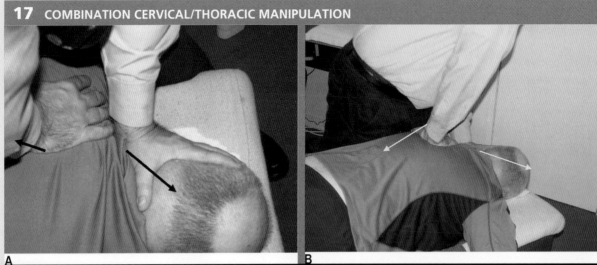

Fig. 17.17 Combination cervical/thoracic manipulation. (A) From a position on the ipsilateral side of the involved segment, cup the patient's ipsilateral occiput in your non-contact hand and contact the transverse process of the thoracic vertebra with the pisiform of your contact hand. (B) The position of both the patient and the manipulating neurologist for the performance of the combination cervical/thoracic manipulation. The thrust is superior to inferior and posterior to anterior along a line of drive following the facet lines of the thoracic vertebra in question.

Indication

This manipulation can be used to address a thoracic vertebra that is fixed in posterior or not moving into rotation. This manipulation can also be used to stimulate the ipsilateral cerebellum and contralateral cortex in relation to the contact.

Contact

The manipulating neurologist contacts the patient's ipsilateral occiput with the palm of the non-contact hand. A pisiform contact is established on the transverse process of the thoracic vertebra in question (Fig. 17.17A).

Patient Position

The patient should be comfortably prone, with their arms at their sides. Roll the patient's head into rotation with the palm of your non-contact hand pushing slightly superiorly and laterally to medially on their occiput. The patient is then asked to relax and take a deep breath in and out and allow their body to relax.

Adjuster's Position

The manipulating neurologist should be positioned standing above and to the side the patient, with their superior hand cupping the patient's occiput and the inferior hand contacting the thoracic vertebra in question (Figs 17.17A and 17.17B).

Thrust

The thrust is a body drop impulse down the contact arm along a line of drive that follows the facet joints of the thoracic vertebra in question. The line of drive should be superior to inferior and posterior to anterior in nature. The non-contact hand applies steady superior and lateral to medial pressure to stabilize the head during the thrust (Figs 17.17A and 17.17B).

Clinical Comments

This manipulation must be performed with the patient relaxed. The manipulating neurologist must concentrate the line of drive of the thrust through the contact. If the manipulator maintains a fairly straight arm when the thrust is given the full body drop component of the manipulation can be utilized, making the manipulation much easier to perform. Asking the patient to exhale just before thrusting can also be helpful.

18 ANALYSIS OF THE TEMPORAL MANDIBULAR JOINT

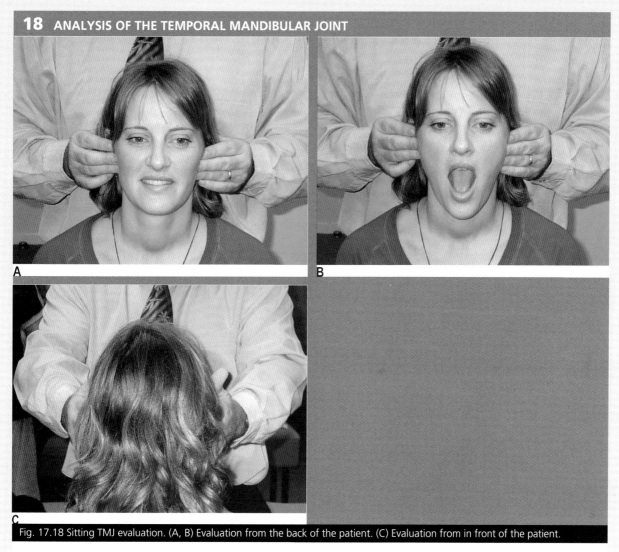

Fig. 17.18 Sitting TMJ evaluation. (A, B) Evaluation from the back of the patient. (C) Evaluation from in front of the patient.

Analysis Technique

Palpation of the temporal mandibular joint (TMJ) bilaterally can give you a very good idea of how the joint is functioning. The fingers should contact the area of the TMJ in order to appreciate both the rotational and translational components of TMJ function. The patient is then asked to open and close their mouth slowly and repeatedly to allow the adjuster the opportunity to evaluate the motion of the TMJ. The translational and rotational components of the TMJ are compared bilaterally for delays or aberrant function including swinging of the mandible to the left or right. The technique can be performed from the back (Figs 17.18A and 17.18B) or from the front (Fig. 17.18C) of the patient.

19 TEMPORAL MANDIBULAR JOINT SITTING TRANSLATION ADJUSTMENT

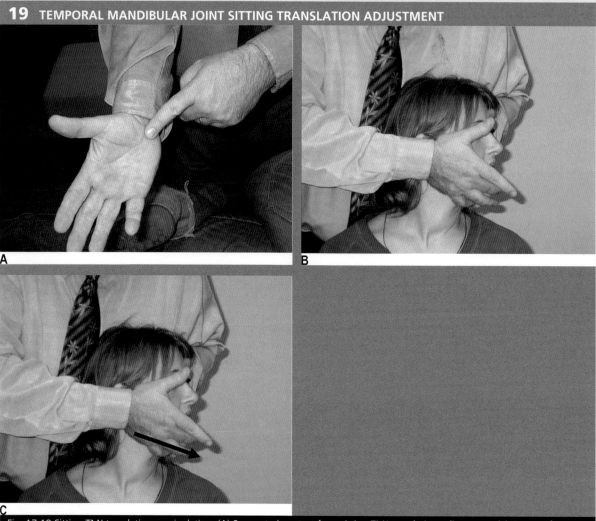

Fig. 17.19 Sitting TMJ translation manipulation. (A) Suggested contact for a sitting TMJ translation adjustment. (B) Contact for a sitting TMJ translation adjustment. (C) Adjuster's position for a sitting TMJ translation adjustment. Note the sternal notch posterior to the contact point.

Indication

This adjustment can be used to address a TMJ that is not translating during opening motion.

Contact

A pisiform contact over the TMJ in question is the most efficient contact for this adjustment. The fifth finger and lateral aspect of the hand should rest lightly on the mandible with the fingers pointing down the jaw line. Skin slack should be taken from superior to inferior and lateral to medial. The contact should be firm but not causing the patient discomfort (Figs 17.19A and 17.19B).

Patient Position

The patient should be sitting comfortably in front of the adjuster, with their head turned to bring the involved TMJ away from the adjuster.

Adjuster's Position

The adjuster should be standing with feet slightly more than shoulder-width apart, knees slightly bent, facing the patient on a 75–80° angle from the patient's head,

on the same side as the contact (Fig. 17.19B). The sternal notch should be posterior to the contact.

Thrust

The thrust is an impulse along the line of the mandible (Fig. 17.19C). The non-thrust hand stabilizes the head and neck to avoid over rotation.

Clinical Comments

TMJ adjusting can be very anxiety provoking for patients and chiropractors alike. This results in ridged stiff hands that cause the patient to 'tighten up'. Taking a moment to remind yourself to relax your hands is very useful. You must also be very watchful not to stick your thumb into the patient's eye as you concentrate on performance of the adjustment. Students are often concerned about the amount of thrust to use when performing a TMJ adjustment. This can be overcome by starting with a light thrust and progressing over two or three thrusts, allowing the force to increase slightly each time until you have developed a feel for the amount of thrust to utilize.

20 TEMPORAL MANDIBULAR JOINT SITTING ROTATIONAL ADJUSTMENT

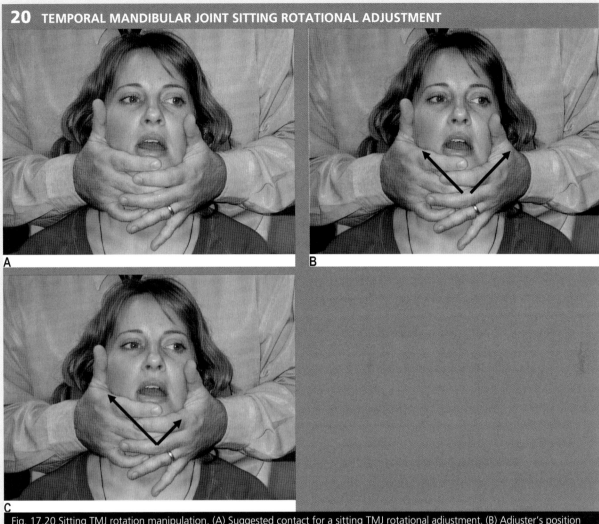

Fig. 17.20 Sitting TMJ rotation manipulation. (A) Suggested contact for a sitting TMJ rotational adjustment. (B) Adjuster's position for a sitting TMJ rotational adjustment. The line of drive in this case is bilateral and equal. Note the sternal notch posterior to the contact point. (C) In this illustration the thrust is dominant to the patient's right TMJ.

Indication

This adjustment can be used to address a TMJ that is not rotating during opening motion.

Contact

A double-handed interlocked finger contact cupping the mandible is the most efficient contact for this adjustment. The palmer aspect of the hand should rest lightly on the mandible with the fingers pointing down the jaw line. Skin slack should be taken from superior to inferior and lateral to medial. The contact should be firm but not causing the patient discomfort (Fig. 17.20A).

Patient Position

The patient should be sitting comfortably in front of the adjuster, with their eyes looking straight ahead. The patient is then asked to open and close their mouth slowly and repeatedly.

Adjuster's Position

The adjuster should be standing with feet slightly more than shoulder-width apart, directly behind the patient (Fig. 17.20A). The sternal notch should be posterior to the contact.

Thrust

The thrust is an impulse along the line of the mandible just as the TMJ begins the rotational component of movement. The thrust can be bilateral and equal or emphasis directed on one side by altering the amount of thrust on each side (Figs 17.20B and 17.20C).

Clinical Comments

TMJ adjusting can be very anxiety provoking for patients and chiropractors alike. This results in ridged stiff hands that cause the patient to 'tighten up'. Taking a moment to remind yourself to relax your hands is very useful. You must also be very watchful not to stick your thumb into the patient's eye as you concentrate on performance of the adjustment. Students are often concerned about the amount of thrust to use when performing a TMJ adjustment. This can be overcome by starting with a light thrust and progressing over two or three thrusts, allowing the force to increase slightly each time until you have developed a feel for the amount of thrust to utilize.

The patient should be reminded to pull their tongue back into their mouth to avoid trapping it between their teeth when the thrust occurs.

21 TEMPORAL MANDIBULAR JOINT SUPINE TRANSLATION ADJUSTMENT

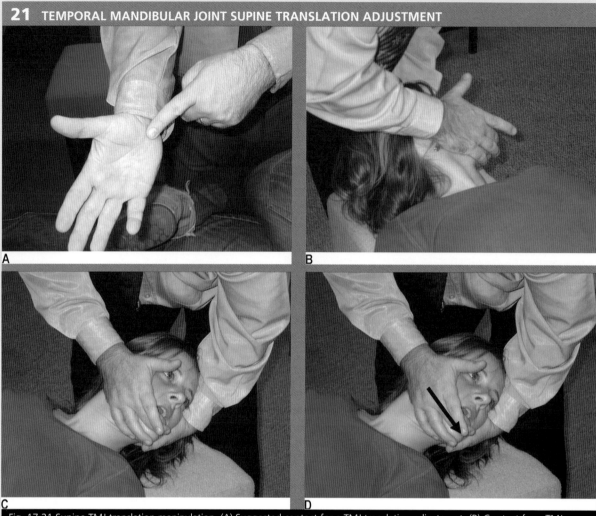

Fig. 17.21 Supine TMJ translation manipulation. (A) Suggested contact for a TMJ translation adjustment. (B) Contact for a TMJ translation adjustment. (C) Adjuster's position for a supine TMJ translation adjustment. Note the sternal notch over the contact point. (D) Line of drive for a supine TMJ translation adjustment. The final resultant is represented by the arrow.

Indication

This adjustment can be used to address a TMJ that is not translating during opening motion.

Contact

A pisiform contact over the TMJ in question is the most efficient contact for this adjustment. The fifth finger and lateral aspect of the hand should rest lightly on the mandible with the fingers pointing down the jaw line. Skin slack should be taken from superior to inferior and lateral to medial. The contact should be firm but not causing the patient discomfort (Figs 17.21A and 17.21B).

Patient Position

The patient should be lying comfortably in the supine position, with their head turned to bring the involved TMJ facing up.

Adjuster's Position

The adjuster should be standing with feet slightly more than shoulder-width apart, knees slightly bent, facing the patient on a 75–80° angle from the patient's head,

on the same side as the contact (Fig. 17.21C). The sternal notch should be over or posterior to the contact.

Thrust

The thrust is an impulse along the line of the mandible (Fig. 17.21D).

Clinical Comments

TMJ adjusting can be very anxiety provoking for patients and chiropractors alike. This results in ridged stiff hands that cause the patient to 'tighten up'. Taking a moment to remind yourself to relax your hands is very useful. You must also be very watchful not to stick your thumb into the patient's eye as you concentrate on performance of the adjustment. Students are often concerned about the amount of thrust to use when performing a TMJ adjustment. This can be overcome by starting with a light thrust and progressing over two or three thrusts, allowing the force to increase slightly each time until you have developed a feel for the amount of thrust to utilize.

22 STERNAL-CLAVICULAR INFERIOR GLIDE ADJUSTMENT

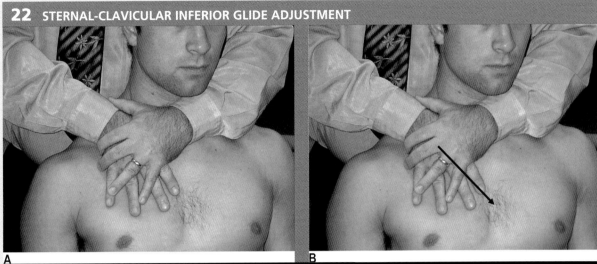

Fig. 17.22 Sternal-clavicular inferior glide manipulation. (A) Pisiform contact for a sternal-clavicular joint fixated in inferior glide motion. (B) Contact, line of drive, and positioning for a sternal-clavicular inferior glide adjustment.

Indication

This adjustment can be used to address a sternal-clavicular joint fixated in downward glide on motion palpation.

Contact

A pisiform contact with the thrust hand contacting the head of the sternum, the non-adjusting hand reinforces the thrusting hand to maintain downward pressure during the thrust so the contact does not slip (Fig. 17.22A).

Patient Position

The patient should be comfortably seated with their arms at their sides. When the adjuster has established his/her contact the patient is then asked to relax and take a deep breath in and out.

Adjuster's Position

The adjuster should be behind and centred to the patient with a gentle pressure on the contact (see Fig. 17.22B).

Thrust

The thrust is an impulse downwards along the joint line.

23 STERNAL-CLAVICULAR SUPERIOR GLIDE ADJUSTMENT

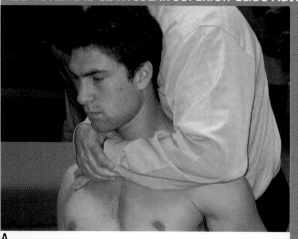 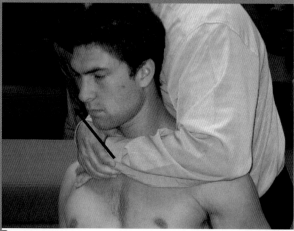

Fig. 17.23 Sternal-clavicular superior glide manipulation. (A) Pisiform contact for a sternal-clavicular joint fixated in superior glide motion. (B) Contact, line of drive, and positioning for a sternal-clavicular superior glide adjustment.

Indication

This adjustment can be used to address a sternal-clavicular joint fixated in superior glide on motion palpation.

Contact

A pisiform contact with the thrust hand contacting the head of the clavicle, the non-adjusting hand re-enforces the thrusting hand to maintain downward pressure during the thrust so the contact does not slip (Fig. 17.23A).

Patient Position

The patient should be comfortably seated with their arms at their sides. When the adjuster has established his/her contact the patient is then asked to relax and take a deep breath in and out.

Adjuster's Position

The adjuster should be behind and centred to the patient with a gentle pressure on the contact (see Fig. 17.23B).

Thrust

The thrust is an impulse upwards along the joint line.

24 SITTING POSTERIOR CAPSULE SHOULDER ADJUSTMENT

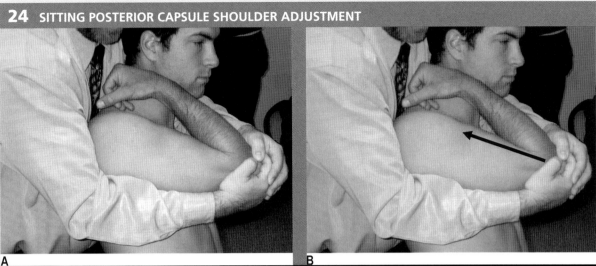

Fig. 17.24 Sitting posterior capsule shoulder manipulation. (A) Suggested contact for a sitting posterior capsule adhesion. (B) The thrust is an impulse along the line of the humerus.

Indication

This adjustment can be used to address a glenohumeral that has posterior joint capsule adhesions or is not moving in posterior glide.

Contact

A double-handed interlocked finger contact cupping the elbow is the most efficient contact for this adjustment. The palmer aspect of the hand should rest lightly on the elbow with the fingers interlocked or overlapped for strength. Skin slack should be taken from inferior to superior and anterior to posterior. The contact should be firm but not causing the patient discomfort (Fig. 17.24A).

Patient Position

The patient should be sitting comfortably in front of the adjuster, with their eyes looking straight ahead.

Adjuster's Position

The adjuster should be standing with feet slightly more than shoulder-width apart, directly behind the patient (Fig. 17.24A). The sternal notch should be posterior to the contact.

Thrust

The humerus is elevated to about 90°. The thrust is an impulse along the line of the humerus (Fig. 17.24B).

Clinical Comments

Shoulder adjusting can be very anxiety provoking for patients and chiropractors alike due to the discomfort often felt by the patient when in the preloaded position. The patient can be comforted by informing them that in most cases the pain will subside in a few minutes following the adjustment.

25 SITTING SUPERIOR CAPSULE AND A/C JOINT ADJUSTMENT

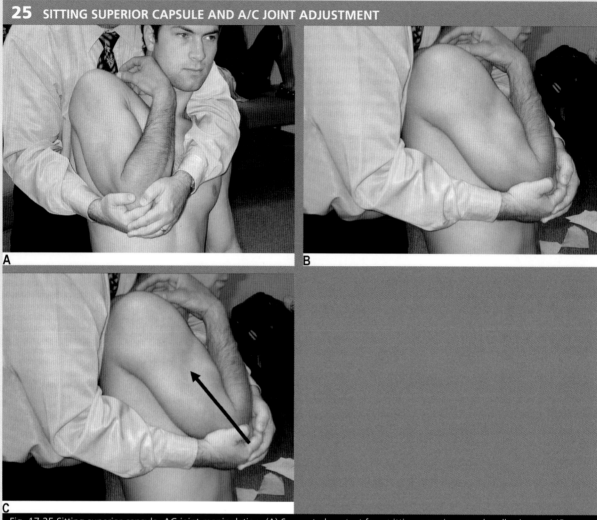

Fig. 17.25 Sitting superior capsule, AC joint manipulation. (A) Suggested contact for a sitting superior capsule adhesion or A/C adjustment. (B, C) Adjuster's position for a sitting superior capsule or A/C joint adjustment. The line of drive in this case is straight up the humerus. Note the sternal notch posterior to the contact point.

Indication

This adjustment can be used to address a glenohumeral or A/C joint that has superior joint capsule adhesions or an A/C joint not moving in superior glide.

Contact

A double-handed interlocked finger contact cupping the elbow is the most efficient contact for this adjustment. The palmer aspect of the hand should rest lightly on the elbow with the fingers interlocked or overlapped for strength. Skin slack should be taken from inferior to superior. The contact should be firm but not causing the patient discomfort (Fig. 17.25A).

Patient Position

The patient should be sitting comfortably in front of the adjuster, with their eyes looking straight ahead.

Adjuster's Position

The adjuster should be standing with feet slightly more than shoulder-width apart, directly behind the patient

(Fig. 17.25A). The sternal notch should be posterior to the contact.

Thrust

The thrust is an impulse along the line of the humerus.

Clinical Comments

Shoulder adjusting can be very anxiety provoking for patients and chiropractors alike due to the discomfort often felt by the patient when in the preloaded position. The patient can be comforted by informing them that in most cases the pain will subside in a few minutes following the adjustment.

26 SITTING FIRST RIB ADJUSTMENT

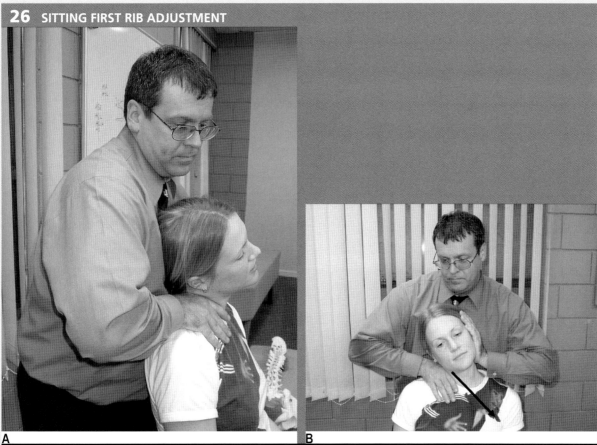

Fig. 17.26 Sitting first rib manipulation. (A) Contact for a right first rib not moving inferiorly. (B) Patient and adjuster position as well as line of drive indicated by the arrow.

Indication

This adjustment can be used to address a first rib that is not moving inferiorly in motion palpation or fixed superior on static palpation.

Contact

The first rib is contacted with the first metacarpal phalangeal joint of the thrusting hand. The support hand cups the contralateral occiput to the contact and applies a steady rostral and lateral to medial force that causes the patient's head to laterally flex towards and rotate away from the contact (see Fig. 17.26A).

Patient Position

The patient should be sitting comfortably facing away from the adjuster with their arms hanging to their sides. When the adjuster has established his/her contact the patient is then asked to relax and let him/herself fall into the adjuster for support.

Adjuster's Position

The adjuster should be behind the patient with the contact centred to his/her body slightly below the sternal notch so the thrust hand is almost parallel with the floor.

Thrust

The thrust is an impulse to the first rib directed through the joint line. The support hand maintains the initial pressure on the head throughout the adjustment but does not counter-thrust.

Clinical Comments

A first rib adjustment may be quite uncomfortable for the patient especially if the attempt is not successful. No more than two attempts should be made during any one visit.

27 POSTERIOR RIB HEAD ADJUSTMENT (ANTERIOR POSITIONING)

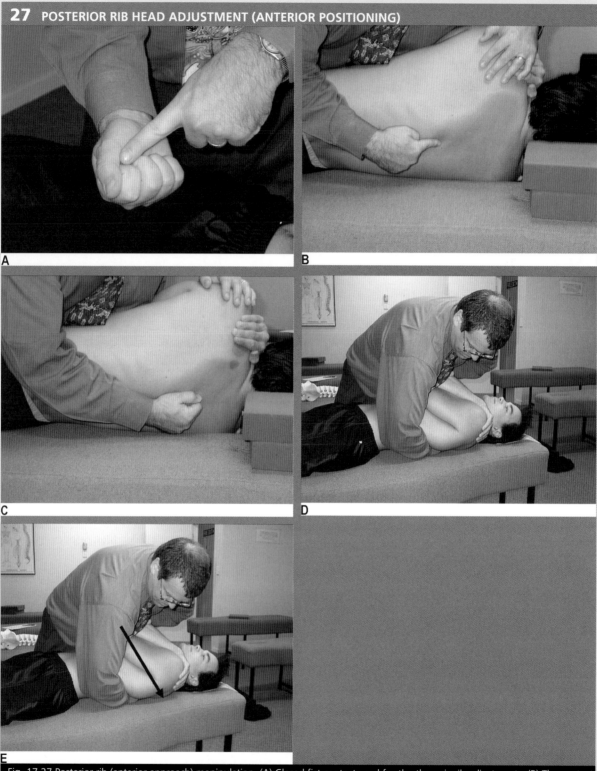

Fig. 17.27 Posterior rib (anterior approach) manipulation. (A) Closed fist contact used for the thoracic rib adjustments. (B) The contact location is identified and the patient is rolled so the contact can be established on the involved rib head. (C) Contact is made for an anterior rib adjustment. (D) The patient is lowered down to the supine position with the contact on the rib head. (E) The arrow indicates the final resultant vector of the thrust.

27 POSTERIOR RIB HEAD ADJUSTMENT (ANTERIOR POSITIONING) continued

Indication

This adjustment addresses a rib head that is not moving into bucket handle or that is fixed posterior on static palpation.

Contact

A closed fist contact with fingers facing upwards is probably the best contact for this adjustment, although many variations of hand configuration may also be used (Fig. 17.27A). The contact is made on the head of the involved rib. The adjuster wraps his/her arm around the patient to contact the rib head in question (Fig. 17.27B).

Patient Position

The patient should be comfortably lying supine with their arms folded across their chest and their legs slightly bent.

Adjuster's Position

The adjuster should be in a fencer stance with the pelvis facing in a forward position. This will allow the body drop thrust to be transmitted along the proper resultant vector with maximum efficiency. The sternal notch (the functional centre of gravity) should be positioned over or posterior to the contact on the spine. The adjuster takes the contact as described above and as illustrated in Figs 17.27C and 17.27D below.

Thrust

The thrust is a body drop with impulse directed through the contact hand in such a manner as to cause the contacted rib head to move anterior and superior (Fig. 17.27E).

Clinical Comments

The most common mistake made when attempting this adjustment is to body drop straight down on your patient and not align your force through the appropriate vector. You may also ask the patient to breath in and out, applying your thrust as the patient breathes out.

28 SITTING RADIAL HEAD ADJUSTMENT

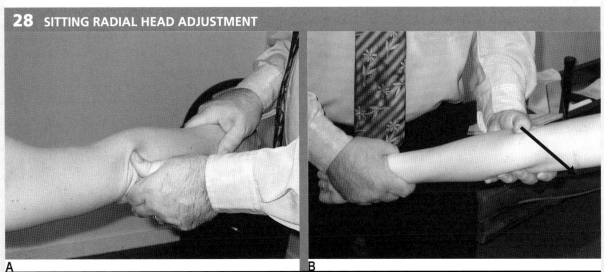

Fig. 17.28 Sitting radial head manipulation. (A) Suggested contact for a sitting radial head joint adjustment. (B) Thrust for a radial head mobilization.

Indication

This adjustment can be used to address a radial head joint that is not moving in internal rotation or is subluxated posteriorly.

Contact

A single-handed thumb contact on the radial head in question just below the joint line is the most efficient contact for this adjustment. Skin slack should be taken into the direction of thrust. The contact should be firm but not causing the patient discomfort (Fig. 17.28A).

Patient Position

The patient should be sitting comfortably in front of the adjuster, with their arm outstretched.

Adjuster's Position

The adjuster should be standing with feet slightly more than shoulder-width apart, beside the patient (Fig. 17.28A).

Thrust

The thrust is an impulse that is initiated just as the elbow comes into full extension (Fig. 17.28B).

29 SITTING CARPAL JOINT ADJUSTMENT

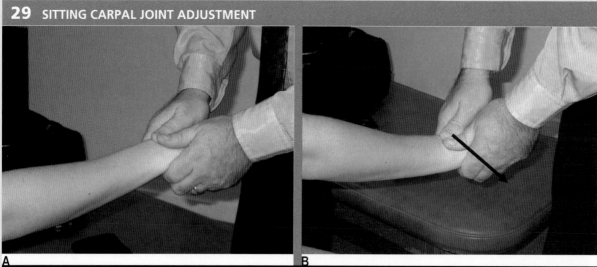

Fig. 17.29 Sitting carpal joint mobilization. (A) Suggested contact for a sitting carpal joint adjustment. (B) Thrust for a carpal joint mobilization.

Indication

This adjustment can be used to address a carpal joint that is not moving in anterior or posterior glide.

Contact

A double-handed reinforced thumb contact gripping the carpal bone in question just below the joint line of the specific bone is the most efficient contact for this adjustment. Skin slack should be taken into the direction of thrust. The contact should be firm but not causing the patient discomfort (Fig. 17.29A).

Patient Position

The patient should be sitting comfortably in front of the adjuster, with their arm outstretched.

Adjuster's Position

The adjuster should be standing with feet slightly more than shoulder-width apart, directly over the patient (Fig. 17.29A).

Thrust

The thrust is an impulse that is initiated just as the wrist comes into full extension (Fig. 17.29B).

30 SUPINE GENERAL MOBILIZATION HIP ADJUSTMENT

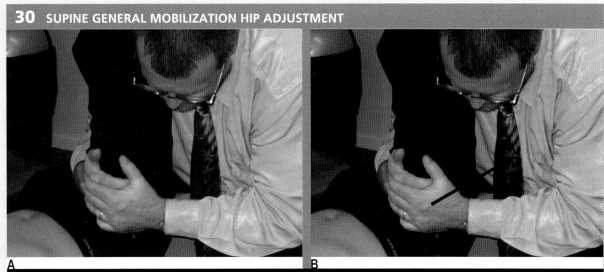

Fig. 17.30 Supine general mobilization of the hip manipulation. (A) Suggested contact for a supine general mobilization hip adjustment. (B) Thrust for a general mobilization of the hip.

Indication

This adjustment can be used to address a hip joint that is not moving in internal or external rotation or not gapping in long axis traction.

Contact

A double-handed interlocking finger contact gripping the leg just above the flexed hip is the most efficient contact for this adjustment. Skin slack should be taken in the direction of thrust, which is superior to inferior. The contact should be firm but not causing the patient discomfort (Fig. 17.30A).

Patient Position

The patient should be lying comfortably in front of the adjuster, with their leg flexed to 90° and resting on the adjuster's shoulder.

Adjuster's Position

The adjuster should be standing with feet slightly more than shoulder-width apart, bent slightly forward (Fig. 17.30A).

Thrust

The thrust is an impulse directed superior to inferior in a manner that will gap the hip joint (Fig. 17.30B).

31 SUPINE LONG AXIS TRACTION/ INTERNAL/EXTERNAL ROTATION HIP ADJUSTMENT

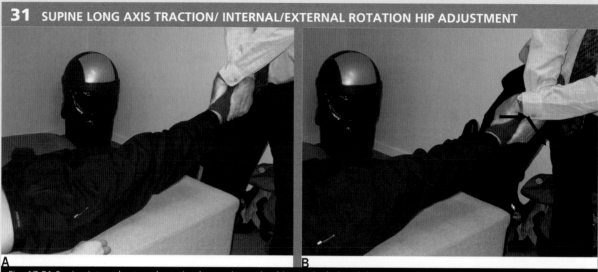

Fig. 17.31 Supine internal external rotation long axis traction hip manipulation. (A) Suggested contact for a supine internal/external rotation or long axis hip adjustment. (B) Thrust for an external rotation fixation of the hip.

Indication

This adjustment can be used to address a hip joint that is not moving in internal or external rotation or not gapping in long axis traction.

Contact

A double-handed cross-handed contact gripping the leg just above the ankle is the most efficient contact for this adjustment. Skin slack should be taken in the direction of thrust, either internal or external rotation or long axis traction. The contact should be firm but not causing the patient discomfort (Fig. 17.31A).

Patient Position

The patient should be lying comfortably in front of the adjuster, with their leg outstretched.

Adjuster's Position

The adjuster should be standing with feet slightly more than shoulder-width apart, directly over the patient (Fig. 17.31A).

Thrust

The thrust is an impulse directed in a rotary fashion that will bring the hip into internal or external rotation or direct long axis traction, whichever is the desired thrust (Fig. 17.31B).

32 SUPINE INTERNAL ROTATION KNEE ADJUSTMENT

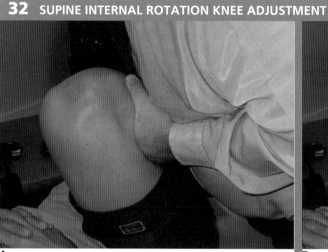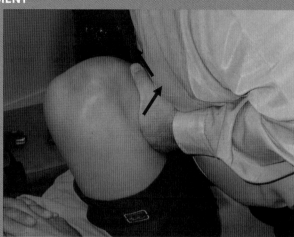

Fig. 17.32 Supine internal rotation knee manipulation. (A) Suggested contact for a supine internal rotation knee adjustment. (B) Thrust for an internal rotation fixation.

Indication

This adjustment can be used to address a knee joint that has anterior joint capsule adhesions or is not moving in internal rotation.

Contact

A single-handed palmer contact cupping the lateral posterior tibia is the most efficient contact for this adjustment. The palmer aspect of the hand should rest lightly on the posterior tibial region. Skin slack should be taken from posterior to anterior and lateral to medial. The contact should be firm but not causing the patient discomfort. The non-thrust hand should be holding the patient's lower leg above the ankle (Fig. 17.32A).

Patient Position

The patient should be lying comfortably in front of the adjuster, with their knee as fully flexed as possible.

Adjuster's Position

The adjuster should be standing with feet slightly more than shoulder-width apart, directly over the patient (Fig. 17.32A). The sternal notch should be at the level of the contact.

Thrust

The thrust is an impulse directed in a rotary fashion that will bring the tibia into internal rotation. The knee is flexed in a bucket handle fashion as the thrust is applied (Fig. 17.32B).

33 SUPINE INTERNAL/EXTERNAL ROTATION KNEE ADJUSTMENT

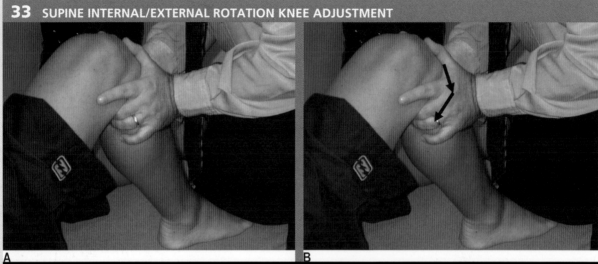

Fig. 17.33 Supine external rotation knee manipulation. (A) Suggested contact for a supine external rotation knee adjustment. (B) Thrust for an external rotation fixation.

Indication

This adjustment can be used to address a knee joint that has anterior joint capsule adhesions or is not moving in internal or external rotation.

Contact

A double-handed palmer 'choke' contact gripping the tibia just below the joint line is the most efficient contact for this adjustment. The palmer aspect of the thrust hand should rest lightly on the anterior tibial region. Skin slack should be taken from anterior to posterior and in the direction of thrust, either internal or external rotation. The contact should be firm but not causing the patient discomfort (Fig. 17.33A).

Patient Position

The patient should be lying comfortably in front of the adjuster, with their knee as comfortably flexed.

Adjuster's Position

The adjuster should be standing with feet slightly more than shoulder-width apart, directly over the patient (Fig. 17.33A). The sternal notch should be at the level of the contact. The adjuster's knee should lock the patient's foot in place with light pressure.

Thrust

The thrust is an impulse directed in a rotary fashion that will bring the tibia into internal or external rotation, whichever is the desired thrust (Fig. 17.33B).

34 SUPINE TALUS/NAVICULAR INTERNAL/EXTERNAL ROTATION ADJUSTMENT

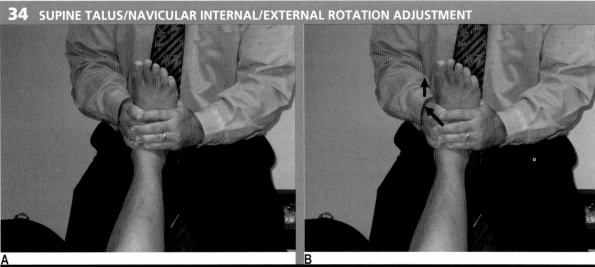

Fig. 17.34 Supine internal/external rotation navicula talar manipulation. (A) Suggested contact for a supine internal/external rotation talar or navicular adjustment. (B) Thrust for an internal rotation fixation of the navicular.

Indication

This adjustment can be used to address a talar or navicular joint that is not moving in internal or external rotation.

Contact

A double-handed reinforced finger contact gripping the navicular or the talus just below their respective joint lines is the most efficient contact for this adjustment. The palmer aspect of the thrust hand should rest lightly on the medial arch region. Skin slack should be taken from anterior to posterior and in the direction of thrust, either internal or external rotation. The contact should be firm but not causing the patient discomfort (Fig. 17.34A).

Patient Position

The patient should be lying comfortably in front of the adjuster, with their leg outstretched.

Adjuster's Position

The adjuster should be standing with feet slightly more than shoulder-width apart, directly over the patient (Fig. 17.34A). The sternal notch should be at the level of the contact.

Thrust

The thrust is an impulse directed in a rotary fashion that will bring the tibia into internal or external rotation, whichever is the desired thrust (Fig. 17.34B).

Contraindications for Manipulation

Manipulation when employed in appropriate circumstances is a safe and effective technique for restoring joint biomechanics and as a form of afferent stimulation. I have outlined several common conditions that may constitute contraindications to manipulation in certain cases; for a more comprehensive description see Beck et al (2004). There are very few situations or conditions where some form of manipulation cannot be performed as a form of stimulus to the neuraxis.

Fractures/Dislocation

There are three basic types of fractures that can be differentiated based largely on the history. In cases of fracture resulting from *direct trauma* the history is usually consistent with injury. In cases of suspected *stress fractures* the history of repetitive microtrauma should be a strong indicator for further imaging studies such as bone scanning. In situations where the injury is inconsistent with injury consideration should be given to the possibility of a *pathological fracture*. In these cases the presence of a pathology in the bone results in a weakened bone structure that fractures in situations that a normal bone would be expected to tolerate.

QUICK FACTS 1	Clinical Indications that May Indicate a Fracture

- Immediate muscle splinting
- Possible haematoma
- Disfiguration
- Unwilling to move
- Tuning fork and X-rays may be useful
- In children fractures that cross or involve the growth plate must be referred for orthopaedic consult

Some common clinical indications that may indicate the presence of a fracture include immediate muscle splinting, especially in cases of vertebral fractures where the splinting is also bilateral, presence of large immediate haematoma, disfiguration of the normal conture of the joint or area, and unwillingness of the patient to move or let someone else move the joint. The application of a tuning fork will usually produce pain in fractures but not in sprains. X-rays may be useful but many fractures will not be evident on X-ray immediately. A final clinical note concerning children with suspected fractures is necessary. In children fractures that cross or involve the growth plate must be referred for orthopaedic consult as soon as possible, as disruption of the growth plate may result in deformation or retardation of bone growth.

Haemarthrosis

Haemarthrosis, which is bleeding inside the capsule or joint space of a joint, can be extremely damaging to the articular surface of the joint. The enzymatic contents of blood and inflammatory response is very destructive to synovial tissues and cartilage. These types of injuries are most commonly caused from tears in intracapsular ligaments, for example the cruciate ligaments of the knee, the vascular portion of the menisci, ruptures of synovial membranes, or fractures that cross the osteochondral junction. In my experience one-third of all acute cases will need orthopaedic surgical reconstruction if the haemarthrosis is present for more then 2 days.

The clinical indications of a haemarthrosis include extreme, immediate swelling of the joint to the point that the joint is held at an angle to relieve some of the pressure within the capsule. The swelling may also have a pulsatile character.

Instability

Instability or *ligament tears* can be acute, chronic, or recurrent in nature and usually result in different degrees of instability which become apparent from minor movement of the joint. This is due to swelling and kinematic dysfunction of the joint due to the dislocation. Usually the direction of causative force relates to the direction of instability and patients are very apprehensive about any movement in the direction of the instability.

It is important to keep in mind that ligament instability may also be caused by infection, inflammatory processes, or autoimmune conditions.

Muscular Tendon Tears

Muscular tendon tears are often associated with degeneration of a tendon due to overuse, old age, or ischaemia. Patients often describe hearing a 'popping' sound prior to loss of strength. Complete or severe tears often result in 'tennis ball' appearing, which is the bunching of muscle proximal to the tear with a significant loss of muscular strength across the joint involved. Rehabilitation can sometimes be effective at restoring reasonable function but surgical reattachment is often necessary.

Acute Compartment Syndrome

Acute compartment syndrome (ACS) most commonly results from infarction or interruption of blood supply to a muscle group from swelling inside muscular fascia or constriction due to a bandage. The forearm flexors, gastrocnemius/soleus, and quadriceps are most commonly involved. ACS may lead to nerve damage and scar tissue formation and often results in contracture of distal digits. The clinical indications include rapid pain escalation beyond what would be expected in cases of sprain or strain and alterations in pulses, colour, and temperature of the affected limb. In cases where pain persists or circulation does not return to normal, surgical decompression may be necessary.

Infection

Infection may be caused by a wide variety of pathogens and conditions. The two most common causes are blood-borne infection from distant focus and direct implantation following trauma. Diabetes is a common systemic disease in peripheral infections. The joint will usually display marked local joint swelling, elevated temperature, and redness. The patient may hold the joint in the position of maximum bursal space for that joint, usually about 70° of flexion as previously described for haemarthrosis. In addition to the joint signs, systemic signs including fever and malaise may be present. Movement or rest will usually not alter symptoms and night pain is common. Most commonly tuberculosis, syphilis, gonococcal and staphylococcal infections target joints. It is important for the patient to seek pharmaceutical treatment immediately because septic arthritis and joint destruction may develop if the condition is left untreated.

Tumours

A variety of *tumours* can involve bones and joints. A brief overview of some of the more common considerations is outlined below.

1. *Metastatic tumours*—In cases of metastatic tumour involvement the primary site must be identified and located.

2. *Multiple myeloma*—This condition most commonly affects long bones and marrow-producing bones including the vertebra.

3. *Ewing's sarcoma*—This condition prefers long bones such as the humerus, radius, and ulna.

4. *Reticular cell carcinoma*—This condition is rare, but prefers the humerus when it does occur

5. *Osteochondroma*—This condition prefers the area around the knee most commonly, followed by the area around the elbow.

6. *Paget's disease*—This condition results in deformation of the bony matrix and changes in bone deposits. It may affect all bones but most commonly the head, jaw, and pelvis are involved.

The clinical indications of tumour involvement may include night pain, unremitting or worsening pain, and pain with no explanation of onset. Commonly the pain of a space-occupying tumour cannot be reproduced by mechanical means.

Arthritides

Some arthritides can result in situations of contraindication to manipulation especially in their reactive or inflammatory phase. Some common arthritides encountered in practice include the following:

1. *Osteoarthritis*—In many cases osteoarthritis is not a contraindication for manipulation; however, it may be contraindicated in severe cases.

2. *Rheumatoid arthritis* (RA)—In addition to pain the process of RA may lead to ligament destruction, including the alar ligaments of the atlas/axis complex; for this reason great care needs to be taken when manipulating patients with a history of RA.

3. *Charcot's (neuropathic) joint*—Destruction of the proprioceptive nerves to a joint result in massive destruction due to denervation of the joint. These joints can become extremely disfigured with relatively no pain to the patient.

4. *Psoriatic arthritis*—This condition is associated with psoriasis of the skin and may also result in severe joint destruction in some cases.

5. *Gout*—This condition usually affects the joints of the hands and feet and in the inflammatory stage may be too painful to manipulate.

Metabolic Disorders

Several metabolic disorders may also be of cause for concern when considering manipulation as a treatment modality. These include the following:

1. *Osteoporosis*—This condition may occur idiopathically, post-trauma, post-immobilization, or as the result of drug therapy with such drugs as HRT and corticosteroids.

2. *Osteopetrosis*—This condition causes bones to become very brittle and manipulation attempts may lead to fractures.

Congenital Anomalies

A variety of congenital anomalies can be considered as contraindications for manipulation or at the very least result in alteration of the manipulation approach applied. Extra bones such as a fabella or segmented patella may interfere with the standard manipulation approach. Pseudo-joints, ossifications, and scar tissue may occur following trauma or surgical interventions that may also result in difficulties when considering manipulation. Several structural deformities such as club foot, pes planus, and pes cavus can also present a manipulative challenge. These congenital anomalies usually coexist with other deformities so check the patients thoroughly before manipulating.

Manipulation Can Produce Complications

Although manipulation is one of the safest treatment interventions, some complications can arise. The most common complications are minor discomfort or stiffness a few hours following the manipulation. Some serious complications have been reported, the most serious being vertebrobasilar or other forms of stroke following cervical spine manipulation.

Vertebrobasilar Strokes (VBS)

Firstly, it must be accepted and understood that VBS following manipulation of the cervical spine can and do occur. The temporal relationship between young healthy patients without apparent osseous or vascular disease attending for manipulation and then suffering this type of rare stroke is well documented (Terrett 2001).

QUICK FACTS 2	Characteristics of Patients who Suffer a VBS or VBS-like Symptoms Following Manipulation

- They are young healthy adults.
- They have uneventful medical or health histories.
- They have no or only a few of the stroke 'risk factors'.
- They cannot be identified a priori by clinical or radiographic exam.
- Women do not appear to be at greater risk.
- Injuries to the vertebral arteries can occur anywhere along their entire path.

The vast majority of cases involve the use of a high-velocity/low-amplitude type of manipulation. The proposed mechanism of injury includes trauma to blood vessel walls which may have had preexisting damage. Alternatively, active pathological processes may have been present and may be exaggerated from the force of the manipulation. Regardless of the mechanism the end results of the manipulation are the following:

- Intimal laceration;
- Subintimal haemorrhages;
- Vessel wall dissections;
- Aneurysms;
- Thrombus formation; and
- Embolus formation.

Any of the above occurrences can result in acute and residual neurological deficit, several types of plegia, or death.

A variety of studies have reported a wide range of incidence findings, ranging from 1 incident per 300,000 manipulations to 1 per 14,000,000 manipulations (Maigne 1972; Cyriax 1978; Hosek et al 1981; Gutmann 1983; Carey 1993). Terrett (2001) examined 255 cases of vertebrobasilar insufficiency (VBI) following spinal manipulation; this investigation revealed that there is no greater risk for any age range, although the greatest number of occurrences was in the range 30–45 years, and there is no greater risk for any sex, although women had the greatest number of occurrences.

Patients who suffer a VBS or VBS-like symptoms display the following characteristics:

- They are young healthy adults;
- They have uneventful medical or health histories;
- They have no or only a few of the stroke 'risk factors';
- They cannot be identified a priori by clinical or radiographic exam;
- Women do not appear to be at greater risk; and
- Injuries to the vertebral arteries can occur anywhere along their entire path.

The symptoms of VBI most commonly found include:

1. Dizziness/vertigo/giddiness/light-headedness;
2. Drop attacks/loss of consciousness;
3. Diplopia (amaurosis fugax);
4. Dysarthria;
5. Dysphagia;
6. Ataxia of gait/falling to one side;
7. Nausea;
8. Numbness of one side of the face and/or body; and
9. Nystagmus.

The five most common presenting complaints in patients who subsequently developed VBI include:

1. Neck pain and or stiffness (42%);
2. Neck pain and headache (18%);
3. Headache (14%);
4. Torticollis (6%); and
5. Low back pain (3%).

If a patient suffers symptoms of VBI, do not adjust them again. Left alone the patient may recover.

Wallenberg and 'Locked in' Syndromes

Two syndromes that may also result from cervical spine manipulation have been identified: Wallenberg syndrome and the 'locked in' syndrome. Wallenberg syndrome (dorsolateral medullary syndrome) is a syndrome of symptoms that results from an injury or dysfunction in the dorsal lateral medulla, which usually is a result of an infarct in blood supply caused by occlusion of the vertebral artery but may also result from occlusion of the posterior inferior cerebellar artery (PICA). The most common symptoms include:

- Gait ataxia, and hypotonia ipsilateral to side of lesion;

QUICK FACTS 3   **Wallenberg Syndrome**

- Gait ataxia, and hypotonia ipsilateral to side of lesion.
- Loss of pain and temperature from the ipsilateral side of the face and loss of corneal reflex on the ipsilateral side
- Loss of pain and temperature from the contralateral body
- Horner's syndrome
- Nystagmus, vertigo, nausea, and vomiting
- Hoarseness, dysphasia, and intractable hiccups.

- Loss of pain and temperature from the ipsilateral side of the face and loss of corneal reflex on the ipsilateral side;
- Loss of pain and temperature from the contralateral body;
- Horner's syndrome;
- Nystagmus, vertigo, nausea, and vomiting; and
- Hoarseness, dysphasia, and intractable hiccups.

The *'locked in' syndrome* can result from the occlusion of the mid-basilar artery, which results from bilateral ventral pontine infarction. The patient will experience a state of total consciousness with or without sensation, and no voluntary movement except vertical eye movement.

Cortical Stimulation

Ipsilateral Cortical Stimulation/Activation in Rehabilitation
- Any complex chore involves both sides of the brain;
- Contralateral cerebellar activation, novel hand, foot movements, vibration;
- Contralateral music, sound, snapping fingers;
- Light stimulation in the contralateral visual field;
- Ipsilateral smell stimulation;
- Watching vertical movement on ipsilateral side;
- OPK to ipsilateral side as therapy; and
- Contralateral TENS to cervical (Ghatan et al 1998).

Ipsilateral Cortical Inhibition in Rehabilitation
- All evoked potentials at reduced amplitude, monitor fatigue;
- Earplugs;
- Blinders;
- Dark glasses; and
- Visualize rather than perform activities.

Right Cortical Stimulation/Activation in Rehabilitation
- Arranging blocks is very right-sided activity;
- Listening to and reading stories, especially with images;
- Listen for double meanings, puns, jokes;
- Holding many possible meanings in mind;
- Functions more as an arbiter, selects the meaning according to the context;
- Summarizing the gist of something, getting the 'bigger picture';
- Look at shapes, lines, crosses, cubes, dots displays;
- Looking at anonymous faces or meeting new people;
- Appraisal of self-worth, attachment, and bonding;

- Look at global activity versus details;
- Knowing where/what objects are in a blurred picture, or from general outlines;
- Seeing links between things at the same time, different places;
- Seeing things as they are, not as they 'should' be, literal rather than interpretive;
- Estimate the time passage;
- Imagine space;
- Tap to flashing lights, target synchronized with memory;
- Trace mazes with eyes, hands, look for object in a picture or maze;
- Map reading;
- Listen for the melody of music, tone, especially with the left ear, especially the lower tones, including heartbeat, digestion;
- Listen to words used to describe the mind: 'think', 'imagine';
- Spatial attention, such as mental rotation of objects while looking at parts;
- Completing words;
- Movement of larger muscles (arm and leg escape, running and fighting);
- Judge time, compare; and
- Recalling letters or words without reference to meaning (Burgund & Marsolek 1997; Epstein et al 1997; Fink et al 1997b; Henry 1997; Lechevalier 1997; Tranel et al 1997).

Left Cortical Stimulation/Activation in Rehabilitation
- Writing is a very left sided function;
- Speaking fluently is more left than right;
- Listen for the rhythm of music, pitch, familiarity, identification;
- Listening with right ear especially the higher tones;
- Reading imageless technical material, imageless concepts;
- Reading sentences with centre-embedded meanings requires more memory;
- Drawing detailed new diagrams or pictures;
- Verbal organizational, interpretational skills;
- Seeing the links between things presented sequentially;
- Seeing similarities between words on paired lists;
- Classification of words, pictures, into categories;
- Word games, deriving small words from larger words, finding a word in a list;
- Number organizational, interpretational skills;
- Counting exercises such as subtracting 7's from 100;
- Paying attention to details of an object;
- Identification of familiar faces, objects, shapes;
- Interpreting incomplete pictures;
- Making stories when details are incomplete, true or false;
- Interpreting things based on a sense of 'should', dependent on past experience;
- Rapid selection of a single meaning;
- Paying attention to details other than the object in view;
- Attention-switching exercises;
- Self-preservation versus species preservation;
- Movement of smaller muscles;
- Recalling meaningful information, or well-practised complex narrative; and
- Silent verb generation activities and cognitive processes leading to the answer 'yes' (Andreasen et al 1995; Herholtz et al 1996; Schumacher et al 1996; Carlsson 1997; Fallgatter et al 1997; Fink et al 1997a,b; Henriques & Davidson 1997; Jennings et al 1997; Lechevalier 1997; Pashek 1997; Wang 1997; Gabrieli et al 1998)

Activation of the Left Supplemental Motor Area

- Read nouns aloud; and
- Attention exercises involving timing such as pushing a button when a light flashes (Harrington et al 1998; Ojemann et al 1998)

Activation of the Left Premotor Area

- Look at tools, name them, picture using them;
- Point with the right hand;
- Non-unique tools; and
- Judging time and comparing it with a standard unit of time, for example pushing a button every time a light does not appear after a predetermined time period (Maquet et al 1996; Grafton et al 1997; Inoue et al 1998).

Activation of Auditory Cortex

Any single frequency of sound activates the most lateral aspects of the auditory cortex and multiple frequencies stimulate the entire auditory cortex (Ottaviani et al 1997).

Frontal Lobe Stimulation/Activation in Rehabilitation

- Generate verb-to-noun list;
- Recall well-practised material;
- Meaningful hand action;
- Pay attention to rhythm (Broca's area);
- Verbal exercises which impose a heavy burden on working memory;
- Cerebellar activation, especially of hands and fingers, which is specific for the dentate nucleus;
- Volitional eye activity or saccadic movement activity to the contralateral side;
- Interpret visual stimuli;
- Listen to complex concepts; and
- Learn new songs (Decety et al 1997; Paradiso et al 1997).

Temporal Lobe Stimulation/Activation in Rehabilitation

- Naming/viewing pictures of new faces or novel experiences;
- Point with the ipsilateral hand;
- Cognitive processes leading to the answer 'yes';
- Read nouns aloud;
- Generate verb-to-noun list;
- Working with or looking at animals produces left medial temporal lobe stimulation;
- Verbs/actions stimulate the left middle temporal gyrus;
- Time and place (long-term episodic memory)—left prefrontal cortex;
- Spatial orientation in remembered places stimulates the right hippocampus and temporal lobe areas;
- Listening and counting, listen for how many times a word is spoken in a sentence, etc.;
- Performing tasks with familiar stimulus;
- Recall visual landmarks which activates spatial memory centres;
- Quarter field stimulation from superior quadrant of contralateral side;
- Listening to music in the contralateral ear;
- Ipsilateral smell stimulation;
- Looking at unknown persons, faces;
- Remember where objects are in the environment;
- Narrative recall and list learning (Berthoz 1997; Grady et al 1997; Henriques & Davidson 1997).

Parietal Lobe Stimulation/Activation in Rehabilitation

- Judge time, compare;
- Trace a maze, initial unskilled attempts;
- Quarter field stimulation from inferior quadrant of contralateral side;
- Remember words and pseudo-words;
- Meaningless hand movements; and
- Attention exercises involving timing such as pushing a button when a light flashes (Decety et al 1997; Pashek 1997; Harrington et al 1998; Schiffer 1998).

Occipital Lobe Stimulation in Rehabilitation

- Spatial orientation; and
- Vertical movement in the respective visual field stimulates the ipsilateral occipital cortex (Tootell et al 1998).

Cerebellar Stimulation/Activation in Rehabilitation

General Cerebellar Stimulation Techniques
- Warming the auditory canal will stimulate the cerebellum on the ipsilateral side;
- Revolve chair to the right will stimulate the cerebellum on the right and vice versa but will also stimulate the vestibular system;
- Passive muscle stretch will stimulate the cerebellum on the ipsilateral side;
- Squeezing a tennis ball will stimulate the cerebellum on the ipsilateral side;
- Alternate passive stretch on ipsilateral side with active stretch of contralateral side;
- Eye movements up to ipsilateral side and down to contralateral side will stimulate the respective cerebellum and not the vestibular system; and
- Pointing with the ipsilateral hand (Inoue et al 1998).

Efferent Copy and Feedback (Medial Cerebellum)
- Gym ball exercises (including limb exercises with resistance etc.);
- Wobble board, wobble sandals, balance mat etc.;
- Gyroscope;
- Bouncing ball against the ground;
- Visual fixation exercises involving head rotation with a monitored focus; and
- Fukuda's marching in place with feedback.

Feedforward and Efferent Copy (Lateral Cerebellum)
- Cognitive processes leading to the answer 'yes';
- Learning a musical instrument;
- Tracing a maze especially the first few attempts;
- Throwing and catching a ball off the wall;
- Tapping to the beat of a metronome or to music;
- Voluntary motor activities;
- Trying to write with the eyes closed (with dominant or non-dominant hand);
- Board games involving strategy and forward planning; and
- Silent generation of verbs and reading nouns out loud (Herholtz et al 1996; Jennings et al 1997; Pashek 1997; Ojemann et al 1998).

Mesencephalic Stimulation/Activation in Rehabilitation

- Eye exercises include alternating focusing on near and then far objects;
- Listening to music and sounds is especially crucial when IML activation level is high;
- Light and visual stimulation especially when IML activation is low; and
- Increase cerebellar activation, especially novel contralateral hand activities.

Mesencephalic Inhibition in Rehabilitation

- Increase frontal activation through BG loops to inhibit mesencephalic activation;
- Increase contralateral mesencephalic activation;
- Patch ipsilateral eye, use contra eye to gaze to ipsilateral eye fields; and
- Wear red/pink-coloured glasses.

Brainstem Stimulation/Activation in Rehabilitation

- Smell, taste food;
- Speech, phonation, 'ah', singing;
- Facial movement, winking;
- Corneal puffs;
- Palatal stimulation, roll gum;
- Jaw exercises; and
- Rectal dilation increases vagal feedback.

Vestibular System Stimulation/Activation in Rehabilitation

The following are Cawthorne-Cooksey exercises for patients with vestibular hypofunction:

A. **In bed**

1. Eye movements—at first slow, then quick
   a. Up and down
   b. From side to side
   c. Focusing on finger moving from 3 ft to 1 ft away from face
2. Head movements—at first slow, then quick; later with eyes closed
   a. Bending forwards and backwards
   b. Turning from side to side

B. **Sitting (in class)**

1. Eye movements (as above)
2. Head movements (as above)
3. Shoulder shrugging and circling
4. Bending forwards and picking up objects from the ground

C. **Standing (in class)**

1. Eye movements (as above)
2. Head movements (as above)
3. Shoulder shrugging and circling
4. Changing from sitting to standing position with eyes open and shut
5. Throwing a small ball from hand to hand (above eye level)
6. Throwing ball from hand to hand under knee
7. Changing from sitting to standing and turning round in between

D. **Moving about (in class)**

1. Circle round centre person who will throw a large ball and to whom it will be returned
2. Walk across room with eyes open and then closed
3. Walk up and down slope with eyes open and then closed
4. Walk up and down steps with eyes open then closed
5. Any game involving stooping and stretching and aiming such as skittles, bowls, or basketball

Diligence and perseverance are required but the earlier and more regularly the exercise regimen is carried out, the faster and more complete will be the return to normal activity (Dix 1979).

Exercises to Improve Postural Stability

There are many different balance exercises that can be used. These exercises are devised to incorporate head movement (vestibular stimulation) or to foster the use of different sensory cues for balance (Herdman et al 1994).

1. The patient stands with his or her feet as close together as possible with both or one hand helping maintain balance by touching a wall if needed. The patient then turns his or her head to the right and to the left horizontally while looking straight ahead at the wall for 1 minute without stopping. The patient takes his or her hand or hands off the wall for longer and longer periods of time while maintaining balance. The patient then tries moving his or her feet even closer together.

2. The patient walks, with someone for assistance if needed, as often as possible (acute disorders).

3. The patient begins to practise turning his or her head while walking. This will make the patient less stable so the patient should stay near a wall as he or she walks.

4. The patient stands with his or her feet shoulder-width apart with eyes open, looking straight ahead at a target on the wall. He or she progressively narrows the base of support from feet apart to feet together to a semi-heel-to-toe position. The exercise is performed first with arms outstretched, then with arms close to the body, and then with arms folded across the chest. Each position is held for 15 seconds before the patient does the next most difficult exercise. The patient practises for a total of 5 to 15 minutes.

5. The patient stands with his or her feet shoulder-width apart with eyes open, looking straight ahead at a target on the wall. The patient progressively narrows his or her base of support from feet apart to feet together to a semi-heel-to-toe-position. The exercise is performed first with arms outstretched, then with arms close to the body, and then the patient tries the next position. The patient practises for a total of 5 to 15 minutes.

6. A headlamp can be attached to the patient's waist or shoulders, and the patient can practise shifting weight to place the light into targets marked on the wall. This home 'biofeedback' exercise can be used with the feet in different positions and with the patient standing on surfaces of different densities.

7. The patient practises standing on a cushioned surface. Progressively more difficult tasks might be hard floor (linoleum, wood), thin carpet, shag carpet, thin pillow, sofa cushion. Graded-density foam can also be purchased.

8. The patient practises walking with a more narrow base of support. The patient can do this first, touching the wall for support or for tactile cues and then gradually touching only intermittently and then not at all.

9. The patient practises turning around while walking, at first making a large circle but gradually making smaller and smaller turns. The patient must be sure to turn in both directions.

10. The patient can practise standing and then walking on ramps, either with a firm surface or with more cushioned surface.

11. The patient can practise maintaining balance while sitting and bouncing on a Swedish ball or while bouncing on a trampoline. This exercise can be incorporated with attempting to maintain visual fixation or a stationary target, thus facilitating adaptation of the otolith-ocular reflexes.

12. Out in the community, the patient can practise walking in a mall before it is open and therefore while it is quiet; can practise walking in the mall while walking in the same direction as the flow of traffic; and can walk against the flow of traffic (Herdman et al 1994).

Exercises to Improve Gaze Stability

Acute Stage (Also Used with Chronic, Uncompensated Patients)

1. A business card or other target with words on it (foveal target) is taped on the wall in front of the patient so he or she can read it. The patient moves his or her head gently back and forth horizontally for 1 minute while keeping the words in focus.

2. This is repeated moving the head vertically for 1 minute.

3. Depending on whether this induces any nausea, the exercise is then repeated using a large pattern such as a checkerboard (full-field stimulus), moving the head horizontally.

4. The exercise with the checkerboard is then repeated moving the head vertically.

The patient should repeat each exercise at least three times a day. The duration of each of the exercises is extended gradually from 1 to 2 minutes. Patients should be cautioned that the exercises may make them feel dizzy or even nauseated but that they should try to persist for the full 1 to 2 minutes of the exercise, resting between exercises.

Subacute Stage

1. The patient holds a business card in front of him or her so that he or she can read it. The patient moves the card and his or her head back and forth horizontally in opposite directions, keeping the words in focus for 1 minute without stopping.

2. This is repeated with vertical head movements and with a large, full-field stimulus.

The duration is gradually extended from 1 to 2 minutes. The patient should repeat each exercise at least three times each day (Herdman et al 1994).

Treatment of Vestibular Hypofunction

1. Increase and alternate the speed of exercises;

2. Perform exercises in various positions and activities (i.e., head movements performed in sitting, then standing, and finally during walking);

3. Perform exercises in situations of decreasing visual and/or somatosensory input (i.e., eyes open to eyes closed);

4. Expose the patient to a variety of task and environmental situations and contexts (i.e., walking in the home to walking at a shopping mall);

5. Trace the alphabet with your foot; and

6. Step forwards and backwards and cross over your legs (Dix 1979; Herdman et al 1994).

Activation of Special Areas

Mesolimbic Stimulation/Activation in Rehabilitation

- Left caudate—look at pleasant scenes; and
- Left amygdala, hippocampus—look at unpleasant scenes.

Unilateral Deafness Treatment Approaches

- Metronome;
- Discrete single-frequency or narrowband sounds;
- Spinal adjusting and stabilization;
- Ear mobilization;
- Occipitalis, suboccipital or neck/shoulder STT;
- Vestibular stimulation;
- Magnesium, ginkgo biloba;
- Feedback or tinnitus retraining therapy; and
- Ear coning.

Sympathetic Tone Inhibition in Rehabilitation

- Red stimuli;
- Warm local area with towels, clothes; and
- TENS.

Correcting Respiratory Aberrancy or Dysfunction

- Respiratory exercises, breathe against a band;
- O_2 canula, mask;
- O_2/CO_2 mix; and
- Concentration or awareness in breathing patterns (Naveen et al 1997).

Peripheral Nerve Dysfunction

- Electrical stimulus such as TENS, microcurrent;

- Cross cord reflexes;
- Homologous columns;
- Homonymous muscle activities, passive;
- Decompress peripheral nerves; and
- Reduce iatrogenesis, teach individual.

Tinnitus
- Ipsilateral light, sound, vibration; and
- Contralateral smell.

Spasm Reduction
- Reduce muscle spasm with less cortical effect by slow stretching the antagonist muscles.

Amygdala and Hippocampal Stimulation
- Visualizing unpleasant stimuli; and
- Narrative recall and list learning (Sass et al 1995; Leask & Crow 1997).

Caudate Stimulus
- Visualizing pleasant stimuli (Leask & Crow 1997).

References

Andreasen NC, O'Leary DS, Cizadlo T et al 1995 II. PET studies of memory: novel versus practiced free recall of word lists. Neuroimaging 2(4):296–305.

Beck RW 2003 Psychoneuroimmunology. In: Beirman R (ed) Handbook of clinical diagnosis. Sydney. p 27–35.

Beck RW, Holt KR, Fox MA et al 2004 Radiographic anomalies that may alter chiropractic intervention strategies found in a New Zealand population. Journal of Manipulative and Physiological Therapeutics 27(9):554–559.

Berthoz A 1997 Parietal and hippocampal contribution to topokinetic and topographic memory. Philosophical Transactions of the Royal Society of London, Series B, Biological Sciences 352(1360):1437–1448.

Burgund ED; Marsolek CJ 1997 Letter-case-specific priming in the right cerebral hemisphere with a form-specific perceptual identification task. Brain and Cognition 35(2):239–258.

Carey PF 1993 A report on the occurrence of cerebrovascular accidents in chiropractic practice. Journal of Canadian Chiropractic Association 37(2):104–106.

Carlsson G 1997 Memory for words and drawings in children with hemiplegic cerebral palsy. Scandinavian Journal of Psychology 38(4):265–273.

Carrick FR 1991 Advanced manipulative techniques and neurological video series. Logan College, St Louis MO.

Carrick FR 1994 Advanced manipulative techniques and neurological video series. Logan College, St Louis MO.

Carrick FR 1997 Changes in brain function after manipulation of the cervical spine. Journal of Manipulative and Physiological Therapeutics 20(8):529–545.

Chiu T, Wright A 1996 To compare the effects of different rates of application of a cervical mobilisation technique on sympathetic outflow to the upper limb in normal subjects. Manual Therapy 1:(4):198–203.

Cyriax J 1978 Textbook of orthopaedic medicine, vol 1 Diagnosis of soft tissue lesions, 7th edn. Bailliere Tindall, London, 165

Decety J, Grezes J, Costes N et al 1997 Brain activity during observation of actions. Influence of action content and subject's strategy. Brain 120(Pt 10):1763–1777.

Dix MR 1979 The rational and technique of head exercises in the treatment of vertigo. Acta Oto-Rhino-Laryngologica Belgica 33:370–384.

Drummond P 1988 Autonomic disturbances in cluster headache. Brain 111:1199–1209.

Drummond PD 1993 The effect of sympathetic blockade on facial sweating and cutaneous vascular responses to painful stimulation of the eye. Brain 116:233–241.

Drummond PD, Lance JW 1984 Facial temperature in migraine, tension-vascular and tension headache. Cephalalgia 4:149–158.

Epstein JN, Conners CK, Erhardt D et al 1997 Asymmetrical hemispheric control of visual-spatial attention in adults with attention deficit hyperactivity disorder. Neuropsychology 11(40):467–473.

Fallgatter AJ, Roesler M, Sitzmann L et al 1997 Loss of functional hemispheric asymmetry in Alzheimer's dementia assessed with near-infrared spectroscopy. Brain Research. Cognitive Brain Research 6(1):67–72.

Fink GR, Halligan PW, Marshall JC et al 1997a Neural mechanisms involved in the processing of global and local aspects of hierarchically organized visual stimuli. Brain 120(Pt 10):1779–1791.

Fink GR, Dolan RJ, Halligan PW et al 1997b Space-based and object-based visual attention: shared and specific neural domains. Brain 120(Pt 11):2013–2028.

Gabrieli JD, Poldrack RA, Desmond JE 1998 The role of the left prefrontal cortex in language and memory. Proceedings of the National Academy of Science USA 95(3):906–913.

Ghatan PH, Hsieh JC, Pettersson KM et al 1998 Coexistence of attention-based facilitation and inhibition in the human cortex. Neuroimage 7(1):23–29.

Grady CL, Van Meter JW, Maisog JM et al 1997 Attention-related modulation of activity in primary and secondary auditory cortex. Neuroreport 8(11):2511–2516.

Grafton ST, Fadiga L, Arbib MA et al 1997 Premotor cortex activation during observation and naming of familiar tools. Neuroimage 6(4):231–236.

Gutmann B 1983 Verletzungen der arteria vertebralis durch manuelle therapie. Manuelle Medizin 21:2–14.

Harrington DL, Haaland KY, Knight RT 1998 Cortical networks underlying mechanisms of time perception. Journal of Neuroscience 18(3):1085–1095.

Henriques JB, Davidson RJ 1997 Brain electrical asymmetries during cognitive task performance in depressed and nondepressed subjects. Biological Psychiatry 42(11):1039–1050.

Henry JP 1997 Psychological and physiological responses to stress: the right hemisphere and the hypothalamo-pituitary-adrenal axis, and inquiry into problems of human bonding. Acta-Physiologica Scandinavica Supplementum 640:10–25.

Herdman SJ, Borello-France DF, Whitney SL 1994 Treatment of vestibular hypofunction. In: Herdman S (ed) Vestibular rehabilitation. FH Davis, Philadelphia,

Herholz K, Thiel A, Wienhard K et al 1996 Individual functional anatomy of verb generation. Neuroimage 3(3 pt 1):185–194.

Holt K, Beck RW, Sexton S 2006 Reflex effects of a spinal adjustment on blood pressure. Proceedings of the Association of Chiropractic Colleges: Research agenda conference, Washington DC.

Hosek RS, Schram SB, Silverman H et al 1981 Cervical manipulation. Journal of American Medical Association 245:922.

Inoue K, Kawashima R, Satoh K et al 1998 PET study of pointing with visual feedback of moving hands. Journal of Neurophysiology 79(1):117–125.

Jennings JM, McIntosh AR, Kapur S et al 1997 Cognitive subtractions may not add up: the interaction between semantic processing and response mode. Neuroimage 5(3):229–239.

Kelly DD, Murphy BA, et al 2000 Use of a mental rotation reaction-time paradigm to measure the efects of upper cervical adjustments on Cortical processing: A pilot study. Journal of Manipulative and Physiological Therapeutics 23(4):246–251.

Knutsen GA 2001 Significant changes in systolic blood pressure post vectored upper cervical adjustment vs resting control groups: A possible effect of the cervicosympathetic and/or pressor reflex. Journal of Manipulative and Physiological Therapeutics 24(2):101–109.

Korr IM 1979 The spinal cord as organiser of disease processes: III. Hyperactivity of sympathetic innervation as a common factor in disease. Journal of the American Osteopathic Association 79(4):232–237.

Leask SJ, Crow TJ 1997 How far does the brain lateralize?: an unbiased method for determining the optimum degree of hemispheric specialization. Neuropsychologia 35(10):1381–1387.

Lechevalier B 1997 (Perception of musical sounds: contributions of position emission tomography). La perception des sons musicaux: apports de la camera a positions. Bulletin de l'Academie nationale de medicine 181(6):1191–1199; discussion 1199–1200

Maigne R 1972 Orthopedic medicine: a new approach to vertebral manipulations. Thomas CC, Springfield, IL: 155, 169

Maquet P, Lejeune H, Pouthas V et al 1996 Brain activation induced by estimation of duration: a PET study. Neuroimage 3(2):119–126.

Naveen KV, Nagarathna R, Nagendra HR et al 1997 Yoga breathing through a particular nostril increases spatial memory scores without lateralized effects. Psychological Reports 81(2):555–561.

Ojemann JG, Neil JM, MacLeod AM et al 1998 Increased functional vascular response in the region of a glioma. Journal of Cerebral Blood Flow and Metabolism 18(2):148–153.

Ottaviani F, DiGirolamo S, Briglia G et al 1997 Tonotopic organization of human auditory cortex and analyzed by SPET. Audiology 36(5):241–248.

Paradiso S, Crespo Facorro B, Andreasen NC et al 1997 Brain activity assessed with PET during recall of work lists and narratives. Neuroreport 8(14):3091–3096.

Pashek GV 1997 A case study of gesturally cued naming in aphasia: dominant versus nondominant hand training. Journal of Communication Disorders 30(5):349–365; quiz 365–366

Sass KJ, Silberfein CM, Platis I et al 1995 Right hemisphere mediation of verbal learning and memory in acquired right hemisphere speech dominant patients. Journal of the International Neuropsychological Society 1(6):554–560.

Sato A 1992 The reflex effects of spinal somatic nerve stimulation on visceral function. Journal of Manipulative and Physiological Therapeutics 15(1):57–61.

Schiffer F 1998 Cognitive activity of the right hemisphere: possible contributions to psychological function. Harvard Review of Psychiatry 4(3):126–138.

Schumacher EH, Lauber E, Awh E et al 1996 PET evidence for an amodal verbal working memory system. Neuroimage 3(2):79–88.

Stephens D, Pollard H, Bilton D et al 1999 Bilateral simultaneous optic nerve dysfunction after periorbital trauma: recovery of vision in association with chiropractic spinal manipulation therapy. Journal of Manipulative and Physiological Therapeutics 22(9):615–621.

Terrett AG 2001 Current concepts in vertebral basilar complications following spinal manipulation. NCIMC Chiropractic Solutions.

Thomas MD, Wood J 1992 Upper cervical adjustments may improve mental function. Journal of Manual Medicine 6:215–216.

Tootell RB, Mendola JD, Hadjikhani NK et al 1998 The representation of the ipsilateral visual field in human cerebral cortex. Proceedings of the National Academy of Science USA 95(3):818–824.

Tranel D, Damasio H, Damasio AR 1997 A neural basis for the retrieval of conceptual knowledge. Neuropsychologia 35(10):1319–1327.

Wang S 1997 Traumatic stress and attachment. Acta Physiologica Scandinavica Supplementum 640:164–169.

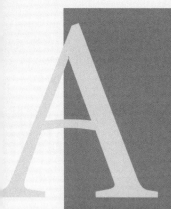

Clinical Case Answers

Case 17.1

17.1.1   Any combination of the following in the appropriate amounts would be beneficial to this woman:

- Writing is a very left-sided function;
- Speaking fluently is more left than right;
- Listen for the rhythm of music, pitch, familiarity, identification;
- Listening with right ear especially the higher tones;
- Reading imageless technical material, imageless concepts;
- Reading sentences with centre-embedded meanings requires more memory;
- Drawing detailed new diagrams or pictures;
- Verbal organizational, interpretational skills;
- Seeing the links between things presented sequentially;
- Seeing similarities between words on paired lists;
- Classification of words, pictures, into categories;
- Word games, deriving small words from larger words, finding a word in a list;
- Number organizational, interpretational skills;
- Counting exercises such as subtracting 7's from 100;
- Paying attention to details of an object
- Identification of familiar faces, objects, shapes;
- Interpreting incomplete pictures;
- Making stories when details are incomplete, true or false;
- Interpreting things based on a sense of 'should', dependent on past experience;
- Rapid selection of a single meaning;
- Paying attention to details other than the object in view;
- Attention-switching exercises;
- Self-preservation versus species preservation;
- Movement of smaller muscles;
- Recalling meaningful information, or well-practised complex narrative;
- Silent verb generation activities and cognitive processes leading to the answer 'yes'; and
- Manipulation to the right side of the body.

Case 17.2

17.2.1   Any of the following would be beneficial to this young man in the appropriate amounts:

General Cerebellar Stimulation Techniques

- Warming the auditory canal will stimulate the cerebellum on the ipsilateral side;
- Revolve chair to the right will stimulate the cerebellum on the right and vice versa but will also stimulate the vestibular system;

- Passive muscle stretch will stimulate the cerebellum on the ipsilateral side;
- Squeezing a tennis ball will stimulate the cerebellum on the ipsilateral side;
- Alternate passive stretch on ipsilateral side with active stretch of contralateral side;
- Eye movements up to ipsilateral side and down to contralateral side will stimulate the respective cerebellum and not the vestibular system; and
- Pointing with the ipsilateral hand.

Efferent Copy and Feedback (Medial Cerebellum)

- Gym ball exercises (including limb exercises with resistance etc);
- Wobble board, wobble sandals, balance mat, etc.;
- Gyroscope;
- Bouncing ball against the ground;
- Visual fixation exercises involving head rotation with a monitored focus; and
- Fukuda's marching in place with feedback.

Feedforward and Efferent Copy (Lateral Cerebellum)

- Cognitive processes leading to the answer 'yes';
- Learning a musical instrument;
- Tracing a maze especially the first few attempts;
- Throwing and catching a ball off the wall;
- Tapping to the beat of a metronome or to music;
- Voluntary motor activities;
- Trying to write with the eyes closed (with dominant or non-dominant hand);
- Board games involving strategy and forward planning;
- Silent generation of verbs and reading nouns out loud;
- Warming the auditory canal will stimulate the cerebellum on the ipsilateral side;
- Revolve chair to the right will stimulate the cerebellum on the right and visa versa but will also stimulate the vestibular system;
- Passive muscle stretch will stimulate the cerebellum on the ipsilateral side;
- Squeezing a tennis ball will stimulate the cerebellum on the ipsilateral side;
- Alternate passive stretch on ipsilateral side with active stretch of contralateral side;
- Eye movements up to ipsilateral side and down to contralateral side will stimulate the respective cerebellum and not the vestibular system; and
- Pointing with the ipsilateral hand.

Functional Neurological Approaches to Patient Management

Introduction

Perhaps the greatest challenge in clinical functional neurology is integrating the theoretical knowledge that one has acquired and results obtained via practical testing into a coherent approach that can be applied to a patient's presentation. This is so challenging because everything that happens to us in our daily lives can in some instances be important clinically and in others not matter in the slightest. Everyday events involving sensory stimulation, deprivation, and learning can effectively weaken synaptic connections in some circumstances and strengthen them in others. Just because structural or functional changes may not initially be detected following clinical examination does not rule out the possibility that important biological changes are never the less occurring. They may simply be below the level of detection with the limited techniques available to us.

In this chapter I will try to highlight the approach that I and other neurologists have taken with a variety of patients that have presented to me or other functional neurologists that have graciously supplied the case details to me for this chapter. In all cases I have tried to present a discussion of why the therapy was applied and the outcome of the treatment when available. Some of the physical examination findings in some cases are not reported as completely as I would have liked, but in real practice one does not always have a complete picture but is expected to move ahead regardless. In this respect I have tried to present the cases as they were presented to me or as they have been recorded in my notes. This should give the reader a better feel for clinical application.

Case 1

Presenting Complaint

TWB is a 17-year-old male who presented with learning disabilities and inability to concentrate.

Past History

When his mother was pregnant, she developed a pulmonary embolus and as a result placenta received less blood. She was subsequently on heparin throughout the rest of the pregnancy. TWB was born 4 weeks premature, at a weight of 1645 g, via an emergency C-section because his heart had stopped, but his lungs were fully developed. TWB reports that he has experienced no trauma to the head nor taken any antibiotics or orthodox medicine. He has experienced no childhood viruses that were out of the ordinary. TWB was evaluated for ADDH when 4 years old by a homeopathic physician, who found him to be within normal limits for his age.

Present History

TWB complains of blurry vision to close objects. He reports that he has not had his eyes checked in the past year. No balance problems were present. His concentration is interrupted every few minutes.

Coordination is not up to par. Spicy and junk food gives him stomach trouble. He reports no headaches. Dizzy feelings are felt occasionally throughout the day. Shoulder and rib pain is occasionally bilaterally. He complains of achy bones lately, and also reports he may have a tendency towards obsessive-compulsive activities. TWB was extremely effected when his parents broke up. He was afraid he would not see his father again. His father believes that he has lost respect for women because of the break-up. TWB's stepfather is verbally abusive towards his mother but not to TWB. It bothered TWB when his mother and stepfather got married.

Physical Exam

- Right pupil response shows TND;
- Visual tracking was dyskinetic with loss of maintained focus;
- Rhomberg's test—patient fell to the left;
- Rapid alternating movements (RAM)—demonstrated left hand uncoordinated compared to right;
- Tandem walking—within normal limits;
- Finger to nose test—patient repeatedly missed target bilaterally but worse with the left hand;
- Single foot standing—showed worse balance on left foot;
- Reflexes—hyperresponsive on right at C5, C6, L4, S1 levels;
- Muscle strength—within normal limits bilaterally in both upper and lower limbs;
- Hearing—within normal limits bilaterally;
- Heart rate—72, normal sinus rhythm;
- Respirations—28 per minute;
- Abdominal examination—negative; and
- Forehead skin temperature—35.5 °C on the left and 34.8 °C on the right.

Diagnosis

A diagnosis of attention deficit hyperactivity disorder (ADHD) secondary to right cortical hemisphericity was made. To confirm the diagnosis follow-up qEEG analysis was undertaken, where a large increase in theta:beta power ratio supported by decrease in absolute beta and high beta power over frontal and central regions particularly the vertex (Cz) was found. However, there was no significant increase in absolute theta power. Typical ADHD has these signs, as well as an increase in absolute theta, which is also present. Therefore the results of this qEEG are consistent with previous history-based diagnosis of ADHD with an associated learning disability. These conclusions were made from linked ears analysis and Laplacian (looking at default report settings enabling determination of power ratios).

Treatment

- Supplementation: omega 3 fish oils, omega 3 cofactors, vitamin B complex, CoQ_{10};
- Breathing exercises to slow down his breathing patterns and increase the pH of his blood;
- Manipulation was applied two times per week to spinal motion segments and peripheral extremity joints on left side of his body that expressed dyskinetic hypomobility;
- Sound therapy involved listening to Mozart 10 minutes per day both ears; and
- Spatial rearrangement exercises involved the task of completing jigsaw puzzles with only his left hand for 10 minutes per day.

Clinical Outcome After 12 Weeks

- Concentration greatly improved;
- Reading ability greatly improved;

- Normal visual tracking;
- Normal Romberg and Fukuda tests; and
- Scored passing grades in all of his end-of-term examinations for the first time in his life.

Prognosis

A follow-up qEEG is planned to document any changes since therapy was instituted. It is expected that TWB will continue to improve in all areas of concern until his full potential is reached.

Discussion

The pattern of signs and symptoms revealed during TWB's functional neurological consultation provide an insight into the possible levels of dysfunction in the longitudinal and horizontal planes of the neuraxis. Localization of the lesion is assisted by a comprehensive knowledge of the afferent and efferent connections throughout the neuraxis and an ability to ascertain the frequency of firing (FOF) and integrity of fuel delivery in different regions and systems. History and examination directed at localizing the symptoms to a specific level of the neuraxis including the following well-defined functional levels is necessary:

- End organ;
- Receptor;
- Peripheral nerve;
- Spinal cord;
- Brainstem;
- Cerebellum;
- Thalamus; and
- Cortex.

Asymmetry or dysfunction in each of these components of the nervous system can directly or indirectly affect various motor, sensory, visceral, and mental functions or indicate a dysfunction in any of these modalities.

Most importantly from a functional neurological perspective, asymmetry or dysfunction in the most influential components of the nervous system should be considered:

1. Vestibulocerebellar system;
2. Autonomic nervous system; and
3. Cerebral neuronal activity.

In the case of TWB he showed signs and symptoms of left cerebellar and right cortical dysfunction. This was expressed in the physical exam by his relative lack of coordination on the left, his pupillary TND on the right, Romberg's test falling to the left, his lack of ability to concentrate, and the hyperresponsiveness of his right-sided reflexes, which indicates increased tone due to decreased activation of the PMRF ipsilaterally.

ADHD is thought to occur as a result of an inability of the individual to maintain attention on a primary task because of an inability to inhibit or suppress motor responses to incoming sensory stimuli (Barkley 1997). Some consistency has been found in people with dysfunctions of the right frontal cortex in that they express great difficulty in suppressing motor responses to incoming sensory stimuli (Sergeant 2000). The right frontal cortex functions in some manner to inhibit inappropriate motor responses in a normal functioning brain. The activity of the right frontal cortex relies heavily on the dentato-ponto-cortical and dentato-rubral-thalamo-cortical pathways. Asymmetric reduction in afferent information to the cerebellum because of asymmetric dysfunctional peripheral afferent pathways may cause diaschisis in functional circuits downstream from the cerebellum, in this case the contralateral cortex. In this case the application of manipulation to increase the afferent stimulus received by the cerebellum and other therapies aimed at increasing the activation of the right frontal cortex were successful in reducing the patient's symptoms and ultimately his state of disability.

Case 2

Past History

RS initially presented to another practitioner with a chief complaint of low back pain. The other practitioner manipulated RS's neck and he immediately felt light-headed and developed a left-sided paraspinal muscle spasm in the cervical spine. RS left the practitioner's office but felt unstable while walking and developed nausea within minutes of leaving. One to two hours following the manipulation RS reported an increase in the nausea and flashing sensations in his left eye. He also reports feeling a sense of mounting confusion. The neck pain and spasm intensified as the night progressed to the point that RS screamed out in pain. At this point he also developed a headache and notes that his body felt cold.

The following day RS reports that he had a persistent headache, nausea, confusion, and visual disturbances in left eye. He also reports that he also developed a tremor in his left hand. RS returned to the initial practitioner and explained his symptoms. The initial practitioner palpates RS and proceeds to adjust the co/occipital region. RS reports no change in symptoms following the adjustment.

RS attended the initial practitioner again the following day and he manipulated C1 bilaterally. RS noted immediate worsening of his symptoms and became increasingly unstable while standing and walking. RS was referred to my clinic for evaluation.

Presenting Symptoms

A left occipital headache, which changed sides occasionally, had been present since the first adjustment. RS still reported light nausea which was exacerbated by walking. He reported his left eye felt dry and larger than the right. The visual field of the left eye remained burred with spotted blacked-out areas noted occasionally. He still had difficulty focusing. RS still felt confused and noticed difficulty forming sentences. He had a noticeable tremor of his left hand that had gradually worsened. He reported a feeling of unsteadiness on his feet and walked with a wide-based gait pattern. Pain was still present in the left cervical region.

Examination Findings

Vital Signs
- BP: 110/70 Rt, 110/90 Lt;
- HR: 66 regular sinus rhythm;
- Temperature: within normal range; and
- Bruit auscultation: negative bilaterally in both carotid and vertebral artery regions.

Neurological Testing
- Eye movements—left end range nystagmus noted, pursuit tracking was non-uniform and interrupted;
- Accommodation was good with concentric, bilateral, pupillary constriction;
- Retinal ophthalmic exam revealed V/A ratios of 1.5/1.0 and normal fundal appearance;
- Visual field challenge revealed equal and concentric fields in both eyes;
- Both eyes showed normal intorsion and extorsion on lateral flexion test;
- Corneal reflexes were present and equal bilaterally;
- Pupillary reflexes showed an increase time to activation and decreased time of fatigue on the left;
- Opticokinetic (OPK) testing revealed dysmetria when tracking from left to right;
- Hearing was good in both ears with vibration centrally localized and air conduction greater than bone conduction bilaterally;
- The patient expressed a mild left-sided pyramidal paresis, and a visible, regular, left-sided hand tremor on observation;

- On Romberg's challenge the patient fell to the left;
- The patient was dysdiadochokinetic on the left when challenged with rapid alternating movements of the hands and overshoot of the left hand on finger to nose testing;
- The patient indicated bilateral and equal sensation to touch in the arms, legs, and hands; extinction test was negative.
- Vibration was felt equally bilaterally in the C5–T1 dermatomes;
- Muscle strength was 5 in all muscles but the left bicep, which was 3;
- Reflexes were all strong and equal with no fatigue;
- Plantar reflex revealed down going toes bilaterally;
- Trigeminal nerve testing revealed an area of decreased sensation to prick in the left medial maxillary area;
- Oral examination revealed increased right-sided scarring on the tongue and a right palatal paresis; tongue strength and protrusion were both good;
- Spinal motion segment dysfunction was noted at the following levels:
  - Rt SI joint
  - L5
  - T5–T7
  - T1–T3
  - C4
  - C2
  - Lt C0
- Paraspinal muscle spasms and trigger points were present on the left from C1 to T1.

Diagnosis

RS presents with the clinical signs of a vestibular-cerebellar dysfunction on the left and right decreased cerebral hemispheric function. The cause of the dysfunction may be vascular or physiological in nature.

Treatment

CT scan of the medulla-pons and cerebellar regions was conducted to rule out vascular damage. The results of these tests were inconclusive. Soft tissue and trigger point therapy was initiated to relieve the soft tissue trigger points. Left-sided manipulation was performed in a graded fashion to restore normal kinematics to his spinal motion segments and peripheral joints. The cervical spine was not manipulated for several weeks into therapy.

The patient was given breathing exercises to improve oxygenation levels. RS was also given omega 3 fish oils, CoQ_{10} and B-complex supplementation to help in neuron repair processes.

Clinical Outcome After 12 Weeks

RS experienced a rapid reduction in his symptoms over the first week of treatment. This was followed by a gradual improvement over the next 8–10 weeks. His gait has returned to normal, he has normal OPK testing results, and his headaches are gone. He still feels that he experiences periods of confusion but these are also becoming less frequent and less severe.

Prognosis

It is my hope that RS will continue to improve until he has returned to his previous state. In my experience about 70% of these types of presentation will return to essentially normal function with continued treatment; however, about 30% of these patients will not return to their previous state despite further treatment.

Discussion

I have included this case for a number of reasons. Firstly, it is important for manipulating practitioners to understand that the manipulations they give are for the most part helpful to the patient; however, they can also hurt the patient when delivered in an inappropriate fashion (Carrick 1997). Secondly, it is important for functional neurologists to know how to handle this type of case because these cases tend to be referred to us for an opinion at some point.

Case 3

CH, RH's mother, accompanied RH to this assessment and related the history.

Previous History

RH was in France where it was proposed she took some marijuana laced with some chemical, which resulted in some form of encephalitis developing. The resulting state of depression led to her attempting suicide by hanging herself. She was hypoxic for approximately 4–6 minutes before she was found and taken down. She has since received a variety of medications that have resulted in various forms of brain insults and has left her in a somewhat catatonic state. Her mother related that she is basically the same temperament and personality that she was previously but now she exhibits the more negative emotional parts of her personality.

Presenting Complaint

Depression and catatonic state.

Examination Findings

RH responded in monosyllables (yes, no, fine) to most questions. She lacked the ability to sustain visual attention for more then 3–5 seconds in both right and left visual fields. Visual tracking was dyskinetic to the left. Her pupil responses were fast and fatiguing on the left. She exhibited anisocoria with the right pupil dilated. She showed good and accurate response to palmar dermatographia bilaterally. She showed no signs of extinction to touch in the C5–8 dermatomes but did to hearing on the left. Her reflexes (C5, C7, L4, S1) were diminished and fatiguing on the left. Heart rate was increased and stomach sounds decreased. No abdominal rigidity was noted. Both hands and feet were cold to touch. She stated her hands were always like this. Muscle strength was good in both hands. She could remember 5 of a 7-digit number immediately but no numbers 2–3 minutes later. RAM revealed a generalized lack of coordination in both hands but worse on the left. During Romberg's test, RH fell to the left repeatedly with eyes closed.

MRI and EEG reports showed findings consistent with anoxia. qEEG results showed a significant increase in beta and high beta over the right hemisphere, particularly central regions and occipital regions. Also present were major but fairly localized right hemisphere dysfunction in particular central to the mid-temporal region. The raw EEG data also revealed what appeared to be an asymmetric 'spindle coma' pattern, which is responsible largely for the significant increase in beta/high beta over the right hemisphere. These findings are consistent with anoxic injury or dysfunction, especially triggered by high doses of barbiturates.

Diagnosis

Generalized cortical dysfunction, mainly involving the right hemisphere, secondary to an acute anoxic episode.

Treatment

Sound therapy was utilized in this case. RH was advised to listen to Mozart or similar music from the left side for 10 minutes per day. Breathing exercises were also instituted to increase her oxygenation levels, initially for 2 minutes twice a day with expansion to 4 times per day after 2 weeks. Manipulation was performed to restore normal motion to the spinal motion segments and peripheral joints on the left side of her body. Supplementation with omega 3 fish oils, CoQ_{10}, Vitamin B complex, and amino acids was also instituted. After 4 weeks of care RH was instructed to look at old photo albums and make up stories about the pictures, then try to recall these stories at various times throughout the day. After 6 weeks of treatment, RH was also given the task of completing jigsaw puzzles with her left hand only.

Clinical Outcome after 12 Weeks

RH has shown remarkable progress considering her presenting state. She now answers in simple sentences instead of one-word replies. Her mother reports that her 'facial expressions look more human'. RH is now showing initiative in performing her daily chores. She does not fall on Romberg testing. qEEG follow-up showed significant changes, including a more normalized alpha pattern over the frontal lobes.

Prognosis

RH will continue to receive therapy employing novel stimuli, manipulation, and supplementation with the hope of further return of function.

Discussion

I think this case demonstrates the incredible ability that the neuraxis has to restore function when given the appropriate conditions. This young woman, who was previously a Rhodes scholar recipient, has undergone a series of traumatic cerebral events, exposing her brain to severe biochemical and physical stresses, but still the brain retains the amazing ability to maintain plasticity and recover.

Case 4

Presenting Complaint

A 47-year-old man, JS, presented with the chief complaint of left foot drop and low back pain centralized over the L5 region.

History

JS was involved in a serious skiing accident 2 years previous where he was paralysed from the waist down for several days. He eventually recovered and experienced no problems until last week when JS was lifting some packages from the trunk of his car. He felt his back snap and immediately felt low back pain over the L5 region. Over the next 2 days he noticed that his left foot was numb and not functioning properly. He also noticed that his ability to concentrate had diminished and his short memory had been affected.

Examination Findings

Vital Signs
- BP: 110/70 Rt, 110/70 Lt;
- HR: 72 regular sinus rhythm;
- Temperature: within normal range; and
- Bruit Auscultation was negative bilaterally in both carotid and vertebral artery regions.

Neurological Testing
- Eye movements—left end range nystagmus noted, pursuit tracking was non-uniform and interrupted;
- Accommodation was good with concentric, bilateral, pupillary constriction;
- Retinal ophthalmic exam revealed V/A ratios of 1.5/1.0 and normal fundal appearance;

- Visual field challenge revealed equal and concentric fields in both eyes;
- Both eyes showed normal intorsion and extorsion on lateral flexion test;
- Corneal reflexes were present and equal bilaterally;
- Pupillary reflexes showed an increase time to activation and decreased time of fatigue on the left;
- OPK testing revealed normal function;
- Hearing was good in both ears with vibration centrally localized and air conduction greater than bone conduction bilaterally;
- The patient expressed a mild right-sided pyramidal paresis;
- On Romberg's challenge the patient fell to the left;
- The patient was dysdiadochokinetic on the left when challenged with rapid alternating movements of the hands and overshoot of the left hand on finger to nose testing;
- The patient indicated bilateral and equal sensation to touch in the arms, legs, and hands with the exception of the dorsum of the left foot and lateral foot areas (L5, S1 dermatomal distributions), which were numb to touch; extinction test was negative;
- Vibration was felt equally bilaterally in the all dermatomes with the exception of the left L5, S1 dermatomes;
- Muscle strength was 5 in all muscles but the left peroneal muscles were at 3;
- Reflexes were all strong and equal with no fatigue with the exception of the left S1 reflex, which was absent;
- Plantar reflex revealed down going toes bilaterally;
- Spinal motion segment dysfunction was noted at the following levels:
  - Lt SI joint
  - L5 bilater.
  - T1–T3
  - C2
  - Lt C0
- Paraspinal muscle spasms and trigger points were present on the left from L1 to L5 and left piriformis trigger points were also noted.

Imaging

Lumbopelvic AP, lateral and oblique radiographs were unremarkable with the exception of mild osteoarthritic degeneration at L5/S1. MRI showed a small disc protrusion at the L5/S1 disc.

Diagnosis

Mild right hemisphericity secondary to spinal root compression at L5/S1.

Treatment

JS received manipulation to address the altered spinal motion units and dysfunctional peripheral joint motion units discovered on examination. He received a natural anti-inflammatory supplement and multivitamins. He was given rib adjustments and breathing exercises to increase his oxygenation.

Clinical Outcome after 12 Weeks

JS is now pain free. The numbness over his left foot still reoccurs from time to time but he feels very pleased with the outcome to date. He was originally scheduled for spinal fusion surgery, which he has now cancelled.

Discussion

This case was included because it demonstrates that simple musculoskeletal problems also respond to functional neurological application. It was also included because it is a good case for illustrating the concept of localizing the problem to the longitudinal level of the lesion. Some of my diagnostic considerations at each longitudinal level in this case included:

- Common peroneal lesion at the hip;
- Common peroneal lesion at the knee;
- Spinal cord compression;
- HMSN;
- Brain lesion;
- Neural insufficiency—canal stenosis;
- L4/5 nerve root lesion;
- Disc protrusion;
- Neurofibroma;
- Metastases;
- Benign tumours; and
- Diabetes peripheral neuropathy.

These considerations were systematically ruled in or out by physical examination findings or further imaging such as MRI.

Case 5

Presenting Complaint

Migraines and balance problems to the point that she falls over.

History

DC is a 57-year-old woman who initially noted the onset of dizziness and left-sided facial weakness 2 weeks prior to presentation. The facial weakness was noted only during migraine headaches that she also had been getting for 2–3 years now. She currently had a headache for the past 3 weeks straight. She experienced high stress in her profession and had been under extremely high stress for the last 6 weeks. She also reported that she fell and injured her neck quite badly 6–7 years previous. She had attended her general practitioner three times over the past 3 weeks with no improvement in symptomatology.

Examination Findings

Vital Signs
- BP: 118/70 Rt, 120/70 Lt;
- HR: 77 regular sinus rhythm;
- Temperature: within normal range; and
- Bruit auscultation was negative bilaterally in both carotid and vertebral artery regions.

Neurological Testing
- Eye movements—right end range nystagmus noted, pursuit tracking was non-uniform and interrupted;
- Accommodation was good with concentric, bilateral, pupillary constriction;
- Retinal ophthalmic exam revealed V/A ratios of 1.5/1.0 and normal fundal appearance;
- Visual field challenge revealed equal and concentric fields in both eyes;
- Both eyes showed normal intorsion and extorsion on lateral flexion test;
- Corneal reflexes were present and equal bilaterally;
- Pupillary reflexes showed an increase time to activation and decreased time of fatigue on the left;
- OPK testing revealed dyskinetic movements and hypermetria of return phase;

- Hearing was good in both ears with vibration centrally localized and air conduction greater than bone conduction bilaterally;
- The patient expressed a mild right-sided pyramidal paresis;
- On Romberg's challenge the patient fell to the left with eyes closed;
- The patient was dysdiadochokinetic on the left when challenged with rapid alternating movements of the hands and overshoot of the left hand on finger to nose testing;
- The patient indicated bilateral and equal sensation to touch in the arms, legs, and hands with the exception of the left hand and arm, which were numb to touch; extinction test was negative;
- Vibration was felt equally bilaterally in the all dermatomes with the exception of the C6 dermatome on the left;
- Muscle strength was 5 in all muscles of the upper and lower extremities;
- Reflexes were all strong and equal with no fatigue; however, the left C5 reflex initiated a tingling sensation in her left arm;
- Plantar reflex revealed down going toes bilaterally;
- Spinal motion segment dysfunction was noted at the following levels:
    - L5 bilater.
    - T1–T3
    - C2
    - Lt C0
- Paraspinal muscle spasms and trigger points were present bilaterally from T1 to T5.

Imaging

- Cervical spine AP, lateral and oblique radiographs were unremarkable. Head MRI was also unremarkable.
- qEEG demonstrated a reduced alpha wave activity over the right frontal cortex.

Differential Diagnosis

- A number of diagnostic possibilities were considered in this case:
- Menière's disease;
- Pre-cervico-oto-ocular syndrome;
- Cervico-oto-ocular syndrome;
- Benign paroxysmal positional vertigo (BPPV);
- Vestibular neuronitis;
- Labyrinthitis;
- Anaemia;
- Carotid sinus hypersensitivity; and
- Vasovagal syncope.

A final working diagnosis of migraine syndrome secondary to right hemisphericity was made and treatment instituted on that basis.

Treatment

Manipulation was performed on the left to remove any dysfunctional spinal motion segments. DC was also given visual exercises to focus on her thumbs of her outstretched arms as she turned from to her left side to stimulate cortical pathways via the vestibular system. DC could not take supplementation due to her aversion to pills although she was placed on a high protein diet. Breathing exercises and rib adjustments were also given to increase her oxygenation.

Clinical Outcome After 12 Weeks

From week 2 of treatment, DC has only had two minor headaches. Her vertigo and dizziness have resolved and she has no numbness or tingling in her arms. qEEG follow-up indicated a balance in alpha wave function.

Discussion

It is possible that her accident several years ago slowly developed a hemispheric dominance of her left cortex. This imbalance may be responsible for initiating her migraines and her vertigo. When asymmetry of function between hemispheres occurs as appears to have happened in this case quite commonly an asymmetrical decrease in the ability of the cortex to excite certain areas of the brainstem including the mesencephalon and other areas namely the pontomedullary reticular formation (PMRF) ensues. This can result in vestibular involvement in the form of vertigo or the sensation of dizziness. The high stress levels that she was experiencing have remained constant so this, although probably a contributing factor, appears not to be involved in the production of her symptoms.

Case 6

Presenting Complaint

AV, an 8-year-old female, presented with unbearable left leg and foot pain without any sensation of touch or pressure, along with depression.

Past History

AV underwent surgery for the removal of ear grommets 9 months prior to presentation. Before administration of the anaesthesia the nurse noted that AV had a rash on her arms and neck. The anaesthetist also noted the rash but thought that it was not an issue of concern. Following the surgery AV developed pain lost motor control of both her legs. She reported to the emergency department and was diagnosed with viral myalgia. Over the next several weeks AV reported to the emergency room several times and was extensively evaluated with no explanation of her pain given other than viral myalgia. She was discharged to her mother's care and sent home.

Present History

AV was still experiencing loss of motor control and chronic pain in both legs but especially the left leg on presentation. Her mother had been carrying her everywhere and carried her into the office today.

Examination Findings

Vital Signs
- BP: 118/70 Rt, 128/70 Lt;
- HR: 72 regular sinus rhythm;
- Temperature: within normal range; and
- Bruit auscultation was negative bilaterally in both carotid and vertebral artery regions.

Neurological Testing
- Eye movements—right end range nystagmus noted, pursuit tracking was non-uniform and interrupted;
- Accommodation was good with concentric, bilateral, pupillary constriction;
- Retinal ophthalmic exam revealed V/A ratios of 2.0/1.0 in the left eye with normal fundal appearance;
- Visual field challenge revealed equal and concentric fields in both eyes;
- Both eyes showed normal intorsion and extorsion on lateral flexion test;
- Corneal reflexes were present and equal bilaterally;
- Pupillary reflexes showed an increase time to activation and decreased time of fatigue on the left;
- OPK testing revealed dyskinetic movements and hypermetria of return phase;

- Hearing was good in both ears with vibration centrally localized and air conduction greater than bone conduction bilaterally;
- Romberg's challenge could not be performed because of non-weight bearing condition of the patient;
- The patient was dysdiadochokinetic on the left when challenged with rapid alternating movements of the hands and overshoot of the left hand on finger to nose testing;
- The patient indicated bilateral and equal sensation to touch in the arms, legs, and hands with the exception of the left leg, which was numb to touch; extinction test was negative;
- Vibration was felt equally bilaterally in all the dermatomes;
- Muscle strength was 4 in all muscles of the upper and lower extremities with the exception of the muscles of the left leg, which could not be tested due to pain;
- Reflexes were all strong and equal with no fatigue;
- Dermatographia was present bilaterally in the legs with gross flare response on the left leg;
- Plantar reflex revealed down going toes bilaterally;
- Spinal motion segment dysfunction was noted at the following levels:
  - L5 bilater.
  - T1–T3
  - C2
  - Lt C0
- Paraspinal muscle spasms and trigger points were present bilaterally from T1 to T5.

Imaging

Cervical spine AP, lateral and oblique radiographs were unremarkable. MRI was also unremarkable.

Diagnosis

Previous medical testing had ruled out meningitis, and tumour as a differential. The diagnosis of complex regional pain syndrome secondary to asymmetric hemispheric function was made.

Treatment

Manipulations were performed initially only on the legs. Eventually manipulations of the entire spine were carried out. Supplementation including omega 3 fish oils, amino acids, and standard multivitamins were instituted. Orthotics were fitted to provide support for her feet, which were highly pronated due to the lack of use. Breathing exercises were introduced. When spasms of pain occurred she was instructed to count backwards from 100 by 7's to increase the activation level of her cortex and inhibit the pain somewhat. This technique appeared to be highly successful. Hot and cold compressed were applied to her legs on a daily basis.

Clinical Outcome After 12 Weeks

AV showed a remarkable recovery with the return of full control of her legs and full weight bearing after 3 weeks of treatment. She still experiences bouts of pain that may last 2–3 hours in duration but has returned to a virtually normal life, attending school and playing soccer.

Discussion

When asymmetry of function between hemispheres occurs as appears to be happening in this case quite commonly a decrease in the ability of the cortex to excite certain areas of the brainstem including the mesencephalon and other areas namely the PMRF ensues. A decreased excitation of the PMRF can result in a decrease in inhibition of the intermediolateral (IML) cell column, which results in increases in sympathetic activity. This can lead to dysautonomia and result in somewhat bizarre symptomatology, including the development of complex regional pain syndrome.

Conclusion

In this chapter I have describe and discussed a few of the cases that I have consulted on over the past year or so. Many other cases involving as diverse a symptomatology as depression, anxiety, obsessive–compulsive disorder, tinnitus, various dystonias, Parkinson's disease, oral dysplasia, dysautonomia, postconcussion syndrome, and ablative stroke have shown a remarkable propensity for improvement when the principles of functional neurology are applied.

References

Barkley RA 1997 Behavioral inhibition, sustained attention and executive functions: constructing a unifying theory of ADHD. Psychological Bulletin 121:65–69.

Carrick FR 1997 Changes in brain function after manipulation of the cervical spine. Journal of Manipulative and Physiological Therapeutics 20(8):529–545.

Sergeant J 2000 The cognitive energetic model: an empirical approach to attention deficit hyperactivity disorder. Neuroscience and Biobehavioral Reviews 24:7–12.

Index

B

M

Ventrolateral thalamic nuclei, 143
Ventromedial group of axons, 149, 152
Vermis, 366, 369, 378
Vertebral column development, 33–6, 35
Vertebral foramina, 176
Vertebral posterior arch defects, 33, 35, 38
Vertebrobasilar strokes (VBS), 492–3
Vertical saccade, 346–8, 349, 363
Vertigo, 386, 393 *see also* Benign paroxysmal positional vertigo (BPPV)
Vessel integrity, 221
Vestibular apparatus, 381, 382–3
Vestibular evoked myogenic potentials (VEMPs), 81
Vestibular neuritis, 391
Vestibular nuclear complex, 383–4, 427
Vestibular system, 381–8
    afferent projections into the, 381–2
    afferent stimulus to the, 386–7
    dysfunction, 390–1, 508–10
    evaluation of output, 387
    functions of the, 386
    integration system of the, 385
    output projections of the, 385–6
    stimulation, 498–500
    vestibular apparatus, 381, 382–3
    vestibular nuclear complex, 383–4, 427
    see also Vestibulocerebellar system
Vestibulo-autonomic reflexes, 211–12, 387–8
Vestibulo-ocular reflexes, 383
Vestibulocerebellar system, 332, 365–91
    advanced functions of the, 388–91
    cerebellar cortex, 373–80
    cerebellum *see* Cerebellum
    disorders, 98
    dysfunction and asymmetry, 102–3
    function and asymmetry, 389–91
Vestibulocochlear nerve (VIII), 97–8, 353–5, 361
Vestibulospinal tract, 168–9
Vestibulosympathetic pathways, 453
Vestibulosympathetic reflex, 388–9

Video nystagmography (VNG), 81
VINDICATES, 77–8
Visceral grey area, 161
Visceral pain, 427
    referred, 218
Visceral sensation modulation, 338
Visceral sensory projections of the vagus nerve, 358
Visceromotor fibres, 211
Visual agnosia, 256, 315
Visual field, 17, 82, 344
    defects, 346
Visual information, 382
Visual receptors, 125–6
Visual striate cortex, 275
Visuospatial sketchpad, 241, 318
Vital signs, 82
Vocal chords, 357

W

Wallenberg's syndrome, 329, 350, 493–4
Wallerian degeneration, 179–80
Watson, James, 423
Werdnig–Hoffman syndrome, 193
Wernicke pupil, 83
Wernicke's aphasia, 256
Wernicke's area, 248, 256
Whiplash, 261
White blood cells (WBC), 396
White matter, spinal cord, 157, 163–5
White rami communicans, 201, 210
'Wind-up,' neurological, 12–13
Wohlfart–Kugelberg–Welander disease, 193
Writer's cramp, 301–2

Z

Zinc finger proteins, 50